Managing Chronic Disorders

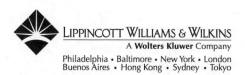

LIPPINCOTT WILLIAMS & WILKINS
A **Wolters Kluwer** Company

Philadelphia • Baltimore • New York • London
Buenos Aires • Hong Kong • Sydney • Tokyo

STAFF

Executive Publisher
Judith A. Schilling McCann, RN, MSN

Editorial Director
H. Nancy Holmes

Clinical Director
Joan M. Robinson, RN, MSN

Senior Art Director
Arlene Putterman

Editorial Project Manager
William Welsh

Clinical Project Manager
Mary Perrong, RN, CRNP, MSN, APRN,BC

Electronic Production Manager
John Macalino

Clinical Editor
Marcy Caplin, RN, MSN; Jane L. Sciarra, RN, CRNP, MSN

Copy Editors
Kimberly Bilotta (supervisor), Scotti Cohn, Tom DeZego, Amy Furman, Kelly Pavlovsky, Dona Perkins, Carolyn Peterson, Dorothy P. Terry, Pamela Wingrod

Designer
Susan Hopkins Rodzewich (book design and project manager)

Digital Composition Services
Diane Paluba (manager), Joyce Rossi Biletz, Donna S. Morris

Manufacturing
Patricia K. Dorshaw (director), Beth J. Welsh

Editorial Assistants
Megan L. Aldinger, Karen J. Kirk, Linda K. Ruhf

Indexer
Barbara Hodgson

MCD010705 — D N O S A J

07 06 05   10 9 8 7 6 5 4 3 2 1

Library of Congress Cataloging-in-Publication Data
Managing chronic disorders.
    p. ; cm.
    Includes bibliographical references and index.
    1. Chronic diseases — Nursing — Handbooks, manuals, etc. I. Lippincott Williams & Wilkins. [DNLM: 1. Chronic Disease — nursing — Handbooks. 2. Patient Education — methods — Handbooks. WY 49 M266 2006]
RT120.C45M36 2006
616'.044—dc22
ISBN 1-58255-442-0 (alk. paper)   2005009339

⬭ Contents

Contributors and consultants

Deborah Berry, RN, MSN, MS, CWOCN
Clinical Nurse Specialist
Franklin Square Hospital Center
Baltimore

Lillian Craig, RN, MSN, FNP-C
Family Nurse Practitioner
Claude (Tex.) Rural Health Clinic
Nursing Instructor
Oklahoma Panhandle State University
Goodwell, Tex.

Shirley Lyon Garcia, RN, BSN
Nursing Program Director
McDowell Technical Community College
Marion, N.C.

Janice Donaldson Hausauer, RN, MS, FNP
Adjunct Assistant Professor
Montana State University College of Nursing
Bozeman

Joy Herzog, RN, ADN
Assistant Director of Nursing Services
Beverly Healthcare of Doylestown, Pa.

Charla K. Hollin, RN, BSN
Nursing Program Director
Rich Mountain Community College
Mena, Ark.

Merita Konstantacos, RN, MSN
Consultant
Clinton, Ohio

Cheryl Laskowski, RN, APRN-BC, DNS
Assistant Professor
University of Vermont Department of Nursing
Burlington

Beryl Stetson, RNC, MSN, CLC, LCCE
Assistant Professor
Raritan Valley Community College
Somerville, N.J.

Elliott Stetson, RN,BC, MSN, CCRN
Staff Nurse
Robert Wood Johnson University Hospital
New Brunswick, N.J.

Mary E. Walker, RN, MSN, CCRN, CCNS
Staff Nurse – Burn Center
U.S. Army Institute of Surgical Research –
    Brooke Army Medical Center
Fort Sam Houston, Tex.
Clinical Instructor
University of Texas Health Science Center,
    Chronic Nursing Department
San Antonio

Foreword

The proper management of chronic disorders is one of the health care professional's most challenging tasks. The sheer size of the disease burden is staggering. According to the Centers for Disease Control and Prevention, chronic disorders cause major limitations in daily living for more than 25 million people in the United States, and recent estimates say that 7 of every 10 Americans who die each year, or more than 1.7 million people, die of a chronic disorder.

Age plays an important role in the development of chronic disease. Approximately 80% of older adults have at least one chronic disorder, and as the population ages, the percentage of people living with chronic disorders is expected to rise. However, chronic disorders aren't the exclusive domain of older adults. Some chronic disorders, such as sickle cell anemia and epilepsy, primarily affect younger populations. Other chronic disorders, such as type 2 diabetes and obesity, are reaching epidemic proportions in children and adolescents because of their sedentary lifestyle and excessive caloric intake.

Not surprisingly, health care professionals from all specialties are finding themselves caring for more and more patients with these devastating diseases. Therefore, we must all be able to spot the telltale signs of chronic disease, know the implications, guide patient care appropriately once a diagnosis has been reached, and be able to help the patient take part in his own care through education that leaves him feeling confident in his ability to help manage his disorder.

Managing Chronic Disorders is a practical, authoritative guide to more than 100 of the most common chronic disorders affecting people across the life span, including chronic obstructive pulmonary disease, diabetes, heart failure, and stroke. The broad spectrum of conditions covered in this important title include psychological disorders, such as depression, alcoholism, attention deficit disorder, and disorders that affect multiple body systems, such as hepatitis, HIV, and rheumatoid arthritis. Pain, which many health care professionals don't view as a chronic disorder, receives special attention because of its debilitating potential.

Managing Chronic Disorders is composed of two parts. Part 1 is a compendium of the most common chronic disorders. Organized in time-saving alphabetical order, the disorders are discussed in detail using a consistent format and a highly visual approach that lends itself to quick reference.

Each entry begins with a definition of the disorder and continues with sections on causes, pathophysiology, assessment findings, diagnosis, complications, treatment, and special considerations that every health care professional should keep in mind. At the end of each entry is a list of applicable patient-teaching aids that can be found either in Part 2 of the book (denoted by an asterisk) or on the accompanying CD-ROM.

In addition to the core text, Part 1 also features four useful graphic icons that call your attention to important points. *Close up* uses detailed illustrations to explain how a disease develops and progresses. These short informational pieces can help you brush up on pathophysiology and enable you to explain difficult topics to your patients.

Collaborative management, which focuses on an interdisciplinary approach to managing chronic disorders, presents vital information on the role of each health care professional to provide quality patient care in a team environment.

Patients with chronic disorders sometimes experience acute exacerbations that worsen their condition. *Acute episode* highlights typical exacerbations and provides critical guidance for treatment.

Proper patient teaching is crucial to the patient's understanding of home management and the necessary lifestyle adjustments that must be made in the face of a chronic disorder. It's equally important for people who occasionally experience an acute exacerbation and need to know how to manage those episodes. *Key teaching points* highlights critical patient-teaching topics for each disorder.

Part 2 of *Managing Chronic Disorders* continues this focus on patient teaching by providing 100 reproducible patient-teaching aids that can supplement the teaching done by nurses and other interdisciplinary team members. The accompanying CD-ROM, which contains all of the patient-teaching aids in Part 2, also contains 280 more aids, including ones on health promotion activities, nutrition, medication administration, and self-management of selected chronic disorders.

Managing Chronic Disorders won't just help you manage your patients—it will also help your patients manage themselves.

Valuable appendices include a handy listing of internet resources for chronic disorders as well as selected references that you can consult for more information.

Managing Chronic Disorders is an organized and comprehensive reference for all health care professionals who wish to confirm, update, and expand their knowledge of this clinically significant subject, and it's a must read for anyone who assists people across the life span in managing their chronic conditions. It's a part of my reference library, and I highly recommend that it become a part of yours.

Patricia E. McDonald, RN, MS, PhD
Assistant Professor of Nursing
Case Western Reserve University, FPB School
   of Nursing
Cleveland

Chronic disorders

Part one

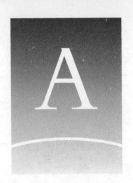

Adrenal hypofunction

Adrenal hypofunction is classified as primary or secondary. Primary adrenal hypofunction or insufficiency, also known as *Addison's disease,* originates within the adrenal gland and is characterized by the decreased secretion of mineralocorticoids, glucocorticoids, and androgens. Secondary adrenal hypofunction is caused by a disorder outside the gland such as impaired pituitary secretion of corticotropin. It's characterized by decreased glucocorticoid secretion.

Primary adrenal hypofunction is relatively uncommon and can occur at any age and in both sexes. Secondary adrenal hypofunction occurs when a patient abruptly stops long-term exogenous steroid therapy or when the pituitary gland is injured by a tumor or by infiltrative or autoimmune processes that occur when circulating antibodies react specifically against adrenal tissue, causing inflammation and infiltration of the cells by lymphocytes. With early diagnosis and adequate replacement therapy, the prognosis for primary and secondary adrenal hypofunction is good.

Adrenal crisis, also known as *addisonian crisis,* is a critical deficiency of mineralocorticoids and glucocorticoids that generally follows acute stress, sepsis, trauma, surgery, or the omission of steroid therapy in patients who have chronic adrenal insufficiency. It's a medical emergency that needs immediate treatment.

Causes

Primary adrenal hypofunction occurs when more than 90% of both adrenal glands are de-

stroyed, an occurrence that typically results from an autoimmune process in which circulating antibodies react specifically against the adrenal tissue. Other causes include tuberculosis (once the chief cause; now responsible for less than 10% of adult cases), bilateral adrenalectomy, hemorrhage into the adrenal gland, neoplasms, and such infections as acquired immunodeficiency syndrome, histoplasmosis, and cytomegalovirus. Rarely, a familial tendency to autoimmune disease predisposes the patient to adrenal hypofunction and other endocrinopathies.

Secondary adrenal hypofunction that results in glucocorticoid deficiency can stem from hypopituitarism (causing decreased corticotropin secretion), abrupt withdrawal of long-term corticosteroid therapy (long-term exogenous corticosteroid stimulation suppresses pituitary corticotropin secretion and results in adrenal gland atrophy), or removal of a nonendocrine, corticotropin-secreting tumor.

Adrenal crisis follows when trauma, surgery, or another physiologic stress exhausts the body's stores of glucocorticoids in a person with adrenal hypofunction.

Pathophysiology

Primary adrenal hypofunction is a chronic condition that results from the partial or complete destruction of the adrenal cortex. (See *Adrenal hypofunction: How it happens.*) It manifests as a clinical syndrome in which the symptoms are associated with deficient production of the adrenocortical hormones, cortisol, aldosterone, and androgens. High levels of corticotropin and

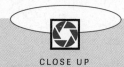

CLOSE UP

Adrenal hypofunction: How it happens

Primary adrenal hypofunction originates within the adrenal gland and is characterized by decreased secretion of mineralocorticoids, glucocorticoids, and androgens and complete or partial destruction of the adrenal cortex.

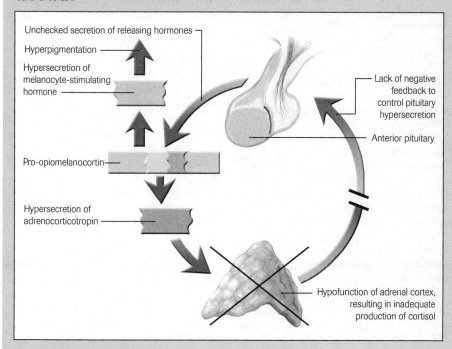

Unchecked secretion of releasing hormones

Hyperpigmentation

Hypersecretion of melanocyte-stimulating hormone

Pro-opiomelanocortin

Hypersecretion of adrenocorticotropin

Lack of negative feedback to control pituitary hypersecretion

Anterior pituitary

Hypofunction of adrenal cortex, resulting in inadequate production of cortisol

corticotropin-releasing hormone accompany the low glucocorticoid levels.

Corticotropin acts primarily to regulate the adrenal release of glucocorticoids (primarily cortisol); mineralocorticoids, including aldosterone; and sex steroids that supplement those produced by the gonads. Corticotropin secretion is controlled by corticotropin-releasing hormone from the hypothalamus and by negative feedback control by the glucocorticoids.

Primary adrenal hypofunction involves all zones of the cortex, causing deficiencies of the adrenocortical secretions, glucocorticoids, androgens, and mineralocorticoids. Usually, cellu-lar atrophy is limited to the cortex, although medullary involvement may occur, resulting in catecholamine deficiency. Cortisol deficiency causes decreased liver gluconeogenesis (the formation of glucose from molecules that aren't carbohydrates). The resulting low blood glucose levels can become dangerously low in patients who take insulin routinely.

Aldosterone deficiency causes increased renal sodium loss and enhances potassium reabsorption. Sodium excretion causes a reduction in fluid volume that leads to hypotension. Patients with primary adrenal hypofunction may have normal blood pressure when supine,

Adrenal crisis

In the patient with adrenal crisis, be alert for such signs and symptoms as profound weakness, fatigue, nausea, vomiting, hypotension, dehydration and, occasionally, high fever followed by hypothermia. If you detect these signs and symptoms, follow the guidelines listed below to prevent vascular collapse, renal shutdown, coma and, possibly, death.

● Monitor the patient's vital signs carefully, especially for hypotension, volume depletion, and other signs of shock (decreased level of consciousness and urine output).

● Promptly administer an I.V. bolus of hydrocortisone. Later, doses are given I.M. or are diluted with dextrose in normal saline solution and given I.V. until the patient's condition stabilizes.

● Monitor the patient for hyperkalemia before treatment and for hypokalemia after treatment (from excessive mineralocorticoid effect).

● Monitor the patient for cardiac arrhythmias, which may be caused by a serum potassium disturbance.

● If the patient also has diabetes, check blood glucose levels periodically because steroid replacement may require insulin dosage adjustments.

● Document the patient's weight and intake and output carefully because he may have volume depletion. Until the onset of mineralocorticoid effect, force fluids to replace excessive fluid loss.

● After the crisis, administer maintenance doses of hydrocortisone, as ordered, to preserve physiologic stability.

but show marked hypotension and tachycardia after standing for several minutes. Low plasma volume and arteriolar pressure stimulate renin release and a resulting increased production of angiotensin II.

Androgen deficiency may decrease hair growth in axillary and pubic areas as well as on the extremities of women. The metabolic ef-

fects of testicular androgens make such hair growth less noticeable in men.

Assessment findings

Primary adrenal hypofunction typically produces such effects as weakness, fatigue, weight loss, and various GI disturbances, such as nausea, vomiting, anorexia, and chronic diarrhea. It usually causes a conspicuous bronze coloration of the skin; the patient appears to be deeply suntanned, especially in the creases of the hands and over the metacarpophalangeal joints, the elbows, and the knees. He may also exhibit a darkening of scars, areas of vitiligo (absence of pigmentation), and increased pigmentation of the mucous membranes, especially the buccal mucosa. Cardiovascular abnormalities associated with primary adrenal-hypofunction include orthostatic hypotension, decreased cardiac size and output, and a weak, irregular pulse. Other clinical effects include decreased tolerance for even minor stress, poor coordination, fasting hypoglycemia (due to decreased gluconeogenesis), and a craving for salty food.

Adrenal hypofunction may also retard axillary and pubic hair growth in females, decrease the libido (from decreased androgen production) and, in severe cases, cause amenorrhea.

Secondary adrenal hypofunction produces similar clinical effects but without hyperpigmentation and possibly no hypotension and electrolyte abnormalities.

Adrenal crisis produces profound weakness, fatigue, nausea, vomiting, hypotension, dehydration and, occasionally, high fever followed by hypothermia. (See *Adrenal crisis*.)

Diagnosis

❍ Decreased plasma cortisol levels confirm adrenal insufficiency.

❍ The corticotropin stimulation test differentiates between primary and secondary adrenal hypofunction. However, the rapid corticotropin stimulation test may be necessary to confirm the diagnosis. A low corticotropin level indicates a secondary disorder, while an elevated level indicates a primary disorder.

❍ The metyrapone test is indicated when secondary adrenal hypofunction is suspected.

(Oral or I.V. metyrapone blocks cortisol production and should stimulate the release of corticotropin from the hypothalamic-pituitary system; in primary adrenal hypofunction, the hypothalamic-pituitary system responds normally and plasma corticotropin levels are high, but because the adrenal glands are destroyed, plasma concentrations of the cortisol precursor 11 deoxycortisol increase, as do urinary 17 hydroxycorticosteroids.)

In a patient with typical symptoms of adrenal crisis, these laboratory findings strongly suggest acute adrenal insufficiency:

○ decreased plasma cortisol level (less than 10 mcg/dl) in the morning, with an even greater decreased level in the evening
○ decreased serum sodium and fasting blood glucose levels
○ increased serum potassium, calcium, and blood urea nitrogen levels
○ elevated hematocrit; increased lymphocyte and eosinophil counts
○ X-rays showing adrenal calcification if the cause is infectious.

Complications
○ Deficient or excessive steroid treatment
○ Hyperpyrexia
○ Profound hypoglycemia
○ Psychotic reactions
○ Shock
○ Ultimate vascular collapse, renal shutdown, coma, and death (if untreated)

Treatment
○ Corticosteroid replacement, usually with cortisone or hydrocortisone (both of which also have a mineralocorticoid effect), is the primary treatment for primary and secondary adrenal hypofunction; it must continue throughout the patient's life.
○ I.V. desoxycorticosterone (a pure mineralocorticoid) or oral fludrocortisone (a synthetic mineralocorticoid) prevent dangerous dehydration and hypotension.

 COLLABORATIVE MANAGEMENT
Care of the patient with adrenal hypofunction involves several members of the interdisciplinary team. The endocrinologist can identify causative factors and pre-

KEY TEACHING POINTS

Teaching about adrenal hypofunction

Remember these key points when teaching your patient about adrenal hypofunction:
● Explain that lifelong steroid therapy is necessary.
● Teach the patient the signs and symptoms of steroid overdose, such as swelling and weight gain, and steroid underdose, such as lethargy and weakness.
● Explain to the patient the importance of keeping physician and laboratory appointments for monitoring test results and drug dose adjustments.
● Advise the patient that infection, injury, or profuse sweating in hot weather may precipitate adrenal crisis.
● Instruct the patient to always carry a medical identification card stating that he takes a steroid and giving the name of the drug and the dosage.
● Teach the patient and his family how to give a hydrocortisone injection.
● Tell the patient to keep an emergency kit available containing hydrocortisone in a prepared syringe for use in times of stress.
● Explain to the patient the importance of taking antacids while on steroids. Antacids will help to decrease the gastric irritation caused by steroids.
● Explain to the patient that physical and emotional stress may necessitate additional cortisone dosage to prevent adrenal crisis. Review stress management techniques, and encourage adequate rest and nutrition.

scribe therapy to control the disorder. The dietitian can counsel the patient on snacks that help prevent hypoglycemia, how to deal with anorexia, and the need for a high-protein, high-carbohydrate diet. The nurse practitioner or a clinical nurse specialist can help the patient reduce his stress level, which helps prevent adrenal crisis. The pharmacist can provide information on pharmacologic therapy and the administration of hydrocortisone injections.

Special considerations
○ Arrange for a high-carbohydrate, high-protein diet that maintains sodium and potassium balances. Tell the patient to make sure a late-morning snack is available in case he becomes hypoglycemic.
○ If the patient is anorexic, suggest six small meals per day to increase caloric intake.
○ Observe the patient receiving steroids for cushingoid signs such as fluid retention around the eyes and face.
○ Watch for fluid and electrolyte imbalances, especially if the patient is receiving mineralocorticoids.
○ Monitor weight and check blood pressure to assess body fluid status.
○ Check for petechiae in patients taking corticosteroids because these patients bruise easily.
○ If the patient receives glucocorticoids alone, observe him for orthostatic hypotension or electrolyte abnormalities, which may indicate a need for mineralocorticoid therapy.
○ Provide patient education. (See *Teaching about adrenal hypofunction,* page 5.)

Applicable patient-teaching aids
○ Learning about corticosteroids
○ Preventing adrenal crisis *
○ Taking your blood pressure *

○ Alcohol addiction

The patient with alcohol addiction experiences a need for the daily intake of large amounts of alcohol for day-to-day functioning. A regular pattern of heavy drinking that's limited to weekends, with periods of sobriety between weekends, also suggests a pattern of abuse. People with these drinking patterns usually show impaired social and occupational functioning.

More than 15% of American adults have a problem with alcohol use, and about 5% to 10% of male and 3% to 5% of female drinkers are alcohol dependent, accounting for about 12.5 million people. Alcohol-related disorders cut across all social and economic groups, involve both sexes, and occur at all stages of the life cycle, beginning as early as elementary school.

Causes
Numerous biological, psychological, and sociocultural factors appear to be involved in alcohol addiction. An offspring of one alcoholic parent is seven to eight times more likely to become an alcoholic than is a peer without such a parent. Biological factors may include genetic or biochemical abnormalities, nutritional deficiencies, endocrine imbalances, and allergic responses.

Psychological factors may include the urge to drink alcohol to reduce anxiety or symptoms of mental illness; the desire to avoid responsibility in familial, social, and work relationships; and the need to bolster self-esteem.

Sociocultural factors include the availability of alcoholic beverages, group or peer pressure, an excessively stressful lifestyle, and social attitudes that approve of frequent drinking.

Pathophysiology
Alcohol is soluble in water and lipids and permeates all body tissues. The liver metabolizes 90% of the alcohol absorbed in the body and is the most severely affected organ with chronic alcohol abuse. Hepatic steatosis followed by hepatic fibrosis is evident days after heavy drinking. Laënnec's cirrhosis may develop after an inflammatory response (alcoholic hepatitis) or in the absence of inflammation, as a consequence of direct activation of lipocytes (Ito cells). With chronic alcohol ingestion, lactic acidosis and excess uric acid is promoted; gluconeogenesis, B-oxidation of fatty acids, and the Krebs cycle are opposed; and hypoglycemia and hyperlipidemia develop. Toxicity of cells occurs through the reduction of mitochondrial oxygenation utilization, depletion of deoxyribonucleic acid, and other actions.

Assessment findings
The patient may report daily or episodic alcohol use to maintain adequate functioning. He may

Signs and symptoms of alcohol withdrawal

Signs and symptoms of alcohol withdrawal may vary in degree from mild (morning hangover) to severe (alcohol withdrawal delirium). Formerly known as *delirium tremens*, alcohol withdrawal delirium is marked by acute distress following abrupt withdrawal after prolonged or massive use.

Signs and symptoms	Mild	Moderate	Severe
Anxiety	Mild restlessness	Obvious motor restlessness and anxiety	Extreme restlessness and agitation with intense fearfulness
Appetite	Impaired appetite	Marked anorexia	Rejection of all food and fluid except alcohol
Blood pressure	Normal or slightly elevated systolic	Usually elevated systolic	Elevated systolic and diastolic
Confusion	None	Variable	Marked confusion and disorientation
GI symptoms	Nausea	Nausea and vomiting	Dry heaves and vomiting
Hallucinations	None	Vague, transient visual and auditory hallucinations and illusions (commonly nocturnal)	Visual and, occasionally, auditory hallucinations, usually of fearful or threatening content; misidentification of people and frightening delusions related to hallucinatory experiences
Seizures	None	Possible	Common
Sleep disturbance	Restless sleep or insomnia	Marked insomnia and nightmares	Total wakefulness
Sweating	Slight	Obvious	Marked hyperhidrosis

also report an inability to discontinue or reduce his alcohol intake. His history may reveal episodes of anesthesia or amnesia (blackouts) and episodes of violence during intoxication, as well as impaired social and familial relationships and impaired performance of occupational responsibilities. If he takes the CAGE questionnaire and gives two or more positive responses, alcohol addiction is indicated.

The patient may report malaise, dyspepsia, mood swings or depression, and an increased incidence of infection. Observe the patient for poor personal hygiene and untreated injuries, such as cigarette burns, fractures, and bruises that the patient can't fully explain.

Watch for secretive or manipulative behavior. When confronted, the patient may deny or rationalize the problem, or he may be guarded or hostile in his response. He may also project anger or feelings of guilt or inadequacy onto others.

After abstinence or reduction of alcohol intake, signs and symptoms of withdrawal—which begin shortly after drinking has stopped and last for 5 to 7 days—may vary. (See *Signs and symptoms of alcohol withdrawal.*)

Diagnosis

❍ A blood alcohol level ranging from 0.08% to 0.10% weight/volume (200 mg/dl) is accepted as the level of intoxication, depending on the

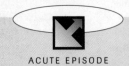

ACUTE EPISODE

Acute intoxication

Acute intoxication is treated symptomatically and may involve respiratory support, fluid replacement, correction of acid-base imbalance, and hypothermia or emergency measures for trauma or GI bleeding. When treating acute intoxication, follow these guidelines:

• Assess the patient's airway, respiratory status, and support respirations, as indicated.

• Monitor the patient's level of consciousness to detect deterioration.

• Assess the patient's heart rate, breath sounds, blood pressure, and temperature frequently.

• Institute seizure precautions.

• Administer medications prescribed to treat the signs and symptoms of withdrawal.

• Prevent aspiration of vomitus by positioning the patient on his side with the head of the bed elevated. A nasogastric tube may be inserted for vomiting.

• Replace fluids and administer I.V. glucose to prevent hypoglycemia.

• Monitor for and correct hypothermia and acidosis.

• Initiate emergency treatment for trauma, infection, or GI bleeding.

• Orient the patient to reality because he may have hallucinations and may try to harm himself or others.

• Maintain a calm environment, minimizing noise and shadows to reduce the incidence of delusions and hallucinations.

• Avoid restraining the patient unless necessary to protect him or others.

state or country. The blood alcohol level in a physically dependent and tolerant drinker may exceed levels that would cause severe dysfunction or death in a nontolerant drinker. (See *Acute intoxication.*)

❍ In severe hepatic disease, the patient may have an increased blood urea nitrogen level and a decreased serum glucose level. Serum ammonia and amylase levels may also be increased.

❍ Urine toxicology studies may help to determine if the patient with alcohol withdrawal delirium or another acute complication abuses other drugs as well.

❍ Liver function studies revealing increased levels of serum cholesterol, lactate dehydrogenase, alanine aminotransferase, aspartate aminotransferase, and creatine kinase may point to liver damage. Elevated serum amylase and lipase levels point to acute pancreatitis.

❍ A hematologic workup can identify anemia, thrombocytopenia, increased prothrombin time, and increased partial thromboplastin time.

Complications
❍ Brain damage
❍ Cardiomyopathy
❍ Cirrhosis of the liver
❍ Death
❍ Depression
❍ Esophageal varices
❍ Hypoglycemia
❍ Malnutrition
❍ Multiple substance abuse
❍ Pancreatitis
❍ Peripheral neuropathy
❍ Pneumonia
❍ Seizure disorder
❍ Suicide and homicide
❍ Wernicke's encephalopathy (see *Complications of alcohol use*)

Treatment
❍ Total abstinence from alcohol is the only effective treatment. Supportive programs that offer detoxification, rehabilitation, and aftercare, including continued involvement in Alcoholics Anonymous, may produce good long-term results.

❍ Aversion, or deterrent, therapy using disulfiram prevents compulsive drinking by producing immediate and potentially fatal distress in the event the patient consumes alcohol up to 2 weeks after taking it.

❍ B-complex vitamin supplements may be given to correct nutritional deficiencies.

Complications of alcohol use

Alcohol can damage body tissues by its direct irritating effects, by changes that take place in the body during its metabolism, by aggravation of existing disease, by accidents occurring during intoxication, and by interactions between the substance and drugs. Such tissue damage can cause these complications:

Cardiopulmonary
- Cardiac arrhythmias
- Cardiomyopathy
- Chronic obstructive pulmonary disease
- Essential hypertension
- Increased risk of tuberculosis
- Pneumonia

Hematologic
- Anemia
- Leukopenia
- Reduced number of phagocytes

Hepatic
- Alcoholic hepatitis
- Cirrhosis
- Fatty liver

GI
- Chronic diarrhea
- Esophageal cancer
- Esophageal varices
- Esophagitis
- Gastric ulcers
- Gastritis
- GI bleeding
- Malabsorption
- Pancreatitis

Neurologic
- Alcoholic dementia
- Alcoholic hallucinosis
- Alcohol withdrawal delirium
- Korsakoff's syndrome
- Peripheral neuropathy
- Seizure disorders
- Subdural hematoma
- Wernicke's encephalopathy

Psychiatric
- Abuse of multiple substances
- Amotivational syndrome
- Depression
- Impaired social and occupational functioning
- Suicide

Other
- Beriberi
- Fetal alcohol syndrome
- Hypoglycemia
- Impaired respiratory diffusion
- Increased incidence of pulmonary infections
- Infertility
- Leg and foot ulcers
- Myopathies
- Prostatitis
- Sexual performance difficulties

○ Naltrexone is an opiate antagonist that prevents the pleasurable effects of increased endorphins produced by increased alcohol intake. Preventing these effects reduces the severity of alcohol cravings, thereby reducing alcohol intake and relapse incidence.

○ Supportive counseling or individual, group, or family psychotherapy provides ongoing support.

 COLLABORATIVE MANAGEMENT Care of the patient with alcohol addiction involves several members of the interdisciplinary team. In addition to the registered nurse, the interdisciplinary team may consist of a social worker to assist with financial and psychosocial issues, a dietitian to optimize nutrition, a physical therapist to teach energy conservation measures, and a drug or alcohol counselor to provide support with abstinence.

Special considerations

○ Assess for signs of inadequate nutrition and dehydration and provide nutritional support and fluid therapy, as indicated.

○ Approach the patient in a nonthreatening way. Limit sustained eye contact. Even if he's verbally abusive, listen attentively and respond with empathy. Explain all procedures.

○ Monitor the patient for signs of depression or impending suicide.

○ For individuals who have lost all contact with family and friends and who have a long history of unemployment, trouble with the law, or other problems associated with alcohol abuse, rehabilitation may i_____ _____ining, sheltered workshops, halfw____ ____er supervised facilities.

○ Refer spouses of alcoh__ children of alcoholics to _

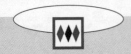
ing in these self-help groups, family members learn to relinquish responsibility for the individual's drinking. Point out that family involvement in rehabilitation can reduce family tensions.
○ Refer adult children of alcoholics to the National Association for Children of Alcoholics.
○ Provide patient education. (See *Teaching about alcohol addiction.*)

Applicable patient-teaching aids
○ Dietary do's and don'ts for cirrhosis *

◌ Alzheimer's disease

Alzheimer's disease is a degenerative disorder of the cerebral cortex, especially the frontal lobe, which accounts for more than one-half of all cases of dementia. Although primarily found in the elderly population, 1% to 10% of cases have their onset in middle age.

Because this is a primary progressive dementia, the prognosis for a patient with this disease is poor.

Causes
The cause of Alzheimer's disease is unknown; however, several factors are implicated in this disease. These include neurochemical factors, such as deficiencies in the neurotransmitter acetylcholine, somatostatin, substance P, and norepinephrine; environmental factors, such as repeated head trauma and exposure to aluminum or manganese; and genetic immunologic factors. Genetic studies show that an autosomal dominant form of Alzheimer's disease is associated with early onset and early death, accounting for about 100,000 deaths per year. A family history of Alzheimer's disease and the presence of Down syndrome are two established risk factors.

Pathophysiology
The brain tissue of patients with Alzheimer's disease exhibits three distinct and characteristic features:
○ neurofibrillatory tangles (fibrous proteins)
○ neuritic plaques (composed of degenerating axons and dendrites)
○ granulovascular changes. (See *Abnormal cellular structures in Alzheimer's disease.*)

   Additional structural changes include cortical atrophy, ventricular dilation, deposition of amyloid (a glycoprotein) around the cortical blood vessels, and reduced brain volume. Also found is a selective loss of cholinergic neurons in the pathways to the frontal lobes and hippocampus, areas that are important for memory and cognitive functions. Examination of the brain after death commonly reveals an atrophic brain, commonly weighing less than 1,000 g (normal, 1,380 g).

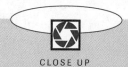

CLOSE UP

Abnormal cellular structures in Alzheimer's disease

How and why neurons die in Alzheimer's disease is largely unknown. The brain tissue of patients with Alzheimer's disease exhibits three distinct and characteristic features: granulovacuolar degeneration, neurofibrillary tangles, and amyloid plaques.

Granulovacuolar degeneration

Granulovacuolar degeneration occurs inside the neurons of the hippocampus. An abnormally high number of fluid-filled spaces (vacuoles) enlarge the cell's body, possibly causing the cell to die.

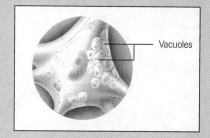

Neurofibrillary tangles

Neurofibrillary tangles are bundles of filaments inside the neuron that abnormally twist around one another. They're found in the brain areas associated with memory and learning (hippocampus), fear and aggression (amygdala), and thinking (cerebral cortex). These tangles may play a role in the memory loss and personality changes that commonly occur in Alzheimer's disease.

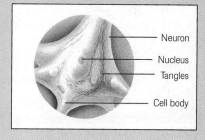

Amyloid plaques

Also called *senile plaques*, amyloid plaques are found outside neurons in the extracellular space of the cerebral cortex and hippocampus. They contain a core of beta amyloid protein surrounded by abnormal nerve endings (neurites).

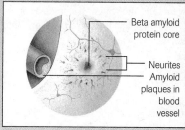

Assessment findings

Initially, the patient undergoes almost imperceptible changes, such as forgetfulness, recent memory loss, difficulty learning and remembering new information, deterioration in personal hygiene and appearance, and an inability to concentrate. Gradually, tasks that require abstract thinking and activities that require judgment become more difficult. Progressive difficulty in communication and severe deterioration in memory, language, and motor function, result in a loss of coordination and an inability to write or speak. Personality changes, such as restlessness and irritability, and nocturnal awakenings are common.

Patients also exhibit loss of eye contact, a fearful look, wringing of the hands, and other signs of anxiety. When a patient with Alzheimer's disease is overwhelmed with anxiety, he becomes dysfunctional, acutely confused, agitated, compulsive, or fearful.

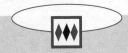

Teaching about Alzheimer's disease

Remember these key points when teaching the patient, family, and caregiver about Alzheimer's disease:

● Teach them about the disease and its treatments, and refer them to social service and community resources for legal and financial advice and support.

● Teach the need for activity and exercise to maintain mobility and help prevent complications.

● Discuss dietary adjustments for patients with restlessness, dysphagia, or coordination problems.

● Emphasize the importance of establishing a daily routine, providing a safe environment, and avoiding overstimulation.

● Instruct the caregiver about self-care, including the importance of adequate rest, good nutrition, and private time.

Eventually, the patient becomes disoriented, and emotional lability and physical and intellectual disability progress.

Diagnosis

○ Alzheimer's disease is diagnosed by ruling out other disorders as the cause for the patient's signs and symptoms. The only true way to confirm Alzheimer's disease is by finding pathological changes in the brain at autopsy.

○ Positron emission tomography shows changes in cerebral cortex metabolism.

○ Computed tomography scan shows evidence of early brain atrophy in excess of that which occurs in normal aging.

○ Magnetic resonance imaging shows no lesion as the cause of the dementia.

○ Electroencephalography shows evidence of slowed brain waves in the later stages of the disease.

○ Cerebral blood flow studies show abnormalities in blood flow.

Complications

○ Aspiration
○ Death
○ Dehydration
○ Injury secondary to violent behavior or wandering
○ Malnutrition
○ Pneumonia and other infections

Treatment

○ No cure or definitive treatment exists for Alzheimer's disease; however, therapy may include:

– N-methyl-D-aspartate receptor antagonist therapy to improve memory and learning in patients with moderate to severe Alzheimer's disease

– cholinesterase inhibitors to help improve memory deficits

– antidepressants to improve mood and reduce irritability

– antipsychotics to treat hallucinations, delusions, aggression, hostility, and uncooperativeness

– anxiolytics to treat anxiety, restlessness, verbally disruptive behavior, and resistance

– antioxidant therapy (vitamin E therapy currently under study), possibly, to delay disease effects

– omega-3 fatty acids (found in fish such as salmon) to reduce risk of Alzheimer's disease

– behavioral interventions (simplifying environment, tasks, routines) to prevent agitation

– effective communication strategies to ensure continued communication between patient and family

– teaching aids, safety needs, and social service and community references to educate caregivers and provide legal and financial advice and support.

 COLLABORATIVE MANAGEMENT
An interdisciplinary approach is crucial in providing care to the patient with Alzheimer's disease. The nurse helps maintain the patient's abilities, compensate for those that he has lost, and supports the caregivers. The neurologist diagnoses the disorder and develops a treatment plan to reduce behavioral problems and complications. Caregivers must be included in planning

treatment because they are most familiar with the patient's specific behaviors and responses and will be the ones providing care. The dietitian helps to maintain nutrition by recommending a dietary plan, style of food preparation, and approach to feeding. The physical therapist helps the patient maintain the highest level of safe independent functioning. The occupation therapist can teach the patient to complete simple tasks such as those involved in activities of daily living. The social worker can guide families and caregivers to appropriate community resources, assist with financial difficulties, and explain advanced directives.

Special considerations

○ Establish an effective communication system with the patient and his family to help them adjust to the patient's altered cognitive abilities.
○ Offer emotional support to the patient and his family.
○ Maintain a calm, structured environment because behavior problems may be worsened by excess stimulation or a change in established routine.
○ Anxiety may cause the patient to become agitated or fearful. Intervene by helping him focus on another activity.
○ Provide the patient with a safe environment. Encourage him to exercise, as ordered, to help maintain mobility.
○ Refer caregivers to social services and community resources for support and legal and financial assistance.
○ Provide patient education. (See *Teaching about Alzheimer's disease*.)

Applicable patient-teaching aids

○ Avoiding burnout: Aid for the caregiver *
○ Planning home care *
○ Preparing for the patient's homecoming *
○ Promoting patient safety *

○ Amyotrophic lateral sclerosis

Commonly called *Lou Gehrig disease*, after the New York Yankees first baseman who died of this disorder, amyotrophic lateral sclerosis (ALS) is the most common of the motor neuron

---

Motor neuron disease

In its final stages, motor neuron disease affects upper and lower motor neuron cells. However, the site of initial cell damage varies according to the specific disease:
● *progressive bulbar palsy:* degeneration of upper motor neurons in the medulla oblongata
● *progressive muscular atrophy:* degeneration of lower motor neurons in the spinal cord
● *amyotrophic lateral sclerosis:* degeneration of upper motor neurons in the medulla oblongata and lower motor neurons in the spinal cord.

---

diseases causing muscular atrophy. Other motor neuron diseases include progressive muscular atrophy and progressive bulbar palsy. Onset usually occurs between ages 40 and 70. A chronic, progressively debilitating disease, ALS may be fatal in less than 1 year or continue for 10 years or more, depending on the muscles affected. More than 30,000 Americans have ALS; about 5,000 new cases are diagnosed each year; and the disease affects three times as many men as women. (See *Motor neuron disease*.)

Causes

The exact cause of ALS is unknown, but about 5% to 10% of cases have a genetic component—an autosomal dominant trait that affects men and women equally.

Several mechanisms have been postulated, including:
○ a slow-acting virus
○ a nutritional deficiency related to a disturbance in enzyme metabolism
○ a metabolic interference in nucleic acid production by the nerve fibers
○ autoimmune disorders that affect immune complexes in the renal glomerulus and basement membrane.

Precipitating factors for acute deterioration include any severe stress, such as myocardial infarction, trauma, viral infections, and physical exhaustion.

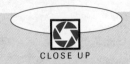

CLOSE UP

ALS: How it happens

Amyotrophic lateral sclerosis (ALS) progressively destroys upper and lower motor neurons (including anterior horn cells of the spinal cord, upper motor neurons of the cerebral cortex, and motor nuclei of the brain stem).

| May begin when glutamate (primary excitatory neurotransmitter of the central nervous system) accumulates to toxic levels at synapses. |

↓

| Affected motor units are no longer innervated; progressive degeneration of axons causes loss of myelin. |

↓

| Nonfunctional scar tissue replaces normal neuronal tissue; denervation leads to muscle fiber atrophy and motor neuron degeneration. |

Pathophysiology

ALS progressively destroys the upper and lower motor neurons. It doesn't affect cranial nerves III, IV, and VI and, therefore, some facial movements, such as blinking, persist. Intellectual and sensory functions aren't affected.

Some researchers believe that glutamate — the primary excitatory neurotransmitter of the central nervous system — accumulates to toxic levels at the synapses. The affected motor units are no longer innervated and progressive degeneration of axons causes loss of myelin. Some nearby motor nerves may sprout axons in an attempt to maintain function but, ultimately, nonfunctional scar tissue replaces normal neuronal tissue. (See *ALS: How it happens*.)

Assessment findings

The patient with ALS develops progressive loss of muscle strength and coordination that eventually interfere with everyday activities. The patient also develops fasciculations, accompanied by atrophy and weakness, especially in the muscles of the feet and the hands; impaired speech; difficulty chewing, swallowing, and breathing; occasionally, choking and excessive drooling; and depression, as a reaction to the disease.

Diagnosis

○ Electromyography shows abnormalities of electrical activity in involved muscles.
○ Muscle biopsy shows atrophic fibers interspersed between normal fibers.
○ Nerve conduction studies show normal results.
○ Computed tomography scan and EEG show normal results and thus rule out multiple sclerosis, spinal cord neoplasm, polyarteritis, syringomyelia, myasthenia gravis, progressive muscular dystrophy, and progressive stroke.

Complications

○ Aspiration
○ Complications of physical immobility
○ Respiratory failure
○ Respiratory infections

Treatment

○ Riluzole, which modulates glutamate activity, may slow the disease progression and increase the quality of life and survival but doesn't reverse or stop disease progression.

○ Baclofen, dantrolene, or diazepam help control spasticity that interferes with activities of daily living.

○ Trihexyphenidyl or amitriptyline may be used for impaired ability to swallow saliva.

○ Quinine therapy may relieve painful leg cramps.

○ Thyrotropin-releasing hormone may temporarily improve motor function (successful only in some patients).

○ Gastrostomy may be needed for nutritional support for patients at risk for aspiration.

○ Devices to assist in breathing at night or mechanical ventilation should be discussed, but the patient's wishes should be respected.

○ Stem-cell therapy, which shows great promise, is being studied.

 COLLABORATIVE MANAGEMENT
An interdisciplinary approach is necessary to maximize patient functioning and reduce the risk of complications. The nurse provides support, education, and cares for the patient during acute exacerbations. If the patient is depressed, a medical social worker or therapist can help provide counseling for this progressive, fatal illness. The physical therapist and occupational therapist assist in promoting the highest level of independent functioning and recommend the use of appliances and assistive devices. The speech therapist helps with communication deficits, assesses for swallowing difficulties, and makes recommendations for gastrostomy tube placement if the patient is at risk for aspiration. The dietitian provides proper nutritional counseling.

Special considerations

○ Remember that because mental status remains intact while progressive physical degeneration takes place, the patient acutely perceives every change that threatens his relationships, career, income, muscle coordination, sexuality, and energy.

○ Implement a rehabilitation program designed to maintain independence as long as possible.

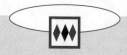

KEY TEACHING POINTS

Teaching about ALS

Remember these key points when teaching your patient and his family or caregiver about amyotrophic lateral sclerosis (ALS):

● Teach the patient how motor neuron degeneration affects muscles and motor function.

● Encourage the patient to exercise to maintain strength in unaffected muscles.

● Describe dietary changes to facilitate swallowing.

● Demonstrate how to operate a wheelchair safely.

● Explain tips for preventing and dealing with complications such as pressure ulcers.

● Assist the patient with developing alternative communication techniques.

● Teach the patient to suction himself if he's unable to handle an increased accumulation of secretions.

● If the patient has a gastrostomy tube, show the patient's family (or the patient if he's still able to feed himself) how to administer tube feedings.

● Discuss directives regarding health care decisions.

○ Help the patient obtain assistive equipment, such as a walker and a wheelchair.

○ Depending on the patient's muscular capacity, assist with bathing, personal hygiene, and transfers from wheelchair to bed.

○ Help establish a regular bowel and bladder routine.

○ To prevent skin breakdown, provide good skin care when the patient is bedridden. Turn him often, keep his skin clean and dry, and use pressure-reducing devices such as an alternating air mattress.

○ If the patient has trouble swallowing, give him soft, solid foods and position him upright during meals.

○ Provide feedings through a gastrostomy or nasogastric tube if he can no longer swallow.

○ Provide emotional support. Prepare the patient and his family for his eventual death, and encourage the start of the grieving process. Patients with ALS may benefit from a hospice program or the local ALS support group chapter.

○ Arrange for a visiting nurse to oversee the patient's status, provide support, and teach the family about the illness. (See *Teaching about ALS,* page 15.)

Applicable patient-teaching aids
○ Choosing the right wheelchair *
○ Coping with a fall from a wheelchair *
○ Giving an intermittent feeding
○ Helping a person into or out of a wheelchair *
○ Learning to communicate without speech *

○ Ankylosing spondylitis

A chronic, usually progressive inflammatory disease, ankylosing spondylitis primarily affects the sacroiliac, apophyseal, and costovertebral joints, along with adjacent soft tissue. The disease (also known as *rheumatoid spondylitis* and *Marie-Strümpell disease*) usually begins in the sacroiliac joints and gradually progresses to the spine's lumbar, thoracic, and cervical regions. Deterioration of bone and cartilage can lead to fibrous tissue formation with eventual fusion of the spine or peripheral joints. Signs and symptoms of ankylosing spondylitis can progress unpredictably, and the disease can go into remission, exacerbation, or arrest at any stage.

Ankylosing spondylitis affects one out of every 10,000 people and affects more males than females. Progressive disease is well recognized in men, but the diagnosis is commonly overlooked or missed in females, who tend to have more peripheral joint involvement. It usually emerges between ages 20 and 40, but it may develop in children younger than age 10.

Causes
Evidence strongly suggests a familial tendency in ankylosing spondylitis. The presence of human leukocyte antigen (HLA)-B27 (positive in more than 90% of patients with this disease)

and circulating immune complexes suggests immunologic activity.

Pathophysiology
Fibrous tissue of the joint capsule is infiltrated by inflammatory cells that erode the bone and fibrocartilage. Repair of the cartilaginous structures begins with the proliferation of fibroblasts, which synthesize and secrete collagen. The collagen forms fibrous scar tissue that eventually undergoes calcification and ossification, causing the joint to fuse or lose flexibility.

Assessment findings
The first indication of ankylosing spondylitis is intermittent lower back pain that's usually most severe in the morning or after a period of inactivity. Other signs and symptoms depend on the disease stage and may include:
○ hip deformity and associated limited range of motion (ROM)
○ kyphosis, occurring in advanced stages, caused by chronic stooping to relieve symptoms
○ mild fatigue; fever, anorexia or weight loss; occasional iritis; aortic insufficiency and cardiomegaly; and upper lobe pulmonary fibrosis and may cause dyspnea (mimics tuberculosis)
○ pain and limited expansion of the chest due to involvement of the costovertebral joints
○ peripheral arthritis possibly involving the shoulders, hips, and knees
○ stiffness and limited motion of the lumbar spine
○ tenderness over the inflammation site.

Diagnosis
○ The presence of HLA-B27 strongly suggests ankylosing spondylitis.
○ Radiologic studies show these characteristic findings: blurring of the bony margins of joints in the early stage, bilateral sacroiliac involvement, patchy sclerosis with superficial bony erosions, eventual squaring of vertebral bodies, and bamboo spine with complete ankylosis.
○ Erythrocyte sedimentation rate and alkaline phosphatase and serum immunoglobulin A levels may be elevated.

O Negative rheumatoid factor helps rule out rheumatoid arthritis, which produces similar symptoms.

Complications
O Fractures
O Iritis
O Reduced functional ability
O Renal impairment or failure

Treatment
O Anti-inflammatory analgesics, such as aspirin, indomethacin, sulfasalazine, and sulindac, are used to control pain and inflammation.
O Tumor necrosis factor inhibitors have been shown to improve symptoms.
O Corticosteroid therapy suppresses the immune system to control various symptoms.
O Cytotoxic drugs that block cell growth have been used in patients who don't respond well to corticosteroids or those who are dependent on high doses of corticosteroids.
O Surgical hip replacement for severe hip involvement.
O Spinal wedge osteotomy to separate and reposition the vertebrae in severe spinal involvement in selected patients only because of the risk of spinal cord damage and the long convalescence involved.

 COLLABORATIVE MANAGEMENT
Care of the patient with ankylosing spondylitis involves several members of the interdisciplinary team. The physical therapist and occupational therapist help the patient maintain function and minimize deformity through good posture, stretching and deep breathing exercises and, in some patients, braces and lightweight supports. Because ankylosing spondylitis is a chronic, progressively crippling condition, a comprehensive treatment plan should also include a social worker, visiting nurse, and dietitian.

Special considerations
O Keep in mind that limited ROM makes simple tasks difficult.
O Offer support and reassurance because ankylosing spondylitis can be an extremely painful and crippling disease.

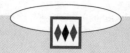

Teaching about ankylosing spondylitis

To minimize deformities, remember these key points when teaching your patient about ankylosing spondylitis:
● Explain the disease process and its treatments.
● Discuss the drugs the patient is taking, including their indications, dosages, and adverse effects.
● Tell the patient to avoid physical activity that places undue stress on the back such as lifting heavy objects.
● Discuss with the patient the need to stand upright; to sit upright in a high, straight chair; and to avoid leaning over a desk.
● Tell the patient to sleep in a prone position on a firm mattress and to avoid using pillows under his neck or knees.
● Advise the patient to avoid prolonged walking, standing, sitting, or driving.
● Demonstrate how to perform regular stretching and deep-breathing exercises.
● Instruct the patient to swim regularly, if he's able.
● Advise the patient to have his height measured every 3 to 4 months to detect a tendency toward kyphosis.
● Recommend vocational counseling to the patient if his job requires standing or prolonged sitting at a desk.
● Discuss the importance of smoking cessation and methods to stop smoking.

O Administer medications as ordered.
O Assess mobility and degree of discomfort frequently. Apply local heat and provide massage to relieve pain.
O Assist with daily exercises as needed to maintain strength and function.
O If treatment includes surgery, provide good postoperative nursing care.

○ Advise the patient to contact the local Arthritis Foundation chapter for a support group.

○ Refer the patient to a smoking-cessation program

○ Provide patient education. (See *Teaching about ankylosing spondylitis,* page 17.)

Applicable patient-teaching aids
○ Learning about corticosteroids
○ Learning about walkers *
○ Protecting your joints *

○ Anorexia nervosa

The key feature of the eating disorder anorexia nervosa is self-imposed starvation, resulting from a distorted body image and an intense, irrational fear of gaining weight, even when the patient is obviously emaciated. A patient with anorexia nervosa is preoccupied with her body size, describes herself as "fat," and commonly expresses dissatisfaction with a particular aspect of her physical appearance. Although the term *anorexia* suggests that the patient's weight loss is associated with a loss of appetite, this is rare.

There are two types of anorexia nervosa: restriction of eating (refusal to eat may be accompanied by compulsive exercise, self-induced vomiting, or abuse of laxatives or diuretics) and binging and purging.

Anorexia nervosa occurs in 5% to 10% of the population; about 90% of those affected are women. This disorder occurs primarily in adolescents and young adults but may also affect older women. The occurrence among males is rising. The prognosis varies but improves if the patient is diagnosed early or if she wants to overcome the disorder and seeks help voluntarily. Mortality ranges from 5% to 15%—the highest mortality associated with a psychiatric disturbance. Death usually results from starvation or suicide.

Causes
No causes of anorexia nervosa have been identified; however, genetic, social, and psychological factors have been implicated. Researchers

in neuroendocrinology are seeking a physiologic cause but have found nothing definite. Clearly, social attitudes that equate slimness with beauty play some role in provoking this disorder; family factors also play a role.

Most theorists believe that refusing to eat is a subconscious effort to exert personal control over one's life. Anorexia nervosa has been associated with other psychiatric disorders, such as obsessive-compulsive disorder, depression, and anxiety.

Pathophysiology
Normally, a physiologic stimulus is responsible for the sensation of hunger. Falling blood glucose levels stimulate the hunger center in the hypothalamus; rising blood fat and amino acid levels promote satiety. Hunger is also stimulated by contraction of an empty stomach and suppressed when the GI tract becomes distended,0 possibly as a result of stimulation of the vagus nerve. Sight, touch, and smell play subtle roles in controlling the appetite center.

In anorexia nervosa, the physiologic stimuli are present but the person has no appetite or desire to eat. Slow gastric emptying or gastric stasis can cause anorexia. High levels of neurotransmitters, such as serotonin (may contribute to satiety), and excess cortisol levels (may suppress hypothalamic control of hunger) have also been implicated as a cause of anorexia.

Assessment findings
The patient's history usually reveals a 25% or greater weight loss for no organic reason, coupled with a morbid dread of being fat and a compulsion to be thin. Such a patient tends to be angry and ritualistic. She may report amenorrhea, infertility, sleep alterations, intolerance to cold, and constipation.

Hypotension and bradycardia may be present. Inspection may reveal an emaciated appearance, with skeletal muscle atrophy, loss of fatty tissue, atrophy of breast tissue, blotchy or sallow skin, lanugo on the face and body, and dryness of scalp hair. If the patient is also bulimic, calluses on the knuckles, and abrasions and scars on the dorsum of the hand may result from tooth injury during self-induced vomiting.

Other signs of vomiting include dental caries and oral or pharyngeal abrasions.

Palpations may disclose painless salivary gland enlargement and bowel distention. Slowed reflexes may occur on percussion. Oddly, the patient usually demonstrates hyperactivity and vigor (despite malnourishment). She may exercise avidly without apparent fatigue.

During psychosocial assessment, the patient may express a morbid fear of gaining weight and an obsession with her physical appearance. Paradoxically, she may also be obsessed with food, preparing elaborate meals for others. Social regression, including poor sexual adjustment and fear of failure, is common. Like bulimia nervosa, anorexia nervosa commonly is associated with depression. The patient may report feelings of despair, hopelessness, and worthlessness, as well as suicidal thoughts.

Diagnosis

○ Hemoglobin level, platelet count, and white blood cell count may be decreased.
○ Bleeding time tends to be prolonged due to thrombocytopenia.
○ Erythrocyte sedimentation rate may be decreased.
○ Serum creatinine, blood urea nitrogen, uric acid, cholesterol, total protein, albumin, sodium, potassium, chloride, calcium, and fasting blood glucose levels may be decreased as a result of malnutrition.
○ Alanine aminotransferase and aspartate aminotransferase may be elevated in severe starvation states.
○ Serum amylase levels may be elevated when pancreatitis isn't present.
○ Serum luteinizing hormone and follicle-stimulating hormone levels may be decreased in females.
○ Triiodothyronine levels may be decreased as a result of a lower basal metabolic rate.
○ Urine may be dilute as a result of the kidneys' impaired ability to concentrate urine.
○ Electrocardiogram (ECG) may reveal non-specific ST interval, prolonged QT interval, and T-wave changes; ventricular arrhythmias may be present. (See *Diagnosing anorexia nervosa*.)

Diagnosing anorexia nervosa

A diagnosis of anorexia nervosa is made when the patient meets these criteria put forth in the *Diagnostic and Statistical Manual of Mental Disorders*, Fourth Edition, Text Revision:

● The patient refuses to maintain body weight over a minimal normal weight for age and height (for example, weight loss leading to maintenance of body weight 15% below that expected); or failure to achieve expected weight gain during a growth period, leading to body weight 15% below that expected.

● The patient experiences intense fear of gaining weight or becoming fat, despite her underweight status.

● The patient has a distorted perception of body weight, size, or shape (that is, the person claims to feel fat even when emaciated or believes that one body area is too fat even when it's obviously underweight).

● In women, absence of at least three consecutive menstrual cycles when otherwise expected to occur.

Reprinted with permission from the *Diagnostic and Statistical Manual of Mental Disorders*, Copyright 2000. American Psychiatric Association.

Complications

○ Amenorrhea
○ Anemia
○ Death
○ Decreased cardiac output
○ Decreased left ventricular muscle mass and chamber size
○ Dehydration
○ Hypotension
○ ECG changes
○ Electrolyte imbalances
○ Esophageal erosion, ulcers, tears, and bleeding
○ Heart failure
○ Increased susceptibility to infection
○ Malnutrition
○ Suicide
○ Tooth and gum erosion and dental caries

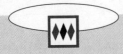

KEY TEACHING POINTS

Teaching about anorexia nervosa

Remember these key points when teaching your patient and her family about anorexia nervosa:
- Explain the disorder and how it affects the body.
- Teach the patient how to keep a food journal, including the types of food eaten, eating frequency, and feelings associated with eating and exercise.
- Advise family members to avoid discussing food with the patient.
- Discuss proper nutrition and long-term weight management.

Treatment

○ Behavior modification may be used such as granting privileges depending on weight gain.
○ Restricted activity for physical reasons, such as arrhythmias, with gradual increase in physical activity when weight gain and stabilization occur
○ Nutritional support, such as vitamin and mineral supplements; a reasonable diet with or without liquid supplements; or subclavian, peripheral, or enteral hyperalimentation (enteral and peripheral routes carry less risk of infection).
○ Group, family, or individual psychotherapy to address the underlying problems of low self-esteem, guilt, anxiety, feelings of hopelessness and helplessness, and depression.

COLLABORATIVE MANAGEMENT
An interdisciplinary approach to care — combining aggressive medical management; nutritional counseling; and individual, group, or family psychotherapy or behavior modification therapy — is most effective in treating anorexia.

Special considerations

○ During hospitalization, regularly monitor vital signs, nutritional status, and intake and output.

○ Weigh the patient daily — before breakfast if possible. Because the patient fears being weighed, vary the weighing routine.
○ Help the patient establish a target weight, and support her efforts to achieve this goal. Expect a weight gain of about 1 lb (0.5 kg) per week.
○ Negotiate an adequate food intake with the patient. Make sure the patient understands that she'll need to comply with this contract or lose privileges.
○ Frequently offer small portions of food or drinks if the patient wants them. Allow the patient to maintain control over the types and amounts of food she eats, if possible.
○ Maintain one-on-one supervision of the patient during meals and for 1 hour afterward to ensure compliance with the dietary treatment program.
○ During an acute anorexic episode, nutritionally complete liquids are more acceptable than solid food because they eliminate the need to choose between foods — something many patients with anorexia find difficult. If tube feedings or other special feeding measures become necessary, fully explain these measures to the patient and be ready to discuss her fears or reluctance; limit the discussion about food itself.
○ If edema or bloating occurs after the patient has returned to normal eating behavior, reassure her that this phenomenon is temporary. She may fear that she's becoming fat and stop complying with the treatment plan.
○ Encourage the patient to recognize and express her feelings freely. If she understands that she can be assertive, she may gradually learn that expressing her true feelings won't result in her losing control or love.
○ Because the patient and her family may need therapy to uncover and correct dysfunctional patterns, refer them to Anorexia Nervosa and Related Eating Disorders, a national information and support organization.
○ Educate the patient and family about anorexia nervosa. (See *Teaching about anorexia nervosa*.)

Applicable patient-teaching aids

○ Learning about daily food choices

Anxiety disorder, generalized

Anxiety is a feeling of apprehension that some describe as an exaggerated feeling of impending doom, dread, or uneasiness. Unlike fear — a reaction to danger from a specific external source — anxiety is a reaction to an internal threat, such as an unacceptable impulse or a repressed thought that's straining to reach a conscious level.

A rational response to a real threat, occasional anxiety is a normal part of life. Overwhelming anxiety, however, can result in generalized anxiety disorder — uncontrollable, unreasonable worry that persists for at least 6 months and narrows perceptions or interferes with normal functioning. Recent evidence indicates that the prevalence of generalized anxiety disorder is greater than previously thought and may be even greater than that of depression.

Causes

Anxiety disorders are thought to result from a combination of genetic, biochemical, neuroanatomic, and psychological factors — plus life experiences.

Generalized anxiety disorder may run in families and have a genetic component. Some believe that an imbalance in neurotransmitters, such as serotonin and dopamine, may play a role. Others theorize that conflict, whether intrapsychic, psychosocial, or interpersonal, promotes an anxiety state.

Pathophysiology

The pathophysiology of generalized anxiety disorder is thought to involve the gamma-aminobutyric (GABA) A receptor-chloride ion channel complex. Benzodiazepines bind two separate GABA-A receptor sites: Type I has broad anatomic distribution, and type II is concentrated in the hippocampus, striatum, and neocortex. Serotonin also appears to have a role in anxiety.

Assessment findings

Signs and symptoms of generalized anxiety disorder vary with the disorder's severity. The patient with mild anxiety may present with mainly

---

Diagnosing generalized anxiety disorder

A diagnosis of generalized anxiety disorder is made when the patient meets these criteria put forth in the *Diagnostic and Statistical Manual of Mental Disorders*, Fourth Edition, Text Revision:
- Excessive worry about a number of events or activities that occurs more days than not for at least 6 months.
- The person finds it difficult to control the worry.
- The anxiety and worry are associated with at least three of these six symptoms:
  − restlessness or feeling keyed up or on edge
  − being easily fatigued
  − difficulty concentrating or mind going blank
  − irritability
  − muscle tension
  − sleep disturbances (difficulty falling or staying asleep or restless, unsatisfying sleep).
- The focus of the anxiety and worry isn't confined to features of an axis I (clinical) disorder.
- The anxiety, worry, or physical symptoms cause clinically significant distress or impairment in social, occupational, or other important areas of functioning.
- The disturbance isn't due to the direct physiologic effects of a substance or a general medical condition and doesn't occur exclusively during a mood disorder, a psychotic disorder, or a pervasive developmental disorder.

Reprinted with permission from the *Diagnostic and Statistical Manual of Mental Disorders*, Copyright 2000. American Psychiatric Association.

---

psychological symptoms, with unusual self-awareness and alertness to the environment. The patient with moderate anxiety may present with selective inattention, but with the ability to concentrate on a single task. The patient with severe anxiety may be unable to concentrate on more than the scattered details of a task; if the patient's in a panic state, he may present with a complete loss of concentration and unintelligible speech.

Other assessment findings of generalized anxiety disorder include signs or symptoms of

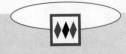

motor tension, including trembling, muscle aches and spasms, headaches, and an inability to relax. Autonomic signs and symptoms, include shortness of breath, tachycardia, sweating, and abdominal complaints. The patient may also present with feelings of apprehension, fear, or anger; may startle easily; and have eating and sleeping difficulties. The medical, psychiatric, and psychosocial histories may fail to identify a specific physical or environmental cause of the anxiety.

Diagnosis

○ The *Diagnostic and Statistical Manual of Mental Disorders,* Fourth Edition, Text Revision, provides the criteria for diagnosing generalized anxiety disorder. (See *Diagnosing generalized anxiety disorder,* page 21.)

○ Laboratory tests exclude organic causes of the patient's signs and symptoms, such as hyperthyroidism, pheochromocytoma, coronary artery disease, supraventricular tachycardia, and Ménière's disease.

○ Complete blood count, white blood cell count and differential, and serum lactate and calcium levels can rule out hypocalcemia.

○ Because anxiety is the central feature of other mental disorders, psychiatric evaluation must rule out phobias, obsessive-compulsive disorders, depression, and acute schizophrenia.

Complications
○ Alcohol and substance abuse
○ Bruxism
○ Depression
○ Headache
○ Impaired social functioning
○ Insomnia
○ Irritable bowel syndrome
○ Panic attacks
○ Phobias

Treatment
○ Benzodiazepines may relieve mild anxiety and improve the patient's ability to cope.

○ Buspirone, an antianxiety drug, causes less sedation and poses less risk of physical and psychological dependence than the benzodiazepines.

○ Selective serotonin reuptake inhibitors may be used to help relieve anxiety.

○ Psychotherapy helps the patient identify and deal with the cause of the anxiety. It also eliminates environmental factors that precipitate an anxious reaction.

○ Relaxation techniques, such as deep breathing, progressive muscle relaxation, focused relaxation, and visualization, may also reduce anxiety.

 COLLABORATIVE MANAGEMENT
Care of the patient with generalized anxiety disorder involves several members of the interdisciplinary team. The physician manages the patient's care. The therapist can help the patient reduce anxiety and learn stress reduction techniques. The nurse reinforces coping strategies and relaxation techniques. The social worker assists with financial and psychosocial issues.

Special considerations
○ Stay with the patient when he's anxious, and encourage him to discuss his feelings.
○ Reduce environmental stimuli and remain calm.

○ Administer antianxiety drugs or tricyclic antidepressants as prescribed, and evaluate the patient's response.

○ Provide patient education. (See *Teaching about generalized anxiety disorder*.)

Applicable patient-teaching aids

○ Performing relaxation breathing exercises *
○ Taking your medication correctly

○ Aortic insufficiency

Aortic insufficiency is the backflow of blood into the left ventricle during diastole. It can result from congenital or acquired conditions. The symptoms range from mild to severe and some people remain asymptomatic for years. It occurs most commonly in males.

Causes

Congenital causes of aortic insufficiency include bicuspid aortic valve and ventricular septal defect (even after repair). It has also been associated with Marfan's syndrome. Aortic insufficiency may also be caused by acquired conditions such as rheumatic fever, syphilis, hypertension, ascending dissecting aortic aneurysm, ankylosing spondylitis, or bacterial endocarditis.

Pathophysiology

Blood flows back into the left ventricle during diastole, causing fluid overload in the ventricle, which dilates and hypertrophies. The excess volume causes fluid overload in the left atrium and, finally, the pulmonary system. Left-sided heart failure and pulmonary edema eventually result.

Pathophysiologic changes in chronic aortic insufficiency result in increased pulmonary vein pressure and cardiac dysfunction, left ventricular dysfunction, inadequate coronary perfusion, a hyperdynamic and tachycardic left ventricle, low diastolic pressure, and regurgitant blood flow through the aortic valve. (See *Understanding aortic insufficiency*.)

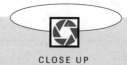

CLOSE UP

Understanding aortic insufficiency

Because of incomplete closure of the semilunar valve, blood flows back into the left ventricle during diastole. This causes fluid overload in the ventricle, which dilates and hypertrophies. The excess volume causes fluid overload in the left atrium and, finally, the pulmonary system. Left-sided heart failure and pulmonary edema eventually result.

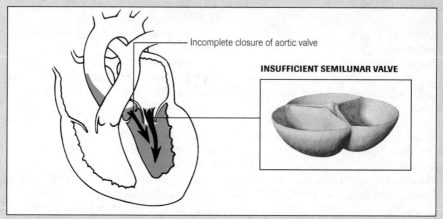

Incomplete closure of aortic valve

INSUFFICIENT SEMILUNAR VALVE

KEY TEACHING POINTS

Teaching about valvular heart disease

Remember these key points when teaching your patient about valvular heart disease:
- Explain normal heart valve function as well as the disease and its treatments.
- Explain the importance of following a low-sodium diet
- Teach about long-term anticoagulation therapy.
- Review activity guidelines.
- Discuss the need for prophylactic antibiotics before surgery and dental work.
- Review signs and symptoms that require medical attention.
- Discuss the need to monitor weight.
- Explain cardiac risk factor modification.

Assessment findings

The patient with chronic aortic insufficiency may be asymptomatic for several years. The most common symptoms are fatigue and dyspnea on exertion. As the disease progresses and heart failure develops, the patient may exhibit cough, orthopnea, paroxysmal nocturnal dyspnea, and palpation and visualization of the apical pulse. Other assessment findings may include:

○ angina
○ cardiac arrhythmias
○ palpitations
○ pulmonary edema
○ pulmonary vein congestion
○ "pulsating" nails beds (Quincke's sign)
○ rapidly rising and collapsing pulses (pulsus bisferiens)
○ S_3 and a diastolic blowing murmur at the left sternal border upon auscultation
○ syncope.

The patient with severe insufficiency may also present with wide pulse pressure.

Diagnosis

○ Cardiac catheterization reveals a reduction in arterial diastolic pressures, aortic regurgitation, other valvular abnormalities, and increased left ventricular end-diastolic pressure.
○ Chest X-rays may show left ventricular enlargement and pulmonary venous congestion.
○ Echocardiography indicates left ventricular enlargement, alterations in mitral valve movement (indirect indication of aortic valve disease), and mitral thickening.
○ Electrocardiography may show sinus tachycardia, left ventricular hypertrophy, and left atrial hypertrophy in severe disease.

Complications

○ Cardiac arrhythmias
○ Endocarditis
○ Heart failure
○ Myocardial ischemia
○ Pulmonary edema
○ Thromboembolism

Treatment

○ Digoxin, a low-sodium diet, diuretics, vasodilators, and angiotensin-converting enzyme inhibitors are used to treat left ventricular failure.
○ Anticoagulants are administered to prevent thrombus formation around diseased or replaced valves.
○ Prophylactic antibiotics are necessary before and after surgery or dental care to prevent endocarditis.
○ Antiarrhythmics may be necessary to treat arrhythmias.
○ Valve replacement with a prosthetic valve may be necessary to control symptoms.

 COLLABORATIVE MANAGEMENT
Care of the patient with aortic insufficiency involves several members of the interdisciplinary team. The nurse plays a crucial role in educating the patient about the disease and its treatments. The dietitian reinforces the need for a low-sodium diet and helps the patient with making proper food choices. The interdisciplinary cardiac rehabilitation team (which may consist of cardiologists, exercise specialists, physical therapists, occupational therapists, dietitians, nurses, and

social workers) provides supervised exercise, education, and cardiac risk modification.

Special considerations

○ Watch closely for signs of heart failure or pulmonary edema and for adverse effects of drug therapy.

○ If the patient has surgery, watch for hypotension, arrhythmias, and thrombus formation. Monitor vital signs, arterial blood gas values, intake and output, daily weight, blood chemistries, chest X-rays, and pulmonary artery catheter readings.

○ Place the patient in an upright position to relieve dyspnea, if indicated.

○ Refer the patient to the American Heart Association for information on vascular heart disease.

○ Arrange for a visiting nurse to see the patient to assess the need for a home health aide or a hospital bed in the home.

○ Provide patient education. (See *Teaching about valvular heart disease.*)

Applicable patient-teaching aids

○ Cutting down on salt *
○ Living with heart failure *
○ Preparing for cardiac catheterization *
○ Preventing infection with antibiotics *
○ Taking anticoagulants *

◯ Aortic stenosis

Aortic stenosis is the narrowing of the aortic valve. It may be classified as acquired or rheumatic and is characterized by the classic triad of angina, syncope, and dyspnea. It occurs most commonly in males.

Causes

Aortic stenosis may be caused by idiopathic fibrosis and calcification, congenital aortic bicuspid valve (associated with coarctation of the aorta), congenital stenosis of the valve cusps, rheumatic fever, and atherosclerosis in elderly patients.

Pathophysiology

In aortic stenosis, increased left ventricular pressure tries to overcome the resistance of the narrowed valvular opening. The added workload increases the demand for oxygen, whereas diminished cardiac output causes poor coronary artery perfusion, ischemia of the left ventricle, and left-sided heart failure. These changes result in abnormal diastolic function, increased oxygen requirement by a hypertrophic myocardium, diminished oxygen delivery secondary to compression of the coronary vessels, systemic vasodilation, arrhythmias, left-sided heart failure, and forced blood flow through the stenotic valve opening. (See *Understanding aortic stenosis,* page 26.)

Assessment findings

The patient with mild aortic stenosis may be asymptomatic. As the disease progresses, the patient may develop dyspnea on exertion and angina. Other findings may include:

○ fatigue, syncope, and palpitations

○ signs and symptoms of left-sided heart failure and pulmonary congestion, paroxysmal nocturnal dyspnea, cough, and orthopnea

○ diminished carotid pulses, pulsus alternans, and cardiac arrhythmias

○ systolic murmur heard at the base of the heart or in the carotid arteries and, possibly, an S_4 on auscultation.

The patient with severe stenosis may develop left ventricular enlargement and heart failure.

Diagnosis

○ Cardiac catheterization reveals a pressure gradient across the valve indicating obstruction and increased left-ventricular end-diastolic pressures.

○ Chest X-rays may reveal valvular calcification, left ventricular enlargement, and pulmonary vein congestion.

○ Echocardiography may reveal a thickened aortic valve and left ventricular wall, possibly coexistent with mitral valve stenosis.

○ Electrocardiography may show left ventricular hypertrophy.

Complications

○ Cardiac arrhythmias
○ Endocarditis
○ Heart failure

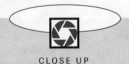

CLOSE UP

Understanding aortic stenosis

Stenosis of the aortic valve results in impedance to forward blood flow. The left ventricle requires greater pressure to open the aortic valve. The added workload increases the demand for oxygen, and diminished cardiac output causes poor coronary artery perfusion, ischemia of the left ventricle, left ventricular hypertrophy, and left-sided heart failure.

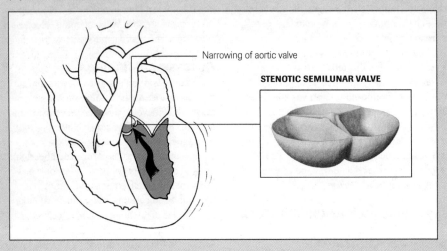

Narrowing of aortic valve

STENOTIC SEMILUNAR VALVE

○ Left ventricular hypertrophy
○ Sudden death

Treatment

○ Digoxin, a low-sodium diet, diuretics, vasodilators, and angiotensin-converting enzyme inhibitors are given to treat left ventricular failure.
○ Nitroglycerin relieves angina.
○ Anticoagulants prevent thrombus formation around diseased or replaced valves.
○ Prophylactic antibiotics must be administered before and after surgery or dental care to prevent endocarditis.
○ Antiarrhythmics may be necessary to treat arrhythmias.
○ Valve replacement with a prosthetic valve or balloon valvuloplasty enlarges the orifice of the stenotic valve.

COLLABORATIVE MANAGEMENT
Care of the patient with aortic stenosis involves several members of the interdisciplinary team. The nurse plays a crucial role in educating the patient about the disease and its treatments. The dietitian reinforces the need for a low-sodium diet and helps the patient with making proper food choices. The interdisciplinary cardiac rehabilitation team (which may consist of cardiologists, exercise specialists, physical therapists, occupational therapists, dietitians, nurses, and social workers) provides supervised exercise, education, and cardiac risk modification.

Special considerations

○ Watch closely for signs of heart failure or pulmonary edema and for adverse effects of drug therapy.

○ If the patient has surgery, watch for hypotension, arrhythmias, and thrombus formation. Monitor vital signs, arterial blood gas values, intake and output, daily weight, blood chemistries, chest X-rays, and pulmonary artery catheter readings.

○ Place the patient in an upright position to relieve dyspnea, if indicated.

○ Refer the patient to the American Heart Association for information on valvular heart disease.

○ Arrange for the visiting nurse to see the patient and assess the need for a home health care aide or a hospital bed in the home.

○ Provide patient education. (See *Teaching about valvular heart disease,* page 24.)

Applicable patient-teaching aids
○ Cutting down on salt *
○ Living with heart failure *
○ Preparing for cardiac catheterization *
○ Preventing infection with antibiotics *
○ Taking anticoagulants *

○ Arterial occlusive disease, chronic

Chronic arterial occlusive disease is the obstruction or narrowing of the lumen of the aorta and its major branches, causing an interruption of blood flow, usually to the legs and feet. This disorder may affect the carotid, vertebral, innominate, subclavian, mesenteric, and celiac arteries. (See *Possible sites of major artery occlusion,* page 28.) Acute arterial occlusion occurs suddenly, often without warning. (*See Acute arterial occlusion,* pages 29 and 30.)

Chronic arterial occlusive disease is more common in males than in females. The prognosis depends on the occlusion's location, the development of collateral circulation to counteract reduced blood flow and, in acute disease, the time elapsed between occlusion and its removal.

Causes
Chronic arterial occlusive disease is a common complication of atherosclerosis. The occlusive mechanism may be endogenous, due to emboli formation or thrombosis, or exogenous, due to trauma or fracture. Predisposing factors include smoking; aging; such conditions as hypertension, hyperlipidemia, and diabetes; and a family history of vascular disorders, myocardial infarction, or stroke.

Pathophysiology
Chronic arterial occlusive disease is almost always the result of atherosclerosis, in which fatty, fibrous plaques narrow the lumen of blood vessels. This occlusion can occur acutely or progressively over 20 to 40 years, with areas of vessel branching, or bifurcation, being the most common sites. The narrowing of the lumens reduces the blood volume that can flow through them, causing arterial insufficiency to the affected area. Ischemia usually occurs after the vessel lumens have narrowed by at least 50%, reducing blood flow to a level at which it no longer meets the needs of tissue and nerves.

Assessment findings
Signs and symptoms of chronic arterial occlusive disease depend on the site of the occlusion. (See *Types of arterial occlusive disease,* page 31.)

Diagnosis
○ Arteriography demonstrates the type (thrombus or embolus), location, and degree of obstruction and the collateral circulation. Arteriography is particularly useful in chronic disease or for evaluating candidates for reconstructive surgery.

○ Doppler ultrasonography and plethysmography are noninvasive tests that show decreased blood flow distal to the occlusion in acute disease.

○ Ophthalmodynamometry helps determine the degree of obstruction in the internal carotid artery by comparing ophthalmic artery pressure to brachial artery pressure on the affected side. More than a 20% difference between pressures suggests insufficiency.

○ EEG and computed tomography scan may be necessary to rule out brain lesions.

(Text continues on page 30.)

Possible sites of major artery occlusion

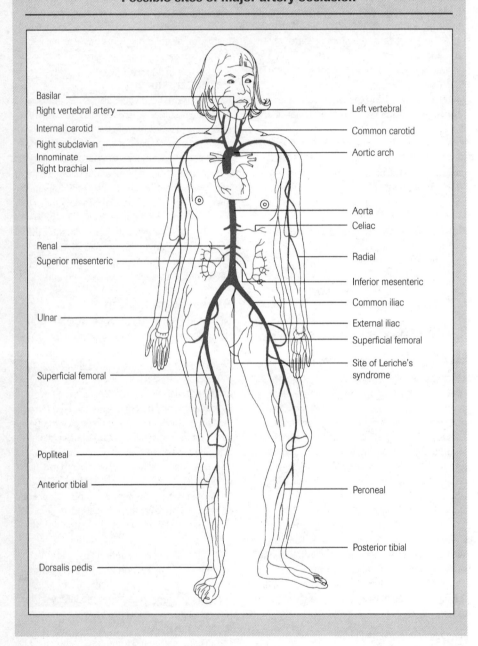

Basilar

Right vertebral artery

Internal carotid

Right subclavian

Innominate

Right brachial

Renal

Superior mesenteric

Ulnar

Superficial femoral

Popliteal

Anterior tibial

Dorsalis pedis

Left vertebral

Common carotid

Aortic arch

Aorta

Celiac

Radial

Inferior mesenteric

Common iliac

External iliac

Superficial femoral

Site of Leriche's syndrome

Peroneal

Posterior tibial

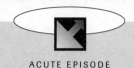

Acute arterial occlusion

Although arterial occlusion is usually chronic, an acute exacerbation can develop, most commonly due to a clot. When caring for a patient with an acute arterial occlusion, follow these guidelines:

● Place the affected limb flat or below the level of the heart.

● Administer thrombolytic or heparin therapy, as prescribed.

● Prepare the patient for possible surgery to restore circulation to the affected area. Possible surgeries include:

– *atherectomy,* in which plaque is excised using a drill or slicing mechanism

– *balloon angioplasty,* in which balloon inflation compresses the obstruction

– *bypass graft,* in which blood flow is diverted through an anastomosed autogenous or Dacron graft past the thrombosed segment

– *embolectomy,* in which a balloon-tipped Fogarty catheter is used to remove thrombotic material from the artery (This procedure is used mainly for mesenteric, femoral, or popliteal artery occlusion.)

– *laser angioplasty,* in which the obstruction is excised and vaporized using hot-tip lasers

– *lumbar sympathectomy,* in which selected nerve fibers are surgically excised, can be used as a possible adjunct to surgery, depending on the condition of the sympathetic nervous system

– *patch grafting,* in which the thrombosed arterial segment is removed and replaced with an autogenous vein or Dacron graft

– *stenting,* in which a mesh of wires that stretch and mold to the arterial wall is inserted to prevent reocclusion (This adjunct follows laser angioplasty or atherectomy.)

– *thromboendarterectomy,* in which the occluded artery is opened and the obstructed thrombus and intimal layer of the arterial wall are removed. (This procedure is usually performed after angiography and commonly used with autogenous vein or Dacron bypass surgery [femoral-popliteal or aortofemoral].)

Preoperative interventions

● Assess the patient's circulatory status by checking for the most distal pulses and by inspecting his skin color and temperature.

● Provide pain relief as needed.

● Administer heparin by continuous I.V. drip, as ordered, using an infusion pump to ensure the proper flow rate.

● Wrap the patient's affected foot in soft cotton batting, and reposition it frequently to prevent pressure on any one area.

● Strictly avoid elevating or applying heat to the affected leg.

● Watch for signs of fluid and electrolyte imbalance, and monitor intake and output for signs of renal failure (urine output less than 30 ml/hour).

● If the patient has carotid, innominate, vertebral, or subclavian artery occlusion, monitor him for signs of stroke, such as numbness in his arm or leg and intermittent blindness.

Postoperatively interventions

● Monitor the patient's vital signs. Continuously assess his bilateral circulatory function by inspecting skin color and temperature and by checking for distal pulses. In charting, compare earlier assessments and observations. Watch closely for signs of hemorrhage (tachycardia and hypotension), and check dressings for excessive bleeding.

● In carotid, innominate, vertebral, or subclavian artery occlusion, assess the patient's neurologic status frequently for changes in level of consciousness or muscle strength and pupil size.

● In mesenteric artery occlusion, connect a nasogastric tube to low intermittent suction. Monitor the patient's intake and output (low urine output may indicate damage to renal arteries during surgery). Check bowel sounds for return of peristalsis. Increased abdominal distention and tenderness may indicate extension of bowel ischemia with resulting gangrene, necessitating further excision, or it may indicate peritonitis.

(continued)

Acute arterial occlusion *(continued)*

● In saddle block occlusion, check distal pulses for adequate circulation. Watch for signs of renal failure and mesenteric artery occlusion (severe abdominal pain) as well as cardiac arrhythmias, which may precipitate embolus formation.
● In iliac artery occlusion, monitor urine output for signs of renal failure from decreased perfusion to the kidneys as a result of surgery. Provide meticulous catheter care.

● In femoral and popliteal artery occlusions, assist the patient with early ambulation, but discourage prolonged sitting.
● After amputation, check the patient's stump carefully for drainage and record its color and amount and the time. Elevate the stump, as ordered, and administer adequate analgesic medication. Because phantom limb pain is common, explain this phenomenon to the patient.

Complications
○ Gangrene, which can lead to limb amputation
○ Impaired nail and hair growth
○ Peripheral or systemic embolism
○ Severe ischemia and necrosis
○ Skin ulceration
○ Stroke or transient ischemic attack

Treatment
○ Supportive measures, such as smoking cessation, hypertension control, stress-management techniques, and mild exercise are appropriate for mild chronic disease.
○ Antiplatelet therapy with ticlopidine or clopidogrel and aspirin may be ordered for carotid artery occlusion.
○ For intermittent claudication of chronic occlusive disease, pentoxifylline and cilostazol may improve blood flow through the capillaries, particularly in patients who are poor candidates for surgery.
○ Surgery may be required to restore circulation to the affected area.
○ Amputation may be necessary if arterial reconstructive surgery fails or if gangrene, persistent infection, or intractable pain develops.
○ Heparin may be prescribed to prevent emboli in embolic occlusion.
○ Bowel resection may be performed after restoration of blood flow for mesenteric artery occlusion.

COLLABORATIVE MANAGEMENT
Care of the patient with arterial occlusive disease involves several members of the interdisciplinary team. The nurse plays a critical role in educating the patient about risk factor modification and proper foot care. The dietitian reinforces the need to follow a diet low in cholesterol and saturated fat and assists the patient in making healthy food choices. The physical therapist assists the patient in developing a walking program.

Special considerations
○ Advise the patient to follow the prescribed medical regimen and to avoid restrictive clothing.
○ Assess for pain and administer analgesics, as indicated.
○ Prevent trauma to the affected extremity.
○ Keep the extremity warm, but avoid the use of heating pads.
○ Advise the patient to stop smoking, and refer him to a smoking-cessation program.
○ Provide comprehensive patient teaching such as proper foot care. (See *Teaching about chronic arterial occlusive disease,* page 32.)

Applicable patient-teaching aids
○ Applying a medicated boot
○ Care and prevention of leg ulcers *
○ Getting ready to go home
○ Learning about heparin *

Types of arterial occlusive disease

Site of occlusion	Signs and symptoms
Aortic bifurcation (saddle block occlusion, a medical emergency associated with cardiac embolization)	• Sensory and motor deficits (muscle weakness, numbness, paresthesia, and paralysis) in both legs • Signs of ischemia (sudden pain and cold, pale legs with decreased or absent peripheral pulses) in both legs
Carotid arterial system • External carotids • Internal carotids	• Absent or decreased pulsation with an auscultatory bruit over the affected vessels • Neurologic dysfunction: transient ischemic attacks (TIAs) due to reduced cerebral circulation producing unilateral sensory or motor dysfunction (transient monocular blindness, and hemiparesis), possible aphasia or dysarthria, confusion, decreased mentation, and headache (These are recurrent features that usually last 5 to 10 minutes but may persist up to 24 hours and may herald a stroke.)
Femoral and popliteal artery (associated with aneurysm formation)	• Gangrene • Intermittent claudication of the calves on exertion • Ischemic pain in feet • Leg pallor and coolness; blanching of the feet on elevation • No palpable pulses in the ankles and feet • Pretrophic pain (heralds necrosis and ulceration)
Iliac artery (Leriche's syndrome)	• Absent or reduced femoral or distal pulses • Impotence • Intermittent claudication of the lower back, buttocks, and thighs, relieved by rest • Possible bruit over femoral arteries
Innominate • Brachiocephalic artery	• Indications of ischemia (claudication) of the right arm • Neurologic dysfunction: signs and symptoms of vertebrobasilar occlusion • Possible bruit over the right side of the neck
Mesenteric artery • Superior (most commonly affected) • Celiac axis • Inferior	• Bowel ischemia, infarct necrosis, and gangrene • Diarrhea • Leukocytosis • Nausea and vomiting • Shock due to massive intraluminal fluid and plasma loss • Sudden, acute abdominal pain
Subclavian artery	• Clinical effects of vertebrobasilar occlusion and exercise-induced arm claudication • Subclavian steal syndrome (characterized by the backflow of blood from the brain through the vertebral artery on the same side as the occlusion, into the subclavian artery distal to the occlusion) • Possibly gangrene (usually limited to the digits)
Vertebrobasilar system • Vertebral arteries • Basilar arteries	• Neurologic dysfunction: TIAs of the brain stem and cerebellum producing binocular visual disturbances, vertigo, dysarthria, and "drop attacks" (falling down without loss of consciousness)

○ Preparing for the patient's homecoming *
○ Taking anticoagulants *

○ Asbestosis

Considered a form of pneumoconiosis, asbestosis is characterized by diffuse interstitial pulmonary fibrosis. Prolonged exposure to airborne particles causes pleural plaques and tumors of the pleura and peritoneum.

Asbestosis may develop 15 to 20 years after regular exposure to asbestos has ended. It's a potent cocarcinogen and increases the smoker's risk of lung cancer. An asbestos worker who smokes is 90 times more likely to develop lung cancer than a smoker who has never worked with asbestos.

Causes

Asbestosis may result from prolonged inhalation of asbestos fibers. People at high risk include workers in the mining, milling, construction, fireproofing, and textile industries. Others at increased risk include those with exposure to asbestos used in paints, plastics, and brake and clutch linings. Asbestos-related diseases develop in families of asbestos workers as a result of exposure to fibrous dust shaken off workers' clothing at home. Exposure to fibrous asbestos dust in deteriorating buildings or in waste piles from asbestos plants also increases the risk of asbestosis.

Pathophysiology

Asbestosis occurs when lung spaces become filled with asbestos fibers. The inhaled asbestos fibers (50 microns or more in length and 0.5 microns or less in diameter) travel down the airway and penetrate respiratory bronchioles and alveolar walls, and the patient coughs in an attempt to expel the fibers. Mucus production and goblet cells are stimulated to protect the airway from the debris and aid in expectoration. Fibers then become encased in a brown, iron-rich proteinlike sheath in sputum or lung tissue, called asbestosis bodies. Chronic irritation by the fibers continues to affect the lower bronchioles and alveoli. The foreign material and inflammation swell airways, and fibrosis develops in response to the chronic irritation. Interstitial fibrosis may develop in lower lung zones, affecting lung parenchyma and the pleurae. Raised hyaline plaques may form in the parietal pleura, the diaphragm, and the pleura adjacent to the pericardium. Hypoxia develops as more alveoli and lower airways are affected.

Assessment findings

The first symptom of asbestosis is usually dyspnea on exertion, typically after 10 years' exposure. Advanced disease also causes a dry cough (may be productive in smokers), chest pain (commonly pleuritic), recurrent respiratory infections, and tachypnea.

Other findings may include basilar crackles (due to air moving through thickened sputum), clubbed fingers (commonly occur due to chronic hypoxia), recurrent respiratory tract infections (occur as pulmonary defense mechanisms begin to fail), and pleural friction rub (due to fibrosis).

Diagnosis

○ Computed tomography scan of lungs also aids in diagnosis.

○ Chest X-rays may show fine, irregular, linear, and diffuse infiltrates. Extensive fibrosis is revealed by a honeycomb or ground-glass appearance. Chest X-rays may also show pleural thickening and calcification, bilateral obliteration of the costophrenic angles and, in later stages, an enlarged heart with a classic "shaggy" border.

○ Pulmonary function studies may identify decreased vital capacity, forced vital capacity (FVC), and total lung capacity; decreased or normal forced expiratory volume in 1 second (FEV_1); a normal ratio, or FEV_1 to FVC; and reduced diffusing capacity for carbon monoxide when fibrosis destroys alveolar walls and thickens the alveolar capillary membrane.

○ Arterial blood gas analysis may reveal decreased partial pressure of arterial oxygen and partial pressure of arterial carbon dioxide from hyperventilation.

Complications

○ Cor pulmonale
○ Malignant mesothelioma
○ Pulmonary fibrosis due to progression of asbestosis
○ Pulmonary hypertension
○ Respiratory failure
○ Right ventricular hypertrophy

Treatment

○ Chest physiotherapy (controlled coughing and postural drainage with chest percussion and vibration) may relieve respiratory signs and symptoms and manage hypoxia and cor pulmonale.

KEY TEACHING POINTS

Teaching about asbestosis

Remember these key points when teaching your patient about asbestosis:

● Explain the disease process and its treatments.

● Teach the patient to prevent infections by avoiding crowds and persons with infections and by receiving influenza and pneumococcal vaccines.

● Explain the importance of increasing fluid intake.

● Discuss prescribed medications and how to take them correctly.

● Demonstrate how to perform bronchial drainage, chest percussion, and vibration.

● Explain the safe use of oxygen in the home.

● Instruct on the prevention of bronchial irritants.

○ Aerosol therapy may be ordered to liquefy mucus, and inhaled mucolytics may be ordered to liquefy and mobilize secretions.

○ The patient's fluid intake should be increased to 3 L/day.

○ Antibiotics may be ordered to treat respiratory tract infections, if necessary.

○ Oxygen administration may be ordered to relieve hypoxia.

○ Diuretics may be prescribed to decrease edema, and digoxin may be prescribed to enhance cardiac output.

○ Salt restriction prevents fluid retention in patients with cor pulmonale.

 COLLABORATIVE MANAGEMENT
Care of the patient with asbestosis involves several members of the interdisciplinary team. The interdisciplinary pulmonary rehabilitation team provides the patient with support, education, and reconditioning exercises. The physical therapist works with the patient to help him regain and maintain muscle strength and functioning. The occupational therapist can teach the patient en-

ergy conservation strategies. The respiratory therapist assesses pulmonary function, provides education on respiratory treatments, and performs chest physiotherapy, postural drainage, and home oxygen therapy, if indicated. The dietitian is crucial in helping the patient maintain an optimal nutritional status.

Special considerations
○ Improve the patient's ventilatory efficiency by encouraging physical reconditioning, energy conservation, and relaxation techniques.
○ Advise the patient to stop smoking, and refer him to a smoking-cessation program.
○ Provide patient education. (See *Teaching about asbestosis,* page 33.)

Applicable patient-teaching aids
○ Gaining mobility with portable oxygen equipment*
○ Learning about immunization for the flu
○ Learning to do controlled coughing exercises *
○ Performing chest physiotherapy (for an adult)
○ Understanding your home oxygen equipment *
○ Using oxygen safely and effectively *

○ Asthma

Asthma is a chronic inflammatory airway disorder characterized by obstruction or narrowing of the airways, which are typically inflamed and hyperresponsive to a variety of stimuli. This widespread but variable airflow obstruction results from bronchospasm, edema of the airway mucosa, and increased mucous production with plugging and airway remolding. Asthma that results from sensitivity to specific external allergens is known as extrinsic. In cases in which the allergen isn't obvious, asthma is referred to as intrinsic. Extrinsic (*atopic*) asthma usually begins in childhood and is accompanied by other manifestations of atopy (type I, immunoglobulin [Ig] E–mediated allergy), such as eczema and allergic rhinitis.

Symptoms usually show a high degree of reversibility, either spontaneously or with treat-

ment, and vary from mild wheezing and dyspnea to life-threatening respiratory failure. (See *Classifying asthma severity*.) Symptoms of bronchial airway obstruction may persist between acute episodes. Asthma may also be classified as a type of chronic obstructive pulmonary disease.

An asthma attack may begin dramatically, with simultaneous onset of many severe symptoms, or insidiously, with gradually increasing respiratory distress. (See *Asthma: Acute exacerbation,* page 36.)

Causes
Allergens that cause extrinsic asthma include pollen, animal dander, house dust or mold, kapok or feather pillows, food additives containing sulfites, and any other sensitizing substance. In intrinsic (*nonatopic*) asthma, no extrinsic allergen can be identified. Most cases are preceded by a severe respiratory infection. Irritants, emotional stress, fatigue, exposure to noxious fumes, and changes in endocrine function, temperature, and humidity may aggravate intrinsic asthma attacks. In many asthmatics, intrinsic and extrinsic asthma coexist.

Several drugs and chemicals may provoke an asthma attack, including aspirin, various nonsteroidal anti-inflammatory drugs (such as indomethacin and mefenamic acid), and tartrazine, a yellow food dye. Exercise may also provoke an asthma attack. In exercise-induced asthma, bronchospasm may follow heat and moisture loss in the upper airways.

Pathophysiology
There are two genetic influences identified with asthma, namely the ability of an individual to develop asthma (atopy) and the tendency to develop hyperresponsiveness of the airways independent of atopy. A locus of chromosome 11 associated with atopy contains an abnormal gene that encodes a part of the IgE receptor. Environmental factors interact with inherited factors to cause asthmatic reactions with associated bronchospasms.

In asthma, bronchial linings overreact to various stimuli, causing episodic smooth muscle spasms that severely constrict the air-

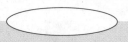

Classifying asthma severity

In adults and children older than age 5 years, asthma is classified by severity using these features:
- frequency, severity, and duration of symptoms
- degree of airflow obstruction: forced expiratory volume in one second (FEV_1) or peak expiratory flow (PEF)
- frequency of nighttime symptoms and the degree that the asthma interferes with daily activities.

Severity can change over time, and even milder cases can become severe in an uncontrolled attack. Long-term therapy depends on whether the patient's asthma is classified as mild intermittent, mild persistent, moder-

ate persistent, or severe persistent. For all patients, quick relief can be obtained by using a short-acting bronchodilator (2 to 4 puffs of short-acting inhaled $beta_2$-adrenergic agonists as needed for symptoms). However, the use of a short-acting bronchodilator more than twice a week in patients with intermittent asthma or daily or increasing use in patients with persistent asthma may indicate the need to initiate or increase long-term control therapy. See the chart below for clinical features of asthma severity before treatment or adequate control of symptoms.

	Daytime symptoms	Nighttime symptoms	Lung function
Step 4 Severe persistent	• Continual symptoms	Frequent	• FEV_1 or PEF ≤ 60% predicted • PEF variability > 30%
Step 3 Moderate persistent	• Daily symptoms	> 1 time per week	• FEV_1 or PEF > 60% to < 80% predicted • PEF variability > 30%
Step 2 Mild persistent	• Symptoms > 2 times per week but < 1 time per day	> 2 times per month	• FEV_1 or PEF ≥ 80% predicted • PEF variability 20% to 30%
Step 1 Mild intermittent	• Symptoms ≤ 2 times per week	≤ 2 times per month	• FEV_1 or PEF ≥ 80% predicted • PEF variability < 20%

Adapted from *Expert Panel Report Guidelines for the Diagnosis and Management of Asthma. Update on Selected Topics 2002*, NIH Publication No. 02-5074, Washington, D.C.: U.S. Department of Health and Human Services, June 2003.

ways. IgE antibodies, attached to histamine-containing mast cells and receptors on cell membranes, initiate intrinsic asthma attacks. When exposed to an antigen, such as pollen, the IgE antibody combines with the antigen.

On subsequent exposure to the antigen, mast cells degranulate and release mediators. Mast cells in the lung interstitium are stimulated to release histamine and leukotrienes. Histamine attaches to receptor sites in the larger bronchi, where it causes swelling in smooth muscles. Mucous membranes become inflamed, irritated, and swollen. The patient may experience dyspnea, prolonged expiration, and an increased respiratory rate.

Leukotrienes attach to receptor sites in the smaller bronchi and cause local swelling of the smooth muscle. Leukotrienes also cause prostaglandins to travel through the bloodstream to the lungs, where they enhance histamine's effect. A wheeze may be audible during coughing—the higher the pitch, the narrower the bronchial lumen. Histamine stimulates the mucous membranes to secrete excessive mucus, further narrowing the bronchial lumen. Goblet cells secrete viscous mucus that's difficult to cough up, resulting in coughing, rhonchi, increased-pitch wheezing, and increased respiratory distress. Mucosal edema and thick-

ACUTE EPISODE

Asthma: Acute exacerbation

If your patient is having an acute asthma attack, act quickly to decrease bronchoconstriction and airway edema and increase pulmonary ventilation. Follow these guidelines:

- First, assess the severity of the attack by checking for progressively worsening shortness of breath, tight and dry cough, wheezing, and chest tightness. Cyanosis, confusion, and lethargy indicate the onset of respiratory failure.
- Assess for tachycardia, tachypnea, and diaphoresis.
- Administer the prescribed treatments and assess the patient's response.
- Place the patient in high Fowler's position and encourage pursed-lip and diaphragmatic breathing. Help him to relax.
- Monitor the patient's vital signs. Developing or increasing tachypnea may indicate worsening asthma or drug toxicity; pulsus paradoxus indicates severe asthma; hypertension may indicate asthma-related hypoxemia.
- Administer humidified oxygen by nasal cannula to ease breathing and to increase the oxygen saturation; adjust oxygen according to vital signs and arterial blood gas levels.

- Anticipate endotracheal intubation and mechanical ventilation if the patient fails to maintain adequate oxygenation.
- Observe the frequency and severity of your patient's cough, and note whether it's productive; then auscultate his lungs, noting adventitious or absent breath sounds.
- If the patient can tolerate postural drainage and chest percussion, perform these procedures to clear secretions.
- Suction an intubated patient as needed.
- Treat dehydration with I.V. fluids until the patient can tolerate oral fluids, to loosen secretions.
    If status asthmaticus develops:
- Monitor the patient closely for respiratory failure.
- Administer oxygen, bronchodilators, epinephrine, corticosteroids, and nebulizer therapies as ordered.
- Intubate and place the patient on mechanical ventilation if the partial pressure of arterial carbon dioxide increases or respiratory failure occurs.

ened secretions further block the airways. (See *Understanding asthma*.)

Assessment findings

In asthma, characteristic wheezing may be accompanied by coarse rhonchi, but fine crackles aren't heard unless associated with a related complication. Between acute attacks, breath sounds may be normal.

The intensity of breath sounds in symptomatic asthma is typically reduced. A prolonged phase of forced expiration is typical of airflow obstruction. Evidence of lung hyperinflation, such as the use of accessory muscles, is particularly common in children.

Diagnosis

○ Pulmonary function studies reveal signs of airway obstruction (decreased peak expiratory flow rates and forced expiratory volume in 1 second), low-normal or decreased vital capacity, and increased total lung and residual capacity. However, pulmonary function studies may be normal between attacks.
○ Pulse oximetry may reveal decreased arterial oxygen saturation.
○ Arterial blood gas (ABG) analysis detects hypoxemia. It also provides the best indication of an attack's severity and guides treatment.
○ Complete blood count with differential reveals increased eosinophil count.
○ Chest X-rays may show hyperinflation with areas of focal atelectasis and can be used to monitor the progress of asthma.

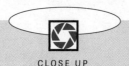

CLOSE UP

Understanding asthma

In asthma, hyperresponsiveness of the airways and bronchospasms occur. These illustrations show how an asthma attack progresses.

● Histamine (H) attaches to receptor sites in larger bronchi, causing swelling of the smooth muscles.

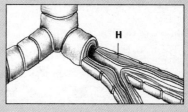

● Leukotrienes (L) attach to receptor sites in the smaller bronchi and cause swelling of smooth muscle there. Leukotrienes also cause prostaglandins to travel through the bloodstream to the lungs, where they enhance histamine's effects.

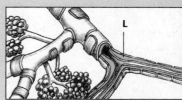

● Histamine stimulates the mucous membranes to secrete excessive mucus, further narrowing the bronchial lumen. On inhalation, the narrowed bronchial lumen can still expand slightly; on exhalation, however, the increased intrathoracic pressure closes the bronchial lumen completely.

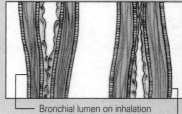

Bronchial lumen on inhalation
Bronchial lumen on exhalation

● Mucus fills lung bases, inhibiting alveolar ventilation. Blood is shunted to alveoli in other parts of the lungs, but it still can't compensate for diminished ventilation.

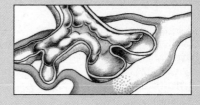

○ Sputum analysis may indicate the presence of Curschmann's spirals (casts of airways), Charcot-Leyden crystals, and eosinophils.
○ Serum IgE levels may increase from an allergic reaction.

○ Skin testing may identify specific allergens. Results read in 1 or 2 days detect an early reaction; after 4 or 5 days, a late reaction.
○ Bronchial challenge testing evaluates the clinical significance of allergens identified by skin testing.

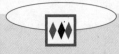

○ Electrocardiography may show sinus tachycardia during an attack.

Complications
○ Pneumonia
○ Respiratory failure
○ Status asthmaticus

Treatment
○ After an acute episode, treatment focuses on identification and avoidance of precipitating factors, such as environmental allergens or irritants.

○ If asthma is known to be caused by a particular antigen, it may be treated by desensitizing the patient through a series of injections of limited amounts of the antigen.

○ Bronchodilators decrease bronchoconstriction, reduce bronchial airway edema, and increase pulmonary ventilation. These include quick-relief agents, such as inhaled short-acting beta$_2$-adrenergic agonists (albuterol), and long-term control agents such as long-acting beta$_2$-adrenergic agonists (salmeterol).

○ Corticosteroids decrease inflammation and edema of airways. Systemic corticosteroids, such as hydrocortisone sodium succinate, are used for acute exacerbations, whereas inhaled corticosteroids, such as fluticasone propionate, are considered the gold standard of long-term asthma control.

○ Mast cell stabilizers, such as nedocromil, block the acute obstructive effects of antigen exposure by inhibiting degranulation of mast cells, thereby preventing the release of chemical mediators responsible for anaphylaxis.

○ Leukotriene modifiers and leukotriene receptor antagonists inhibit potent bronchoconstriction and inflammatory effects of cysteinyl leukotrienes and can also act as adjunctive therapy to avoid high-dose inhaled corticosteroids.

○ Anticholinergic bronchodilators, such as ipratropium bromide, block acetylcholine, another chemical mediator.

○ Low-flow humidified oxygen can be ordered to treat dyspnea and hypoxemia.

○ Relaxation exercises such as yoga increase circulation and can help the patient recover from an asthma attack.

 COLLABORATIVE MANAGEMENT
Care of the patient with asthma involves several members of the interdisciplinary team. The allergy and asthma specialist or pulmonologist identifies causative factors and prescribes therapy to help control attacks. The respiratory therapist performs spirometric and pulmonary function testing, oxygen therapy, and breathing treatments. The dietitian assists with special dietary needs and teaches the patient about proper nutrition.

Special considerations

○ Monitor the patient's respiratory status to detect baseline changes, to assess his response to treatment, and to prevent acute exacerbation and detect complications.

○ Auscultate the lungs frequently, noting the degree of wheezing and quality of air movement.

○ Review ABG levels, pulmonary function test results, and pulse oximetry readings.

○ If the patient is taking systemic corticosteroids, observe for complications, such as elevated blood glucose levels and friable skin and bruising. Cushingoid effects resulting from long-term use of corticosteroids may be minimized by alternate-day dosage or the use of prescribed inhaled corticosteroids.

○ If the patient is taking corticosteroids by inhaler, watch for signs of candidal infection in the mouth and pharynx. Using an extender device and rinsing the mouth afterward may prevent this.

○ Observe the patient's anxiety level. Keep in mind that measures that reduce hypoxemia and breathlessness should help relieve anxiety.

○ Keep the room temperature comfortable and use an air conditioner or a fan in hot, humid weather.

○ Control exercise-induced asthma by instructing the patient to use a bronchodilator or cromolyn 30 minutes before exercise. Also instruct him to use pursed-lip breathing while exercising.

○ Advise the patient to stop smoking, and refer him to a smoking-cessation program.

○ Provide patient education. (See *Teaching about asthma.*)

Applicable patient-teaching aids

○ Avoiding asthma triggers *
○ Avoiding infection *
○ Caring for aerosol equipment
○ Controlling an asthma attack *
○ Exercising safely *
○ Learning about corticosteroids
○ Making a medication clock *
○ Overcoming shortness of breath
○ Performing chest physiotherapy (for an adult)
○ Performing exercises for healthier lungs and easier breathing
○ Performing relaxation breathing exercises *
○ Preparing for pulmonary function tests *
○ Using an oral inhaler *
○ Using breathing devices

○ Atrial fibrillation

Atrial fibrillation is defined as chaotic, asynchronous, electrical activity in atrial tissue. It results from the firing of multiple impulses from numerous ectopic pacemakers in the atria and is characterized by the absence of P waves and an irregularly irregular ventricular response.

When a number of ectopic sites in the atria initiate impulses, depolarization can't spread in an organized manner. Small sections of the atria are depolarized individually, resulting in the atrial muscle quivering instead of contracting. On an electrocardiogram (ECG), uneven baseline fibrillatory waves appear rather than clearly distinguishable P waves.

Like atrial flutter, atrial fibrillation results in a loss of atrial kick. The rhythm may be sustained (occurs suddenly). It can either be preceded by or be the result of premature atrial contractions. (See *Recognizing atrial fibrillation,* page 40.)

Causes

Atrial fibrillation can occur with rheumatic heart disease, valvular heart disease (especially mitral valve disease), hyperthyroidism, pericarditis, coronary artery disease, acute myocardial infarction, hypertension, cardiomyopathy, atrial septal defects, chronic obstructive pulmonary disease, and following cardiac surgery.

The rhythm may also occur in a healthy person who smokes or drinks coffee or alcohol or who's fatigued and under stress. Certain drugs, such as aminophylline and digoxin, may contribute to the development of atrial fibrillation. Endogenous catecholamine released during exercise may also trigger the arrhythmia.

Pathophysiology

The atrioventricular (AV) node protects the ventricles from the 400 to 600 erratic atrial impuls-

Recognizing atrial fibrillation

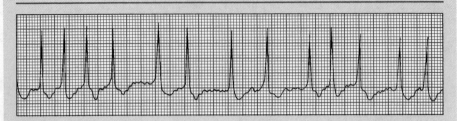

Rhythm
- Atrial: Irregularly irregular
- Ventricular: Irregularly irregular

Rate
- Atrial: Almost indiscernible, usually above 400 beats/minute, and far exceeding ventricular rate because most impulses aren't conducted through the atrioventricular junction
- Ventricular: Usually 100 to 150 beats/minute but can be below 100 beats/minute

P wave
- Absent
- Replaced by baseline fibrillatory waves that represent atrial tetanization from rapid atrial depolarizations

PR interval
- Indiscernible

QRS complex
- Duration and configuration usually normal

T wave
- Indiscernible

QT interval
- Not measurable

Other
- Atrial rhythm may vary between fibrillatory line and flutter waves, called *atrial fib-flutter.*
- May be difficult to differentiate atrial fibrillation from multifocal atrial tachycardia.

es that occur each minute by acting as a filter and blocking some of the impulses. The ventricles respond only to impulses conducted through the AV node, hence the characteristic, wide variation in R-R intervals. When the ventricular response rate drops below 100, atrial fibrillation is considered controlled. When the ventricular rate exceeds 100, the rhythm is considered uncontrolled.

The loss of atrial kick from atrial fibrillation can result in the subsequent loss of approximately 20% of normal end-diastolic volume. Combined with the decreased diastolic filling time associated with a rapid heart rate, clinically significant reductions in cardiac output can result. In uncontrolled atrial fibrillation, the patient may develop heart failure, myocardial ischemia, or syncope.

In atrial fibrillation, neither atrium contracts as a whole. As a result, blood may pool on the atrial wall and mural thrombi may form. Thrombus formation places the patient at risk for emboli or stroke.

Assessment findings
The patient with atrial fibrillation may present with a radial pulse rate that's slower than the apical pulse rate because weaker contractions may not produce a palpable peripheral pulse. Other findings may include an irregularly irregular pulse rhythm with a normal or abnormal heart rate. The patient with a new onset of atrial fibrillation and a rapid ventricular rate may present with hypotension and lightheadedness. (See *Rapid atrial fibrillation.*)

The patient with chronic atrial fibrillation may be asymptomatic

Diagnosis

○ ECG reveals the following characteristics of atrial fibrillation:

– Rhythm: Atrial and ventricular rhythms are grossly irregular, typically described as irregularly irregular.

– Rate: The atrial rate is almost indiscernible and usually exceeds 400 beats/minute. The ventricular rate usually varies, typically from 100 to 150 beats/minute but can be below 100 beats/minute.

– P wave: The P wave is absent. Erratic baseline f waves appear in place of P waves.

– PR interval: Indiscernible.

– QRS complex: Duration and configuration are usually normal.

– T wave: Indiscernible.

– QT interval: Not measurable.

Complications

○ Heart failure

○ Pulmonary, cerebral, or other thromboembolic events

○ Thrombus formation

Treatment

○ Immediate cardioversion is performed if the patient is unstable with a ventricular rate greater than 150 beats/minute.

○ Calcium channel blockers, beta-adrenergic blockers, amiodarone, or digoxin may be prescribed, according to Advanced Cardiac Life Support protocol, if the patient is stable.

○ Anticoagulation therapy reduces the risk of thromboembolism and may be ordered.

○ Radiofrequency catheter ablation therapy may be performed to terminate the arrhythmia in a patient with refractory atrial fibrillation uncontrolled by drugs.

○ Vagal maneuvers or carotid sinus massage in the patient with acute onset atrial fibrillation may slow the ventricular response but won't convert the arrhythmia.

COLLABORATIVE MANAGEMENT
Care of the patient with atrial fibrillation involves several members of the

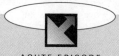

ACUTE EPISODE

Rapid atrial fibrillation

If your patient is hemodynamically unstable and has rapid atrial fibrillation with a ventricular rate greater than 150 beats/minute, notify the physician, prepare for immediate cardioversion, and follow these steps:

● Connect the patient to cardiac and oxygen saturation monitors.

● Have suction and endotracheal intubation equipment at the bedside.

● Make sure the patient has a patent I.V. line.

● Sedate the patient, as ordered.

● Set the defibrillator to the synchronous mode, attach the leads, and check the patient's cardiac rhythm.

● Check for synchronous markers on the R waves.

● Set the energy level as ordered by the physician, usually to 100 joules, and place the conductor pads on the patient's chest (or apply sufficient gel to the paddles).

● Place the paddles on the chest at the sternum and apex.

● Press the CHARGE button and tell everyone to stand clear.

● After checking that everyone is clear, deliver the shock.

● Observe the monitor for the patient's heart rhythm.

● If further shocks are necessary, resynchronize the defibrillator and progressively use energy levels as ordered.

● Monitor cardiac rhythm and cardiopulmonary status after cardioversion.

interdisciplinary team. The nurse plays a key role in educating the patient about controlling symptoms, medications, and lifestyle changes. The home care nurse monitors the patient in the community and communicates findings to the physician. The social worker can help the patient with financial issues. The dietitian educates the patient about sodium and fat dietary

KEY TEACHING POINTS

Teaching about atrial fibrillation

Remember these key points when teaching your patient about atrial fibrillation:

- Explain normal cardiac conduction and what happens in atrial fibrillation.
- Discuss the patient's medications, how he should take them, and adverse effects to report.
- Stress the importance of strict compliance with the prescribed medications.
- If your patient is taking anticoagulants, discuss their proper use, precautions to take, and appropriate follow-up care measures. Also review dietary precautions.
- Tell the patient to immediately report pulse rate changes, syncope or dizziness, chest pain, and signs and symptoms of heart failure, such as dyspnea and peripheral edema.

---

restrictions and advises the patient on high vitamin K foods to avoid when taking anticoagulant therapy.

Special considerations

○ During hospitalization, if the patient isn't on a cardiac monitor, be alert for an irregular pulse and differences in the radial and apical pulse rates.

○ Administer drugs, as ordered, and prepare to assist with cardioversion, as indicated.

○ Assess for symptoms of decreased cardiac output and heart failure.

○ If drug therapy is used, monitor serum drug levels and observe the patient for evidence of toxicity.

○ Watch for signs of hypoperfusion, such as hypotension, reduced level of consciousness, and diminished urine output.

○ Teach the patient to take his radial pulse and advise him to notify the physician if he experiences chest pain, palpitations, lightheadedness, or dyspnea.

○ If the patient is taking anticoagulants, explain safety precautions (such as using an elec-

tric razor) and dietary changes (foods high in vitamin K may interfere with warfarin).

○ Provide patient education. (See *Teaching about atrial fibrillation*.)

Applicable patient-teaching aids

○ Learning about an electrocardiogram *
○ Taking anticoagulants *
○ Taking your medication correctly

◯ Attention deficit hyperactivity disorder

The patient with attention deficit hyperactivity disorder (ADHD) has difficulty focusing his attention or engaging in quiet, passive activities, or both. Although the disorder is present at birth, diagnosis before age 4 or 5 is difficult unless the child shows severe symptoms. Some patients aren't diagnosed until adulthood. Other patients have an attention deficit without hyperactivity; these patients are less likely to be diagnosed and treated. Males are three times more likely to be affected than females.

Causes

ADHD is thought to be a physiologic brain disorder with a familial tendency. Some studies indicate that it may result from disturbances in neurotransmitter levels in the brain due to reduced blood flow in the striated area of the brain.

Pathophysiology

The pathophysiology of ADHD isn't fully understood. Because psychostimulants (which facilitate the release of dopamine) and noradrenergic tricyclics are used to control symptoms of ADHD, it's thought that certain areas of the brain associated with attention are lacking in neural transmission. The neurotransmitters dopamine and norepinephrine have been linked to ADHD. The areas of the brain believed to be involved are the frontal and prefrontal areas.

Assessment findings

ADHD is indicated by hyperactivity that's present over a long period, in at least two settings (such as home and school), and is accompanied by easy distractibility. Impulsive, emotionally labile, explosive, or irritable behavior is possible. Although the patient may be highly intelligent, his school or work performance patterns are sporadic, and he may jump from one partly completed project, thought, or task to another.

In a younger child, signs and symptoms include an inability to wait in line, remain seated, wait his turn, or concentrate on one activity until its completion. An older child or an adult may be described as impulsive, easily distracted and, possibly, inattentive, prone to daydreaming, and disorganized.

Diagnosis

○ Most children are referred for evaluation by the school.

○ Diagnosis of this disorder usually begins by obtaining data from several sources, including the parents, teachers, and the child himself. Complete psychological, medical, and neurologic evaluations rule out other problems. Then the child undergoes tests that measure impulsiveness, attention, and the ability to sustain a task. The combined findings portray a clear picture of the disorder and the areas of support the child will need.

Complications

○ Emotional and social complications
○ Poor nutrition

Treatment

○ Behavior modification, coaching, external structure, use of planning and organizing systems, and supportive psychotherapy help the patient cope with the disorder.

○ Stimulants are the most commonly used agents to relieve symptoms of ADHD; they may sometimes be used in combination with antipsychotics.

○ Other drugs, including tricyclic antidepressants, mood stabilizers, and beta-adrenergic blockers, sometimes help control symptoms.

 COLLABORATIVE MANAGEMENT
Care of the patient with ADHD involves several members of the inter-

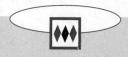

KEY TEACHING POINTS

Teaching about ADHD

Remember these key points when teaching your patient and his family about attention deficit hyperactivity disorder (ADHD):

● Explain the cause and treatment of ADHD.
● Describe the prescribed medications, including their names, dosages, actions, adverse effects, and special instructions.
● Discuss behavioral management techniques such us giving the child immediate and consistent consequences for his behaviors.
● Talk with the family about the effects of having a child with ADHD.
● Discuss resources that are available for support and education.

disciplinary team, which includes parents, teachers, and therapists as well as the patient and the physician. Ideally, the treatment team identifies the symptoms to be managed, selects appropriate medication, and then tracks the patient's symptoms carefully to determine the effectiveness of the medication.

Special considerations

○ Work with the individual to develop external structure and controls.

○ Set realistic expectations and limits because the patient with ADHD is easily frustrated (which leads to decreased self-control).

○ Remain calm and consistent.

○ Keep instructions short and simple.

○ Provide praise, rewards, and positive feedback whenever possible.

○ Provide patient education. (See *Teaching about ADHD*.)

Applicable patient-teaching aids

○ Giving children medication by mouth *

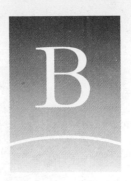

Basal cell carcinoma

Basal cell carcinoma, also known as *basal cell epithelioma,* is a slow-growing, destructive skin tumor. Three types of basal cell carcinoma occur: nodulo-ulcerative lesions, superficial basal cell carcinoma, and sclerosing basal cell carcinoma. If caught and treated early, it has a cure rate of 95%. Regular follow-up is required as new sites of basal cell carcinoma occur.

Basal cell carcinoma is the most common form of cancer in the United States, accounting for 75% of all skin cancers. It usually occurs in persons older than age 40. It's most prevalent in blond, fair-skinned males and is the most common malignant tumor affecting whites.

Causes

Prolonged sun exposure is the most common cause of basal cell carcinoma; however, arsenic ingestion, radiation exposure, burns, and immunosuppression are other possible causes.

Pathophysiology

Although the pathogenesis of basal cell carcinoma is uncertain, some experts now hypothesize that it originates when, under certain conditions, undifferentiated basal cells become carcinomatous instead of differentiating into sweat glands, sebum, and hair. (See *How basal cell carcinoma develops.*)

Noduloulcerative lesions, known as "rodent ulcers," rarely metastasize; however, if untreated, they can spread to vital areas and become infected or cause massive hemorrhage if they invade large blood vessels. Superficial basal cell carcinomas are usually chronic and don't tend to invade other areas. Superficial basal cell carcinomas are related to ingestion of or exposure to arsenic-containing compounds. Sclerosing basal cell carcinomas occur on the head and neck.

Assessment findings

Noduloulcerative lesions usually occur on the face, particularly the forehead, eyelid margins, and nasolabial folds. In early stages, these lesions are small, smooth, pinkish, and translucent papules. Telangiectatic vessels cross the surface, and the lesions are occasionally pigmented. (The pigmented form is a brown-black lesion that must be differentiated from malignant melanoma.) As the lesions enlarge, their centers become depressed and their borders become firm and elevated. Ulceration and local invasion eventually occur.

Superficial basal cell carcinomas are multiple lesions that commonly occur on the chest and back. They're oval or irregularly shaped, lightly pigmented plaques, with sharply defined, slightly elevated threadlike borders. Due to superficial erosion, these lesions appear scaly and have small, atrophic areas in the center that resemble psoriasis or eczema.

Sclerosing basal cell carcinomas are waxy, sclerotic lesions with yellow to white plaques without distinct borders. Occurring on the head and neck, sclerosing basal cell epitheliomas typically look like small patches of scleroderma.

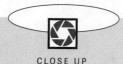

CLOSE UP

How basal cell carcinoma develops

Basal cell carcinoma is thought to originate when undifferentiated basal cells become carcinomatous instead of differentiating into sweat glands, sebum, and hair. The most common cancer, basal cell carcinoma begins as a papule, enlarges, and develops a central crater. Usually, it spreads only locally.

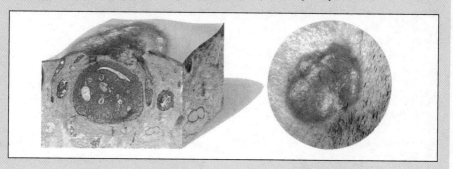

Diagnosis

◯ Incisional or excisional biopsy and histologic study help determine the tumor type and histologic subtype.

Complications

◯ Disfigurement
◯ Hemorrhage
◯ Infection
◯ Metastasis

Treatment

◯ Curettage and electrodesiccation removes small lesions; offers good cosmetic results for small lesions.

◯ Topical 5-fluorouracil is commonly used for superficial lesions; produces marked local irritation or inflammation in the involved tissue but no systemic effects.

◯ Microscopically controlled surgical excision (such as Moh's micrographic surgery) carefully removes recurrent lesions until a tumor-free plane is achieved; after removal of large lesions, skin grafting may be required.

◯ Irradiation is used for tumor locations that require it and for elderly or debilitated patients who might not withstand surgery.

◯ Cryosurgery with liquid nitrogen freezes and kills the cells.

◯ Chemosurgery generally is necessary for persistent or recurrent lesions; it consists of periodic applications of a fixative paste (such as zinc chloride) and subsequent removal of fixed pathologic tissue.

 COLLABORATIVE MANAGEMENT
Care of the patient with basal cell carcinoma involves several members of the interdisciplinary team. The registered nurse provides education and screening and monitors for adverse effects of therapy. The dietitian makes sure that the patient is receiving adequate nutrition and hydration. The oncologist and dermatologist diagnose the disorder and determine the treatment plan and the surgeon excises tumors.

Special considerations

◯ Provide the patient with frequent small meals that are high in protein. Suggest "blenderized" foods or liquid protein supple-

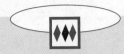

ments if the lesion has invaded the oral cavity and caused eating problems.

❍ Monitor for complications of treatment.

❍ Provide emotional support for patients with disfigurement.

❍ Provide the patient with resources and support services.

❍ Provide patient education. (See *Teaching about basal cell carcinoma*.)

Applicable patient-teaching aids
❍ Changing a dry dressing
❍ Minimizing sun exposure *

Bipolar disorder

Marked by severe pathologic mood swings from hyperactivity and euphoria to sadness and depression, bipolar disorders involve various symptom combinations. Type I bipolar disorder is characterized by alternating episodes of mania and depression, whereas type II is characterized by recurrent depressive episodes and occasional mild manic (hypomanic) episodes. In some patients, bipolar disorder assumes a seasonal pattern, marked by a cyclic relation between the onset of the mood episode and a particular 60-day period of the year.

The American Psychiatric Association estimates that 0.4% to 1.2% of adults experience bipolar disorder. This disorder affects women and men equally and is more common in higher socioeconomic groups. It can begin any time after adolescence, but onset usually occurs between ages 20 and 35; about 35% of patients experience onset between ages 35 and 60. Before the onset of overt symptoms, many patients with bipolar disorder have an energetic and outgoing personality with a history of wide mood swings.

Bipolar disorder recurs in 80% of patients; as they grow older, the episodes recur more frequently and last longer. This illness is associated with a significant mortality; 20% of patients commit suicide, many just as the depression lifts.

Causes

The cause of bipolar disorder is unclear, but hereditary, biological, and psychological factors may play a part. There appears to be an autosomal dominant inheritance found in genetic studies. The incidence of bipolar disorder among relatives of affected patients is higher than in the general population and highest among maternal relatives (the closer the relationship, the greater the susceptibility). Evidence also suggests that bipolar disorder is linked to an X chromosome.

Although certain biochemical changes accompany mood swings, it isn't clear whether these changes cause the mood swings or result from them. Also, patients with mood disorders have a defect in the way the brain handles certain neurotransmitters.

New data suggest that changes in the circadian rhythms that control hormone secretion, body temperature, and appetite may contribute to the development of bipolar disorder.

Emotional or physical trauma, such as bereavement, disruption of an important relationship, or a serious accidental injury, may precede the onset of bipolar disorder; however, bipolar disorder commonly appears without identifiable predisposing factors.

Manic episodes may follow a stressful event, but they're also associated with antidepressant therapy and childbirth. Major depressive episodes may be precipitated by chronic physical illness, psychoactive drug dependence, psychosocial stressors, and childbirth. Other familial influences, especially the early loss of a parent, parental depression, incest, or abuse, may predispose a person to depressive illness. (See *Cyclothymic disorder.*)

Pathophysiology

Biochemical changes occur in people with bipolar disorder. In mania and depression, intracellular sodium concentration increases during illness and returns to normal with recovery. Alterations in neurotransmitters may also play a role. Low levels of the chemicals dopamine and norepinephrine, for example, have been linked to depression, whereas excessively high levels of these chemicals are associated with mania. Changes in the concentration of acetylcholine and serotonin may also play a role. Although neurobiologists have yet to prove that these chemical shifts cause bipolar disorder, it's widely assumed that most antidepressant medications work by modifying these neurotransmitter systems.

Assessment findings

Signs and symptoms vary widely, depending on whether the patient is experiencing a manic or depressive episode.

During the assessment interview, the manic patient typically appears grandiose, euphoric, expansive, or irritable with little control over activities and responses. He may describe hyperactive or excessive behavior, including elaborate plans for numerous social events, efforts to renew old acquaintances by telephoning friends at all hours of the night, buying sprees, or promiscuous sexual activity.

Cyclothymic disorder

A chronic mood disturbance of at least 2 years' duration, cyclothymic disorder involves numerous episodes of hypomania or depression that aren't of sufficient severity or duration to qualify as a major depressive episode or a bipolar disorder.

Cyclothymia commonly starts in adolescence or early adulthood. Beginning insidiously, this disorder leads to persistent social and occupational dysfunction.

Signs and symptoms
In the hypomanic phase, the patient may experience insomnia, hyperactivity, inflated self-esteem, increased productivity and creativity, rapid speech, physical restlessness, and overinvolvement in pleasurable activities, including an increased sexual drive. Depressive symptoms may include insomnia, feelings of inadequacy, decreased productivity, social withdrawal, loss of libido, loss of interest in pleasurable activities, lethargy, slow speech, and crying.

Diagnosis
A number of medical disorders (for example, endocrinopathies, such as Cushing's syndrome, stroke, brain tumors, and head trauma) and drug overdose can produce a similar pattern of mood alteration. These organic causes must be ruled out before making a diagnosis of cyclothymic disorder.

The patient's activities may have a bizarre quality, such as dressing in colorful or strange garments, wearing excessive makeup, or giving advice to passing strangers. He often expresses an inflated sense of self-esteem, ranging from uncritical self-confidence to marked grandiosity, which may be delusional.

Accelerated and pressured speech, frequent changes of topic, and flight of ideas are also common features of the manic phase. The patient is easily distracted and responds rapidly to external stimuli, such as background noise or a ringing telephone.

Physical examination of the manic patient may reveal signs of malnutrition and poor personal hygiene. He may also report sleeping and eating deficiencies, as well as an increase in physical activity.

Hypomania can be recognized by three classic symptoms: euphoric but unstable mood, pressured speech, and increased motor activity. The hypomanic patient may appear elated, easily distracted, highly energetic, hyperactive, talkative, irritable, impatient, or impulsive.

The patient who experiences a depressive episode may report a loss of self-esteem, overwhelming inertia, social withdrawal, and feelings of hopelessness, apathy, or self-reproach. He may believe that he is wicked and deserves to be punished. His growing sadness, guilt, negativity, and fatigue place extraordinary burdens on his family.

During the assessment interview, the patient may speak and respond slowly. He may complain of difficulty concentrating or thinking clearly but usually isn't obviously disoriented or intellectually impaired.

Physical examination may reveal reduced psychomotor activity, lethargy, low muscle tonus, weight loss, slowed gait, and constipation. The patient may also report sleep disturbances (falling asleep, staying asleep, or early morning awakening), sexual dysfunction, headaches, chest pains, and heaviness in the limbs.

The patient's concerns about his health may become hypochondriacal. He may also develop suicidal idealization (possibly with homicidal idealization), especially as his depression begins to lift and his energy levels rise.

Diagnosis
○ The diagnosis of bipolar disorder is confirmed when the patient meets criteria documented in the *Diagnostic and Statistical Manual of Mental Disorders,* Fourth Edition, Text Revision. (See *Diagnosing bipolar disorders.*)
○ Physical examination and laboratory tests, such as endocrine function studies, rule out

medical causes of the mood disturbances, including intra-abdominal neoplasm, hypothyroidism, heart failure, cerebral arteriosclerosis, parkinsonism, psychoactive drug abuse, brain tumor, and uremia.
○ Review of the medications prescribed for other disorders may point to drug-induced depression or mania.

Complications
○ Emotional and social consequences
○ Exhaustion
○ Nutritional deficits
○ Sleep disturbances
○ Sexually transmitted disease
○ Suicide

Treatment
○ Lithium relieves and prevents manic episodes. It curbs the accelerated thought processes and hyperactive behavior without producing the sedating effect of antipsychotic drugs.
○ Anticonvulsants, such as carbamazepine, valproic acid, and clonazepam, are used either alone or with lithium to treat mood disorders. Carbamazepine and divalproex are effective in many patients who are lithium-resistant.
○ Electroconvulsive therapy is effective in treating severe depression.
○ Antidepressants are used to treat depressive symptoms but they may trigger a manic episode.

 COLLABORATIVE MANAGEMENT
Care of the patient with bipolar disorder involves an interdisciplinary approach. The psychiatrist diagnoses the disorders and determines the treatment plan. The dietitian assures adequate nutrition and hydration. The physical therapist can assist in monitoring activity during the manic phase and devise an appropriate activity plan during the depressed stage. The occupational therapist can provide appropriate diversionary activities. Therapists provide individual and group therapy.

Special considerations
For the manic patient:

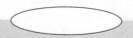

Diagnosing bipolar disorders

Use these criteria from the *Diagnostic and Statistical Manual of Mental Disorders,* Fourth Edition, Text Revision, for the diagnosis of a patient with bipolar disorder.

For a manic episode
● A distinct period of abnormally and persistently elevated, expansive, or irritable mood lasting at least 1 week (or any duration if hospitalization is needed).
● During the mood disturbance period, at least three of these symptoms must have persisted (four, if the mood is only irritable) and have been present to a significant degree:
– inflated self-esteem or grandiosity
– decreased need for sleep
– more talkative than usual or pressured to keep talking
– flight of ideas or subjective experience that thoughts are racing
– distractibility
– increased goal-directed activity or psychomotor agitation
– excessive involvement in pleasurable activities that have a high potential for painful consequences.
● The symptoms don't meet the criteria for a mixed episode.
● The mood disturbance is sufficiently severe to cause one of these to occur:
– marked impairment in occupational functioning or in usual social activities or relationships with others
– hospitalization to prevent harm to self or others
– evidence of psychotic features.
● The symptoms aren't due to the direct physiologic effects of a substance or a general medical condition.

For a hypomanic episode
● A distinct period of abnormally and persistently elevated, expansive, or irritable mood lasting at least 4 days that's clearly different from the usual nondepressed mood.
● During the mood disturbance period, at least three of these symptoms must have persisted (four, if the mood is only irritable) and have been present to a significant degree:
– inflated self-esteem or grandiosity
– decreased need for sleep

– more talkative than usual or pressured to keep talking
– flight of ideas or subjective experience that thoughts are racing
– distractibility
– increased goal-directed activity or psychomotor agitation
– excessive involvement in pleasurable activities that have a high potential for painful consequences.
● The episode is associated with an unequivocal change in functioning that's uncharacteristic of the person when not symptomatic.
● Others can recognize the disturbance in mood and the change in functioning.
● The episode isn't severe enough to markedly impair social or occupational functioning or to necessitate hospitalization to prevent harm to self or others. No psychotic features are evident.
● The symptoms aren't due to the direct physiologic effects of a substance or a general medical condition.

For a bipolar I single manic episode
● The presence of only one manic episode and no past major depressive episodes.
● The manic episode isn't better accounted for by schizoaffective disorder and isn't superimposed on schizophrenia, schizophreniform disorder, delusional disorder, or psychotic disorder not otherwise specified.

For a bipolar I disorder, most recent episode hypomanic
● The person is currently (or was most recently) in a hypomanic episode.
● The person previously had at least one manic episode or mixed episode.
● The mood symptoms cause clinically significant distress or impairment in social, occupational, or other important areas of functioning.
● The first two exacerbations of the mood episode (above) aren't better accounted for by schizoaffec-

(continued)

Diagnosing bipolar disorders *(continued)*

tive disorder and aren't superimposed on schizophrenia, schizophreniform disorder, delusional disorder, or psychotic disorder not otherwise specified.

For a bipolar I disorder, most recent episode manic
● The person is currently (or was most recently) in a manic episode.
● The person previously had at least one major depressive episode, manic episode, or mixed episode.
● The first two exacerbations of mood episode (above) aren't better accounted for by schizoaffective disorder and aren't superimposed on schizophrenia, schizophreniform disorder, delusional disorder, or psychotic disorder not otherwise specified.

For a bipolar I disorder, most recent episode mixed
● The person is currently (or was most recently) in a mixed episode.
● The person previously had at least one major depressive episode, manic episode, or mixed episode.
● The first two exacerbations of mood episode (above) aren't better accounted for by schizoaffective disorder and aren't superimposed on schizophrenia, schizophreniform disorder, delusional disorder, or psychotic disorder not otherwise specified.

For a bipolar I disorder, most recent episode depressed
● The person is currently (or was most recently) in a major depressive episode.
● The person previously had at least one manic episode or mixed episode.
● The first two exacerbations of mood episode (above) aren't better accounted for by schizoaffective disorder and aren't superimposed on schizo-

phrenia, schizophreniform disorder, delusional disorder, or psychotic disorder not otherwise specified.

For a bipolar I disorder, most recent episode unspecified
● Criteria, except for duration, are currently (or most recently) met for a manic, hypomanic, mixed, or major depressive episode.
● The person previously had at least one manic episode or mixed episode.
● The mood symptoms cause clinically significant distress or impairment in social, occupational, or other important areas of functioning.
● The first two exacerbations of mood episode (above) aren't better accounted for by schizoaffective disorder and aren't superimposed on schizophrenia, schizophreniform disorder, delusional disorder, or psychotic disorder not otherwise specified.
● The first two exacerbations of mood episode (above) aren't due to the direct physiologic effects of a substance or a general medical condition.

For a bipolar II disorder
● The presence (or history) of one or more major depressive episodes.
● The presence (or history) of at least one hypomanic episode.
● The patient has never had a manic episode or a mixed episode.
● The first two exacerbations of mood episode (above) aren't better accounted for by schizoaffective disorder and aren't superimposed on schizophrenia, schizophreniform disorder, delusional disorder, or psychotic disorder not otherwise specified.
● The symptoms cause clinically significant distress or impairment in social, occupational, or other important areas of functioning.

○ Monitor serum lithium levels and adjust drug dosage, as ordered, to maintain levels within a narrow therapeutic range.

○ Encourage the manic patient to eat and provide a diet that's high in calories, carbohydrates, and liquids.

○ As the patient's symptoms subside, encourage him to assume responsibility for personal care.

○ Provide emotional support, maintain a calm environment, and set realistic goals for behavior.

○ Provide diversionary activities suited to a short attention span; firmly discourage the patient if he tries to overextend himself.

○ Provide structured activities involving large motor movements to expend surplus energy.

○ Reduce or eliminate group activities during acute manic episodes.

○ When necessary, reorient the patient to reality.

○ Set limits in a calm, clear, and self-confident manner for the manic patient's demanding, hyperactive, manipulative, and acting-out behaviors.

○ Listen to requests attentively and with a neutral attitude. Avoid power struggles if a patient tries to put you on the spot for an immediate answer. Explain that you'll seriously consider the request and will respond later.

○ Encourage solitary activities such as writing out one's thoughts.

○ Collaborate with other staff members to provide consistent responses to the patient's manipulative or acting-out behaviors.

○ Watch for early signs of frustration (when the patient's anger escalates from verbal threats to hitting an object). Tell the patient firmly that threats and hitting are unacceptable. Explain that these behaviors show that he needs help to control his behavior. Inform him that the staff will help him move to a quiet area to help him control his behavior, so he won't hurt himself or others.

○ Alert the staff team promptly when acting-out behavior escalates. It's safer to have help available before you need it than to try controlling an anxious or frightened patient by yourself.

○ When the incident is over and the patient is calm and in control, discuss his feelings with him and offer suggestions on how to prevent a recurrence.

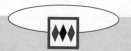

KEY TEACHING POINTS

Teaching about bipolar disorder

Remember these key points when teaching your patient about bipolar disorder:

● Explain the disorder and its treatments.

● Discuss medication administration, dosage, and possible adverse effects.

● Reinforce the importance of continuing the prescribed medication regimen and keeping follow-up appointments.

● If the patient is taking lithium, tell him to temporarily stop the medication and notify the physician if signs or symptoms of toxicity, such as diarrhea, abdominal cramps, vomiting, unsteadiness, drowsiness, muscle weakness, polyuria, or tremors, occur.

○ Provide patient education. (See *Teaching about bipolar disorder.*)

For the depressed patient:

○ Provide continual positive reinforcement to improve self-esteem.

○ Provide a structured routine, including activities to boost his self-confidence and promote interaction with others (for example, group therapy).

○ Keep reassuring the patient that his depression will lift.

○ Encourage the patient to talk or to write down his feelings if he's having trouble expressing them.

○ Listen attentively and respectfully; allow the patient time to formulate thoughts if he seems sluggish.

○ To prevent possible self-injury or suicide, remove harmful objects (such as glass, belts, rope, or bobby pins) from the patient's environment, observe him closely, and strictly supervise his medications. Institute suicide precautions as dictated by facility policy.

○ If necessary, assist the patient with personal hygiene measures.

○ Encourage him to eat, or feed him if necessary. If he's constipated, add high-fiber foods to his diet; offer small, frequent meals; and encourage physical activity.

○ If the patient is taking an antidepressant, watch for signs of mania.

Applicable patient-teaching aids
○ Coping with depression

○ Bladder cancer

Bladder tumors can develop on the surface of the bladder wall (benign or malignant papillomas) or grow within the bladder wall (generally more virulent) and quickly invade underlying muscles. Ninety percent of bladder tumors are transitional cell carcinomas, arising from the transitional epithelium of mucous membranes. Less common are adenocarcinomas, epidermoid carcinomas, squamous cell cancers, sarcomas, tumors in bladder diverticula, and carcinoma in situ. Bladder cancer is the most common cancer of the urinary tract.

Causes
Certain environmental carcinogens, such as 2-naphthylamine, benzidine, tobacco, and nitrates, predispose people to transitional cell tumors. Thus, workers in certain industries (rubber workers, weavers and leather finishers, aniline dye workers, hairdressers, petroleum workers, and spray painters) are at high risk for such tumors. The period between exposure to the carcinogen and development of symptoms is about 18 years.

Squamous cell cancer of the bladder is most common in geographic areas where schistosomiasis is endemic. It's also associated with chronic bladder irritation and infection (for example, from kidney stones, indwelling urinary catheters, and cystitis caused by cyclophosphamide).

Bladder tumors are most prevalent in men older than age 50 and are more common in densely populated industrial areas.

Pathophysiology
Transitional cells and squamous cells line the bladder. The majority of bladder cancers start in the transitional cells; only a small percent arise from the squamous cells. Cancer that arises from cells in the bladder lining often recurs. Superficial bladder tumors may grow through the lining and invade the muscular layer of the bladder as well as neighboring structures, such as the prostate (in men) and the uterus and vagina (in women). At this point, cancer cells may be found in the lymph nodes close by and may spread to organs, such as the lungs, liver, or bones. (See *How bladder cancer develops*.)

Assessment findings
In early stages, approximately 25% of patients with bladder tumors have no symptoms. Commonly, the first sign is gross, painless, intermittent hematuria (in many cases, with clots in the urine). Many patients with invasive lesions have suprapubic pain after voiding. Other signs and symptoms include bladder irritability, urinary frequency, nocturia, and dribbling.

Diagnosis
○ Cystoscopy and biopsy confirm bladder cancer. A bimanual examination may be performed during cystoscopy if the patient has received anesthesia to determine whether the bladder is fixed to the pelvic wall.

○ Urinalysis can detect blood in the urine and malignant cytology.

○ Excretory urography can identify a large, early stage tumor or an infiltrating tumor, delineate functional problems in the upper urinary tract, assess hydronephrosis, and detect rigid deformity of the bladder wall.

○ Retrograde cystography evaluates bladder structure and integrity. Test results help to confirm the diagnosis.

○ Pelvic arteriography can reveal tumor invasion into the bladder wall.

○ Computed tomography scan reveals the thickness of the involved bladder wall and detects enlarged retroperitoneal lymph nodes.

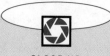

CLOSE UP

How bladder cancer develops

Bladder tumors can develop on the surface of the bladder wall or grow within the bladder wall and quickly invade underlying muscle. Most bladder tumors (90%) are transitional cell carcinomas, arising from the transitional epithelium of mucous membranes. They may also result from malignant transformation of benign papillomas. This illustration shows a bladder carcinoma infiltrating the bladder wall.

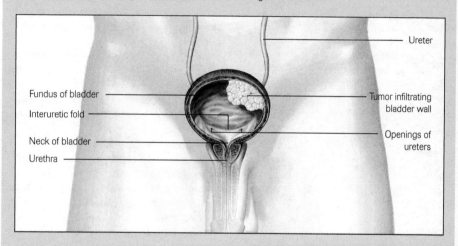

Ureter

Fundus of bladder

Tumor infiltrating bladder wall

Interuretic fold

Neck of bladder

Openings of ureters

Urethra

○ Ultrasonography can detect metastasis beyond the bladder and can distinguish a bladder cyst from a tumor.

○ I.V. pyelogram evaluates the upper urinary tract for tumors or blockage.

Complications

○ Bone metastasis

○ Problems resulting from tumor invasion of contiguous viscera

Treatment

○ Transurethral (cystoscopic) resection and fulguration (electrical destruction) are performed to remove superficial bladder tumors when the tumor hasn't invaded the muscle.

○ Intravesicular chemotherapy, most commonly with thiotepa, doxorubicin, mitomycin, or Bacille Calmette-Guérin immunotherapy, is also used for superficial tumors (especially those that occur in many sites) and to prevent tumor recurrence.

○ Segmental bladder resection is performed to remove a full-thickness section of the bladder for tumors too large to be treated through a cystoscope and for tumors that aren't near the bladder neck or ureteral orifices.

○ Bladder instillation of thiotepa, mitomycin-C, or doxorubicin after transurethral resection may also help control such tumors.

○ Radical cystectomy is the treatment of choice for infiltrating bladder tumors.

○ External beam therapy to the bladder may precede cystectomy.

○ Surgery involves removal of the bladder with perivesical fat, lymph nodes, urethra, the prostate and seminal vesicles (in males), and the uterus and adnexa (in females) with urinary

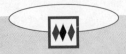

KEY TEACHING POINTS

Teaching about bladder cancer

Remember these key points when teaching your patient and his family about bladder cancer:

● Teach the patient about the disease process and its treatments.

● Discuss the importance of increasing fluid intake and monitoring urine output.

● Teach the patient and his family about care of the urinary stoma and appliances.

● Advise the patient with a urinary stoma that he may participate in most activities, except for heavy lifting and contact sports.

● Review signs and symptoms of complications, such as urinary tract infection, skin breakdown, and cancer recurrence, that should be reported to the physician immediately.

● Emphasize the importance of regular follow-up care.

---

diversion, such as an ileal conduit, ureterostomy, nephrostomy, vesicostomy, ileal bladder, ileal loop, and sigmoid conduit.

○ Treatment of advanced bladder cancer includes cystectomy to remove the tumor, radiation therapy, and systemic chemotherapy with such drugs as doxorubicin, methotrexate, vinblastine, and cisplatin.

○ Investigational treatments include photodynamic therapy and intravesicular administration of interferon-alpha and tumor necrosis factor.

 COLLABORATIVE MANAGEMENT
Care of the patient with bladder cancer involves several members of the interdisciplinary team. The nurse provides support, education, and care of the patient following surgery, chemotherapy, and other procedures. The surgeon performs resection and urinary diversion. The oncologist makes recommendations and supervises the administration of chemotherapy and radiation therapy.

An enterostomal therapist provides counseling and education before and after surgery about appliances and care of the stoma and promotes self-care. The social worker can assist the patient with obtaining supplies and helps with seeking financial assistance, if appropriate.

Special considerations

○ Before surgery, refer the patient to an enterostomal therapist, to provide education, to assist in selecting a stoma site, and to teach self-care.

○ After surgery, encourage the patient to look at the stoma to promote healthy adjustment to his new body image.

○ To obtain a specimen for culture and sensitivity testing, catheterize the patient using sterile technique.

○ Arrange for follow-up with a home health care nurse, who will help coordinate and monitor the patient's care after discharge.

○ Select a skin barrier that contains synthetics and little or no karaya (which urine tends to destroy) to ensure a good skin seal.

○ Check the ostomy pouch frequently to make sure that the skin seal remains intact.

○ Keep the skin around the stoma clean and free from irritation.

○ Refer all high-risk people — for example, chemical workers and people with a history of benign bladder tumors or persistent cystitis — for periodic cytologic examinations; they should also be instructed about the danger of disease-causing agents.

○ Refer patients with ostomies to such support organizations as the American Cancer Society and the United Ostomy Association.

○ Provide patient education. (See *Teaching about bladder cancer.*)

Applicable patient-teaching aids

○ Applying an ostomy pouch *
○ Caring for your nephrostomy tube *
○ Caring for your urinary stoma
○ Controlling the side effects of chemotherapy *
○ Draining an ostomy pouch

○ Learning about bladder-instilled chemo-therapy
○ Learning about cystoscopy *
○ Preparing for a kidney-ureter-bladder X-ray
○ Preparing for excretory urography
○ Preparing for renal ultrasonography
○ Removing an ostomy pouch *

○ Breast cancer

Breast cancer is the most common cancer affecting women and the second leading cause of death in women after lung cancer. Most breast cancer deaths occur in women age 50 and older; however, it may develop any time after puberty. It occurs in men, but rarely.

The 5-year survival rate for localized breast cancer has improved because of earlier diagnosis and the variety of treatments now available. According to the most recent data, mortality continues to decline in White women and, for the first time, is also declining in Black women younger than age 50.

Causes

The cause of breast cancer isn't known, but its high incidence in women implicates estrogen.

Certain predisposing factors are clear; women at high risk include those who have a family history of breast cancer, particularly first-degree relatives (mother, sister). Other women at high risk include those who:
○ have long menstrual cycles or began menses early (before age 12) or menopause late (after age 55)
○ have taken hormonal contraceptives
○ used hormone replacement therapy for more than 5 years
○ took diethylstilbestrol to prevent miscarriage
○ have never been pregnant
○ were first pregnant after age 30
○ have had unilateral breast cancer
○ have had ovarian cancer—particularly at a young age
○ were exposed to low-level ionizing radiation.

Recently, scientists have discovered the BRCA1 and BRCA2 genes. Mutations in these genes are thought to be responsible for approximately 5% of breast cancers. However, these discoveries have made genetic predisposition testing an option for women at high risk for breast cancer.

Lifestyle related risk factors for breast cancer include obesity, lack of physical activity, and alcohol use.

Pathophysiology

Breast cancer occurs more commonly in the left breast than the right and more commonly in the outer upper quadrant. Growth rates vary. Theoretically, slow-growing breast cancer may take up to 8 years to become palpable at 1 cm in size. It spreads by way of the lymphatic system and the bloodstream, through the right side of the heart to the lungs, and eventually to the other breast, the chest wall, liver, bone, and brain.

The estimated growth rate of breast cancer is referred to as "doubling time," or the time it takes the malignant cells to double in number. Survival time for breast cancer is based on tumor size and spread; the number of involved nodes is the single most important factor in predicting survival time. Breast cancer is classified by histologic appearance and location of the lesion. (See *Cellular progression of breast cancer,* page 56.)

These histologic classifications should be coupled with a staging or nodal status classification system for a clearer understanding of the extent of the cancer. The most commonly used system for staging cancer, both before and after surgery, is the TNM staging (tumor size, nodal involvement, metastatic progress) system.

Assessment findings

Warning signals of possible breast cancer include:
○ a lump or mass in the breast (a hard, stony mass is usually malignant)
○ change in symmetry or size of the breast
○ change in skin, thickening, scaly skin around the nipple, dimpling, edema (peau d'orange), or ulceration

CLOSE UP

Cellular progression of breast cancer

Breast cancer may be classified as invasive or non-invasive. Invasive tumor cells, which make up 90% of all breast cancers, break through duct walls and encroach on other breast tissues. Noninvasive tumor cells remain confined to the duct in which they originate.

Breast cancer can also be classified by histologic appearance and the lesion's location as follows:
- *adenocarcinoma* — arising from the epithelium
- *intraductal* — developing within the ducts (includes Paget's disease)

- *infiltrating* — occurring in parenchymal tissue
- *inflammatory* (rare) — rapidly growing and causing overlying skin to become edematous, inflamed, and indurated
- *lobular carcinoma in situ* — involving lobes of glandular tissue
- *medullary or circumscribed* — enlarging rapidly.

Breast cancer originates in the epithelial lining of the breast. This illustration shows the intraductal changes, with transformation of benign cells to atypical cells to malignant cells.

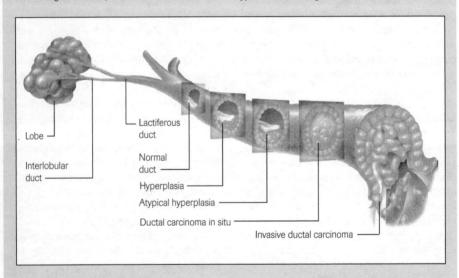

Lobe

Interlobular duct

Lactiferous duct

Normal duct

Hyperplasia

Atypical hyperplasia

Ductal carcinoma in situ

Invasive ductal carcinoma

○ change in skin temperature (a warm, hot, or pink area; suspect cancer in a nonlactating woman older than childbearing age until proved otherwise)
○ unusual drainage or discharge (A spontaneous discharge of any kind in a non-breast-feeding, nonlactating woman warrants thorough investigation, as does any discharge produced by breast manipulation [greenish black, white, creamy, serous, or bloody].)

○ change in the nipple, such as itching, burning, erosion, or retraction
○ pain (not usually a symptom of breast cancer unless the tumor is advanced, but it should be investigated)
○ bone metastasis, pathologic bone fractures, and hypercalcemia
○ edema of the arm.

Diagnosis

○ Clinical breast examination followed by immediate evaluation of any abnormality is the most reliable method of detecting breast cancer.

○ Mammography can reveal a tumor that's too small to palpate.

○ Ultrasonography can distinguish between a fluid-filled cyst and solid mass.

○ Chest X-rays can pinpoint metastases in the chest.

○ Scans of the bone, brain, liver, and other organs can detect distant metastases.

○ Fine needle aspiration and excisional biopsy provide cells for histologic examination that may confirm the diagnosis.

○ Serum alkaline phosphatase levels and liver function studies can detect distant metastases.

○ Hormonal receptor assay can determine if the tumor is estrogen or progesterone dependent. (This test guides decisions to use therapy that blocks the action of the estrogen hormone that supports tumor growth.)

○ Sentinel lymph-node biopsy, performed during surgery, identifies and samples the sentinel lymph node closest to the breast tumor and is used as a prognostic indicator.

Complications

○ Central nervous system effects
○ Infection
○ Metastasis
○ Recurrence
○ Respiratory effects

Treatment

○ The choice of therapy depends on the stage of the disease, the woman's age and menopausal status, and the disfiguring effects of the surgery.

○ Surgery involves lumpectomy and dissection of the axillary lymph nodes (leaves the breast intact), simple mastectomy (removes the breast but not the lymph nodes or pectoral muscles), modified radical mastectomy (removes the breast and the axillary lymph nodes), or radical mastectomy (removes the breast, pectoralis major and minor, and the axillary lymph nodes).

○ Reconstructive breast surgery, including the insertion of breast implants or a transverse rectus abdominis musculocutaneous flap, can be performed at the same time as mastectomy or it can be planned for a later date.

○ Chemotherapy, involving various cytotoxic drug combinations, is used as either adjuvant or primary therapy, depending on several factors, including the TNM staging and estrogen receptor status. The most commonly used drugs are cyclophosphamide, fluorouracil, methotrexate, doxorubicin, vincristine, and paclitaxel.

○ Antiestrogens tamoxifen, toremifene, or fulvestrant are given to bind to the estrogen receptors and inhibit estrogen-mediated tumor growth in breast tissue. Tamoxifen is the adjuvant treatment of choice for postmenopausal patients with positive estrogen receptor status and reduces the risk of breast cancer in women at high risk.

○ The selective estrogen receptor modulator raloxifene is being compared to tamoxifen in clinical trials to determine if it's more effective in preventing prevent breast cancer with fewer adverse effects than tamoxifen.

○ Aromatase inhibitors, anastrozole and letrozole, are used to treat primary postmenopausal women with metastatic breast cancer.

○ Estrogen, progesterone, androgen, or antiandrogen aminoglutethimide therapy may also be used to treat metastatic breast cancer.

○ Monoclonal antibody therapy is used to treat women with metastatic disease.

○ Peripheral stem cell therapy is an option, but it's rarely used for advanced breast cancer.

○ Primary radiation therapy before or after tumor removal is effective for small tumors in early stages with no evidence of distant metastasis; it's also used to prevent or treat local recurrence. Presurgical radiation to the breast in inflammatory breast cancer helps make tumors more surgically manageable.

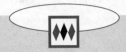

Teaching about breast cancer

Remember these key points when teaching your patient about breast cancer:

- Explain the disorder and its treatments.
- Teach about self-care activities to combat the adverse effects of chemotherapy, hormonal therapy, and radiation therapy.
- For the woman undergoing surgery, explain the procedure and perioperative considerations, such as preparation for surgery, pain after surgery, and coping with emotional distress.
- Discuss measures to prevent lymphedema with the woman who has had a mastectomy.
- Instruct the patient about breast prostheses.
- Discuss cancer-screening guidelines and demonstrate breast self-examination.
- Refer the patient to the American Cancer Society's Reach to Recovery group for instruction, emotional support and counseling, and a list of area stores that sell prostheses.

 COLLABORATIVE MANAGEMENT
Care of the patient with breast cancer involves several members of the interdisciplinary team. The nurse explains the disease process and treatment options, coordinates the health care team, monitors the patient's response to treatment, and educates the patient regarding self-care. The surgeon discusses the surgical options with the patient and performs the selected procedure. The medical oncologist and radiation oncologist make recommendations about the use of chemotherapy and radiation therapy, respectively, and monitor the treatment course. The dietitian helps the patient to maintain proper nutrition during treatment. The physical therapist helps the woman maintain range of motion in the affected arm and reduce lymphedema. The social worker assists with problems related to health insurance, finances, and work. Volunteers who have survived breast cancer can provide emotional support.

Special considerations

○ Explain the surgical procedure to the patient and tell her what to expect in the postoperative period.

○ Assess the patient's feelings about her illness, and determine what she knows about it and what she expects. Assess her coping strategies and consult social services as needed.

○ Advise the patient to ask her physician about reconstructive surgery. In many cases, reconstructive surgery may be planned before the mastectomy.

For postoperative care, perform the following:

○ Inspect the dressing and report bleeding promptly.

○ Measure and record the amount of drainage; also note the color. Expect drainage to be bloody during the first 4 hours and afterward to become serous.

○ Check circulatory status (blood pressure, pulse, respirations, and bleeding).

○ Monitor intake and output for at least 48 hours after general anesthesia.

○ Prevent lymphedema of the arm, which may occur following surgery that involves lymph node manipulation. Avoid drawing blood, starting an I.V., giving an injection, or taking a blood pressure on the affected side because these activities increase the chances of developing lymphedema.

○ Inspect the incision and encourage the patient and her partner to look at her incision as soon as possible.

○ Give psychological and emotional support.

○ Explain that breast surgery doesn't interfere with sexual function and that the patient may resume sexual activity as soon as she desires after surgery.

○ Listen to the patient's concerns, offer support, and refer her to an appropriate organization such as the American Cancer Society's Reach to Recovery, which offers caring and sharing groups to help breast cancer patients in the hospital and at home.

○ For patients receiving chemotherapy, discuss proper nutrition and mouth care to help relieve discomfort from mouth sores.

○ Discuss possible complications from chemotherapy or radiation therapy; also discuss the follow-up regimen.

○ For patients with lymphedema, discuss proper skin care and daily exercises for the affected arm.

○ Advise patients with breast implants to report discomfort, change in size or shape of the implant, or palpable lumps.

○ Consider palliative care for the patient with metastatic disease. Assess the need for pain management and nutritional support, and discuss with the patient and her family the need for hospice care.

○ Provide patient education. (See *Teaching about breast cancer*.)

Applicable patient-teaching aids

○ Caring for a Jackson-Pratt drain
○ Caring for your hair and scalp during cancer treatment *
○ Controlling the side effects of chemotherapy *
○ Coping with depression
○ Dressing with confidence after a mastectomy *
○ Examining your breasts
○ Exercising to strengthen your arm and shoulder
○ Minimizing hair loss from chemotherapy
○ Preparing for needle aspiration of the breast *
○ Preventing infections after mastectomy

○ Bronchitis, chronic

A form of chronic obstructive pulmonary disease (COPD), chronic bronchitis is inflammation of the bronchi caused by irritants or infection. In this disorder, hypersecretion of mucus and a chronic productive cough last for 3 months of the year and occur for at least 2 consecutive years. The distinguishing characteristic of bronchitis is airflow obstruction.

COPD affects an estimated 17 million Americans, and its prevalence is rising. It af-

fects more men than women and more Whites than Blacks.

Causes

Common causes of chronic bronchitis include exposure to irritants, cigarette smoking, genetic predisposition, exposure to organic or inorganic dusts, exposure to noxious gases, and respiratory tract infection. Respiratory infections can trigger acute exacerbations, and respiratory failure can occur.

Pathophysiology

Chronic bronchitis occurs when irritants are inhaled for a prolonged time. The irritants inflame the tracheobronchial tree, leading to increased mucus production and a narrowed or blocked airway. As the inflammation continues, changes in the cells lining the respiratory tract result in resistance of the small airways and severe ventilation-perfusion ($\dot{V}/\dot{Q}$) imbalance, which decreases arterial oxygenation.

Chronic bronchitis results in hypertrophy and hyperplasia of the mucous glands, increased goblet cells, ciliary damage, squamous metaplasia of the columnar epithelium, and chronic leukocytic and lymphocytic infiltration of bronchial walls. Hypersecretion of the goblet cells blocks the free movement of the cilia, which normally sweep dust, irritants, and mucus away from the airways. With mucus and debris accumulating in the airway, the defenses are altered, and the individual is prone to respiratory tract infections. (See *Understanding chronic bronchitis,* page 60.)

Additional effects include widespread inflammation, airway narrowing, and mucus within the airways. Bronchial walls become inflamed and thickened from edema and accumulation of inflammatory cells, and the effects of smooth muscle bronchospasm further narrow the lumen. Airways become obstructed and closure occurs, especially on expiration. The gas is then trapped in the distal portion of the lung. Hypoventilation occurs, leading to a $\dot{V}/\dot{Q}$ mismatch and resultant hypoxemia.

Hypoxemia and hypercapnia occur secondary to hypoventilation. Pulmonary vascular

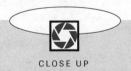

CLOSE UP

Understanding chronic bronchitis

In chronic bronchitis, irritants inflame the tracheobronchial tree over time, leading to increased mucus production and a narrowed or blocked airway. As the inflammation continues, goblet and epithelial cells hypertrophy. Because the natural defense mechanisms are blocked, the airways accumulate debris in the respiratory tract.

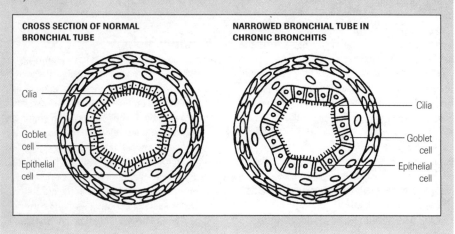

CROSS SECTION OF NORMAL BRONCHIAL TUBE

Cilia

Goblet cell

Epithelial cell

NARROWED BRONCHIAL TUBE IN CHRONIC BRONCHITIS

Cilia

Goblet cell

Epithelial cell

resistance increases as inflammatory and compensatory vasoconstriction in hypoventilated areas narrows the pulmonary arteries. Increased pulmonary vascular resistance leads to increased afterload of the right ventricle. With repeated inflammatory episodes, scarring of the airways occurs, and permanent structural changes develop.

Patients with chronic bronchitis have a diminished respiratory drive. The resulting chronic hypoxia causes the kidneys to produce erythropoietin, which stimulates excessive red blood cell production and leads to polycythemia. Although hemoglobin levels are high, the amount of reduced (not fully oxygenated) hemoglobin in contact with oxygen is low; therefore, cyanosis occurs.

Assessment findings

The patient with chronic bronchitis may have a history of smoking and frequent upper respiratory tract infections. He may also have a productive cough that's initially prevalent in the winter months but eventually becomes a year-round problem with increasingly severe episodes. The patient may develop weight gain due to edema, as well as progressively worsening dyspnea that takes increasingly longer to subside.

Physical examination may reveal a cyanotic appearance and the use of accessory muscles for breathing, tachypnea, pedal edema, and jugular vein distention. Auscultation may reveal wheezing, prolonged expiratory time, and rhonchi. The patient's symptoms may worsen with decompensation and acute respiratory failure. (See *Acute respiratory failure.*)

Diagnosis

○ Chest X-rays may show hyperinflation and increased bronchovascular markings.

○ Pulmonary function studies indicate increased residual volume, decreased vital capacity and forced expiratory flow, and normal static compliance and diffusing capacity.

○ Arterial blood gas analysis reveals decreased partial pressure of arterial oxygen and normal or increased partial pressure of arterial carbon dioxide.

○ Sputum analysis may reveal many microorganisms and neutrophils.

○ Electrocardiography may show atrial arrhythmias; peaked P waves in leads II, III, and aV_F; and, occasionally, right ventricular hypertrophy.

Complications
○ Acute respiratory failure
○ Cor pulmonale
○ Heart failure
○ Pulmonary hypertension

Treatment
○ Smoking cessation and avoidance of air pollutants are the most effective treatments.

○ Antibiotics can be used to treat recurring infections.

○ Bronchodilators may relieve bronchospasms and facilitate mucociliary clearance.

○ Adequate hydration liquefies secretions and chest physiotherapy mobilizes secretions.

○ Ultrasonic or mechanical nebulizers loosen and mobilize secretions.

○ Corticosteroids may be given to combat inflammation.

○ Diuretics may be used to reduce edema.

○ Oxygen may be necessary to treat hypoxia.

 COLLABORATIVE MANAGEMENT
Care of the patient with chronic bronchitis involves several members of the interdisciplinary team. The nurse typically coordinates the interdisciplinary team while providing education and therapeutic interventions. The physician diagnoses and directs the medical care, and a nurse practitioner may assist in care management. The physical therapist devises a program to promote muscle reconditioning and prevent further loss of muscle strength and tone. The occupational

ACUTE EPISODE

Acute respiratory failure

Acute respiratory failure in the patient with chronic bronchitis is an emergency. If your patient's respiratory status deteriorates, proceed as follows:

● Prepare the patient and his family for transfer to the intensive care unit.

● Administer an antibiotic, a bronchodilator, an anxiolytic and, possibly, a steroid, as ordered.

● Administer oxygen at concentrations to maintain a partial pressure of arterial oxygen of at least 50 to 60 mm Hg, and monitor for improved breathing using nasal prongs or a Venturi mask.

● For significant respiratory acidosis, a bidirectional positive-pressure airway mask or mechanical ventilation through an endotracheal or tracheostomy tube may be necessary.

● Anticipate high-frequency ventilation if the patient doesn't respond to conventional mechanical ventilation.

● If the patient is retaining carbon dioxide, encourage him to cough and deep breathe with pursed lips.

● If the patient is alert, have him use an incentive spirometer; if he's intubated and lethargic, turn him every 1 to 2 hours.

● Use postural drainage and chest physiotherapy to help clear the patient's secretions.

● If the patient is intubated, suction his trachea using sterile technique, as needed, after hyperoxygenation. Observe him for a change in the quantity, consistency, or color of his sputum. Provide humidification to liquefy the secretions.

● Observe the patient closely for respiratory arrest. Auscultate for breath sounds and monitor arterial blood gases for changes.

● Monitor serum electrolyte levels and correct imbalances.

● Monitor intake and output and daily weight.

● Monitor for cardiac arrhythmias.

therapist teaches energy conservation techniques. The respiratory therapist performs pulmonary function tests, coordinates the use of

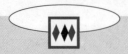

Teaching about chronic bronchitis

Remember these key points when teaching your patient and his family about chronic bronchitis:

• Explain the disease process and its treatments.

• Discuss the importance of not smoking and avoiding other bronchial irritants, such as secondhand smoke, allergens, pollution, aerosol sprays, and adverse weather conditions.

• Advise the patient to avoid crowds and people with known infections and to obtain influenza and pneumococcal immunizations.

• Warn the patient that exposure to blasts of cold air may precipitate bronchospasm; suggest that he avoid cold, windy weather or that he cover his mouth and nose with a scarf or mask if he must go outside.

• Explain all medications, including their indications, dosages, adverse effects, and special considerations.

• Demonstrate how to use a metered dose inhaler.

• Demonstrate the proper use of safe home oxygen therapy.

• Teach the patient and his family how to perform postural drainage and chest physiotherapy.

• Discuss the importance of drinking plenty of fluids to liquefy secretions.

○ Assess the patient for changes in baseline respiratory function.

○ Evaluate sputum quality and quantity, restlessness, increased tachypnea, and altered breath sounds.

○ As needed, perform chest physiotherapy, including postural drainage as well as chest percussion and vibration for involved lobes, several times daily.

○ Weigh the patient three times weekly, and assess for edema.

○ Provide the patient with a high-calorie, protein-rich diet. Offer small, frequent meals to conserve the patient's energy and prevent fatigue.

○ Make sure the patient receives adequate fluids (at least 3 qt [3 L] per day) to loosen secretions.

○ Schedule respiratory therapy at least 1 hour before or after meals. Provide mouth care after bronchodilator inhalation therapy.

○ Discuss safety tips for patients with home oxygen therapy.

○ Assess the patient's respiratory status during activities of daily living, reinforce energy conservation techniques, and evaluate the need for equipment in the home, such as a shower chair.

○ Provide patient education. (See *Teaching about chronic bronchitis.*)

Applicable patient-teaching aids

○ Caring for aerosol equipment

○ Learning about immunization for the flu

○ Learning to do controlled coughing exercises *

○ Performing chest physiotherapy (for an adult)

○ Preparing for pulmonary function tests *

○ Preventing infection with proper hand washing *

○ Using an oral inhaler *

○ Using an oral roto inhaler

oxygen, performs breathing treatments, and teaches the patient coughing and breathing techniques. The dietitian assesses the patient's nutritional status and makes recommendations to maintain body weight and muscle mass. The social worker can aid in obtaining medical equipment and with financial difficulties.

Special considerations

○ If the patient smokes, encourage him to stop. Provide him with smoking-cessation resources or counseling if necessary.

⬭ Buerger's disease

Buerger's disease (sometimes called *thromboangiitis obliterans*) — an inflammatory, nonatheromatous occlusive condition — impairs circulation to the legs, feet and, occasionally, the hands. It causes segmental lesions and subsequent thrombus formation in the small and medium arteries (and sometimes the veins), resulting in decreased blood flow to the feet and legs. This disorder may produce ulceration and, eventually, gangrene. Incidence is highest among men of Jewish ancestry, ages 20 to 40, who smoke heavily.

Causes

Although the cause of Buerger's disease is unknown, a definite link to smoking has been found, suggesting a hypersensitivity reaction to nicotine. It may also be associated with a history of Raynaud's disease and may occur in people with autoimmune disease.

Pathophysiology

Buerger's disease is caused by vasculitis, an inflammation of blood vessels, primarily of the hands and feet. Polymorphonuclear leukocytes infiltrate the walls of small and medium-sized arteries and veins. Thrombi develop in the vascular lumen, eventually occluding and obliterating portions of the small vessels, resulting in decreased blood flow to the feet and legs. This diminished blood flow may produce pain, ulceration and, eventually, gangrene.

Assessment findings

Buerger's disease typically produces intermittent claudication of the instep, which is aggravated by exercise and relieved by rest. During exposure to low temperature, the feet initially become cold, cyanotic, and numb; later, they redden, become hot, and tingle. Associated signs and symptoms may include impaired peripheral pulses and migratory superficial thrombophlebitis.

Diagnosis

◯ Doppler ultrasonography may show diminished circulation in the peripheral vessels.
◯ Plethysmography detects decreased circulation in the peripheral vessels.
◯ Arteriography locates lesions and rules out atherosclerosis.

Complications

◯ Gangrene
◯ Muscle atrophy
◯ Painful fingertip ulcerations if the hands are affected
◯ Ulceration

Treatment

◯ An exercise program that uses gravity to fill and drain blood vessels may relieve symptoms.
◯ In severe disease, a lumbar sympathectomy may be performed to increase blood supply to the skin.
◯ Amputation may be considered for nonhealing ulcers, intractable pain, or gangrene.
◯ Aspirin and vasodilators may be used to promote circulation.

 COLLABORATIVE MANAGEMENT
Care of the patient with Buerger's disease involves several members of the interdisciplinary team. The nurse provides education and referrals to smoking cessation programs. The physical therapist provides debridement and rehabilitation for the patient who has undergone amputation. The social worker can refer the patient for job retraining if his occupation contributed to the disorder or if he can no longer perform his job due to amputation.

Special considerations

◯ Strongly urge the patient to discontinue smoking permanently to enhance the effectiveness of treatment and refer him to a self-help group to stop smoking.
◯ If the patient has ulcers and gangrene, enforce bed rest, use a padded footboard or bed cradle to prevent pressure from bed linens, and protect his feet with soft padding.

KEY TEACHING POINTS

Teaching about Buerger's disease

Remember these key points when teaching your patient about Buerger's disease:
- Teach the patient about the disease process and its treatments.
- Warn the patient to avoid precipitating factors, such as emotional stress, exposure to extreme temperatures, and trauma.
- Teach proper foot care, especially the importance of wearing well-fitting shoes and cotton or wool socks.
- Discuss the importance of smoking cessation and methods to stop smoking.
- Discuss signs and symptoms that require immediate medical attention, such as the development of ulcers and worsening pain.
- Discuss care of the stump and prosthesis, if the patient had an amputation.

○ Provide emotional support.
○ If necessary, refer the patient for psychological counseling to help him cope with restrictions imposed by this chronic disease.
○ If the patient has undergone amputation, assess rehabilitative needs, especially regarding changes in body image.
○ Provide patient education. (See *Teaching about Buerger's disease.*)

Applicable patient-teaching aids
○ Care and prevention of leg ulcers *
○ Learning about walkers *
○ Wrapping your above-the-knee stump
○ Wrapping your below-the-knee stump

○ Bulimia nervosa

The essential features of the eating disorder bulimia nervosa include eating binges followed by feelings of guilt, humiliation, and self-deprecation. (See *Characteristics of patients with bulimia nervosa.*) These feelings cause the patient to engage in self-induced vomiting, use laxatives or diuretics, follow a strict diet, or fast to overcome the effects of the binges. Unless the patient spends an excessive amount of time bingeing and purging, bulimia nervosa is seldom incapacitating. However, electrolyte imbalances (metabolic alkalosis, hypochloremia, and hypokalemia) and dehydration can occur, increasing the risk of physical complications.

Bulimia nervosa usually begins in adolescence or early adulthood and can occur simultaneously with anorexia nervosa. It affects nine women for every man. Nearly 2% of adult women meet the diagnostic criteria for bulimia nervosa; 5% to 15% have some symptoms of the disorder.

Causes
The cause of bulimia nervosa is unknown, but psychosocial factors may contribute to its development. These factors include family disturbance or conflict, sexual abuse, maladaptive learned behavior, struggle for control or self-identity, cultural overemphasis on physical appearance, and parental obesity. Bulimia nervosa is associated with depression, anxiety, phobias, and obsessive-compulsive disorder. Eating disorders are most prevalent in affluent cultural groups and are essentially unknown in cultural groups where poverty and malnutrition are prevalent. In developing countries, almost no cases of eating disorders have been recognized.

Pathophysiology
Bulimia nervosa is often accompanied by fluid and electrolyte imbalances. Hypokalemia, hyponatremia, and hypochloremia may occur. The use of enemas and laxatives may produce diarrhea, resulting in metabolic acidosis. Frequent vomiting, however, may cause metabolic alkalosis.

Reduced levels of cholecystokinin, an intestinal hormone, have been found in patients with bulimia nervosa. Aberrations in the hypothalamic-pituitary-adrenal pathway have also been noted. Patients with bulimia nervosa may also have reduced serotonin and satiety levels.

Characteristics of patients with bulimia nervosa

Recognizing the patient with bulimia nervosa isn't always easy. Unlike patients with anorexia, patients with bulimia nervosa don't deny that their eating habits are abnormal, but they commonly conceal their behavior out of shame. If you suspect bulimia nervosa, watch for these features:
- chronic depression
- difficulty expressing feelings such as anger
- difficulty with impulse control
- exaggerated sense of guilt
- feelings of alienation
- impaired social or occupational adjustment
- low tolerance for frustration
- recurrent anxiety
- self-consciousness.

Diagnosing bulimia nervosa

Use these criteria from the *Diagnostic and Statistical Manual of Mental Disorders,* Fourth Edition, Text Revision, for the diagnosis of a patient with bulimia nervosa. Both of the behaviors listed below must occur at least twice per week for 3 months:
- recurrent episodes of binge eating (rapid consumption of a large amount of food in a discrete period of time and a feeling of lack of control over eating behavior during the eating binges)
- recurrent inappropriate compensatory behavior to prevent weight gain (self-induced vomiting; misuse of laxatives, diuretics, enemas or other medications; fasting; excessive exercise).

Reprinted with permission from the *Diagnostic and Statistical Manual of Mental Disorders,* Copyright 2000. American Psychiatric Association.

Assessment findings

The history of a patient with bulimia nervosa is characterized by episodes of binge eating that may occur up to several times per day. The patient commonly repairs a binge-eating episode during which she continues eating until abdominal pain, sleep, or the presence of another person interrupts it. The preferred food is usually sweet, soft, and high in calories and carbohydrate content.

The patient with bulimia nervosa may appear thin and emaciated. Typically, however, although her weight frequently fluctuates, it usually stays within normal limits—through the use if diuretics, laxatives, vomiting, and exercise.

Overt clues to bulimia nervosa include hyperactivity, peculiar eating habits or rituals, frequent weighing, and distorted body image.

The patient with bulimia nervosa may complain of abdominal and epigastric pain caused by acute gastric dilation. She may also have amenorrhea. Repetitive vomiting may cause painless swelling of the salivary glands, hoarseness, throat irritation or lacerations, and dental erosion. The patient may also exhibit calluses on the dorsum of the hand, resulting from tooth injury during self-induced vomiting.

The patient with bulimia commonly is perceived by others as a "perfect" student, mother, or career woman; an adolescent may be distinguished for participation in competitive activities such as sports. However, the patient's psychosocial history may reveal an exaggerated sense of guilt, symptoms of depression, childhood trauma (especially sexual abuse), parental obesity, and unsatisfactory sexual relationships.

Diagnosis

❍ The diagnosis of bulimia nervosa is made when the patient meets criteria put forth in the *Diagnostic and Statistical Manual of Mental Disorders,* Fourth Edition, Text Revision. (See *Diagnosing bulimia nervosa.*)
❍ The Beck Depression Inventory may identify coexisting depression.
❍ Serum electrolyte studies may show elevated bicarbonate, decreased potassium, and decreased sodium levels.

Teaching about bulimia nervosa

Remember these key points when teaching your patient about bulimia nervosa:
● Teach about the disorder and its treatments.
● Teach the patient how to keep a food journal to monitor treatment progress.
● Explain the risks of laxative, emetic, and diuretic abuse for the patient.
● Teach the patient to be assertive to allow her to gain control over her behavior and achieve a realistic and positive self-image.
● Discuss the prescribed drugs, how to take them, dosages, and possible adverse effects.
● Tell the patient taking a tricyclic antidepressant to take the drug with food and to avoid consuming alcoholic beverages; exposing herself to sunlight, heat lamps, or tanning salons; and discontinuing the medication unless she has notified the physician.

Complications

○ Arrhythmias
○ Cardiac failure
○ Dehydration
○ Dental caries
○ Electrolyte and acid-base imbalances
○ Erosion of tooth enamel
○ Esophageal tears
○ Gastric rupture
○ Gum infections
○ Intestinal mucosal damage
○ Parotitis
○ Sudden death
○ Suicide

Treatment

○ Psychotherapy concentrates on interrupting the binge-purge cycle and helping the patient regain control over her eating behavior.
○ Inpatient or outpatient treatment includes behavior modification therapy, which may take place in highly structured psychoeducational group meetings.
○ Cognitive behavioral therapy, group therapy, and family therapy, which address the eating disorder as a symptom of unresolved conflict, may help the patient understand the basis of her behavior and teach her self-control strategies.
○ Antidepressant drugs may be used as an adjunct to psychotherapy.
○ Self-help groups may be helpful, such as Overeaters Anonymous or a drug rehabilitation program if the patient has a concurrent substance abuse problem.

COLLABORATIVE MANAGEMENT
Care of the patient with bulimia nervosa involves several members of the interdisciplinary team. The nurse establishes a therapeutic relationship with the patient to help her take responsibility for her actions. The therapist helps the patient stop the binge-purge cycle through individual or group therapy. The dietitian provides education about healthy eating and assesses the patient's nutritional status.

Special considerations

○ Supervise the patient during mealtimes and for a specified period after meals (usually 1 hour).
○ Set a time limit for each meal.
○ Provide a pleasant, relaxed environment for eating.
○ Using behavior modification techniques, reward the patient for satisfactory weight gain.
○ Establish a contract with the patient, specifying the amount and type of food to be eaten at each meal.
○ Encourage the patient to recognize and express her feelings about her eating behavior.
○ Maintain an accepting and nonjudgmental attitude, controlling your reactions to the patient's behavior and feelings.
○ Encourage the patient to talk about stressful issues, such as achievement, independence, socialization, sexuality, family problems, and control.
○ Identify the patient's elimination patterns.
○ Assess the patient's suicide potential.

○ Refer the patient and her family to the American Anorexia and Bulimia Association and to Anorexia Nervosa and Related Eating Disorders for additional information and support.

○ Provide patient education. (See *Teaching about bulimia nervosa*.)

Applicable patient-teaching aids
○ Learning about daily food choices

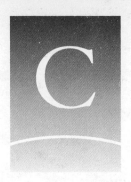

Cardiomyopathy, dilated

Dilated cardiomyopathy results from extensively damaged myocardial muscle fibers. (See *Understanding dilated cardiomyopathy*.) This disorder is primarily a disorder of the ventricular myocardium, but it also interferes with myocardial metabolism and grossly dilates all four chambers of the heart, giving the heart a globular appearance and shape. Hypertrophy may be present.

Dilated cardiomyopathy leads to intractable heart failure, arrhythmias, and emboli. Because this disease isn't usually diagnosed until it's in the advanced stages, the patient's prognosis is generally poor. Dilated cardiomyopathy occurs in 2 of every 100 people and affects all ages and sexes. It's most common in adult men.

Causes

The cause of most cardiomyopathies is unknown. (See *Comparing cardiomyopathies*, pages 70 and 71.) Occasionally, dilated cardiomyopathy results from myocardial destruction by toxic, infectious, or metabolic agents, such as certain viruses, endocrine and electrolyte disorders, and nutritional deficiencies. Other causes include muscle disorders (myasthenia gravis, progressive muscular dystrophy, and myotonic dystrophy), infiltrative disorders (hemochromatosis and amyloidosis), sarcoidosis and, possibly, genetic factors.

Cardiomyopathy may also be a complication of alcoholism. In such cases, it may improve with abstinence from alcohol but recurs when the patient resumes drinking.

Researchers suspect a link between viral myocarditis and subsequent dilated cardiomyopathy, especially after infection with poliovirus, coxsackievirus B, influenza virus, or human immunodeficiency virus.

Metabolic cardiomyopathies are related to endocrine and electrolyte disorders and nutritional deficiencies. Thus, dilated cardiomyopathy may develop in patients with hyperthyroidism, pheochromocytoma, beriberi (thiamine deficiency), or kwashiorkor (protein deficiency). Cardiomyopathy may also result from rheumatic fever, especially among children with myocarditis.

Antepartal or postpartal cardiomyopathy may develop during the last trimester or within months after delivery. Its cause is unknown, but it occurs most frequently in multiparous women older than age 30, particularly those with malnutrition or preeclampsia.

Pathophysiology

Dilated cardiomyopathy results from extensively damaged myocardial muscle fibers. Consequently, there's reduced contractility in the left ventricle. As systolic function declines, stroke volume, ejection fraction, and cardiac output fall. As end-diastolic volumes rise, pulmonary congestion may occur. The elevated end-diastolic volume is a compensatory response to preserve stroke volume despite a reduced ejection fraction. The sympathetic nervous system is also stimulated to increase heart rate and contractility. The kidneys are stimulated to retain sodium and water to maintain cardiac output, and vasoconstriction also occurs as the renin-angiotensin system is stimulated. When

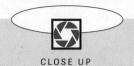

CLOSE UP

Understanding dilated cardiomyopathy

Extensively damaged myocardial muscle fibers reduce contractility of the left ventricle. As systolic function declines, stroke volume, ejection fraction, and cardiac output fall. The sympathetic nervous system is stimulated to increase heart rate and contractility. The kidneys are stimulated to retain sodium and water to maintain cardiac output, and vasoconstriction also occurs as the renin-angiotensin system is stimulated.

When compensatory mechanisms can no longer maintain cardiac output, the heart begins to fail. Left ventricular dilation occurs as venous return and systemic vascular resistance rise. Eventually, the atria also dilate as more work is required to pump blood into the full ventricles. Cardiomegaly occurs as a consequence of dilation of the atria and ventricles.

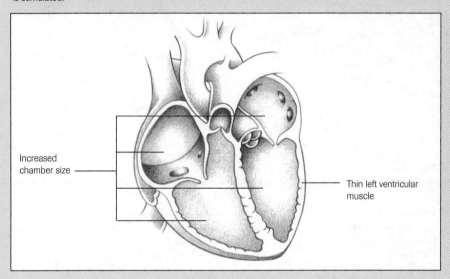

Increased chamber size

Thin left ventricular muscle

these compensatory mechanisms can no longer maintain cardiac output, the heart begins to fail. Left ventricular dilation occurs as venous return and systemic vascular resistance rise. Eventually, the atria also dilate as more work is required to pump blood into the full ventricles. Cardiomegaly occurs as a consequence of dilation of the atria and ventricles. Blood pooling in the ventricles increases the risk of mural thrombi.

Assessment findings

In dilated cardiomyopathy, the patient develops signs of heart failure—both left-sided (short-ness of breath, orthopnea, dyspnea on exertion, paroxysmal nocturnal dyspnea, fatigue, dizziness, and an irritating dry cough) and right-sided (peripheral edema, hepatomegaly, jugular vein distention, and weight gain). Dilated cardiomyopathy also produces peripheral cyanosis and sinus tachycardia or atrial fibrillation in some patients secondary to a low cardiac output. Auscultation reveals diffuse apical impulses, pansystolic murmur (mitral and tricuspid insufficiency secondary to cardiomegaly and weak papillary muscles), and S_3 and S_4 gallop rhythms.

Comparing cardiomyopathies

Cardiomyopathies include a variety of structural or functional abnormalities of the ventricles. They're grouped into three main pathophysiologic types — dilated, hypertrophic, and restrictive. These conditions may lead to heart failure by impairing myocardial structure and function.

Normal heart   **Dilated cardiomyopathy**

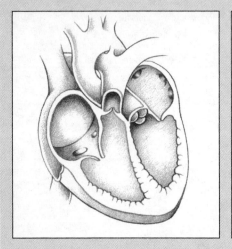   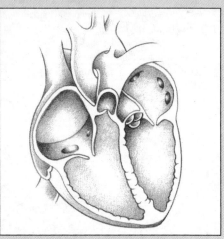

Ventricles	● Greatly increased chamber size
	● Thinning of left ventricular muscle
Atrial chamber size	● Increased
Myocardial mass	● Increased
Ventricular inflow resistance	● Normal
Contractility	● Decreased
Possible causes	● Cardiotoxic effects of drugs or alcohol
	● Chemotherapy
	● Drug hypersensitivity
	● Hypertension
	● Ischemic heart disease
	● Peripartum syndrome related to toxemia
	● Valvular disease
	● Viral or bacterial infection

Decreased cardiac output also leads to worsening renal function, which produces decreased renal perfusion and reduced urine output.

Diagnosis

○ Diagnosis requires elimination of other possible causes of heart failure and arrhythmias.
○ Electrocardiography (ECG) and angiography rule out ischemic heart disease; ECG may also

Hypertrophic cardiomyopathy	Restrictive cardiomyopathy
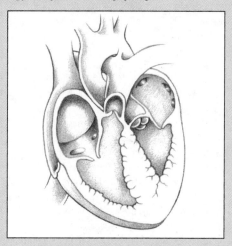	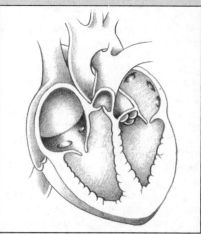
• Normal right and decreased left chamber size • Left ventricular hypertrophy • Thickened interventricular septum (hypertrophic obstructive cardiomyopathy [HOCM])	• Decreased ventricular chamber size • Left ventricular hypertrophy
• Increased on left	• Increased
• Increased	• Normal
• Increased	• Increased
• Increased or decreased	• Decreased
• Autosomal dominant trait (HOCM) • Hypertension • Obstructive valvular disease • Thyroid disease	• Amyloidosis • Hemochromatosis • Infiltrative neoplastic disease • Sarcoidosis

show biventricular hypertrophy, sinus tachycardia, atrial enlargement and, in 20% of patients, atrial fibrillation and bundle-branch block.

○ Chest X-ray shows cardiomegaly—usually affecting all heart chambers—and may demonstrate pulmonary congestion, pleural or pericardial effusion, or pulmonary vein hypertension.

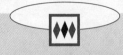

Teaching about dilated cardiomyopathy

Remember these key points when teaching your patient and his family about dilated cardiomyopathy:
- Explain how dilated cardiomyopathy affects heart muscle and circulation.
- Discuss signs and symptoms of the disease.
- Discuss signs and symptoms of complications, such as a weight gain of 3 or more pounds over 1 to 2 days indicating heart failure, that require immediate medical attention.
- Teach about sodium and fluid restrictions.
- Discuss the patient's medications, dosages, how to take them, and their adverse effects.
- Emphasize the need to avoid alcohol and smoking.
- Explain preoperative and postoperative care to the patient undergoing heart surgery.
- Teach the family cardiopulmonary resuscitation.

○ Chest computed tomography scan or echocardiography identifies left ventricular thrombi, global hypokinesia, and degree of left ventricular dilation.
○ Nuclear heart scans, such as multiple-gated acquisition and ventriculography, show heart enlargement, lung congestion, heart failure, and decreased movement or functioning of the heart.
○ Troponin I and troponin II may help differentiate ischemic heart disease from dilated cardiomyopathy.
○ B-type natriuretic peptide assay determines the severity of heart failure.

Complications
○ Arrhythmias
○ Heart failure
○ Sudden death
○ Systemic or pulmonary embolization

Treatment
○ Treat the underlying cause, if it can be identified.
○ Angiotensin-converting enzyme (ACE) inhibitors are a first-line therapy to reduce afterload through vasodilation.
○ Diuretics, taken with ACE inhibitors, reduce fluid retention.
○ Potassium supplements may be administered for patients on loop diuretics.
○ Digoxin may be used to improve myocardial contractility.
○ Hydralazine and isosorbide dinitrate may be given in combination to produce vasodilation.
○ Beta-adrenergic blockers may be used for the patient with New York Heart Association (NYHA) class II or III heart failure.
○ Antiarrhythmics, such as amiodarone, are used cautiously to control arrhythmias.
○ An implantable cardioverter-defibrillator may be inserted to treat ventricular arrhythmias and for prophylaxis (due to the high incidence of sudden death in the patient with NYHA class III or IV heart failure).
○ Cardioversion may be used to convert atrial fibrillation to sinus rhythm.
○ A pacemaker may be necessary to correct arrhythmias.
○ Anticoagulants reduce the risk of emboli.
○ A biventricular pacemaker is inserted for cardiac resynchronization therapy if symptoms of dilated cardiomyopathy continue despite optimal medication therapy, the patient is classified as NYHA class III or IV heart failure, QRS duration is 0.13 second or more, or ejection fraction is 35% or less.
○ Revascularization, such as coronary artery bypass graft surgery, is performed if dilated cardiomyopathy is due to ischemia.
○ Valvular repair or replacement is performed if dilated cardiomyopathy is due to valve dysfunction.
○ Heart transplantation may be recommended in the patient refractory to medical therapy.
○ Lifestyle modifications (such as smoking cessation; low-fat, low-cholesterol, low-sodium diet; physical activity; and abstinence from alcohol) can reduce symptoms and improve quality of life.

COLLABORATIVE MANAGEMENT
Care of the patient with dilated cardiomyopathy involves several members of the interdisciplinary team. The nurse plays a key role in educating the patient about controlling symptoms, medication therapy, and lifestyle modification. The home care nurse monitors the patient in the community and communicates findings to the physician. The social worker can help the patient with financial concerns. The dietitian educates the patient about the importance of restricting sodium and helps him make proper food choices. The physical therapist can help the patient plan an activity program to improve his functional status. The occupational therapist teaches the patient energy conservation techniques.

Special considerations

○ Monitor for signs of progressive failure (increasing crackles and dyspnea and increased jugular vein distention) and compromised renal perfusion (oliguria, elevated blood urea nitrogen and creatinine levels, and electrolyte imbalances).
○ Weigh the patient daily.
○ If the patient is receiving vasodilators, check his blood pressure and heart rate, as appropriate.
○ If the patient is receiving diuretics, monitor for signs of resolving congestion (decreased crackles and dyspnea) or too vigorous diuresis.
○ Check the serum potassium level for hypokalemia, especially if therapy includes digoxin.
○ Offer support and let the patient express his feelings because therapeutic restrictions and an uncertain prognosis usually cause profound anxiety and depression.
○ Encourage the patient's family members to learn cardiopulmonary resuscitation.
○ Consider hospice referral for the patient with end-stage disease.
○ Provide patient education. (See *Teaching about dilated cardiomyopathy.*)

Applicable patient-teaching aids

○ Cutting down on salt *
○ Learning about ACE inhibitors *
○ Learning about beta-adrenergic blockers *
○ Learning about digoxin *
○ Living with heart failure *
○ Helping your pacemaker help you *
○ Maintaining a safe level of activity

○ Cardiomyopathy, hypertrophic

Hypertrophic cardiomyopathy, also called *idiopathic hypertrophic subaortic stenosis,* is the primary disease of cardiac muscle. It's characterized by disproportionate, asymmetrical thickening of the interventricular septum, particularly in the left ventricle's free wall. In this disorder, cardiac output may be low, normal, or high, depending on whether stenosis is obstructive or nonobstructive. If cardiac output is normal or high, hypertrophic cardiomyopathy may go undetected for years; low cardiac output may lead to potentially fatal heart failure.

The disease course varies. Some patients progressively deteriorate; others remain stable for years. Most patients have obstructive disease, resulting from effects of ventricular septal hypertrophy and the movement of the anterior mitral valve leaflet into the outflow tract during systole. Eventually, left ventricular dysfunction, from rigidity and decreased compliance, causes pump failure. This disorder affects 2 to 5 of every 1,000 people.

Causes

Despite being designated as idiopathic, in almost all cases, hypertrophic cardiomyopathy may be inherited as a non-sex-linked autosomal dominant trait.

Pathophysiology

Hypertrophic cardiomyopathy primarily affects diastolic function. The hypertrophied ventricle becomes stiff, noncompliant, and unable to relax during ventricular filling. Consequently, ventricular filling is reduced and left ventricular filling pressure rises, causing a rise in left atrial and pulmonary vein pressures and leading to venous congestion and dyspnea. Ventricular filling time is further reduced as a compensatory response to tachycardia leading to low cardiac output. If papillary muscles become hyper-

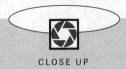

CLOSE UP

Understanding hypertrophic obstructive cardiomyopathy

Hypertrophic obstructive cardiomyopathy affects diastolic function. The left ventricle and intraventricular septum hypertrophy and become stiff, noncompliant, and unable to relax during ventricular filling. Ventricular filling decreases and left ventricular filling pressure rises, causing a rise in left atrial and pulmonary vein pressures. This leads to rapid, forceful contractions of the left ventricle and impaired relaxation. The forceful ejection of blood draws the anterior leaflet of the mitral valve to the intraventricular septum. This causes early closure of the outflow tract, decreasing ejection fraction.

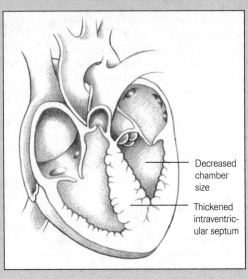

Decreased chamber size

Thickened intraventricular septum

trophied and don't close completely during contraction, mitral insufficiency occurs.

The features of hypertrophic obstructive cardiomyopathy include asymmetrical left ventricular hypertrophy; hypertrophy of the intraventricular septum; rapid, forceful contractions of the left ventricle; impaired relaxation; and obstruction to left ventricular outflow. The forceful ejection of blood draws the anterior leaflet of the mitral valve to the intraventricular septum. This causes early closure of the outflow tract, decreasing ejection fraction. Moreover, intramural coronary arteries are abnormally small and may not be sufficient to supply the hypertrophied muscle with enough blood and oxygen to meet the increased needs of the hyperdynamic muscle. (See *Understanding hypertrophic obstructive cardiomyopathy*.)

Assessment findings

Reduced inflow and subsequent low output may produce angina pectoris, arrhythmias, dys-

pnea, orthopnea, fatigue, syncope, heart failure, and death. Auscultation reveals a harsh midsystolic ejection murmur along the left sternal border and at the apex. Palpation reveals a peripheral pulse with a characteristic double impulse (pulsus biferiens) and, with atrial fibrillation, an irregular pulse.

Diagnosis

○ Echocardiography is the most useful test for diagnosing hypertrophic cardiomyopathy. It shows increased thickness of the intraventricular septum and abnormal motion of the anterior mitral leaflet during systole, which occludes left ventricular outflow in obstructive disease.
○ Cardiac catheterization reveals elevated left ventricular end-diastolic pressure and, possibly, mitral insufficiency.
○ Electrocardiography usually shows left ventricular hypertrophy, T-wave inversion, left anterior hemiblock, Q waves in precordial and

inferior leads, ventricular arrhythmias and, possibly, atrial fibrillation.

Complications
- Arrhythmias
- Heart failure
- Pulmonary hypertension
- Sudden death
- Systemic or pulmonary embolization

Treatment
- Beta-adrenergic blockers, such as propranolol, slow the heart rate and increase ventricular filling by relaxing the obstructing muscle, thereby reducing angina, syncope, dyspnea, and arrhythmias.
- Calcium channel blockers verapamil or diltiazem can reduce septal stiffness and elevated diastolic pressures.
- Cardioversion is used to treat atrial fibrillation arrhythmia and, because of the high risk of systemic embolism, anticoagulant therapy is initiated until fibrillation subsides.
- Antiarrhythmics may be necessary to suppress ventricular arrhythmias.
- An implantable-cardioverter defibrillator may be necessary to prevent sudden death in a patient with potentially lethal arrhythmias.
- Ventricular myotomy (resection of the hypertrophied septum) or ventricular myectomy (removal of the hypertrophied septum) alone or combined with mitral valve replacement may ease outflow tract obstruction and relieve symptoms.
- Heart transplantation may be performed for intractable symptoms.

COLLABORATIVE MANAGEMENT
Care of the patient with hypertrophic cardiomyopathy involves several members of the interdisciplinary team. The nurse plays a critical role in educating the patient about controlling symptoms, medication therapy, and lifestyle modification. Home health care nurses monitor the patient in the community and communicate findings to the health care provider. The social worker can help the patient with financial concerns. The dietitian educates the patient about the importance of restricting sodium and losing weight

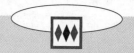

Teaching about hypertrophic cardiomyopathy

Remember these key points when teaching your patient and his family about hypertrophic cardiomyopathy:
- Explain the way hypertrophic cardiomyopathy affects the heart muscle and circulation.
- Discuss signs and symptoms of the disease.
- Explain complications that require immediate medical attention, such as heart failure.
- Because syncope or sudden death may follow well-tolerated exercise, warn against strenuous physical activity such as running.
- Warn the patient not to stop taking propranolol abruptly; doing so may increase myocardial demands.
- Discuss dietary restrictions, including calorie and sodium reduction.
- Tell the patient to discuss antibiotic prophylaxis for subacute infective endocarditis with his health care provider, before dental work or surgery.
- Prepare the patient for heart surgery, if indicated.
- Because sudden cardiac arrest is possible, urge the patient's family to learn cardiopulmonary resuscitation.

(if overweight) and helps him make proper food choices. The physical therapist helps the patient plan an activity program to improve his functional status. The occupational therapist teaches the patient energy conservation techniques.

Special considerations
- Because syncope or sudden death may follow exercise, advise the patient to avoid strenuous physical activity.
- Administer medications as prescribed.
Remember: Avoid nitroglycerin, digoxin, and diuretics because they can worsen obstruction.

○ To determine the patient's tolerance for an increased dosage of propranolol, take his pulse to check for bradycardia. Also take his blood pressure while he's supine and standing; a drop in blood pressure greater than 10 mm Hg when he's standing may indicate orthostatic hypotension.

○ Administer antibiotic prophylaxis for subacute infective endocarditis before dental work or surgery.

○ Provide psychological support.

○ If the patient has a prolonged hospitalization, be flexible with visiting hours and encourage occasional weekends away from the hospital, if possible.

○ Refer the patient for psychosocial counseling to help him and his family accept his restricted lifestyle and poor prognosis. If the patient has end-stage disease, consider a hospice referral.

○ Consider family screening because of the possible genetic component.

○ If the patient is a child, have his parents arrange for him to continue his studies in the health care facility.

○ Provide patient education. (See *Teaching about hypertrophic cardiomyopathy,* page 75.)

Applicable patient-teaching aids

○ Cutting down on salt *
○ Helping your pacemaker help you *
○ Living with heart failure *
○ Maintaining a safe level of activity

○ Cardiomyopathy, restrictive

Restrictive cardiomyopathy, a disorder of the myocardial musculature, is characterized by restricted ventricular filling (the result of left ventricular hypertrophy) and endocardial fibrosis and thickening. If severe, it's irreversible.

Restrictive cardiomyopathy is rare. It's most common in children and young adults. Africans, South Americans, and East Indians are at increased risk.

Causes

Primary restrictive cardiomyopathy is of unknown etiology. However, restrictive cardiomyopathy syndrome, a manifestation of amyloidosis, results from infiltration of amyloid into the intracellular spaces in the myocardium, endocardium, and subendocardium. It may also result from hemochromatosis.

Pathophysiology

Restrictive cardiomyopathy is characterized by stiffness of the ventricle caused by left ventricular hypertrophy and endocardial fibrosis and thickening, thus reducing the ability of the ventricle to relax and fill during diastole. Moreover, the rigid myocardium fails to contract completely during systole. As a result, cardiac output falls. (See *Understanding restrictive cardiomyopathy.*)

Assessment findings

Because restrictive cardiomyopathy lowers cardiac output and leads to heart failure, it also leads to fatigue, dyspnea, orthopnea, chest pain, generalized edema, liver engorgement, peripheral cyanosis, pallor, S_3 or S_4 gallop rhythms, and systolic murmurs of mitral and tricuspid insufficiency.

Diagnosis

○ In advanced stages, chest X-ray shows massive cardiomegaly (affecting all four chambers of the heart), pericardial effusion, and pulmonary congestion.

○ Echocardiography, computed tomography scan, or magnetic resonance imaging rules out constrictive pericarditis as the cause of restricted filling by detecting increased left ventricular muscle mass and differences in end-diastolic pressures between the ventricles.

○ Electrocardiography may show low-voltage complexes, hypertrophy, atrioventricular conduction defects, or arrhythmias.

○ Arterial pulsation reveals blunt carotid upstroke with small volume.

○ Cardiac catheterization shows increased left ventricular end-diastolic pressure and rules out constrictive pericarditis as the cause of restricted filling.

○ A heart muscle biopsy may be performed to confirm the diagnosis of restrictive cardiomyopathy.

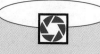

CLOSE UP

Understanding restrictive cardiomyopathy

Restrictive cardiomyopathy is characterized by stiffness of the ventricle caused by left ventricular hypertrophy and endocardial fibrosis and thickening, thus reducing the ability of the ventricle to relax and fill during diastole. The rigid myocardium fails to contract completely during systole. As a result, cardiac output falls.

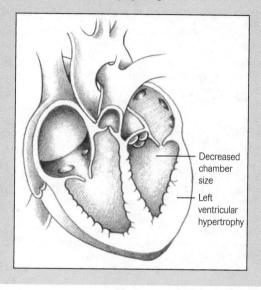

Decreased chamber size

Left ventricular hypertrophy

Complications
○ Arrhythmias
○ Heart failure
○ Sudden death
○ Systemic or pulmonary embolization

Treatment
○ Although no therapy currently exists for restricted ventricular filling, cardiac glycosides, diuretics, and a restricted sodium diet are beneficial because they ease the symptoms of heart failure.
○ Oral vasodilators — such as isosorbide dinitrate, prazosin, and hydralazine — may control intractable heart failure.
○ Anticoagulant therapy may be necessary to prevent thrombophlebitis in the patient on prolonged bed rest.
○ Steroids or chemotherapy may help with the underlying disease process.
○ A heart transplant may be considered in the patient with poor myocardial functioning.

○ Deferoxamine may be used to bind iron in restrictive cardiomyopathy that results from hemochromatosis.

 COLLABORATIVE MANAGEMENT
Care of the patient with restrictive cardiomyopathy involves several members of the interdisciplinary team. The nurse plays a key role in educating the patient about controlling symptoms, medication therapy, and lifestyle modification. Home health care nurses monitor the patient in the community and communicate findings to the health care provider. The social worker can help the patient with financial concerns. The dietitian educates the patient about the importance of restricting sodium and helps him make proper food choices. The physical therapist can help the patient plan an activity program to improve his functional status. The occupational therapist teaches the patient energy conservation techniques.

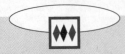

Teaching about restrictive cardiomyopathy

Remember these key points when teaching your patient and his family about restrictive cardiomyopathy:

● Explain how restrictive cardiomyopathy affects heart muscle and circulation.

● Discuss signs and symptoms of the disease.

● Discuss signs and symptoms of complications, such as a weight gain of 3 or more pounds over 1 to 2 days indicating heart failure, that require immediate medical attention.

● Teach about sodium and fluid restrictions and to document and report weight gain.

● Discuss the patient's medications, dosages, how to take them, and adverse effects.

● Teach the patient to watch for and report signs of digoxin toxicity, such as anorexia, nausea, vomiting, and yellow vision.

● Explain preoperative and postoperative care to the patient undergoing heart surgery.

Special considerations

○ Monitor the patient's heart rate and rhythm, blood pressure, urine output, and pulmonary artery pressure readings to help guide treatment.

○ Encourage the patient to express his fears. Give psychological support as needed; a poor prognosis may cause profound anxiety and depression.

○ Refer the patient for psychosocial counseling, as necessary, for assistance in coping with his restricted lifestyle.

○ Provide appropriate diversionary activities for the patient restricted to prolonged bed rest.

○ Consider a hospice referral for the patient with end-stage disease.

○ Provide patient education. (See *Teaching about restrictive cardiomyopathy.*)

Applicable patient-teaching aids

○ Cutting down on salt *

○ Learning about digoxin *

○ Living with heart failure *

○ Maintaining a safe level of activity

Carpal tunnel syndrome

Carpal tunnel syndrome, a form of repetitive stress injury, is the most common of the nerve entrapment syndromes. It results from compression of the median nerve at the wrist, within the carpal tunnel. (See *Understanding carpal tunnel syndrome.*) This compression neuropathy causes sensory and motor changes in the median distribution of the hand.

Carpal tunnel injury is five times more common in women than in men. It usually occurs in women between ages 30 and 60 and poses a serious occupational health problem. Any strenuous use of the hands—sustained grasping, twisting, or flexing—aggravates this condition.

Causes

Many conditions can cause the contents or structure of the carpal tunnel to swell and press the median nerve against the transverse carpal ligament. Such conditions include rheumatoid arthritis, flexor tenosynovitis (commonly associated with rheumatic disease), nerve compression, pregnancy, renal failure, menopause, diabetes mellitus, acromegaly, edema following Colles' fracture, hypothyroidism, amyloidosis, myxedema, benign tumors, tuberculosis, and other granulomatous diseases. Another source of damage to the median nerve is dislocation or acute sprain of the wrist. Assembly-line workers and packers and people who repeatedly use poorly designed tools are most likely to develop this disorder.

Pathophysiology

The carpal bones and the transverse carpal ligament form the carpal tunnel. Inflammation or fibrosis of the tendon sheaths that pass through the carpal tunnel usually causes edema and compression of the median nerve. This compression neuropathy causes sensory and motor changes in the median distribution of the hands,

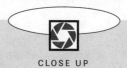

CLOSE UP

Understanding carpal tunnel syndrome

The carpal bones and transverse carpal ligament form the carpal tunnel. Inflammation or fibrosis of the tendon sheaths that pass through the carpal tunnel causes compression and edema of the median nerve. The myelin sheath begins to thin and degenerate. This compression neuropathy causes sensory and motor changes in the median distribution of the hands, initially impairing sensory transmission to the thumb, index finger, second finger, and inner aspect of the third finger.

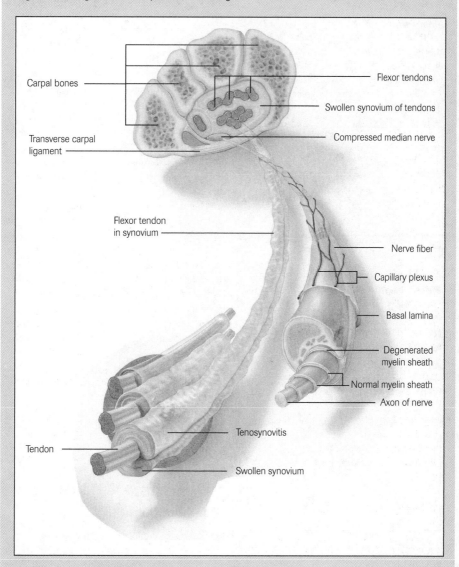

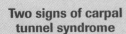

Two signs of carpal tunnel syndrome

Two simple tests — for Tinel's sign and for Phalen's sign — confirm the diagnosis of carpal tunnel syndrome. These tests elicit symptoms confirming that certain wrist movements compress the median nerve, causing pain, burning, numbness, or tingling in the hand and fingers.

Tinel's sign
Percuss the transverse carpal ligament (lying over the median nerve where the patient's palm and wrist meet). If the patient feels discomfort, such as numbness or tingling, shooting into the palm and fingers, the patient has Tinel's sign — positive evidence of carpal tunnel syndrome.

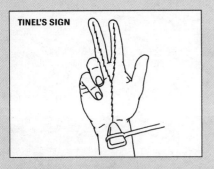

TINEL'S SIGN

Phalen's sign
Flex the patient's wrist for about 30 seconds. If the patient feels subsequent pain or numbness in the hands or fingers, the patient has Phalen's sign — positive evidence of carpal tunnel syndrome.

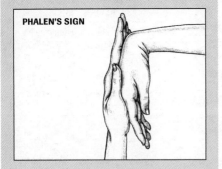

PHALEN'S SIGN

initially impairing sensory transmission to the thumb, index finger, second finger, and inner aspect of the third finger.

Assessment findings
The patient with carpal tunnel syndrome usually complains of weakness, pain, burning, numbness, or tingling in the hands affecting the thumb, forefinger, middle finger, and half of the fourth finger. The patient is unable to clench her hand into a fist, her nails may be atrophic, and her skin may be dry and shiny.

Because of vasodilation and venous stasis, symptoms are typically worse at night and in the morning. The pain may spread to the forearm and, in severe cases, as far as the shoulder or neck. The patient can usually relieve such pain by shaking or rubbing his hands vigorously or dangling her arms at her side.

Diagnosis
○ Physical examination reveals decreased sensation to light touch or pinpricks in the affected fingers.
○ Thenar muscle atrophy occurs in about one-half of all cases of carpal tunnel syndrome, but it's usually a late sign.
○ Tinel's sign reveals tingling over the median nerve on light percussion.
○ Phalen's wrist-flexion test (holding the forearms vertically and allowing both hands to drop into complete flexion at the wrists for 1 minute) reproduces symptoms of carpal tunnel syndrome. (See *Two signs of carpal tunnel syndrome*.)
○ A compression test supports the diagnosis of carpal tunnel syndrome when a blood pressure cuff inflated above systolic pressure on the forearm for 1 to 2 minutes elicits pain and paresthesia along the distribution of the median nerve.
○ Electromyography and nerve conduction velocity detect a median nerve motor conduction delay of more than 5 milliseconds.

Complications
○ Compression
○ Neural ischemia

○ Permanent nerve damage with loss of movement and sensation
○ Tendon inflammation

Treatment
○ Conservative treatment should be tried first; the patient's wrist may be splinted in neutral extension for 1 to 2 weeks in order to let the hand rest.
○ Nonsteroidal anti-inflammatory drugs usually provide symptomatic relief.
○ Hydrocortisone and lidocaine injection of the carpal tunnel may provide significant but temporary relief.
○ If a definite link has been established between the patient's occupation and the development of repetitive stress injury, the patient should make ergonomic modifications to the work environment or may have to seek other work.
○ Effective treatment may also require correction of an underlying disorder.
○ Surgical decompression of the nerve by resecting the entire transverse carpal tunnel ligament or by using endoscopic surgical techniques is used when conservative treatment fails.
○ Neurolysis (freeing of the nerve fibers) may also be necessary.

 COLLABORATIVE MANAGEMENT
Care of the patient with carpal tunnel syndrome involves several members of the interdisciplinary team. The nurse explains the condition and provides postoperative care. The physical therapist teaches the patient how to perform exercises for the elbow and shoulder following surgery. The occupational therapist teaches the patient how to modify work habits to reduce symptoms.

Special considerations
○ Administer mild analgesics as needed.
○ If the patient's dominant hand has been impaired, she may need help with eating and bathing.
○ After surgery, monitor the patient's vital signs, and regularly check the color, sensation, and motion of the affected hand.

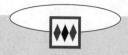

KEY TEACHING POINTS

Teaching about carpal tunnel syndrome

Remember these key points when teaching your patient and her family about carpal tunnel syndrome:
• Teach the patient about the disease process and its treatments
• Explain the relationship between repetitive wrist activity and carpal tunnel syndrome.
• Discuss modifying work habits and the workplace to reduce symptoms.
• Demonstrate strengthening and stretching exercises for the wrist, hand, and fingers.
• Explain the prescribed medications, their indications, dosages, and adverse effects.
• Explain the surgical procedure and postoperative care, if indicated.
• Provide discharge instructions following surgery on incision care and signs and symptoms to report to the physician.
• Teach the patient how to apply a splint and to perform gentle range-of-motion exercises.

○ Suggest occupational counseling for the patient who has to change jobs because of repetitive stress injury.
○ Provide patient education. (See *Teaching about carpal tunnel syndrome*.)

Applicable patient-teaching aids
○ Exercises for patients with carpal tunnel syndrome
○ Relieving symptoms of carpal tunnel syndrome *

○ Cataract

The most common cause of correctable vision loss, a cataract is a gradually developing opacity of the lens or lens capsule of the eye. Cataracts commonly occur bilaterally, with each progressing independently. Exceptions are traumatic cataracts, which are usually unilateral, and congenital cataracts, which may remain stationary. The prognosis is generally good; surgery improves vision in 95% of affected people. (See *Comparing methods of cataract removal.*) Cataracts occur as part of the aging process and are most prevalent in people older than age 70.

Causes

Cataracts have various causes. Senile cataracts develop in elderly patients, probably because of degenerative changes in the chemical state of lens proteins.

Congenital cataracts occur in neonates as genetic defects or as a sequela of maternal rubella during the first trimester. The neonate acquires cataracts through autosomal dominant inheritance, which will occur even if only one parent passes it along. Fifty percent of children in such families are affected.

Traumatic cataracts develop after a foreign body injures the lens with sufficient force to allow aqueous or vitreous humor to enter the lens capsule. Trauma may also dislocate the lens. Complicated cataracts develop as secondary effects in patients with uveitis, glaucoma, or retinitis pigmentosa, or in the course of a systemic disease, such as diabetes, hypoparathyroidism, or atopic dermatitis. They can also result from exposure to ionizing radiation or infrared rays.

Toxic cataracts result from drug or chemical toxicity with prednisone, ergot alkaloids, dinitrophenol, naphthalene, phenothiazine, or pilocarpine or from extended exposure to ultraviolet rays.

Pathophysiology

Pathophysiology may vary with each form of cataract. Senile cataracts show evidence of protein aggregation, oxidative injury, and increased pigmentation in the center of the lens. In traumatic cataracts, phagocytosis of the lens or inflammation may occur when a lens ruptures. The mechanism of a complicated cataract varies with the disease process; for example, in diabetes, increased glucose in the lens causes it to absorb water.

Typically, cataract development goes through four stages:
○ immature—the lens isn't totally opaque
○ mature—the lens is completely opaque and vision loss is significant
○ hypermature—the lens proteins deteriorate, causing peptides to leak through the lens capsule; glaucoma may develop if intraocular fluid outflow is obstructed
○ tumescent—the lens is filled with water; may lead to glaucoma.

Assessment findings

Characteristically, the patient with a cataract experiences painless, gradual blurring and loss of vision. As the cataract progresses, the normally black pupil appears hazy, and when a mature cataract develops, the white lens may be seen through the pupil. Some patients complain of a blinding glare from headlights while driving at night; others complain of poor reading vision, and of an unpleasant glare or poor vision in bright sunlight. The patient with a central opacity may report better vision in dim light than in bright light.

Diagnosis

○ Indirect ophthalmoscopy and slit-lamp examination show a dark area in the normally homogeneous red reflex.
○ Visual acuity test confirms vision loss.

Complications
Cataract complications
○ Blindness
○ Glaucoma

Surgical complications
○ Blindness
○ Glaucoma
○ Hyphema (hemorrhage into the eye's anterior chamber)
○ Infection
○ Loss of vitreous humor
○ Retinal detachment
○ Vitreous-block glaucoma
○ Wound dehiscence from loosening of sutures and flat anterior chamber or iris prolapse into the wound

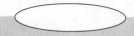

Comparing methods of cataract removal

Cataracts can be removed by intracapsular or extracapsular techniques.

Intracapsular cataract extraction

When performing intracapsular cataract extraction, the surgeon makes a partial incision at the superior limbus arc. He then removes the lens using specially designed forceps or a cryoprobe, which freezes and adheres to the lens to facilitate its removal.

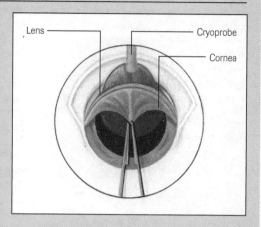

Extracapsular cataract extraction

When performing extracapsular cataract extraction, the surgeon may use irrigation and aspiration or phacoemulsification. If he uses irrigation and aspiration, he makes an incision at the limbus, opens the anterior lens capsule with a cystotome, and exerts pressure from below to express the lens. He then irrigates and suctions the remaining lens cortex.

During phacoemulsification, the surgeon uses an ultrasonic probe to break the lens into minute particles, which are aspirated by the probe.

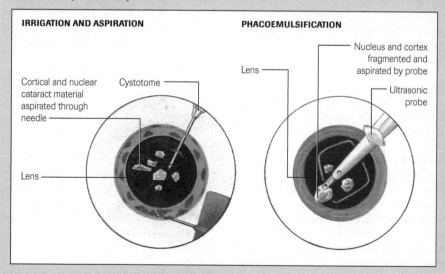

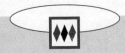

Teaching about cataracts

Remember these key points when teaching your patient and his family about cataracts:

● Teach the patient about the disorder and its treatments.

● Tell the patient what to expect in the postoperative period.

● Urge the patient to protect his eye from accidental injury at night by wearing a plastic or metal shield with perforations; a shield or glasses should be worn for protection during the day.

● Demonstrate how to administer antibiotic ointment or drops.

● Advise the patient to watch for the development of complications, such as a sharp pain in the eye (uncontrolled by analgesics) as a result of hyphema or clouding in the anterior chamber (which may herald an infection), and to report them to the physician immediately.

● Caution the patient about activity restrictions.

● Explain that the majority of patients need either corrective reading glasses or a corrective contact lens, which will be fitted sometime between 4 and 6 weeks after surgery. Tell the patient who hasn't had an intraocular lens implanted that he may be given temporary aphakic cataract glasses.

Treatment

○ Extracapsular cataract extraction removes the anterior lens capsule and cortex, leaving the posterior capsule intact. It's typically performed by using phacoemulsification to fragment the lens with ultrasonic vibrations, then aspirating the pieces. A posterior chamber extraocular lens (IOL) is implanted where the patient's own lens used to be.

○ Intracapsular cataract extraction removes the entire lens within the intact capsule by cryoextraction, in which the moist lens sticks to an extremely cold metal probe for easy and safe extraction. This procedure is rarely performed today. (An IOL may be placed in the anterior or posterior chamber after lens removal; alternatively, a contact lens or aphakic glasses may be used to enhance vision.)

○ Laser surgery may be performed after an extracapsular cataract extraction to restore visual acuity when a secondary membrane forms in the posterior lens capsule that has been left intact.

○ Discission and aspiration may still be used in children with soft cataracts.

○ Contact lenses or lens implantation after surgery improves visual acuity, binocular vision, and depth perception.

COLLABORATIVE MANAGEMENT
Care of the patient with a cataract involves several members of the interdisciplinary team. The ophthalmologist monitors the cataracts and recommends their removal at the appropriate time. A low-vision specialist can provide assistive devices to the patient with reduced vision to allow him to work and perform activities of daily living. The nurse provides presurgical and postsurgical education.

Special considerations

○ Discuss safety measures and interventions that may be useful to help the patient with daily activities before cataract surgery and for those patients with reduced vision who choose not to have surgery. Interventions include removing throw rugs, keeping furniture in place (instruct family members not to move furniture without informing the patient), and using contrasting colors on stair treads.

○ Perform routine postoperative care.

○ Apply an eye shield or eye patch postoperatively, as ordered.

○ Because the patient will be discharged after he recovers from anesthesia, remind him to return for a checkup the next day, and warn him to avoid activities that increase intraocular pressure such as straining.

○ Provide patient education. (See *Teaching about cataracts.*)

Applicable patient-teaching aids

○ Administering eyedrops

○ Removing and applying an eye shield *

◯ Celiac disease

Celiac disease (also known as *idiopathic steatorrhea, nontropical sprue, gluten enteropathy,* and *celiac sprue*) is characterized by poor food absorption and intolerance of gluten, a protein in wheat and wheat products. Malabsorption in the small bowel results from atrophy of the villi and a decrease in the activity and amount of enzymes in the surface epithelium. The prognosis is good with treatment (eliminating gluten from the patient's diet), but residual bowel changes may persist in adults.

Celiac disease affects twice as many females as males and occurs more commonly among relatives, especially siblings. This disease primarily affects whites and those of European ancestry. In the United States, it affects 1 out of every 4,700 persons.

Causes

Celiac disease results from environmental factors and a genetic predisposition, but the exact mechanism is unknown. A strong association exists between the disease and two human leukocyte antigen haplotypes, DR3 and DQw2. It may also be autoimmune in nature.

Many diseases and conditions are associated with celiac disease, including anemia, lactose intolerance, skin disorders such as dermatitis herpetiformis (a burning, itching, blistering rash), type 1 diabetes mellitus, thyroid disease, Down syndrome, unexplained infertility or miscarriage, osteoporosis or osteopenia, and autoimmune disorders, such as rheumatoid arthritis and systemic lupus erythematosus.

Pathophysiology

In celiac disease, an intramucosal enzyme defect produces an inability to digest gluten. Ingestion of gluten causes injury to the villi in the upper small intestine, leading to a decreased surface area. Atrophy of intestinal villi leads to malabsorption of fat, carbohydrates, and protein as well as loss of calories, fat-soluble vitamins (A, D, and K), calcium, and essential minerals and electrolytes. Hematologic effects include normochromic, hypochromic, or macrocytic anemia due to poor absorption

of folate, iron, and vitamin B_{12} and to hypoprothrombinemia from jejunal loss of vitamin K.

Celiac disease also results in inflammatory enteritis, leading to osmotic diarrhea and secretory diarrhea. Resulting tissue toxicity produces rapid cell turnover, increases epithelial lymphocytes, and damages surface epithelium of the small bowel.

Assessment findings

Celiac disease produces clinical effects on many body systems:

◯ GI signs and symptoms include diarrhea, steatorrhea, abdominal distention due to flatulence, stomach cramps, weakness, anorexia and, occasionally, increased appetite without weight gain.

◯ Musculoskeletal signs and symptoms include osteomalacia, osteoporosis, tetany, and bone pain (especially in the lower back, rib cage, and pelvis).

◯ Neurologic signs and symptoms include peripheral neuropathy, seizures, or paresthesia.

◯ Dermatologic signs and symptoms include dry skin, eczema, psoriasis, dermatitis herpetiformis, and acne rosacea; also, generalized fine, sparse, prematurely gray hair; brittle nails; and localized hyperpigmentation on the face, lips, or mucosa (may result from deficiency of sulfur-containing amino acids).

◯ Endocrine signs and symptoms include amenorrhea, hypometabolism and, possibly, with severe malabsorption, adrenocortical insufficiency.

◯ Psychosocial signs and symptoms include mood changes and irritability.

Diagnosis

◯ Esophagogastroduodenoscopy revealing histologic changes seen on small-bowel biopsy specimens—a mosaic pattern of alternating flat and bumpy areas on the bowel surface and an irregular, blunt, and disorganized network of blood vessels — confirms the diagnosis.

◯ Alkaline phosphatase level may be elevated, indicating bone loss.

◯ Cholesterol and albumin levels are low, possibly reflecting malabsorption and malnutrition.

◯ Liver enzymes may be mildly elevated and abnormal blood clotting may also be noted.

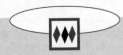

KEY TEACHING POINTS

Teaching about celiac disease

Remember these key points when teaching your patient and his family about celiac disease:

• Explain the disease process and its treatments.

• Explain the necessity of a gluten-free diet to the patient (and to his parents, if the patient is a child); suggest substituting corn or rice for wheat, barley, rye, and oats as well as foods made from these grains, such as breads and baked goods.

• Because many foods contain hidden sources of gluten, teach the patient to read food labels carefully.

• Discuss complications (such as dehydration, electrolyte imbalances, and bleeding) and signs and symptoms that require immediate medical attention.

• Review medications the patient is taking, as well as their dosages, adverse effects, and special considerations.

• Discuss safety measures to prevent fractures and bleeding.

• Advise the patient to contact the Gluten Intolerance Group or the Celiac Disease Foundation for information and support.

○ Complete blood count may reveal normochromic, hypochromic, or macrocytic anemia due to poor absorption of folate, iron, and vitamin B_{12}.

○ Antibody blood tests useful in screening for celiac disease include antiendomysial antibody (immunoglobulin [Ig] A), antitransglutaminase (IgA), antigliadin (IgA and IgG), and total serum IgA. Combined, these antibodies provide a sensitive and specific indicator for the presence of celiac disease.

Complications

○ Anemia
○ Bleeding disorders
○ Bone pain
○ Compression fractures (adults)
○ Malnutrition
○ Osteomalacia
○ Osteoporosis
○ Rickets (children)
○ Small bowel ulcers (may perforate or bleed)
○ Tetany
○ Vitamin D deficiency

Treatment

○ Treatment requires the elimination of gluten from the patient's diet for life.

○ Dietary supplements may include iron, vitamin B_{12}, and folic acid.

○ Electrolyte replacement (by I.V. infusion, if necessary) may be necessary to reverse electrolyte imbalance.

○ I.V. fluid replacement corrects dehydration.

○ Corticosteroids treat accompanying adrenal insufficiency.

○ Vitamin K is administered for hypoprothrombinemia.

COLLABORATIVE MANAGEMENT
Care of the patient with celiac disease involves several members of the interdisciplinary team. The dietitian plays a key role in making dietary recommendations, providing dietary information, and monitoring nutritional status and weight loss. The nurse provides education about nutrition, fluid replacement, and skin care. Physical and occupational therapy assist in reducing activity tolerance in the patient who's weakened.

Special considerations

○ Provide a diet free from wheat, barley, rye, and oats as well as foods made from these grains, such as breads and baked goods. Depending on individual tolerance, the diet initially consists of proteins and gradually expands to include other foods. In the early stages, offer small, frequent meals to counteract anorexia.

○ Assess the patient's acceptance and understanding of the disease, and encourage regular reevaluation.

○ Observe the patient's nutritional status and progress by daily calorie counts and weight checks.

○ Evaluate the patient's tolerance to new foods.

○ Assess the patient's fluid status: record intake, urine output, and number of stools (may exceed 10 per day). Watch for signs of dehydration, such as dry skin and mucous membranes and poor skin turgor.

○ Check serum electrolyte levels. Watch for signs of hypokalemia (weakness, lethargy, rapid pulse, nausea, and diarrhea) and low calcium levels (impaired blood clotting, muscle twitching, and tetany).

○ Monitor prothrombin time, hemoglobin level, and hematocrit. Protect the patient from bleeding and bruising.

○ Use the Z-track method to give iron I.M. If the patient can tolerate oral iron, give it between meals, when absorption is best. Dilute oral iron preparations, and give them through a straw to prevent staining teeth.

○ Protect the patient with osteomalacia from injury by assisting with ambulation, as necessary.

○ Provide patient education. (See *Teaching about celiac disease.*)

Applicable patient-teaching aids
○ Choosing iron-rich foods *

◯ Cerebral palsy

The most common cause of crippling in children, cerebral palsy (CP) is a group of neuromuscular disorders resulting from prenatal, perinatal, or postnatal central nervous system damage. Although nonprogressive, these disorders may become more obvious as an affected infant grows older. Three major types of CP occur — spastic, athetoid, and ataxic — sometimes in mixed forms. Spastic CP is the most common type of CP, affecting about 50% of CP patients. Athetoid CP affects about 20% of CP patients, ataxic CP accounts for another 10% of these patients, and the remaining 20% of patients have mixed CP, with a combination of symptoms.

Motor impairment may be minimal (sometimes apparent only during physical activities such as running) or severely disabling. Associated defects, such as seizures, speech disor-

ders, and mental retardation, are common. The prognosis varies; in cases of mild impairment, proper treatment may make a near-normal life possible.

CP is slightly more common in males than in females. For every 1,000 births, 2 to 4 neonates are affected. Incidence is slightly higher in premature neonates (anoxia plays the greatest role in contributing to CP) and in neonates who are small for their gestational age.

Causes
See *Causes of cerebral palsy,* for a description of the causes of CP.

Pathophysiology
In the early stages of brain development, a lesion or abnormality causes structural and functional defects that in turn cause impaired motor

---

Causes of cerebral palsy

Conditions that result in cerebral anoxia, hemorrhage, or other damage are probably responsible for cerebral palsy (CP).

● *Prenatal conditions that may increase risk of CP:* maternal infection (especially rubella), maternal drug ingestion, radiation, anoxia, toxemia, maternal diabetes, abnormal placental attachment, malnutrition, and isoimmunization

● *Perinatal and birth difficulties that increase the risk of CP:* forceps delivery, breech presentation, placenta previa, abruptio placentae, metabolic or electrolyte disturbances, abnormal maternal vital signs from general or spinal anesthetic, prolapsed cord with delay in delivery of head, premature birth, prolonged or unusually rapid labor, and multiple birth (especially infants born last in a multiple birth)

● *Infection or trauma during infancy:* poisoning, severe kernicterus resulting from erythroblastosis fetalis, brain infection, head trauma, prolonged anoxia, brain tumor, cerebral circulatory anomalies causing blood vessel rupture, and systemic disease resulting in cerebral thrombosis or embolus.

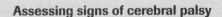

Assessing signs of cerebral palsy

Each type of cerebral palsy (CP) is manifested by specific signs. This chart highlights the major signs and symptoms associated with each type of CP. The manifestations reflect impaired upper motor neuron function and disruption of the normal stretch reflex.

Type of CP	Signs and symptoms
Ataxic CP (due to impairment of the extrapyramidal tract)	• Disturbed balance • Hypoactive reflexes • Incoordination (especially of the arms) • Lack of leg movement during infancy • Muscle weakness • Nystagmus • Sudden or fine movements impossible (due to ataxia) • Tremor • Wide gait as the child begins to walk
Athetoid CP (due to impairment of the extrapyramidal tract)	• Difficulty with speech due to involuntary facial movements • Increasing severity of movements during stress; decreased with relaxation and disappearing entirely during sleep • Involuntary movements usually affecting arms more severely than legs, including: – dystonia – grimacing – sharp jerks – wormlike writhing
Spastic CP (due to impairment of the pyramidal tract [most common type])	• Hyperactive deep tendon reflexes • Increased stretch reflexes • Muscle contraction in response to manipulation • Muscle weakness • Rapid alternating muscle contraction and relaxation • Tendency toward contractures • Typical walking on toes with a scissors gait, crossing one foot in front of the other • Underdevelopment of affected limbs
Mixed CP	• Ataxic and athetoid movements (resulting in severe impairment) • Spasticity and athetoid movements

function or cognition. Even though the defects are present at birth, problems may not be apparent until months later, when the axons have become myelinated and the basal ganglia are mature.

Assessment findings

The patient with cerebral palsy develops signs and symptoms of the disorder shortly after birth, including excessive lethargy or irritability, high-pitched cry, poor head control, and a weak sucking reflex. Other physical findings include delayed motor development; abnormal head circumference, typically smaller than normal for age; abnormal postures, such as leg straightening with toes down when the child is placed on his back and holding the head higher than normal when prone due to arching of back; abnormal reflexes; and abnormal muscle tone. (See *Assessing signs of cerebral palsy.*)

Diagnosis

○ Magnetic resonance imaging and computed tomography scan can reveal structural or congenital abnormalities.

○ Developmental screening reveals a delay in achieving milestones.

○ Vision and hearing screening demonstrates a degree of impairment.

○ EEG identifies the source of seizure activity.

Complications

○ Contractures

○ Dental problems

○ Language and perceptual problems

○ Malnutrition

○ Mental retardation

○ Muscle atrophy

○ Respiratory difficulties, including aspiration from poor gag and swallowing reflexes

○ Seizure disorders

○ Skin breakdown and ulcer formation

○ Speech, hearing, and vision problems

Treatment

○ Braces or splints and special appliances, such as adapted eating utensils and a low toilet seat with arms, help the child with CP perform activities independently.

○ An artificial urinary sphincter may be indicated for the incontinent child who can use the hand controls.

○ Range-of-motion (ROM) exercises minimize contractures.

○ Orthopedic surgery may be indicated to correct contractures. Botulinum toxin has been shown to reduce or delay the need for surgery.

○ Phenytoin, phenobarbital, or another anticonvulsant may be used to control seizures.

○ Muscle relaxants or neurosurgery may be required to decrease spasticity.

COLLABORATIVE MANAGEMENT
CP can't be cured, but proper treatment by an interdisciplinary team can help affected children reach their fullest potential within the limitations set by this disorder. Such treatment requires a comprehensive and cooperative effort involving physicians, nurses, teachers, psychologists, and the child's family. Rehabilitation includes physical, occupational, and speech therapy to maintain or improve functional abilities.

Home care is usually possible. Children with milder forms of CP should attend a regular school; severely afflicted children may need

Teaching about cerebral palsy

Remember these key points when teaching the parents of a child with cerebral palsy:

● Explain the disorder and its treatments.

● Explain all medications, including dosages, adverse effects, and special considerations.

● Discuss how to perform a daily skin inspection and massage.

● Teach the parents how to feed the child to reduce the risk of aspiration and facilitate swallowing.

● Demonstrate correct use of assistive devices.

● Encourage parents to set realistic individual goals.

● Stress the child's need to develop peer relationships; advise the parents against being overprotective.

● Teach the parents how to identify and deal with family stress.

● Refer the parents to supportive community organizations. For more information, tell them to contact United Cerebral Palsy.

special classes. Psychological counseling can help the parents deal with the stress that caring for a child with a chronic illness can create as well as unreasonable guilt about their child's handicap.

Special considerations

○ Speak to the child slowly and distinctly. Encourage him to ask for things he wants. Listen patiently and don't rush him.

○ Plan a high-calorie diet that's adequate to meet the child's high-energy needs.

○ During meals, maintain a quiet, unhurried atmosphere with few distractions. The child should be encouraged to feed himself and may need special utensils and a chair with a solid footrest. Teach him to place food far back in his mouth to facilitate swallowing.

○ Encourage the child to chew food thoroughly, drink through a straw, and suck on lollipops

to develop the muscle control needed to mini-mize drooling.
○ Allow the child to wash and dress indepen-dently, assisting only as needed.
○ Give all care in an unhurried manner; other-wise, muscle spasticity may increase.
○ Encourage the family to participate in the care plan so they can continue it at home.
○ Care for associated hearing or vision distur-bances, as necessary.
○ Give frequent mouth and dental care, as necessary.
○ Reduce muscle spasms that increase postop-erative pain by moving and turning the child carefully after surgery; provide analgesics as needed.
○ After orthopedic surgery, provide cast care.
○ Provide the parents with education and guid-ance. (See *Teaching about cerebral palsy*.)

Applicable patient-teaching aids
○ Avoiding burnout: Aid for the caregiver *
○ Performing active range-of-motion exer-cises *
○ Understanding seizures and your child

⊂⊃ Cervical cancer

One of the most common cancers of the female reproductive system, cervical cancer is classi-fied as either preinvasive or invasive.

Preinvasive carcinoma ranges from minimal cervical dysplasia, in which the lower third of the epithelium contains abnormal cells, to car-cinoma in situ, in which the full thickness of epithelium contains abnormally proliferating cells (also known as *cervical intraepithelial neo-plasia*). Preinvasive carcinoma is curable 75% to 90% of the time with early detection and proper treatment. If untreated (and depending on the form in which it appears), it may progress to in-vasive cervical cancer.

In invasive carcinoma, cancer cells pene-trate the basement membrane and can spread directly to contiguous pelvic structures or dis-seminate to distant sites by lymphatic routes.

In almost all cases of cervical cancer (95%), the histologic type is squamous cell carcinoma, which varies from well-differentiated cells to highly anaplastic spindle cells. Only 5% are

adenocarcinomas. Usually, invasive carcinoma occurs between ages 30 and 50; it occurs rarely in patients younger than age 20.

Causes
Although the cause of cervical cancer is un-known, several predisposing factors have been related to its development: frequent intercourse at a young age (younger than age 16), multiple sexual partners, multiple pregnancies, exposure to sexually transmitted diseases (particularly genital human papillomavirus), and smoking.

Pathophysiology
Preinvasive cervical carcinoma produces mini-mal cervical dysplasia in the lower third of ep-ithelium. Eventually, abnormal cells involve all of the epithelium and progress to the stromal tissue of the cervix. The cancer cells spread di-rectly to nearby structures, such as the rectum, pelvic wall, vagina, and bladder. Metastasis oc-curs through the lymph system to the lungs, mediastinal and supraclavicular nodes, bone, and liver.

Assessment findings
Preinvasive cervical carcinoma produces no symptoms or other clinically apparent changes. Early invasive cervical carcinoma causes ab-normal vaginal bleeding, persistent vaginal discharge, and postcoital pain and bleeding. Advanced invasive cervical carcinoma pro-duces pelvic pain, vaginal leakage of urine and feces from a fistula, anorexia, weight loss, and anemia.

Diagnosis
○ Cytologic examination (Papanicolaou [Pap] smear) can detect cervical cancer before clini-cal evidence appears.
○ Colposcopy, performed following abnormal cervical cytology, detects the presence and ex-tent of preclinical lesions requiring biopsy and histologic examination.
○ Staining may identify areas for biopsy when the smear shows abnormal cells but there's no obvious lesion.
○ Lymphangiography, cystography, and scans can detect metastasis. (See *Staging cervical can-cer*.)

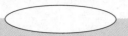

Staging cervical cancer

Cervical cancer treatment decisions depend on accurate staging. The International Federation of Gynecology and Obstetrics defines cervical cancer stages as follows.

Stage 0
Carcinoma in situ, intraepithelial carcinoma

Stage I
Cancer confined to the cervix (extension to the corpus should be disregarded); T1, N0, M0
STAGE IA — preclinical malignant lesions of the cervix (diagnosed only microscopically); T1, N0, M0
STAGE IA1 — minimal microscopically evident stromal invasion
STAGE IA2 — lesions detected microscopically, measuring 5 mm or less from the base of the epithelium, either surface or glandular, from which it originates; lesion width shouldn't exceed 7 mm
STAGE IB — lesions measuring more than 5 mm deep and 7 mm wide, whether seen clinically or not (preformed space involvement shouldn't alter the staging but should be recorded for future treatment decisions); T1b, N0, M0

Stage II
Extension beyond the cervix but not to the pelvic wall; the cancer involves the vagina but hasn't spread to the lower third; T2, N0, M0

STAGE IIA — no obvious parametrial involvement
STAGE IIB — obvious parametrial involvement

Stage III
Extension to the pelvic wall; on rectal examination, no cancer-free space exists between the tumor and the pelvic wall; the tumor involves the lower third of the vagina; this includes all cases with hydronephrosis or nonfunctioning kidney; T3, N0, M0
STAGE IIIA — no extension to the pelvic wall
STAGE IIIB — extension to the pelvic wall and hydronephrosis, nonfunctioning kidney, or both

Stage IV
Extension beyond the true pelvis or involvement of the bladder or the rectal mucosa
STAGE IVA — spread to adjacent organs
STAGE IVB — spread to distant organs

Complications
○ Bowel obstruction
○ Cystitis
○ Distant metastases
○ Proctitis
○ Renal failure
○ Ureterovaginal or vesicovaginal fistula
○ Vaginal stenosis

Treatment
○ Total excisional biopsy, cryosurgery, laser destruction, conization (and frequent Pap smear follow-up) or, rarely, hysterectomy may be performed to treat preinvasive cervical cancer.
○ Radical hysterectomy and radiation therapy (internal, external, or both) may be used to treat invasive squamous cell cancer.

○ Chemotherapy may be used alone or in combination with radiation therapy in treating cervical cancer. Cisplatin and fluorouracil are the agents used.

 COLLABORATIVE MANAGEMENT
Care of the patient with cervical cancer involves several members of the interdisciplinary team. The nurse educates the patient about the disease process, treatments, and self-care following surgery, radiation therapy, or chemotherapy. The enterostomal therapist provides education about stoma care for the patient who has had radical surgery. A therapist can help with such issues as relationships and sexuality. The physician and oncologist recommend and carry out the treatment regimen, assisted by the surgeon and radiation oncologist, as needed.

Teaching about cervical cancer

Remember these key points when teaching your patient and her family about cervical cancer:

● Explain the disease and its predisposing factors.

● Explain all procedures (such as excisional biopsy, cryosurgery, laser therapy or surgery) and aftercare.

● Tell the patient who has had excisional biopsy, cryosurgery, or laser therapy to expect a discharge or spotting for about 1 week after these procedures. Advise her not to douche, use tampons, or engage in sexual intercourse during this time.

● Tell the patient to watch for and report signs of infection following any procedures or surgery.

● Stress the need for a follow-up Papanicolaou smear and a pelvic examination within 3 to 4 months after these procedures and periodically thereafter.

● Advise the patient receiving radiation therapy or chemotherapy to avoid people who are sick.

● Tell the patient that the internal radiation applicator will be inserted in the operating room under general anesthesia and that the radioactive material (such as radium or cesium) will be loaded into it when she's back in her room.

● Explain to the patient that she'll have less contact with staff and visitors while the radiation implant is in place and that she'll require a private room.

● Teach the patient who has received radiation therapy to use a vaginal dilator to prevent vaginal stenosis and to facilitate vaginal examinations and sexual intercourse.

● Reassure the patient that this disease and its treatment shouldn't radically alter her lifestyle or prohibit sexual intimacy.

Special considerations

○ If you assist with a biopsy, cryosurgery, or laser therapy, drape and prepare the patient as for a routine Pap smear and pelvic examination and explain the procedure to her.

○ Provide postoperative care if the patient has had a hysterectomy.

○ Watch for and immediately report signs or symptoms of complications, such as bleeding, abdominal distention, severe pain, and breathing difficulties.

○ Administer analgesics, prophylactic antibiotics, and subcutaneous heparin, as ordered.

○ Encourage deep-breathing and coughing exercises.

For radiation therapy:

○ Find out if the patient is to have internal or external therapy, or both. Usually, internal radiation therapy is the first procedure.

○ Prepare the patient for the internal radiation procedure. Internal radiation requires a 2- to 3-day hospital stay, bowel preparation, a povidone-iodine vaginal douche, a clear liquid diet, insertion of an indwelling urinary catheter, and nothing by mouth the night before the implantation.

○ Remember that safety precautions—time, distance, and shielding—begin as soon as the radioactive source is in place. Organize the time you spend with the patient to minimize your exposure to radiation.

○ Encourage the patient to lie flat and limit movement while the radiation implant is in place. If she prefers, elevate the head of the bed slightly.

○ Check vital signs every 4 hours; watch for skin reaction, vaginal bleeding, abdominal discomfort, or evidence of dehydration.

○ Make sure the patient can reach everything she needs without stretching or straining.

○ If ordered, administer a tranquilizer to help the patient relax and remain still.

○ Inform visitors of safety precautions, and hang a sign listing these precautions on the patient's door.

○ Provide patient education. (See *Teaching about cervical cancer.*)

Applicable patient-teaching aids

○ Learning about an internal radiation implant
○ Preparing for a pelvic exam
○ Understanding conization

⟳ Cholelithiasis, chronic

Cholelithiasis, stones or calculi (gallstones) in the gallbladder, results from changes in bile components. Cholelithiasis is the fifth leading cause of hospitalization among adults and accounts for 90% of all gallbladder and duct diseases.

Cholelithiasis is a common health problem, affecting about 1 out of 1,000 people. The prognosis is usually good with treatment unless infection occurs, in which case the prognosis depends on the disease's severity and response to antibiotics.

One out of every 10 patients with gallstones develops choledocholithiasis, or gallstones in the common bile duct (sometimes called *common duct stones*). This occurs when stones passed out of the gallbladder lodge in the hepatic and common bile ducts and obstruct the flow of bile into the duodenum. Prognosis is good unless infection occurs.

In most cases, gallbladder and bile duct diseases occur in people who are older than age 40, with prevalence greater in women and Native Americans.

Causes

Cholelithiasis results from changes in bile components. They arise during periods of sluggishness in the gallbladder due to pregnancy, hormonal contraceptives, diabetes mellitus, celiac disease, cirrhosis of the liver, and pancreatitis.

Pathophysiology

The presence of stones or calculi in the gallbladder results from changes in bile components. Gallstones are made of cholesterol, calcium bilirubinate, or a mixture of cholesterol and bilirubin pigment. (See *Understanding gallstone formation,* page 94.)

Assessment findings

Chronic cholelithiasis may possibly produce no symptoms. However, the patient may complain of:

○ pain beginning in the right upper quadrant, which may radiate to the back, between the shoulders, or to the front of the chest (may be so severe that the patient seeks emergency department care)
○ pain following meals rich in fats
○ pain at night that suddenly awakens the patient.

Other possible findings include recurring fat intolerance, biliary colic, belching, flatulence, indigestion, diaphoresis, nausea, vomiting, chills, low-grade fever, jaundice (if a stone obstructs the common bile duct), and clay-colored stools (with choledocholithiasis)

Diagnosis

○ Ultrasonography is the test of choice to detect gallstones.
○ Abdominal computed tomography scan or ultrasound reflects stones in the gallbladder.
○ Percutaneous transhepatic cholangiography, done under fluoroscopic control, distinguishes between gallbladder or bile duct disease and cancer of the pancreatic head in patients with jaundice.
○ Endoscopic retrograde cholangiopancreatography (ERCP) visualizes the biliary tree after insertion of an endoscope down the esophagus into the duodenum, cannulation of the common bile and pancreatic ducts, and injection of contrast medium.
○ HIDA scan of the gallbladder detects obstruction of the cystic duct.
○ Oral cholecystography shows stones in the gallbladder and biliary duct obstruction.
○ Total bilirubin, urine bilirubin, and alkaline phosphatase levels support the diagnosis of gallstones when they're elevated.
○ White blood cell count is slightly elevated during a cholecystitis attack.
○ Elevated serum amylase levels suggest acute pancreatitis rather than gallbladder disease as the cause of abdominal pain.

Complications

○ Cholangitis
○ Cholecystitis
○ Choledocholithiasis
○ Gallstone ileus
○ Peritonitis

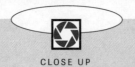

CLOSE UP

Understanding gallstone formation

Abnormal metabolism of cholesterol and bile salts plays an important role in gallstone formation. The liver makes bile continuously. The gall bladder concentrates and stores it until the duodenum signals it needs it to help digest fat. Changes in the composition of bile may allow gallstones to form. Changes to the absorptive ability of the gallbladder lining may also contribute to gallstone formation.

Too much cholesterol

Certain conditions, such as age, obesity, and estrogen imbalance, cause the liver to secrete bile that's abnormally high in cholesterol or lacking the proper concentration of bile salts.

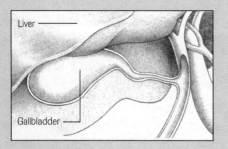

Liver

Gallbladder

Inside the gallbladder

When the gallbladder concentrates this bile, inflammation may occur. Excessive reabsorption of water and bile salts makes the bile less soluble. Cholesterol, calcium, and bilirubin precipitate into gallstones.

Fat entering the duodenum causes the intestinal mucosa to secrete the hormone cholecystokinin, which stimulates the gallbladder to contract and empty. If a stone lodges in the cystic duct, the gallbladder contracts but can't empty.

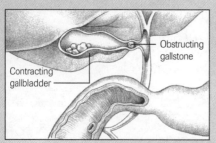

Obstructing gallstone

Contracting gallbladder

Jaundice, irritation, inflammation

If a stone lodges in the common bile duct, the bile can't flow into the duodenum. Bilirubin is absorbed into the blood and causes jaundice.

Biliary narrowing and swelling of the tissue around the stone can also cause irritation and inflammation of the common bile duct.

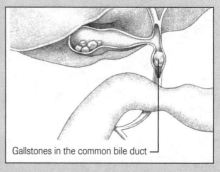

Gallstones in the common bile duct

Up the biliary tree

Inflammation can progress up the biliary tree into any of the bile ducts. This causes scar tissue, fluid accumulation, cirrhosis, portal hypertension, and bleeding.

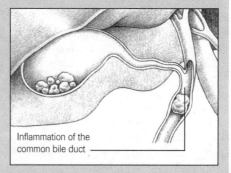

Inflammation of the common bile duct

Treatment
○ Surgery is the treatment of choice and may include open or laparoscopic cholecystectomy, cholecystectomy with operative cholangiography and, possibly, exploration of the common bile duct.

○ Electrohydraulic shock wave lithotripsy can be used to fragment gallstones if they're few in number; it may be used with ursodeoxycholic acid to improve dissolution.

○ Other treatments include a low-fat diet to prevent attacks and vitamin K for itching, jaundice, and bleeding tendencies due to vitamin K deficiency.

○ A nonsurgical treatment for choledocholithiasis involves placement of a catheter through the percutaneous transhepatic cholangiographic route.

○ Chenodeoxycholic acid, which dissolves radiolucent stones, provides an alternative for patients who are poor surgical risks or who refuse surgery.

 COLLABORATIVE MANAGEMENT
Care of the patient with chronic cholelithiasis involves several members of the interdisciplinary team. The physician or nurse practitioner monitors the patient's symptoms and evaluates medical interventions. When pain becomes more severe or frequent, the physician or nurse practitioner makes a referral to a surgeon for possible cholecystectomy. The nurse provides ongoing education and symptom management. A dietitian recommends an appropriate diet and, possibly, a weight-loss program.

Special considerations
○ Provide postoperative care to the patient who has had surgery.

○ Monitor and record intake and output, including T-tube drainage.

○ Evaluate the location, duration, and character of any pain. Administer adequate medication to relieve pain, especially before such activities as deep breathing and ambulation, which increase pain.

○ After surgery, monitor the patient's vital signs for signs of bleeding, infection, or atelectasis; administer analgesics as ordered.

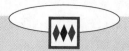

KEY TEACHING POINTS

Teaching about chronic cholelithiasis

Remember these key points when teaching your patient and his family about chronic cholelithiasis:

● Explain the disease process and its treatments.

● If the patient is having surgery, tell him what to expect in the preoperative and postoperative periods.

● Teach the patient who will be discharged with a T tube how to perform dressing changes and routine skin care.

● At discharge, advise the patient who has had surgery against heavy lifting or straining for 6 weeks.

● Discuss signs and symptoms of biliary colic, such as pain, belching, and nausea.

● Instruct the patient about cholelithiasis and other complications that require medical attention.

● Explain that food restrictions are unnecessary unless the patient has an intolerance to a specific food or some underlying condition (such as diabetes, atherosclerosis, or obesity) that requires such restriction.

● Teach about medications the patient will be taking, including their dosages, adverse effects, and special considerations.

● Reinforce the importance of follow-up care to detect recurrent gallstones.

○ Provide the patient with a low-fat diet, if fatty foods trigger an attack. (This is especially important for patients with chronic disease or those who don't plan on having surgery.)

○ Provide patient education. (See *Teaching about chronic cholelithiasis.*)

Applicable patient-teaching aids
○ Caring for your T-tube
○ Preparing for ERCP *
○ Treating and preventing respiratory tract infections *

Chronic fatigue syndrome

Sometimes called *chronic Epstein-Barr virus* or *myalgic encephalomyelitis,* chronic fatigue syndrome (CFS) is typically marked by debilitating fatigue, neurologic abnormalities, and persistent symptoms that suggest chronic mononucleosis. It may develop within a few hours and can last for 6 months or more. It commonly occurs in adults younger than age 45, primarily in females.

Causes

The cause of CFS is unknown, but researchers suspect that it may be found in human herpes virus-6 or in other herpesviruses, enteroviruses, or retroviruses. Recent studies have shown that inflammation of nervous system pathways, acting as an immune or autoimmune response, may play a role as well. CFS may also be associated with a reaction to viral illness that's complicated by dysfunctional immune response and by other factors that may include gender, age, genetic disposition, prior illness, stress, and environment.

Pathophysiology

CFS is a condition characterized by an abnormal immune response and hormonal alterations as a result of infectious agents or environmental factors. It may be the result of an autoimmune response producing inflammation of the nervous system. Autoantibodies, immune complexes, and abnormal immunoglobulins have been noted in some patients with CSF. This disorder may also follow a viral infection that's complicated by a dysfunctional immune system. In the majority of patients, however, no disease process has been identified to cause CFS.

Assessment findings

The characteristic symptom of CFS is prolonged, typically overwhelming fatigue that isn't relieved by rest and is severe enough to restrict activities of daily living by at least 50%; this fatigue is commonly associated with a varying complex of other symptoms that are similar to those of many infections, including myalgia and cephalgia.

Diagnosis

○ Because the cause and nature of CFS are still unknown, no single test unequivocally confirms its presence. (See *Diagnosing chronic fatigue syndrome.*)

Complications

○ Social and occupational impairment

Treatment

○ There's no known curative treatment for CFS.
○ Symptomatic treatment may involve the use of medications to treat depression, anxiety, pain, discomfort, and fever.
○ Antiviral drugs, such as acyclovir, and selected immunomodulating agents, such as I.V. gamma globulin, Ampligen, and transfer factor, reduce symptoms.

Diagnosing chronic fatigue syndrome

Chronic fatigue syndrome is characterized by:
• new or relapsing fatigue that isn't the result of ongoing exertion or alleviated by rest and reduces occupational, educational, social, or personal activities or efforts
• four or more of the following symptoms, occurring for 6 months or more:
— headaches of a new pattern or severity
— multiple joint pain without redness or swelling
— muscle pain
— nonrefreshing sleep
— postexertional malaise lasting 24 hours or longer
— self-reported impairment in short-term memory
— sore throat
— tender cervical or axillary nodes.

COLLABORATIVE MANAGEMENT
Care of the patient with CFS involves several members of the interdisciplinary team. The nurse educates the patient, assists with self-care, and offers support. The physical therapist helps maintain muscle strength and tone. The dietitian assesses the patient's nutritional status and helps the patient chose a well-balanced diet that's high in vitamins and minerals. The social worker can provide assistance with finances and occupational problems. The therapist can help the patient cope with this debilitating disorder and any psychosocial problems that it creates.

Special considerations
○ Some patients may benefit from avoiding environmental irritants and certain foods.
○ Because patients with CFS may benefit from supportive contact with others who share this disease, refer the patient to the Chronic Fatigue Syndrome Association for information and to local support groups.
○ Patients may also benefit from psychological counseling.
○ Provide patient education. (See *Teaching about chronic fatigue syndrome.*)

Applicable patient-teaching aids
○ Learning about daily food choices
○ Taking your medication correctly

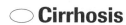 Cirrhosis

Cirrhosis is a chronic hepatic disease characterized by diffuse destruction and fibrotic regeneration of hepatic cells. As necrotic tissue yields to fibrosis, this disease alters liver structure and normal vasculature, impairs blood and lymph flow, and ultimately causes hepatic insufficiency. The prognosis is better in noncirrhotic forms of hepatic fibrosis, which cause minimal hepatic dysfunction and don't destroy liver cells.

Causes
Laënnec's cirrhosis, also known as *portal cirrhosis, nutritional cirrhosis,* and *alcoholic cirrhosis,* is the most common type of cirrhosis. It occurs in 30% to 50% of cirrhotic patients, up to

90% of whom have a history of alcoholism. Liver damage results from malnutrition, especially of dietary protein, and chronic alcohol ingestion. Fibrous tissue forms in portal areas and around central veins.

Biliary cirrhosis results from injury or prolonged obstruction. Postnecrotic *(posthepatitic)* cirrhosis stems from various types of hepatitis. Pigment cirrhosis may result from disorders such as hemochromatosis. Cardiac cirrhosis (rare) refers to liver damage caused by right-sided heart failure. Idiopathic cirrhosis has no known cause. Noncirrhotic fibrosis may result from schistosomiasis or congenital hepatic fibrosis or may be idiopathic.

Pathophysiology
Cirrhosis begins with hepatic scarring or fibrosis. The scar begins as an increase in extracellular matrix components—fibril-forming collagens, proteoglycans, fibronectin, and hyaluronic acid. The site of collagen deposition

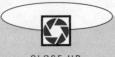

CLOSE UP

Understanding cirrhosis

Cirrhosis is a chronic liver disease characterized by widespread destruction of hepatic cells. The destroyed cells are replaced by fibrotic cells in a process called fibrotic regeneration. As necrotic tissue yields to fibrosis, regenerative nodules form, and the liver parenchyma undergo extensive and irreversible fibrotic changes. The disease alters normal liver structure and vasculature, impairs blood and lymphatic flow and, ultimately, causes hepatic insufficiency.

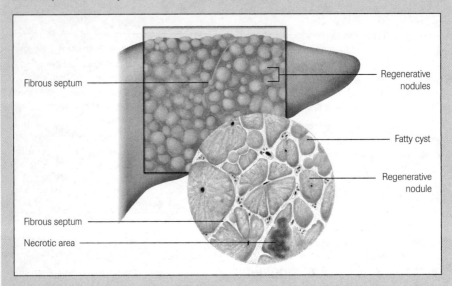

Fibrous septum

Regenerative nodules

Fatty cyst

Regenerative nodule

Fibrous septum

Necrotic area

varies with the cause. Hepatocyte function is eventually impaired as the matrix changes. Fat-storing cells are believed to be the source of the new matrix components. Contraction of these cells may also contribute to disruption of the lobular architecture and obstruction of the flow of blood or bile. Cellular changes producing bands of scar tissue also disrupt the lobular structure. (See *Understanding cirrhosis*.)

Assessment findings

In the early stages of cirrhosis, cirrhosis is marked by vague indications, including:
○ anorexia
○ constipation
○ diarrhea
○ dull abdominal ache

○ indigestion
○ nausea
○ vomiting.

In later stages, signs and symptoms result from hepatic insufficiency and portal hypertension and may include:
○ central nervous system — progressive signs or symptoms of hepatic encephalopathy, such as lethargy, mental changes, slurred speech, asterixis (flapping tremor), peripheral neuritis, paranoia, hallucinations, extreme obtundation, and coma
○ endocrine system — testicular atrophy, menstrual irregularities, gynecomastia, and loss of chest and axillary hair

○ hematologic system—bleeding tendencies (nosebleeds, easy bruising, and bleeding gums) and anemia

○ hepatic system—jaundice, hepatomegaly, ascites, edema of the legs, hepatic encephalopathy, and hepatorenal syndrome

○ respiratory system—pleural effusion and limited thoracic expansion due to abdominal ascites, interfering with efficient gas exchange and leading to hypoxia

○ skin—severe pruritus, extreme dryness, poor tissue turgor, abnormal pigmentation, spider angiomas, palmar erythema, and possibly jaundice

○ miscellaneous—musty breath, enlarged superficial abdominal veins, muscle atrophy, pain in the right upper abdominal quadrant that worsens when the patient sits up or leans forward, palpable liver or spleen, temperature of 101° to 103° F (38.3° to 39.4° C); and bleeding from esophageal varices that results from portal hypertension.

Diagnosis

○ Liver biopsy, the definitive test for cirrhosis, detects destruction and fibrosis of hepatic tissue.

○ Liver scan shows abnormal thickening and a liver mass.

○ Cholecystography and cholangiography visualize the gallbladder and the biliary duct system, respectively.

○ Splenoportal venography visualizes the portal vein system.

○ Percutaneous transhepatic cholangiography differentiates extrahepatic from intrahepatic obstructive jaundice and discloses hepatic pathology and the presence of gallstones.

○ Laboratory findings reveal decreased white blood cell count, hemoglobin level and hematocrit, albumin, serum electrolyte levels (sodium, potassium, chloride, and magnesium), and cholinesterase; elevated levels of globulin, serum ammonia, total bilirubin, alkaline phosphatase, serum aspartate aminotransferase, serum alanine aminotransferase, and lactate dehydrogenase and increased thymol turbidity; prolonged prothrombin and partial thrombo-plastin times; and deficiencies of folic acid, iron, and vitamins A, B_{12}, C, and K.

Complications

○ Ascites

○ Bleeding esophageal varices; acute GI bleeding

○ Coagulopathy

○ Hepatic encephalopathy

○ Jaundice

○ Liver failure

○ Portal hypertension

○ Renal failure

○ Respiratory compromise

Treatment

○ Treatment is designed to remove or alleviate the underlying cause of cirrhosis, if it can be identified.

○ High-calorie and moderate- to high-protein diet may benefit the patient, but the development of hepatic encephalopathy mandates restricted protein intake.

○ Sodium is usually restricted to 200 to 500 mg/day. Fluids are usually restricted to 1 to 1½ qt (1 to 1.5 L)/day.

○ Tube feedings or total parenteral nutrition may be necessary if the patient's condition continues to deteriorate.

○ Supplemental vitamins—A, B complex, D, and K—may be given to compensate for the liver's inability to store them. Vitamin B_{12}, folic acid, and thiamine may be given for deficiency anemia.

○ Rest, moderate exercise, and avoidance of exposure to infections and toxic agents are essential.

○ Vasopressin may be prescribed for esophageal varices.

○ Diuretics may be given for edema; however, they require careful monitoring because fluid and electrolyte imbalance may precipitate hepatic encephalopathy.

○ Lactulose is given to treat encephalopathy.

○ Antibiotics are used to decrease intestinal bacteria and reduce ammonia production, which causes encephalopathy.

○ Blood products or vitamin K may be given to treat coagulopathy.

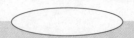

Portal hypertension and esophageal varices

Portal hypertension – elevated pressure in the portal vein – occurs when blood flow meets increased resistance. It's a common result of cirrhosis, but may also stem from mechanical obstruction and occlusion of the hepatic veins (Budd-Chiari syndrome). As portal pressure rises, blood backs up into the spleen and flows through collateral channels to the venous system, bypassing the liver. Consequently, portal hypertension produces splenomegaly with thrombocytopenia, dilated collateral veins (esophageal varices, hemorrhoids, or prominent abdominal veins), and ascites. Nevertheless, in many patients, the first sign of portal hypertension is bleeding from esophageal varices – dilated tortuous veins in the submucosa of the lower esophagus. Bleeding esophageal varices commonly cause massive hematemesis, requiring emergency treatment to control hemorrhage and prevent hypovolemic shock.

Diagnosis and treatment

The following procedures help diagnose and correct esophageal varices.

● Endoscopy identifies the ruptured varix as the bleeding site and excludes other potential sources in the upper GI tract.

● Angiography may aid diagnosis, but is less precise than endoscopy.

● Vasopressin infused into the superior mesenteric artery may temporarily stop bleeding. When angiography is unavailable, vasopressin may be infused by I.V. drip, or diluted with 5% dextrose in water (except in patients with coronary vascular disease), but this route is usually less effective.

● A Minnesota or Sengstaken-Blakemore tube may also help control hemorrhage by applying pressure on the bleeding site. Iced saline lavage through the tube may help control bleeding.

The use of vasopressin or a Minnesota or Sengstaken-Blakemore tube is a temporary measure, especially in the patient with a severely deteriorated liver. Fresh blood and fresh frozen plasma,

if available, are preferred for blood transfusions to replace clotting factors. Treatment with lactulose promotes elimination of old blood from the GI tract, which combats excessive ammonia production and accumulation.

Appropriate surgical bypass procedures include portosystemic anastomosis, splenorenal shunt, and mesocaval shunt. A portacaval or a mesocaval shunt decreases pressure within the liver as well as reduces ascites, plasma loss, and risk of hemorrhage by directing blood from the liver into collateral vessels. Emergency shunts carry a mortality of 25% to 50%. Clinical evidence suggests that the portosystemic bypass doesn't prolong the patient's survival time; however, he will eventually die of hepatic coma rather than of hemorrhage.

Patient care

Care for the patient who has portal hypertension with esophageal varices focuses on careful monitoring for signs and symptoms of hemorrhage and subsequent hypotension, compromised oxygen supply, and altered level of consciousness (LOC).

● Monitor the patient's vital signs, urine output, and central venous pressure to determine fluid volume status.

● Assess the patient's LOC often.

● Provide emotional support and reassurance in the wake of massive GI bleeding, which is always a frightening experience.

● Keep the patient as quiet and comfortable as possible, but remember that tolerance of sedatives and tranquilizers may be decreased because of liver damage.

● Clean the patient's mouth, which may be dry and flecked with dried blood.

● Carefully monitor the patient with a Minnesota or Sengstaken-Blakemore tube in place for persistent bleeding in gastric drainage, signs of asphyxiation from tube displacement, proper inflation of balloons, and correct traction to maintain tube placement.

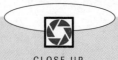

CLOSE UP

Circulation in portal hypertension

As portal vein pressure rises, blood backs up into the spleen and flows through collateral channels to the venous system, bypassing the liver and resulting in esophageal varices.

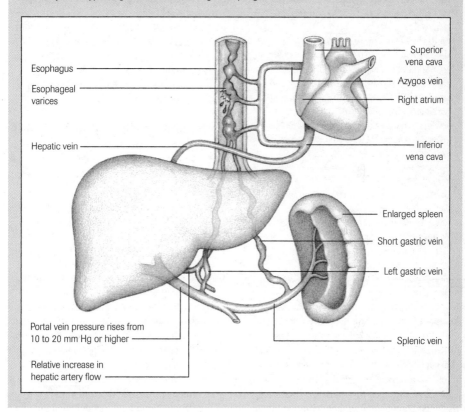

○ Low-protein diets are controversial and are rarely necessary in chronic conditions because of the underlying protein-calorie malnutrition.
○ Paracentesis and infusions of salt-poor albumin, in addition to fluid and salt restrictions, may alleviate ascites.
○ Surgical procedures include treatment of varices by upper endoscopy with banding or sclerosis, splenectomy, esophagogastric resection, and splenorenal or portacaval anastomosis to relieve portal hypertension. (See *Portal*

hypertension and esophageal varices. Also see *Circulation in portal hypertension.*)

 COLLABORATIVE MANAGEMENT
Care of the patient with cirrhosis involves several members of the interdisciplinary team. The nurse provides psychosocial support and teaches the patient to reduce further liver damage and to provide self-care. The physician diagnoses and manages the disorder. The social worker supports the family, refers the patient to support groups

Teaching about cirrhosis

Remember these key points when teaching your patient and his family about cirrhosis:

- Explain the disease process and its treatments.
- Discuss measures to reduce the risk of bleeding, such as warning the patient against taking nonsteroidal anti-inflammatory drugs, straining at stool, and blowing his nose or sneezing too vigorously. Suggest using an electric razor and soft toothbrush.
- Tell the patient that rest and good nutrition will conserve energy and decrease metabolic demands on the liver.
- Urge the patient to eat small, frequent high-calorie meals.
- Stress the need to avoid infections and abstain from alcohol. Refer the patient to Alcoholics Anonymous, if necessary.
- Explain the need to avoid sedatives and acetaminophen.

---

for drug and alcohol abuse, and explores financial concerns. The dietitian assesses nutritional status and devises an appropriate nutritional plan for the patient. The physical therapist may devise an activity program to maintain muscle strength and tone and prevent deconditioning while the occupational therapist teaches energy conservation skills. The drug and alcohol counselor can help the patient abstain from drinking and provide support.

Special considerations

○ Check the patient's skin, gums, stools, and vomitus regularly for bleeding. Apply pressure to injection sites to prevent bleeding.
○ Observe the patient closely for signs of behavioral or personality changes. Report increasing stupor, lethargy, hallucinations, or neuromuscular dysfunction. Awaken him periodically to determine his level of conscious-

ness. Watch for asterixis, a sign of developing hepatic encephalopathy.

○ To assess fluid retention, weigh the patient and measure abdominal girth at least daily, inspect his ankles and sacrum for dependent edema, and accurately record intake and output. Carefully evaluate the patient before, during, and after paracentesis; this drastic loss of fluid may induce shock.

○ To prevent skin breakdown associated with edema and pruritus, tell the patient to avoid using soap when bathing; instead, tell him to use lubricating lotion or moisturizing agents.

○ Provide patient education. (See *Teaching about cirrhosis.*)

Applicable patient-teaching aids

○ Avoiding excessive bleeding *
○ Dietary do's and don'ts for cirrhosis *
○ How to detect — and prevent — infection *
○ Preparing for a liver biopsy
○ Preventing infection with proper hand washing *

◯ Colorectal cancer

Colorectal cancer is the third most common visceral malignant neoplasm. Incidence is equally distributed between men and women. Colorectal malignant tumors are almost always adenocarcinomas. About one-half of these are sessile lesions of the rectosigmoid area; the rest are polypoid lesions.

Colorectal cancer tends to progress slowly and remains localized for a long time. Consequently, it's potentially curable in about 90% of patients if early diagnosis allows resection before nodal involvement. With improved diagnosis, the overall 5-year survival rate is about 60% for adjacent organ or nodal spread, and greater than 90% for early localized disease. (See *Staging colorectal cancer.*)

Causes

The exact cause of colorectal cancer is unknown, but studies showing concentration in areas of higher economic development suggest a relationship to diet (excess saturated animal fat).

The primary risk factor is age, with most cases (more than 90%) diagnosed in people older than age 50. Other factors that magnify the risk of developing colorectal cancer include:
○ familial polyposis (cancer almost always develops by age 50)
○ history of colon polyps
○ history of inflammatory bowel disease
○ other diseases of the digestive tract.

Pathophysiology

The majority of lesions in the colon are moderately differentiated adenocarcinomas. These lesions are slow growing and the patient typically remains asymptomatic for a long time. Lesions in the rectum and sigmoid and descending colon grow circumferentially and constrict the intestinal lumen, whereas those in the ascending colon tend to be large and palpable. (See *How colorectal cancer develops,* page 104.)

Signs and symptoms of colorectal cancer result from local obstruction and, in later stages, from direct extension to adjacent organs (bladder, prostate, ureters, vagina, sacrum) and distant metastasis (usually liver). On the right side of the colon (which absorbs water and electrolytes), early tumor growth causes no signs of obstruction because the tumor tends to grow along the bowel rather than surround the lumen, and the fecal content in this area is normally liquid. On the left side, a tumor causes signs of an obstruction in its early stages because stools in this area are of a formed consistency.

Assessment findings

In the early stages, signs and symptoms are typically vague and depend on the anatomic location and function of the bowel segment containing the tumor. Later signs and symptoms usually include pallor, cachexia, ascites, hepatomegaly, and lymphangiectasis.

On the right side of the colon, early tumor growth causes no signs of obstruction. It may, however, cause black, tarry stools; anemia; and abdominal aching, pressure, or dull cramps. As disease the progresses, the patient develops weakness, fatigue, exertional dyspnea, vertigo and, eventually, diarrhea, obstipation, anorexia,

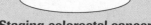

Staging colorectal cancer

Named for pathologist Cuthbert Dukes, the Dukes cancer classification system assigns tumors to four stages. These stages (with substages) reflect the extent of bowel-mucosa and bowel-wall infiltration, lymph node involvement, and metastasis.

Stage A
Malignant cells are confined to the bowel mucosa, and the lymph nodes contain no cancer cells. Treated promptly, about 90% of these patients remain disease-free 5 years later.

Stage B
Malignant cells extend through the bowel mucosa but remain within the bowel wall. The lymph nodes are normal. In substage B2, all bowel wall layers and immediately adjacent structures contain malignant cells, but the lymph nodes remain normal. About 63% of patients with substage B2 survive for 5 or more years. Duke's B is a composite of better (T3, N0, M0) and worse (T4, N0, M0) prognostic groups.

Stage C
Malignant cells extend into the bowel wall and the lymph nodes. In substage C2, malignant cells extend through the entire thickness of the bowel wall and into the lymph nodes. The 5-year survival rate for patients with stage C disease is about 25%. Duke's C is a composite of any T, N1, M0; and any T, N2, M0.

weight loss, vomiting, and other signs or symptoms of intestinal obstruction. In addition, a tumor on the right side may be palpable.

On the left side, a tumor commonly causes rectal bleeding (in many cases ascribed to hemorrhoids), intermittent abdominal fullness or cramping, and rectal pressure. As the disease progresses, the patient develops obstipation, diarrhea, or "ribbon" or pencil-shaped stools and, possibly, pain relief from passage of stool or flatus. At this stage, bleeding from the colon

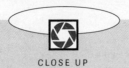

CLOSE UP

How colorectal cancer develops

Most lesions of the large bowel are moderately differentiated adenocarcinomas. These tumors tend to grow slowly and produce no symptoms for long periods. Tumors in the rectum and sigmoid and descending colon grow circumferentially and constrict the intestinal lumen. Tumors in the ascending colon are usually large and palpable.

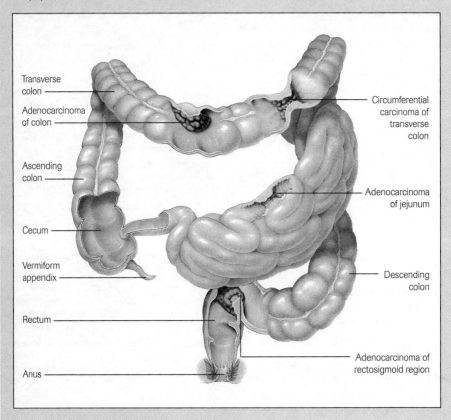

becomes obvious, with dark or bright red blood in the feces and mucus in or on the stools (advanced stage).

With a rectal tumor, the first symptom is a change in bowel habits, in many cases beginning with an urgent need to defecate on arising (morning diarrhea) or obstipation alternating with diarrhea. Other signs are blood or mucus in stool and a sense of incomplete evacuation.

Late in the disease, pain begins as a feeling of rectal fullness that later becomes a dull, and sometimes constant, ache confined to the rectum or sacral region.

Diagnosis
⊙ Biopsy verifies colorectal cancer.
⊙ Digital rectal examination can detect almost 15% of colorectal cancers.

○ Fecal occult blood test can detect blood in stools. However, it's commonly negative in patients with colon cancer.

○ Proctoscopy and sigmoidoscopy detect up to 66% of colorectal cancers.

○ Colonoscopy permits visual inspection (and photographs) of the colon up to the ileocecal valve and gives access for polypectomies and biopsies of suspected lesions.

○ Computed tomography scan helps to detect areas affected by metastasis.

○ Barium X-ray, using a dual contrast with air, can locate lesions that are undetectable manually or visually. Barium examination should follow endoscopy or excretory urography because the barium sulfate interferes with these tests.

○ Carcinoembryonic antigen, though not specific or sensitive enough for early diagnosis, is helpful in monitoring patients before and after treatment to detect metastasis or recurrence.

Complications
○ Abdominal distention
○ Anemia
○ Intestinal obstruction

Treatment
○ Surgery is the most effective treatment of colorectal cancer; the type of surgery depends on the location of the tumor:

– *Cecum and ascending colon* — right hemicolectomy (for advanced disease) may include resection of the terminal segment of the ileum, cecum, ascending colon, and right half of the transverse colon with corresponding mesentery

– *Proximal and middle transverse colon* — right colectomy to include transverse colon and mesentery corresponding to midcolic vessels, or segmental resection of transverse colon and associated midcolic vessels

– *Sigmoid colon* — surgery is usually limited to sigmoid colon and mesentery

– *Upper rectum* — anterior or low anterior resection (newer method, using a stapler, allows for resections much lower than were previously possible)

– *Lower rectum* — abdominoperineal resection and permanent sigmoid colostomy.

○ Chemotherapy is indicated for patients with metastasis, residual disease, or a recurrent inoperable tumor. Medications used in such treatment commonly include fluorouracil with leucovorin, irinotecan, and oxaliplatin.

○ Radiation therapy induces tumor regression and may be used before or after surgery or combined with chemotherapy, especially fluorouracil.

 COLLABORATIVE MANAGEMENT Care of the patient with colorectal cancer involves several members of the interdisciplinary team. The surgeon performs surgery based on the location and stage of the cancer. The oncologist recommends and supervises the administration of chemotherapy. The nurse educates the patient about preoperative and postoperative expectations and stoma care and helps the patient manage symptoms related to chemotherapy. The enterostomal therapist teaches the patient and family about care of and adjustment to the stoma. The social worker can help with financial issues and in obtaining supplies. The dietitian can assist with nutritional issues and management of GI symptoms such as flatus.

Special considerations
Before surgery
○ Monitor the patient's diet modifications, laxatives, enemas, and antibiotics, which are used to clean the bowel and to decrease abdominal and perineal cavity contamination during surgery.

○ Arrange for a consultation with an enterostomal therapist or wound and ostomy care nurse.

○ Arrange a postsurgical visit from a recovered ostomate.

After surgery
○ Consult with an enterostomal therapist to help set up a regimen for the patient.

○ Encourage the patient to look at the stoma and participate in its care as soon as possible.

○ Allow the patient to shower or bathe as soon as the incision heals.

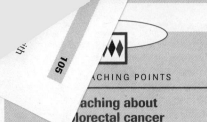

...ACHING POINTS

...aching about
...lorectal cancer

Remember these key points when teaching your patient and his family about colorectal cancer:
● Teach about the disease process and its treatments.
● If the patient is having a colostomy, teach him and his family about the procedure and care of a colostomy and skin.
● Explain risk factors for colorectal cancer and how to reduce or eliminate them.
● Explain to the patient's family the importance of their positive reactions to the patient's adjustment.
● If appropriate, instruct the patient with a sigmoid colostomy to irrigate his colostomy.
● Discuss any dietary restrictions.
● Tell the patient to avoid heavy lifting.
● Recommend a structured, gradually progressive exercise program to strengthen abdominal muscles.
● Reinforce the importance of yearly screening and testing to detect recurrence of colorectal cancer.
● Review signs and symptoms of complications, such as intestinal obstruction and anemia.

○ If appropriate, refer the patient to a home health care agency for follow-up care and counseling.
○ Suggest sexual counseling for male patients; most are impotent after an abdominoperineal resection.
○ Provide patient education. (See *Teaching about colorectal cancer.*)

Applicable patient-teaching aids
○ Applying an ostomy pouch *
○ Caring for your hair and scalp during cancer treatment *
○ Controlling the side effects of chemotherapy *
○ Coping with depression
○ Irrigating your colostomy
○ Minimizing hair loss from chemotherapy
○ Preparing for sigmoidoscopy or a colonoscopy *
○ Testing for blood in your stool

○ Coronary artery disease

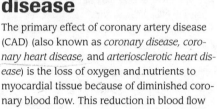

The primary effect of coronary artery disease (CAD) (also known as *coronary disease, coronary heart disease,* and *arteriosclerotic heart disease*) is the loss of oxygen and nutrients to myocardial tissue because of diminished coronary blood flow. This reduction in blood flow can also lead to acute coronary syndromes, such as unstable angina and acute myocardial infarction. The goal of treatment in patients with angina is to either reduce myocardial oxygen demand or increase oxygen supply.

CAD is the leading cause of death in the United States. According to the American Heart Association, someone in the United States suffers a coronary heart event approximately every 29 seconds, and someone dies from such an event approximately every 60 seconds.

Causes
Atherosclerosis is the usual cause of CAD. Risk factors include family history, male gender, age (risk increased in those age 65 or older), hypertension, obesity, smoking, diabetes mellitus, stress, sedentary lifestyle, high serum cholesterol (particularly high low-density lipoprotein [LDL] cholesterol) or triglyceride levels, low high-density lipoprotein cholesterol levels, high blood homocysteine levels, menopause and, possibly, infections producing inflammatory responses in the artery walls.

Uncommon causes of reduced coronary artery blood flow include dissecting aneurysms, infectious vasculitis, syphilis, and congenital defects in the coronary vascular system. Coronary artery spasms may also impede blood flow.

Pathophysiology
Fatty, fibrous plaques progressively narrow the coronary artery lumina, reducing the volume of

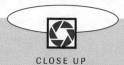

Atherosclerotic plaque development

The coronary arteries are made of three layers: intima (the innermost layer); media (the middle layer), and adventitia (the outermost layer).

Fibrous plaque and lipids progressively narrow the lumen and impede blood flow to the myocardium.

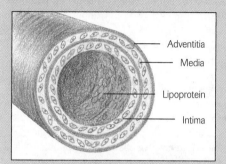

Adventitia
Media
Lipoprotein
Intima

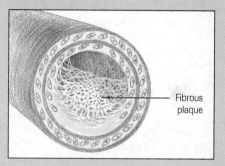

Fibrous plaque

Damaged by risk factors, a fatty streak begins to build up on the intimal layer.

The plaque continues to grow and, in advanced stages, may become a complicated calcified lesion that may rupture.

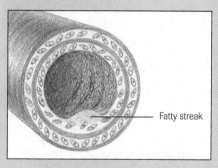

Fatty streak

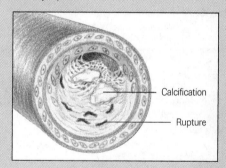

Calcification
Rupture

blood that can flow through them and leading to myocardial ischemia. (See *Atherosclerotic plaque development*.)

As atherosclerosis progresses, luminal narrowing is accompanied by vascular changes that impair the ability of the diseased vessel to dilate. This causes a precarious balance between myocardial oxygen supply and demand, threatening the myocardium beyond the lesion. When oxygen demand exceeds what the diseased vessel can supply, localized myocardial ischemia results.

Myocardial cells become ischemic within 10 seconds of a coronary artery occlusion. Transient ischemia causes reversible changes at the cellular and tissue levels, depressing myocardial function. Untreated, this can lead to tissue injury or necrosis. Within several minutes, oxygen deprivation forces the myocardium to shift from aerobic to anaerobic metabolism, leading to the accumulation of lactic acid and reduction of cellular pH.

The combination of hypoxia, reduced energy availability, and acidosis rapidly impairs left

Types of angina

There are four types of angina:
- *Stable angina:* pain is predictable in frequency and duration and is relieved by rest and nitroglycerin.
- *Unstable angina:* pain increases in frequency and duration and is more easily induced; it indicates a worsening of coronary artery disease that may progress to myocardial infarction.
- *Prinzmetal's or variant angina:* pain is caused by spasm of the coronary arteries; it may occur spontaneously and may not be related to physical exercise or emotional stress.
- *Microvascular angina:* impairment of vasodilator reserve causes angina-like chest pain in a person with normal coronary arteries.

ventricular function. The strength of contractions in the affected myocardial region is reduced as the fibers shorten inadequately, resulting in less force and velocity. Moreover, wall motion is abnormal in the ischemic area, resulting in less blood being ejected from the heart with each contraction. Restoring blood flow through the coronary arteries restores aerobic metabolism and contractility. However, if blood flow isn't restored, myocardial infarction (MI) results.

Assessment findings

The classic symptom of CAD is angina. Anginal pain is usually described as a burning, squeezing, or tight feeling in the substernal or precordial chest that may radiate to the left arm, neck, jaw, or shoulder blade and be accompanied by nausea, vomiting, fainting, sweating, or cool extremities. (See *Types of angina.*) Typically, the patient clenches his fist over his chest or rubs his left arm when describing the pain. Anginal episodes most often follow physical exertion, but may also follow emotional excitement, exposure to cold, or a large meal. (See *Acute myocardial infarction.*)

Diagnosis

○ The patient history—including the frequency and duration of angina and the presence of associated risk factors—is crucial in evaluating CAD.

○ Electrocardiogram (ECG) during angina may show ischemia and, possibly, arrhythmias such as premature ventricular contractions. ECG is apt to be normal when the patient is pain-free. Arrhythmias may occur without infarction, secondary to ischemia.

○ Treadmill or exercise stress test may provoke chest pain and ECG signs of myocardial ischemia; myocardial perfusion imaging with thallium-201, Cardiolite, or Myoview during treadmill exercise detects ischemic areas of the myocardium, visualized as "cold spots."

○ Coronary angiography reveals coronary artery stenosis or obstruction, possible collateral circulation, and the arteries' condition beyond the narrowing.

○ Stress echocardiography may show wall motion abnormalities.

○ Electron-beam computed tomography identifies calcium within arterial plaque; the more calcium seen, the higher the likelihood of CAD.

Complications

○ Arrhythmias
○ Heart failure
○ Ischemic cardiomyopathy
○ MI

Treatment

○ Nitrates, such as nitroglycerin (given sublingually, orally, transdermally, or topically in ointment form), are given to dilate coronary arteries and improve blood supply to the heart.

○ Aspirin, glycoprotein IIb-IIIa inhibitors, and antithrombin drugs may be used to reduce the risk of blood clots.

○ Beta-adrenergic blockers may be used to decrease heart rate and lower the heart's oxygen use.

○ Calcium channel blockers may be administered to relax the coronary arteries and all systemic arteries, reducing the heart's workload.

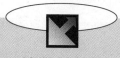

Acute myocardial infarction

If your patient has an acute myocardial infarction (MI) (ST-segment elevation MI or non–ST-segment elevation MI), follow these recommendations established by the American College of Cardiology and the American Heart Association Task Force on Practice Guidelines:

● Assess the patient in the emergency department within 10 minutes of symptom onset because 50% of deaths occur within 1 hour of symptom onset.

● Administer oxygen by nasal cannula to increase oxygenation.

● Give sublingual nitroglycerin to relieve chest pain, unless the patient's systolic blood pressure is less than 90 mm Hg. Morphine is given to relieve chest pain.

● Aspirin, given every day indefinitely, is recommended to inhibit platelet aggregation.

● Initiate continuous cardiac monitoring to detect arrhythmias and ischemia.

● If chest pain lasts at least 30 minutes and symptoms started within the past 12 hours, start I.V fibrinolytic therapy in the patient with ST-segment elevation MI. Following fibrinolytic therapy, begin an infusion of I.V. heparin to promote coronary artery patency.

● Percutaneous transluminal coronary angioplasty (PTCA) may be necessary to revascularize narrowed or blocked coronary arteries.

● Glycoprotein IIb/IIIa receptor blocking agents are administered to inhibit platelet aggregation, as adjunct therapy with PTCA in non–ST-segment elevation MI.

● Limit the patient's physical activity for the first 12 hours to reduce cardiac workload.

● Keep emergency supplies, such as medications to treat arrhythmias, transcutaneous pacing patches or a transvenous pacemaker, and a defibrillator, readily available.

● Begin an infusion of I.V. nitroglycerin for 24 to 48 hours to reduce afterload and preload and relieve chest pain, unless contraindicated.

● Initiate early I.V. beta-adrenergic blockers followed by oral therapy to reduce myocardial oxygen requirements, unless contraindicated

● Administer angiotensin-converting enzyme inhibitors to reduce afterload and preload and prevent remodeling, unless contraindicated. (Begin in ST-segment elevation MI 6 hours after admission or when stable.)

● Magnesium sulfate is recommended for 24 hours to correct hypomagnesemia, if needed.

● The patient with spontaneous or provoked myocardial ischemia following acute MI may require angiography and possible PTCA or surgical revascularization.

● Before discharge, the patient undergoes exercise testing to determine the adequacy of medical therapy and provide an exercise prescription.

● Teach the patient about the importance of following a cardiac risk modification program, which should include weight control; a low-fat, low cholesterol diet; smoking cessation; and regular exercise.

● If the patient has an abnormal fasting lipid profile, he'll require lipid-lowering agents.

○ Angiotensin-converting enzyme inhibitors, diuretics, or other medications may be used to lower blood pressure.

○ Percutaneous transluminal coronary angioplasty may be performed during cardiac catheterization to compress fatty deposits and relieve occlusion in patients with no calcification and partial occlusion

○ Laser angioplasty corrects occlusion by vaporizing fatty deposits.

○ A stent may be placed in the artery to act as a scaffold to hold the artery open.

○ Drug-eluting stent placement, currently under clinical trials, may hold a reopened artery open. It may also be used to minimize the risk of in-stent restenosis.

Teaching about coronary artery disease

Remember these key points when teaching your patient and his family about coronary artery disease (CAD):

● Explain the disease process and its treatments.

● Review the complications of CAD, such as myocardial infarction, and when to seek immediate medical attention.

● Help the patient recognize his cardiac risk factors and to devise a plan of lifestyle modifications, such as exercise, dietary restrictions, stress reduction, weight control, and smoking cessation.

● Discuss the signs and symptoms of angina as well as how to prevent and treat it.

● If the patient is scheduled for surgery, explain the procedure to him and his family; give them a tour of the intensive care unit and introduce them to the staff.

● Explain medications the patient is taking, including their names, dosages, frequencies, adverse effects, and special considerations.

○ Rotational atherectomy removes arterial plaque with a high-speed burr.

○ Coronary artery bypass graft (CABG) surgery may be necessary with obstructive lesions.

○ Minimally invasive coronary artery bypass surgery, also known as *keyhole surgery,* is an alternative to CABG.

○ Coronary brachytherapy, which involves delivering beta or gamma radiation into the coronary arteries, may be used in patients who have undergone stent implantation in a coronary artery but then developed such problems as diffuse in-stent restenosis.

○ Lifestyle modifications — including dietary restrictions, smoking cessation, regular exercise, maintaining an ideal body weight, and

stress reduction — can reduce further progression of CAD.

○ Control of hypertension and elevated serum cholesterol or triglyceride levels (with antilipemics) and measures to minimize platelet aggregation and the danger of blood clots (with aspirin or other antiplatelet agents) are other preventive measures.

 COLLABORATIVE MANAGEMENT

The care of the patient with CAD involves several members of the interdisciplinary team. The nurse educates the patient about CAD, lifestyle changes, controlling symptoms, and drug therapy. The nurse coordinates the many facets of the patient's care. Home health care nurses monitor the patient in the community and communicate findings to the physician. The dietitian educates the patient about the importance of following dietary restrictions to lower serum LDL levels and control hypertension. The interdisciplinary cardiac rehabilitation team, which may consist of cardiologists, exercise specialists, physical therapists, occupational therapists, dietitians, nurses, and social workers, provides supervised exercise, education, and cardiac risk modification.

Special considerations

○ During anginal episodes, monitor the patient's blood pressure and heart rate. Take an ECG during anginal episodes and before administering nitroglycerin or other nitrates. Record duration of pain, amount of medication required to relieve it, and accompanying symptoms.

○ Keep nitroglycerin available for immediate use. Instruct the patient to call immediately whenever he feels chest, arm, or neck pain.

○ Before cardiac catheterization, explain the procedure to the patient.

○ After catheterization, monitor the catheter site for bleeding, check for distal pulses, and make sure the patient drinks plenty of fluids.

○ After surgery, monitor the patient's blood pressure, intake and output, breath sounds, chest tube drainage, and ECG, watching for signs of ischemia and arrhythmias. Also, observe for and treat chest pain and possible dye reactions. Give chest physiotherapy and guide the patient in the removal of secretions through deep breathing, coughing, and expectoration of mucus.

○ Provide patient education. (See *Teaching about coronary artery disease.*)

Applicable patient-teaching aids

○ Cutting down on cholesterol *
○ Cutting down on salt *
○ Exercising safely *
○ Learning about ACE-inhibitors *
○ Learning about beta-adrenergic blockers *
○ Maintaining a safe level of activity
○ Preparing for cardiac catheterization *
○ Resuming sex after a heart attack
○ Taking anticoagulants *
○ Taking nitroglycerin *
○ Taking your pulse *
○ Warming up before exercise *

⊂ Crohn's disease

Crohn's disease, also known as *regional enteritis and granulomatous colitis,* is an inflammation of any part of the GI tract (usually the proximal portion of the colon or, less commonly, the terminal ileum) that extends through all layers of the intestinal wall. It may also involve regional lymph nodes and the mesentery. Granulomas are usually surrounded by normal mucosa; when these lesions are present in multiples, they're commonly referred to as skip lesions. The surface of the inflamed GI tract usually has a cobblestone appearance, which is different from alternating areas of inflammation and fissure crevices.

Crohn's disease is most prevalent in adults ages 20 to 40. Its incidence has risen steadily over the past 50 years; it now affects 7 out of every 100,000 people. It's more common in Whites than in Blacks or Asians.

Causes

Although the exact cause of Crohn's disease is unknown, autoimmune and genetic factors are thought to play a role. Up to 5% of those with the disease have one or more affected relatives. However, a pattern of Mendelian inheritance

hasn't been identified. Lymphatic obstruction and infection may be contributing factors.

Pathophysiology

Whatever the cause of Crohn's disease, inflammation spreads slowly and progressively. Enlarged lymph nodes block lymph flow in the submucosa. Lymphatic obstruction leads to edema, mucosal ulceration and fissures, abscesses and, sometimes, granulomas. Mucosal ulcerations are called "skipping lesions" because they aren't continuous, as in ulcerative colitis.

Oval, elevated patches of closely packed lymph follicles — called *Peyer's patches* — develop in the lining of the small intestine. Subsequent fibrosis thickens the bowel wall and causes stenosis, or narrowing of the lumen. The serous membrane becomes inflamed (serositis), inflamed bowel loops adhere to other diseased or normal loops, and diseased bowel segments become interspersed with healthy ones. Finally, diseased parts of the bowel become thicker, narrower, and shorter. (See *Bowel changes in Crohn's disease,* page 112.)

Assessment findings

Clinical effects may be mild and nonspecific, initially; they vary according to the location and extent of the lesion. Chronic symptoms, which are more typical of the disease, are more persistent and less severe; they include diarrhea (four to six stools per day) with pain in the right lower abdominal quadrant, steatorrhea (excess fat in feces), marked weight loss and, rarely, clubbing of fingers. The patient may complain of weakness and fatigue. The patient may also present with acute inflammatory signs and symptoms that mimic appendicitis, including steady, colicky pain in the right lower quadrant; cramping; tenderness; flatulence; nausea; fever; diarrhea; bleeding (usually mild but may be massive); and bloody stools.

Diagnosis

○ Biopsy, which is required for a definitive diagnosis, reveals granulomas in up to one-half of all specimens.

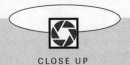

CLOSE UP

Bowel changes in Crohn's disease

As Crohn's disease progresses, fibrosis thickens the bowel wall and narrows the lumen. Narrowing — or stenosis — can occur in any part of the intestine and cause varying degrees of intestinal obstruction. At first, the mucosa may appear normal, but as the disease progresses it takes on a "cobblestone" appearance as shown.

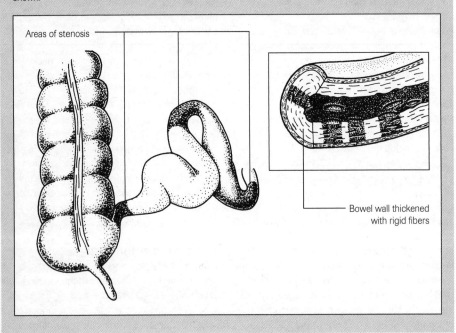

Areas of stenosis

Bowel wall thickened with rigid fibers

○ Fecal occult test reveals minute amounts of blood in stools.
○ Small bowel X-ray shows irregular mucosa, ulceration, and stiffening.
○ Barium enema reveals the string sign (segments of stricture separated by normal bowel) and, possibly, fissures and narrowing of the bowel.
○ Sigmoidoscopy and colonoscopy reveal patchy areas of inflammation (helps to rule out ulcerative colitis), with cobblestone-like mucosal surface. With colon involvement, ulcers may be seen.

○ Blood tests reveal increased white blood cell count and erythrocyte sedimentation rate and decreased potassium, calcium, magnesium, and hemoglobin levels, as well as B_{12} deficiency.

Complications
○ Anal fistula
○ Bowel perforation
○ Fistulas to the bladder or vagina or to the skin in an old scar area
○ Fluid imbalances
○ Intestinal obstruction
○ Intra-abdominal abscesses

○ Nutrient deficiencies (from poor digestion and malabsorption of bile salts and vitamin B_{12})

○ Perineal abscess

Treatment

○ Medications, such as 5-aminosalicylate, may be prescribed to control the inflammatory process.

○ Corticosteroids and immunomodulators may be prescribed if 5-aminosalicylate isn't effective or in patients with severe Crohn's disease.

○ Total parenteral nutrition may be necessary to maintain nutritional status while resting the bowel in debilitated patients.

○ Antibiotics may be prescribed if abscesses or fistulas occur.

○ Infliximab (an antibody to tumor necrosis factor-alpha, an immune chemical that promotes inflammation) may be prescribed.

○ Lifestyle changes, such as physical rest, dietary restrictions (specific foods vary from person to person), and elimination of dairy products for patients who are lactose intolerant, should accompany treatment.

○ Surgery may be necessary to correct bowel perforation, massive hemorrhage, fistulas, or acute intestinal obstruction.

○ Colectomy with ileostomy is necessary in many patients with extensive disease of the large intestine and rectum.

 COLLABORATIVE MANAGEMENT
The care of the patient with Crohn's disease involves several members of the interdisciplinary team. The patient's physician or gastroenterologist manages the patient's care. The surgeon may be consulted if the patient has extensive disease or complications. The nurse provides education, monitors fluid and electrolyte balance, provides skin care, and monitors for complications. The dietitian ensures adequate nutrition, monitors for malabsorption, and recommends nutritional therapy. If stress is clearly an aggravating factor, a therapist may help in the identification of life stressors and assist the patient in learning stress-reduction techniques.

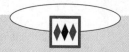

KEY TEACHING POINTS

Teaching about Crohn's disease

Remember these key points when teaching your patient and his family about Crohn's disease:

● Teach about the disease process, including its symptoms, complications, and treatments.

● Explain the importance of adequate rest.

● Stress the need for a severely restricted diet.

● Help the patient identify sources of stress and stress-reducing practices.

● Teach about prescribed medications, including their names, dosages, frequencies, adverse effects, and special considerations.

● Discuss warning signs of complications that require immediate medical attention.

● If the patient is having surgery, explain surgical procedures and refer him to an enterostomal therapist.

● Explain post ileostomy self-care and lifestyle modifications.

● Refer the patient to a support group, such as the Crohn's and Colitis Foundation of America.

Special considerations

○ Record fluid intake and output (including the amount of stool), and weigh the patient daily. Watch for dehydration and maintain fluid and electrolyte balance.

○ Be alert for signs of intestinal bleeding (bloody stools); check stools daily for occult blood.

○ Check hemoglobin level and hematocrit regularly. Give iron supplements and blood transfusions, as ordered.

○ Provide good patient hygiene and mouth care if the patient is restricted to nothing by mouth.

○ After each bowel movement, give good skin care.

○ Observe the patient for fever and pain or pneumaturia, which may signal bladder fistula. Abdominal pain and distention and fever may

indicate intestinal obstruction. Watch for stools from the vagina and an enterovaginal fistula.
○ Before ileostomy, arrange for a visit by an enterostomal therapist.
○ Provide preoperative and postoperative care.
○ After surgery, provide meticulous stoma care, and teach it to the patient and his family.
○ Following ileostomy, offer reassurance and emotional support.
○ Discuss the importance of rest periods throughout the day, especially during disease exacerbations.
○ Teach the patient stress-management techniques and recommend follow-up counseling if appropriate.
○ Provide patient education. (See *Teaching about Crohn's disease,* page 113.)

Applicable patient-teaching aids
○ Applying an ostomy pouch *
○ Draining an ostomy pouch
○ Performing relaxation breathing exercises *
○ Removing an ostomy pouch *

○ Cushing's syndrome

Cushing's syndrome is a cluster of clinical abnormalities caused by excessive levels of adrenocortical hormones (particularly cortisol) or related corticosteroids and, to a lesser extent, androgens and aldosterone. Its unmistakable signs include rapidly developing adiposity of the face (moon face), neck, and trunk and purple striae on the skin.

Cushing's syndrome is more common in females than in males and occurs primarily between ages 25 and 40.

The annual incidence of endogenous cortisol excess in the United States is two to four cases per 1 million people per year. The incidence of Cushing's syndrome resulting from exogenous administration of cortisol is uncertain, but it's known to be much greater than that of endogenous types. The prognosis for endogenous Cushing's syndrome is guardedly favorable with surgery; however, morbidity and mortality are high without treatment. About 50% of individuals with untreated Cushing's syndrome die within 5

years of onset as a result of overwhelming infection, suicide, complications from generalized arteriosclerosis (coronary artery disease), and severe hypertensive disease.

Causes
In approximately 70% of patients, Cushing's syndrome results from excessive production of corticotropin and consequent hyperplasia of the adrenal cortex. Overproduction of corticotropin may stem from pituitary hypersecretion (Cushing's disease), a corticotropin-producing tumor in another organ (particularly bronchogenic or pancreatic cancer), or excessive administration of exogenous glucocorticoids.

In the remaining 30% of patients, Cushing's syndrome results from a cortisol-secreting adrenal tumor, which is usually benign. In infants, the usual cause of Cushing's syndrome is adrenal carcinoma.

Pathophysiology
Cushing's syndrome is caused by prolonged exposure to excess glucocorticoids. (See *Cushing's syndrome: How it happens.*) It can be exogenous, resulting from chronic glucocorticoid or corticotropin administration, or endogenous, resulting from increased cortisol or corticotropin secretion. Cortisol excess results in anti-inflammatory effects and excessive catabolism of protein and peripheral fat to support hepatic glucose production. The mechanism may be corticotropin dependent (elevated plasma corticotropin levels stimulate the adrenal cortex to produce excess cortisol), or corticotropin independent (excess cortisol is produced by the adrenal cortex or exogenously administered). Excess cortisol suppresses the hypothalamic-pituitary-adrenal axis, also present in ectopic corticotropin-secreting tumors, such as tumors in the lung, thymus gland, or pancreas.

Assessment findings
Cushing's syndrome induces changes in multiple body systems, depending on the adrenocortical hormone involved, and may include the following:

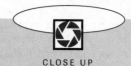

Cushing's syndrome: How it happens

Endogenous Cushing's syndrome results from prolonged exposure to excess glucocorticoids, which can be caused by a pituitary tumor that results in increased production of adrenocorticotropic hormone (ACTH), a non-pituitary ACTH-secreting tumor, or an adrenal tumor. Exogenous Cushing's syndrome results from excessive administration of glucocorticoids.

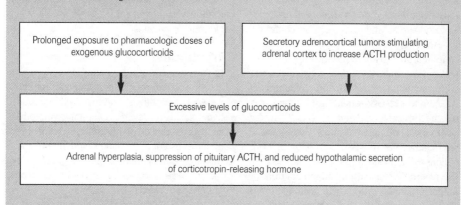

Prolonged exposure to pharmacologic doses of exogenous glucocorticoids

Secretory adrenocortical tumors stimulating adrenal cortex to increase ACTH production

Excessive levels of glucocorticoids

Adrenal hyperplasia, suppression of pituitary ACTH, and reduced hypothalamic secretion of corticotropin-releasing hormone

○ Cardiovascular system—hypertension due to sodium and water retention, left ventricular hypertrophy, and capillary weakness due to protein loss, which leads to bleeding, petechiae, and ecchymosis

○ Central nervous system (CNS)—irritability and emotional lability, ranging from euphoric behavior to depression or psychosis; and insomnia

○ Endocrine and metabolic systems—diabetes mellitus, with decreased glucose tolerance, fasting hyperglycemia, and glycosuria

○ GI system—peptic ulcer, resulting from increased gastric secretions and pepsin production, and decreased gastric mucus

○ Immune system—increased susceptibility to infection due to decreased lymphocyte production and suppressed antibody formation; and decreased resistance to stress (Suppressed inflammatory response may mask even a severe infection.)

○ Musculoskeletal system—muscle weakness due to hypokalemia or to loss of muscle mass from increased catabolism; pathologic fractures due to decreased bone mineral; and skeletal growth retardation in children

○ Renal and urologic systems—sodium and secondary fluid retention, increased potassium excretion, inhibited antidiuretic hormone secretion, and ureteral calculi from increased bone demineralization with hypercalciuria

○ Reproductive system—increased androgen production with clitoral hypertrophy, mild virilism, sexual dysfunction (both sexes), and amenorrhea or oligomenorrhea

○ Skin—purplish striae; fat pads above the clavicles, over the upper back (buffalo hump), on the face (moon face), and throughout the trunk, with slender arms and legs; little or no scar formation; poor wound healing; and acne and hirsutism in females.

Diagnosis

○ Initially, diagnosis of Cushing's syndrome requires determination of plasma steroid levels. In people with healthy hormone balance, plasma cortisol levels are higher in the morning and decrease gradually throughout the day (diurnal variation). In patients with Cushing's syndrome, cortisol levels don't fluctuate and typically remain consistently elevated; 24-hour urine sample demonstrates elevated free cortisol levels.

○ Low-dose dexamethasone suppression test confirms the diagnosis of Cushing's syndrome. Salivary cortisol levels collected at midnight (usually performed on an outpatient basis) are elevated and are the most sensitive confirmatory test.

○ A high-dose dexamethasone suppression test can determine if Cushing's syndrome results from pituitary dysfunction (Cushing's disease). In this test, dexamethasone suppresses plasma cortisol levels, and urinary 17-hydroxycorticosteroid (17-OHCS) and 17-ketogenic steroid levels fall to 50% or less of basal levels. Failure to suppress these levels indicates that the syndrome results from an adrenal tumor or a nonendocrine, corticotropin-secreting tumor. This test can produce false-positive results.

○ In a stimulation test, administration of metyrapone, which blocks cortisol production by the adrenal glands, tests the ability of the pituitary gland and the hypothalamus to detect and correct low levels of plasma cortisol by increasing corticotropin production. The patient with Cushing's disease reacts to this stimulus by secreting an excess of plasma corticotropin as measured by levels of urinary 17-OHCS. If the patient has an adrenal or a nonendocrine corticotropin-secreting tumor, the pituitary gland—which is suppressed by the high cortisol levels — can't respond normally, so steroid levels remain stable or fall.

○ Ultrasound, computed tomography (CT) scan, or angiography localizes adrenal tumors; CT scan and magnetic resonance imaging of the head may identify pituitary tumors.

Complications

○ Diabetes mellitus
○ Dyslipidemia
○ Heart failure
○ Hirsutism
○ Hypertension
○ Impaired glucose tolerance
○ Increased susceptibility to infections
○ Ischemic heart disease
○ Menstrual disturbances
○ Metastasis of malignant tumors
○ Osteoporosis and pathologic fractures
○ Peptic ulcer
○ Psychiatric problems, ranging from mood swings to frank psychosis
○ Sexual dysfunction
○ Slow wound healing
○ Ureteral calculi

Treatment

○ Partial or complete hypophysectomy or pituitary irradiation may be performed for pituitary-dependent Cushing's syndrome with adrenal hyperplasia and severe cushingoid symptoms, such as psychosis, poorly controlled diabetes mellitus, osteoporosis, and severe pathologic fractures. If the patient doesn't respond to either of these therapies, bilateral adrenalectomy may be performed.

○ Excision of nonendocrine corticotropin-producing tumors is necessary, followed by drug therapy (for example, with mitotane, metyrapone, or aminoglutethimide) to decrease cortisol levels if symptoms persist.

○ Aminoglutethimide and ketoconazole, which decrease cortisol levels, may be ordered for the patient with cushingoid symptoms.

○ Aminoglutethimide — alone or in combination with metyrapone — may be useful in treating the patient with metastatic adrenal carcinoma.

○ Control hypertension, edema, diabetes, and cardiovascular manifestations and prevent infection before surgery in the patient with cushingoid symptoms.

○ Glucocorticoid administration on the morning of surgery can help prevent acute adrenal hypofunction during surgery.

○ Cortisol therapy is essential during and after surgery, to help the patient tolerate the physiologic stress imposed by removal of the pituitary gland or adrenal glands. If normal cortisol-production resumes, steroid therapy may be gradually tapered and eventually discontinued. However, bilateral adrenalectomy or total hypophysectomy mandates lifelong steroid replacement therapy to correct hormonal deficiencies.

COLLABORATIVE MANAGEMENT

Care of the patient with Cushing's syndrome involves several members of the interdisciplinary team. The endocrinologist typically manages the patient's care. The nurse educates the patient about the disorder, takes measures to prevent infection and injury, monitors for and corrects fluid and electrolyte imbalances, and provides emotional support. The dietitian assesses the nutritional status of the patient, monitors the patient's weight, and recommends a low-calorie diet that's high in protein, vitamin C, and calcium and low in sodium. The physical therapist helps the patient develop an exercise program to prevent deconditioning and muscle wasting and to promote bone development. The occupational therapist teaches the patient energy conservation techniques. The social worker assesses the patient's financial resources and support systems.

Special considerations

Patients with Cushing's syndrome require painstaking assessment and vigorous supportive care:

○ Frequently monitor vital signs, especially blood pressure. Carefully observe the hypertensive patient who also has cardiac disease.

○ Check laboratory reports for hypernatremia, hypokalemia, hyperglycemia, and glycosuria.

○ Because the cushingoid patient is likely to retain sodium and water, check for edema, and monitor daily weight and intake and output carefully. To minimize weight gain, edema, and hypertension, ask the dietary department to provide a diet that's high in protein and potassium but low in calories, carbohydrates, and sodium.

○ Watch for infection — a particular problem in Cushing's syndrome.

○ If the patient has osteoporosis and is bedridden, perform passive range-of-motion exercises carefully because of the severe risk of pathologic fractures.

○ Remember, Cushing's syndrome produces emotional lability. Document incidents that upset the patient, and try to prevent such situations from occurring. Help him get the physical and mental rest he needs — by sedation if necessary. Offer support to the patient who's emotionally labile throughout the difficult testing period.

After bilateral adrenalectomy and pituitary surgery:

○ Be sure to report wound drainage or temperature elevation to the patient's physician immediately. Use strict sterile technique in changing the patient's dressings.

○ Administer analgesics and replacement steroids, as ordered.

○ Monitor urine output, and check vital signs carefully, watching for signs of shock (decreased blood pressure, increased pulse rate, pallor, and cold, clammy skin). To counteract shock, give vasopressors and increase the rate of I.V. fluids, as ordered. Because mitotane, aminoglutethimide, and metyrapone decrease mental alertness and produce physical weakness, assess neurologic and behavioral status, and warn the patient of adverse CNS effects. Also watch for severe nausea, vomiting, and diarrhea.

○ Check laboratory reports for hypoglycemia due to removal of the source of cortisol, a hormone that maintains blood glucose levels.

○ Check for abdominal distention and return of bowel sounds after adrenalectomy.

○ Check regularly for signs of adrenal hypofunction — orthostatic hypotension, apathy, weakness, fatigue — indicators that steroid replacement is inadequate.

○ In the patient undergoing pituitary surgery, check for and immediately report signs of increased intracranial pressure (confusion, agitation, changes in level of consciousness, nausea, and vomiting). Watch for hypopituitarism.

Provide comprehensive teaching to help the patient cope with lifelong treatment:

○ Advise the patient to take replacement steroids with antacids or meals, to minimize gastric irritation. (Usually, it's helpful to take two-thirds of the dosage in the morning and the remaining one-third in the early afternoon to mimic diurnal adrenal secretion.)

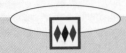

Teaching about Cushing's syndrome

Remember these key points when teaching your patient and his family about Cushing's syndrome:

- Teach about the disease process, including its symptoms, complications, and treatments.
- Explain the importance of adequate rest.
- Help the patient identify sources of stress and stress-reduction techniques.
- Teach about prescribed medications, including their names, indications, dosages, adverse effects, and special considerations.
- Reinforce the need for lifelong steroid replacement.
- Instruct the patient to watch closely for signs and symptoms of inadequate steroid dosage (fatigue, weakness, dizziness) and of overdosage (severe edema, weight gain). Emphatically warn against abrupt discontinuation of steroid dosage because this may produce a fatal adrenal crisis.
- Discuss warning signs and symptoms of complications (such as adrenal crisis, fluid retention, hypokalemia, and infection) that require immediate medical attention and interventions to prevent further complications.
- If the patient is having surgery, explain the surgical procedure and what to expect before and after surgery.
- Tell the patient to carry a medical identification card.
- Instruct the patient to immediately report physiologically stressful situations such as infections, because increased dosages of prescribed medications may be necessary.

○ Tell the patient to carry a medical identification card and to immediately report physiologically stressful situations such as infections, which necessitate increased dosage.

○ Instruct the patient to watch closely for signs of inadequate steroid dosage (fatigue, weakness, dizziness) and of overdosage (severe edema, weight gain). Emphatically warn against abrupt discontinuation of steroid therapy because this may produce a fatal adrenal crisis.
○ Provide patient education. (See *Teaching about Cushing's syndrome.*)

Applicable patient-teaching aids
○ Avoiding infection *
○ Cutting down on salt *
○ How to detect — and prevent — infection *

◯ Cystic fibrosis

Cystic fibrosis is a generalized dysfunction of the exocrine glands that affects multiple organ systems. It's characterized by chronic airway infection leading to bronchiectasis, bronchiolectasis, exocrine pancreatic insufficiency, intestinal dysfunction, abnormal sweat gland function, and reproductive dysfunction.

Cystic fibrosis accounts for almost all cases of pancreatic enzyme deficiency in children. Transmitted as an autosomal recessive trait, it's the most common fatal genetic disease in white children.

Cystic fibrosis is a chronic disease accompanied by many complications. With improvements in treatment over the past decade, the average life expectancy has risen from age 16 to age 32. In the United States, the incidence of cystic fibrosis is highest in Whites of northern European ancestry (1 in 2,000 live births) and lowest in Blacks (1 in 17,000 live births), Native Americans, and Asians. The disease occurs equally in both sexes.

Causes
The responsible gene is on chromosome 7q; it encodes a membrane-associated protein called the cystic fibrosis transmembrane regulator (CFTR). The exact function of CFTR remains unknown, but it appears to help regulate chloride and sodium transport across epithelial membranes.

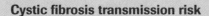

Cystic fibrosis transmission risk

The chance that a relative of a person with cystic fibrosis or a person with no family history will carry the cystic fibrosis gene appears in the chart below.

Relative of affected person	Carrier chance
Brother or sister	2 in 3 (67%)
Niece or nephew	1 in 2 (50%)
Aunt or uncle	1 in 3 (33%)
First cousin	1 in 4 (25%)
No known family history	**Carrier chance**
Whites	1 in 25 (4%)
Blacks	1 in 65 (1.5%)
Asians	1 in 150 (0.67%)

Causes of cystic fibrosis include:
○ abnormal coding found on as many as 350 CFTR alleles
○ autosomal recessive inheritance. (See *Cystic fibrosis transmission risk*.)

Pathophysiology

Most cases of cystic fibrosis arise from the mutation that affects the genetic coding for a single amino acid, resulting in a protein (the CFTR) that doesn't function properly. The CFTR resembles other transmembrane transport proteins, but it lacks the phenylalanine in the protein produced by normal genes. This regulator interferes with cyclic adenosine monophosphate (cAMP)–regulated chloride channels and transport of other ions by preventing adenosine triphosphate from binding to the protein or by interfering with activation by protein kinase. (See *Cystic fibrosis: How it happens,* page 120.)

The mutation affects volume-absorbing epithelia (in the airways and intestines), salt-absorbing epithelia (in sweat ducts), and volume-secretory epithelia (in the pancreas). The clinical effects of cystic fibrosis, aberrations in sweat gland, respiratory, and GI function, may become apparent soon after birth or may take years to develop. The lack of phenylalanine leads to dehydration, increasing the viscosity of mucus-gland secretions and leading to obstruction of glandular ducts. Cystic fibrosis has a varying effect on electrolyte and water transport.

Respiratory symptoms reflect obstructive changes in the lungs. These changes stem from thick, tenacious secretions in the bronchioles and alveoli and eventually lead to severe atelectasis and emphysema.

The GI effects of cystic fibrosis occur mainly in the intestines, pancreas, and liver. Obstruction of the pancreatic ducts and resulting deficiency of trypsin, amylase, and lipase prevent the conversion and absorption of fat and protein in the GI tract. The undigested food is then excreted in frequent, bulky, foul-smelling, pale stools with a high fat content. The inability to absorb fats results in a deficiency of fat-soluble vitamins (A, D, E, and K), leading to clotting problems, retarded bone growth, and delayed sexual development.

In the pancreas, fibrotic tissue, multiple cysts, thick mucus and, eventually, fat replace

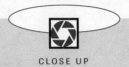

Cystic fibrosis: How it happens

Cystic fibrosis typically arises from a mutation in the genetic coding of a single amino acid found in a protein called cystic fibrosis transmembrane regulator (CFTR). This protein, which is involved in the transportation of chloride and other ions across cell membranes, resembles other transmembrane transport proteins but lacks phenylalanine (an essential amino acid in protein produced by normal genes) and therefore doesn't function properly

Mutation in coding of amino acid

Interference with cyclic adenosine monophosphate (cAMP)–regulated chloride channels and transport of other ions by preventing adenosine triphosphate from binding to the CFTR protein or by interfering with activation by protein kinase

Epithelial dysfunction in airways and intestines (volume-absorbing epithelia), sweat ducts (salt-absorbing epithelia), and pancreas (volume-secretory epithelia)

Dehydration, increased viscosity of mucus secretions, and obstruction of glandular ducts

the acini (small, saclike swellings normally found in this gland), producing symptoms of pancreatic insufficiency: insufficient insulin production, abnormal glucose tolerance, and glycosuria.

Assessment findings

In cystic fibrosis, respiratory symptoms reflect obstructive changes in the lungs: a dry, nonproductive paroxysmal cough; dyspnea; and tachypnea. Children with cystic fibrosis display a barrel chest, cyanosis, and clubbing of the fingers and toes due to chronic hypoxia. Auscultation reveals crackles (due to thick secretions) and wheezes (due to constricted airways).

In the neonate with cystic fibrosis, a possible early symptom is meconium ileus. He also develops signs and symptoms of intestinal ob-

struction, such as abdominal distention, vomiting, constipation, dehydration, and electrolyte imbalance; also in the neonate, prolonged neonatal jaundice.

The infant with cystic fibrosis way show signs of failure to thrive, such as poor weight gain, poor growth, distended abdomen, thin extremities, and sallow skin with poor turgor.

Other common findings in the patient with cystic fibrosis include frequent, bulky, foulsmelling, and pale stools with a high fat content; weight gain; poor growth; ravenous appetite; distended abdomen; thin extremities; sallow skin with poor turgor due to malabsorption; and dehydration and fluid and electrolyte imbalances.

Diagnosis

○ The Cystic Fibrosis Foundation has developed certain criteria for a definitive diagnosis: two sweat tests (to detect elevated sodium chloride levels) using a pilocarpine solution (a sweat inducer) and one of the following: presence of an obstructive pulmonary disease, confirmed pancreatic insufficiency or failure to thrive, and a family history of cystic fibrosis.

○ Chest X-rays indicate early signs of obstructive lung disease.

○ Stool specimen analysis indicates the absence of trypsin, suggesting pancreatic insufficiency.

The following test results may support the diagnosis:

○ Deoxyribonucleic acid testing locates the presence of the Delta F 508 deletion (found in about 70% of patients with cystic fibrosis, although the disease can cause more than 100 other mutations). It allows prenatal diagnosis in families with a previously affected child.

○ Pulmonary function tests reveal decreased vital capacity, elevated residual volume due to air entrapments, and decreased forced expiratory volume in 1 second.

○ Liver enzyme tests may reveal hepatic insufficiency.

○ Sputum culture reveals organisms such as *Staphylococcus* and *Pseudomonas.*

○ Serum albumin measurement helps assess nutritional status.

○ Serum electrolytes may show hypochloremia and hyponatremia.

Complications

○ Arthritis
○ Atelectasis
○ Biliary disease
○ Bronchiectasis
○ Cardiac arrhythmias and cor pulmonale
○ Clotting problems
○ Death
○ Dehydration
○ Delayed sexual development; azoospermia in males, secondary amenorrhea in females
○ Diabetes
○ Distal intestinal obstructive syndrome
○ Electrolyte imbalances

○ Gastroesophageal reflux disease
○ Hepatic disease, including cirrhosis, portal hypertension, and esophageal varices
○ Malnutrition
○ Nasal polyps
○ Pneumonia
○ Potentially fatal shock
○ Rectal prolapse
○ Retarded bone growth
○ Sinusitis

Treatment

○ The type of treatment depends on the organ systems involved.

○ Salt supplements and salty foods are necessary to combat electrolyte losses in sweat.

○ Oral pancreatic enzymes with meals and snacks offset pancreatic enzyme deficiencies.

○ The patient's diet should be low in fat, but high in protein and calories. It should be supplemented with water-miscible, fat-soluble vitamins (A, D, E, and K).

○ Chest physiotherapy, postural drainage, and breathing exercises should be performed several times daily to aid removal of secretions from lungs.

○ Aerosol therapy includes intermittent nebulizer treatments before postural drainage to loosen secretions.

○ Dornase alfa or DNase (recombinant human deoxyribonuclease), genetically engineered pulmonary enzymes given by aerosol nebulizer, help thin airway mucus, improving lung function and reducing the risk of pulmonary infection.

○ Inhaled beta-adrenergic agonists are given to control airway constriction.

○ Sodium-channel blockers may decrease sodium reabsorption from secretions and improve viscosity.

○ Uridine triphosphate stimulates chloride secretion by a non-CFTR.

○ Recombinant alpha-antitrypsin counteracts excessive proteolytic activity produced during airway inflammation.

○ Gene therapy is being studied to introduce normal CFTR into affected epithelial cells.

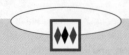

○ Transplantation of heart or lungs may be considered in some patients with severe organ failure.

 COLLABORATIVE MANAGEMENT
An interdisciplinary approach is vital to helping the child with cystic fibrosis lead as normal a life as possible. The nurse educates the child and his family about cystic fibrosis and helps them learn self-care techniques to maintain optimum functioning and reduce exacerbations. The dietitian assesses the patient's nutrition, monitors his weight, and makes dietary recommendations. The physical therapist helps the child maintain muscle strength and tone and prevent deconditioning. The occupational therapist teaches the patient energy-conservation techniques. The respiratory therapist assesses pulmonary function, provides pulmonary treatments, and educates the child and his family about pulmonary function in cystic fibrosis, its breathing treatments, and reducing the risk of pulmonary complications. The social worker can assess the family's financial resources and support systems.

Special considerations

○ Refer the patient who wants to start a family (or the parents of an affected child) for genetic counseling so they can discuss family planning issues or prenatal diagnosis options.
○ Be aware that some patients have recently undergone lung transplants to reduce the effects of the disease.
○ Provide patient education. (See *Teaching about cystic fibrosis*.)

Applicable patient-teaching aids

○ Caring for aerosol equipment
○ Giving children medication by mouth *
○ Improving digestion with pancreatic enzymes
○ Performing chest physiotherapy in cystic fibrosis
○ Performing exercises for healthier lungs and easier breathing
○ Performing forced expiratory technique
○ Preparing for pulmonary function tests *
○ Using an oral inhaler with a holding chamber

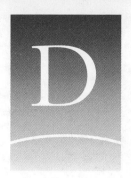

Depression, major

Also known as *unipolar disorder,* major depression is a syndrome of persistently sad, dysphoric mood, accompanied by disturbances in sleep and appetite, lethargy, and an inability to experience pleasure (anhedonia). Depression occurs in up to 18 million U.S. residents, affecting all racial, ethnic, and socioeconomic groups. It affects both sexes, but occurs more commonly in women.

About one-half of all depressed patients experience a single episode and recover completely; the rest have at least one recurrence. (See *Diagnosing major depression,* page 124.) Major depression can profoundly alter social, family, and occupational functioning. Suicide — which can occur when the patient's feelings of worthlessness, guilt, and hopelessness are so overwhelming that the patient no longer considers life worth living — is the most serious consequence of major depression. Nearly twice as many women as men attempt suicide, but men are far more likely to succeed.

Causes

The multiple causes of depression aren't completely understood. Current research suggests possible genetic, familial, biochemical, physical, psychological, and social causes. Psychological causes may include feelings of helplessness and vulnerability, anger, hopelessness and pessimism, guilt, and low self-esteem. They may be related to abnormal character and behavior patterns and troubled personal relationships. In many patients, the history identifies a specific personal loss or severe stressor that probably interacts with the person's predisposition to provoke major depression.

Depression may be secondary to a specific medical condition — for example, endocrine disorders, such as diabetes and Cushing's syndrome; neurologic diseases, such as Parkinson's and Alzheimer's diseases; cancer (especially of the pancreas); viral and bacterial infections, such as influenza and pneumonia; cardiovascular disorders, such as heart failure; pulmonary disorders, such as chronic obstructive lung disease; musculoskeletal disorders, such as degenerative arthritis; GI disorders, such as irritable bowel syndrome; genitourinary problems, such as incontinence; collagen vascular diseases, such as lupus; and anemias.

Drugs prescribed for medical and psychiatric conditions as well as many commonly abused substances can also cause depression. Examples include antihypertensives, psychotropics, opioid and nonopioid analgesics, antiparkinsonian drugs, numerous cardiovascular medications, oral antidiabetics, antimicrobials, steroids, chemotherapeutic agents, cimetidine, and alcohol.

Pathophysiology

The exact pathophysiology of major depression isn't clearly understood. It's thought that changes occur in the receptor-neurotransmitter relationships in the limbic system. Serotonin, involved in the processing of emotions and thoughts, is one of the neurotransmitters thought to play a role in the development of depression. Other neurotransmitters that may be involved include norepinephrine and dopamine.

Diagnosing major depression

A patient is diagnosed with major depression when she fulfills the following criteria for a single major depressive episode put forth in the *Diagnostic and Statistical Manual of Mental Disorders*, Fourth Edition, Text Revision:

● At least five of the following symptoms must have been present during the same 2-week period and must represent a change from previous functioning; one of these must be either depressed mood or loss of interest in previously pleasurable activities:

– depressed mood (irritable mood in children and adolescents) most of the day, nearly every day, as indicated by either subjective account or observation by others

– markedly diminished interest or pleasure in all, or almost all, activities most of the day, nearly every day

– significant weight loss or weight gain when not dieting or decrease or increase in appetite nearly every day (in children, consider failure to make expected weight gains)

– insomnia or hypersomnia nearly every day

– psychomotor agitation or retardation nearly every day

– fatigue or loss of energy nearly every day

– feelings of worthlessness or excessive or inappropriate guilt nearly every day

– diminished ability to think or concentrate, or indecisiveness, nearly every day

– recurrent thoughts of death, recurrent suicidal ideation without a specific plan, a suicide attempt, or a specific plan for committing suicide.

● The symptoms don't meet criteria for a mixed episode.

● The symptoms cause clinically significant distress or impairment in social, occupational, or other important areas of functioning.

● The symptoms aren't due to the direct physiologic effects of a substance or a general medical condition.

● The symptoms aren't better accounted for by bereavement, the symptoms persist for longer than 2 months, or the symptoms are characterized by marked functional impairment, morbid preoccupation with worthlessness, suicidal ideation, psychotic symptoms, or psychomotor retardation.

Reprinted with permission from the *Diagnostic and Statistical Manual of Mental Disorders*, Copyright 2000. American Psychiatric Association.

Assessment findings

The primary features of major depression are a predominantly sad mood and a loss of interest or pleasure in daily activities. The patient may complain of feeling "down in the dumps," express doubts about self-worth or ability to cope, or simply appear unhappy and apathetic. The patient may also report feeling angry or anxious. Symptoms tend to be more severe than those caused by dysthymic disorder, which is a milder, chronic form of depression. (See *Dysthymic disorder*.) Other common signs include difficulty concentrating or thinking clearly, distractibility, and indecisiveness. Anergia, fatigue, and insomnia or other sleep disturbances are common as well. The patient may also experi-

ence anhedonia, which is the inability to experience pleasure.

The patient may report an increase or decrease in appetite, a lack of interest in sexual activity, constipation, or diarrhea. He may also experience reduced psychomotor activity.

Diagnosis

○ A patient is diagnosed with major depression when she fulfills the criteria set forth in the *Diagnostic and Statistical Manual of Mental Disorders,* Fourth Edition, Text Revision.

○ Psychological tests, such as the Beck Depression Inventory, support the diagnosis and may help determine the onset, severity, duration, and progression of depressive symptoms.

○ Toxicology screening may suggest drug-induced depression.

Complications
○ Profound alteration of social, family, and occupational functioning
○ Suicide

Treatment
○ Selective serotonin reuptake inhibitors (SSRIs) are effective first-line antidepressant drugs for the treatment of depression.
○ Tricyclic antidepressants (TCAs) are also a class of antidepressant drugs that may be used to treat depression; however, they have more adverse effects than SSRIs.
○ Monoamine oxidase (MAO) inhibitors are prescribed for patients with atypical depression (for example, depression marked by an increased appetite and need for sleep, rather than anorexia and insomnia) and for some patients who fail to respond to TCAs.
○ Maprotiline, trazodone, and bupropion may also be used.
○ Electroconvulsive therapy is considered in particularly severe or drug-resistant depression.
○ Short-term psychotherapy is also effective in treating major depression.

 COLLABORATIVE MANAGEMENT Care of the patient with major depression involves several members of the interdisciplinary team. A psychiatrist diagnoses the depression and determines the treatment plan. The nurse provides education, develops a therapeutic relationship, and monitors the patient for suicide risk. The dietitian assures adequate nutrition and hydration; provides the patient taking MAO inhibitors a diet free from tyramine, caffeine, and tryptophan; and educates the patient and his family about foods to be avoided. The physical therapist assists in planning activity according to the patient's energy level. The occupational therapist can provide appropriate diversionary activities. A therapist provides individual, family, or group psychotherapy.

Dysthymic disorder

Dysthymic disorder is characterized by a chronic dysphoric mood (irritable mood in children) that persists at least 2 years in adults and 1 year in children and adolescents. It typically begins in childhood, adolescence, or early adulthood and causes only mild social or occupational impairment. In adults, it's more common in women; in children and adolescents, it's equally common in both sexes.

Signs and symptoms
During periods of depression, the patient may experience poor appetite or overeating, insomnia or hypersomnia, low energy or fatigue, low self-esteem, poor concentration or difficulty making decisions, and feelings of hopelessness.

Diagnosis
Dysthymic disorder is confirmed when the patient exhibits at least two of the signs or symptoms listed above nearly every day, with intervening normal moods lasting no more than 2 months during a 2-year period.

Special considerations
○ Share your observations of the patient's behavior with him. For instance, you might say, "You're sitting all by yourself, looking very sad. Is that how you feel?" Because the patient may think and react sluggishly, speak slowly and allow ample time for him to respond.
○ Avoid feigned cheerfulness. However, don't hesitate to laugh with the patient and point out the value of humor.
○ Show the patient he's important by listening attentively and respectfully, preventing interruptions, and avoiding judgmental responses.
○ Provide a structured routine, including noncompetitive activities, to build the patient's self-confidence and encourage interaction.
○ Urge the patient to join group activities and to socialize.

Suicide prevention guidelines

When your patient is diagnosed with major depression, keep in mind the following guidelines.

Assess for clues to suicide
Be alert for the patient's suicidal thoughts, threats, and messages; describing a suicide plan; hoarding medication; talking about death and feelings of futility; giving away prized possessions; and changing behavior, especially as depression begins to lift.

Provide a safe environment
Check patient areas and correct dangerous conditions, such as exposed pipes, windows without safety glass, and access to the roof or balconies.

Remove dangerous objects
Take away potentially dangerous objects, such as belts, razors, suspenders, light cords, glass, knives, nail files and clippers, and metal and hard plastic objects.

Consult with staff
Recognize and document both verbal and nonverbal suicidal behaviors; keep the physician informed; share data with all staff members; clarify the patient's specific restrictions; assess risk and plan for observation; clarify day and night staff responsibilities and the frequency of consultations.

Observe the suicidal patient
Be alert when the patient is taking medication or using the bathroom (to prevent hanging or other injury). Assign the patient to a room near the nurses' station and with another patient. Continuously observe the acutely suicidal patient.

Maintain personal contact
Help the suicidal patient feel that he isn't alone or without resources or hope. Encourage continuity of care and consistency of primary nurses. Building emotional ties to others is the ultimate technique for preventing suicide.

○ Inform the patient that he can help ease depression by expressing his feelings, participating in pleasurable activities, and improving grooming and hygiene.
○ Ask the patient if he thinks of death or suicide. Such thoughts signal an immediate need for consultation and assessment. Failure to detect suicidal thoughts early may encourage the patient to attempt suicide. The risk of suicide increases as the depression lifts. (See *Suicide prevention guidelines.*)
○ If the patient is too depressed to take care of himself, help him with personal hygiene. Encourage him to eat, or feed him if necessary.
○ If the patient is constipated, add high-fiber foods to his diet; offer small, frequent meals; and encourage physical activity and fluid intake.
○ Help the patient to recognize distorted perceptions that may contribute to his depression.

After the patient learns to recognize depressive thought patterns, he can consciously begin to substitute self-affirming thoughts.
○ Make sure that the patient taking an MAO inhibitor doesn't eat cheese, sour cream, pickled herring, liver, canned figs, raisins, bananas, avocados, chocolate, soy sauce, fava beans, yeast extracts, meat tenderizers, coffee, cola drinks, and beer, Chianti, or sherry because these foods contain tyramine, which when taken with MAO inhibitors, can result in a life-threatening hypertensive crisis.
○ Provide patient education. (See *Teaching about major depression.*)

Applicable patient-teaching aids
○ Coping with depression

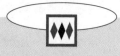

KEY TEACHING POINTS

Teaching about major depression

Remember these key points when teaching your patient about major depression:
- Explain the disorder and its treatments.
- Inform the patient that antidepressants may take several weeks to produce an effect.
- Teach about prescribed antidepressants, including their indications, dosages, and adverse effects.
- Tell the patient to inform his primary health care provider if he's taking antidepressant drugs.
- Suggest sugarless gum or hard candy to relieve dry mouth for medications that produce strong anticholinergic effects, such as amitriptyline and amoxapine.
- Warn the patient taking sedating antidepressants (for example, amitriptyline and trazodone) to avoid

activities that require alertness, including driving and operating mechanical equipment, until the medications' effects on his central nervous system (CNS) are known.
- Caution the patient taking a selective serotonin reuptake inhibitor (SSRI) or tricyclic antidepressant to avoid drinking alcoholic beverages or taking other CNS depressants during therapy. Educate the patient and his family about the potential risk of suicidal ideation, which is associated with the use of SSRI antidepressants, particularly in children and adolescents
- If the patient is taking an MAO inhibitor, emphasize that he must avoid foods that contain tyramine, caffeine, or tryptophan.

Diabetes mellitus

Diabetes mellitus (DM) is a chronic disease of absolute or relative insulin deficiency or resistance characterized by disturbances in carbohydrate, protein, and fat metabolism. A leading cause of death by disease in the United States, this syndrome is a contributing factor in about 50% of myocardial infarctions and about 75% of strokes. It's also a causative factor in renal failure and peripheral vascular disease, and it's the leading cause of new blindness.

DM occurs in four forms classified by etiology: type 1, type 2, other specific types, and gestational diabetes mellitus (GDM). Impaired glucose tolerance and impaired fasting glucose are now referred to as pre-diabetes and are considered risk factors for diabetes and cardiovascular disease. Type 1 is further subdivided into immune-mediated diabetes and idiopathic diabetes. Children and adolescents with type 1 immune-mediated diabetes rapidly develop ketoacidosis, but most adults with this type experience only modest fasting hyperglycemia unless they develop an infection or experience

another stressor. Patients with type 1 idiopathic diabetes are prone to ketoacidosis.

Most patients with type 2 diabetes have insulin resistance with varying degrees of insulin secretory defects. The "other specific types" category includes people who have diabetes as a result of a genetic defect, endocrinopathies, or exposure to certain medications or chemicals. GDM occurs during pregnancy. In this type of diabetes, glucose tolerance levels usually return to normal after delivery. Patients with prediabetes have higher-than-normal blood glucose levels, but the levels aren't high enough to meet the diagnostic criteria for type 2 diabetes.

DM affects an estimated 6% of U.S. residents, about one-half of whom are undiagnosed. Incidence is greater in females and rises with age. Type 2 accounts for 90% of cases. (See *Understanding diabetes mellitus*, page 128.)

Causes

In Type 1 diabetes, pancreatic beta-cell destruction or a primary defect in beta-cell function results in failure to release insulin and ineffective glucose transport. Type 1 immune-mediated di-

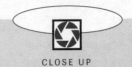

Understanding diabetes mellitus

Diabetes mellitus affects the way the body uses food to make the energy for life. It's the result of absolute or relative insulin deficiency or resistance. It has two primary forms: type 1 and type 2.

Type 1 diabetes

● Pancreas makes little or no insulin.
● In genetically susceptible patients, a triggering event (possibly a viral infection) causes production of autoantibodies against the beta cells of the pancreas.
● Resultant destruction of beta cells leads to a decline in and ultimate lack of insulin secretion.
● Insulin deficiency leads to hyperglycemia, enhanced lipolysis, and protein catabolism. These occur when more than 90% of beta cells have been destroyed.

Type 2 diabetes

● Genetic factors are significant, and onset is accelerated by obesity and a sedentary lifestyle. The pancreas produces some insulin, but it's either too little or ineffective.
● The following factors contribute to its development:
– impaired insulin secretion
– inappropriate hepatic glucose production
– peripheral insulin receptor insensitivity.

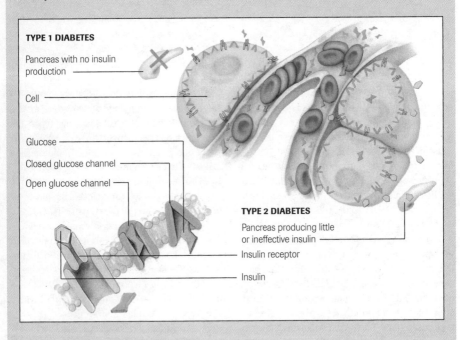

abetes is caused by cell-mediated destruction of pancreatic beta cells. The rate of beta-cell destruction is usually higher in children than in adults. The idiopathic form of type 1 diabetes

has no known cause. Patients with this form have no evidence of autoimmunity and don't produce insulin.

In type 2 diabetes, beta cells release insulin, but receptors are insulin-resistant and glucose transport is variable and ineffective. Risk factors for type 2 diabetes include:

○ obesity (even an increased percentage of body fat primarily in the abdominal region); risk decreases with weight and drug therapy
○ lack of physical activity
○ history of GDM
○ hypertension
○ Black, Hispanic, Pacific Islander, Asian American, Native American origin
○ strong family history of diabetes
○ age over 45
○ high-density lipoprotein cholesterol levels of less than 35 mg/dl or triglyceride levels of greater than 250 mg/dl
○ impaired glucose tolerance or impaired fasting glucose (pre-diabetes).

The "other specific types" of DM result from various conditions (such as a genetic defect of the beta cells or endocrinopathies) or from use of or exposure to certain medications or chemicals. GDM is considered present whenever a patient has any degree of abnormal glucose during pregnancy. This form may result from weight gain and increased levels of estrogen and placental hormones, which antagonize insulin.

Insulin transports glucose into the cell for use as energy and storage as glycogen. It also stimulates protein synthesis and free fatty acid storage in the fat deposits. Insulin deficiency compromises the body tissues' access to essential nutrients for fuel and storage.

Pathophysiology

In persons genetically susceptible to type 1 diabetes, a triggering event, possibly a viral infection, causes production of autoantibodies against the beta cells of the pancreas. The resultant destruction of the beta cells leads to a decline in and ultimate lack of insulin secretion. Insulin deficiency leads to hyperglycemia, enhanced lipolysis (decomposition of fat), and protein catabolism. These characteristics occur when more than 90% of the beta cells have been destroyed.

Type 2 diabetes mellitus is a chronic disease caused by one or more of the following factors: impaired insulin secretion, inappropriate hepatic glucose production, or peripheral insulin receptor insensitivity. Genetic factors are significant, and onset is accelerated by obesity and a sedentary lifestyle. Again, added stress can be a pivotal factor.

Gestational diabetes mellitus occurs when a woman not previously diagnosed with diabetes shows glucose intolerance during pregnancy. This may occur if placental hormones counteract insulin, causing insulin resistance. Gestational diabetes mellitus is a significant risk factor for the future occurrence of type 2 diabetes mellitus.

Assessment findings

The most common symptom of diabetes is fatigue from energy deficiency and a catabolic stage. Insulin deficiency causes hyperglycemia, which pulls fluid from body tissues, causing polyuria, dehydration, polydipsia, dry mucous membranes, poor skin turgor and, in most patients, unexplained weight loss. Other signs and symptoms may include anorexia and occasional polyphagia. Electrolyte imbalances may lead to muscle cramps, irritability, and emotional lability. The patient with peripheral neuropathy may experience numbness or pain in the hands and feet. The patient with autonomic neuropathy may develop gastroparesis (leading to delayed gastric emptying and a feeling of nausea and fullness after meals), nocturnal diarrhea, impotence, and orthostatic hypotension.

In diabetic ketoacidosis (DKA) and hyperosmolar hyperglycemic nonketotic syndrome (HHNS), dehydration may lead to hypovolemia and shock. (See *Understanding the difference between DKA and HHNS,* page 130.)

Diagnosis

○ According to the American Diabetes Association (ADA), DM can be diagnosed if any of the following exist:
– symptoms of diabetes (polyuria, polydipsia, and unexplained weight loss) plus a random (nonfasting) blood glucose level greater than or

Understanding the difference between DKA and HHNS

Diabetic ketoacidosis (DKA) and hyperosmolar hyperglycemic nonketotic syndrome (HHNS), both acute complications associated with diabetes, share some similarities, but they're two distinct conditions. Use the flowchart below to help determine which condition your patient is experiencing.

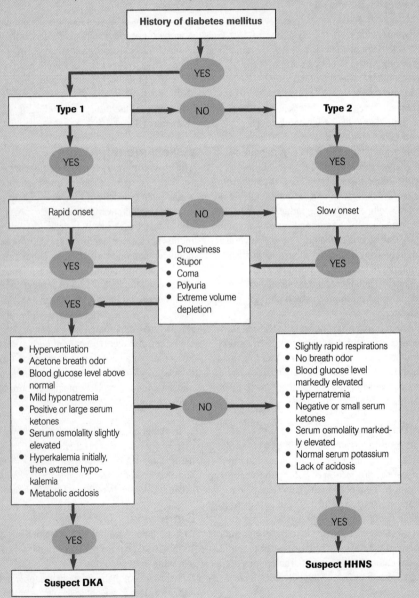

equal to 200 mg/dl accompanied by symptoms of diabetes.
– a fasting blood glucose level (no caloric intake for at least 8 hours) greater than or equal to 126 mg/dl.
– a plasma glucose value in the 2-hour sample of the oral glucose tolerance test greater than or equal to 200 mg/dl. This test should be performed after a glucose load dose of 75 g of anhydrous glucose.
○ The fasting plasma glucose test or the oral glucose tolerance test may be used to make the diagnosis of diabetes. The ADA recommends the fasting plasma glucose test because it's easier and faster to perform and less expensive than the oral glucose tolerance test. (See *Classifying blood glucose levels*.) If results are questionable, the diagnosis should be confirmed by a repeat test on a different day. The ADA also recommends the following testing guidelines:
– Test every 3 years: people age 45 or older without symptoms
– Test immediately: people with the classic symptoms
– Frequent testing for patients in high-risk groups: Individuals with impaired glucose tolerance may have normal blood glucose levels unless challenged by a glucose load. If the 2-hour blood glucose level is 200 mg/dl or above, the person tested would be diagnosed with diabetes.
○ Ophthalmologic examination that may detect diabetic retinopathy.
○ Other diagnostic and monitoring tests include blood testing for glycosylated hemoglobin (A_{1c}), which reflects serum glucose levels over a 3-month period, and urinalysis for acetone.

Complications
○ Chronic renal failure
○ DKA
○ Dyslipidemia
○ Excessive weight gain
○ HHNS
○ Impaired resistance to infection

Classifying blood glucose levels

The American Diabetes Association classifies fasting blood glucose levels as follows:
● Normal: less than 100 mg/dl
● Impaired fasting glucose: 100 to 125 mg/dl
● Diabetes: 126 mg/dl or more, confirmed by repeat test on another day.

○ Macrovascular disease, including coronary, peripheral, and cerebral artery disease
○ Microvascular disease, including retinopathy, nephropathy, and neuropathy
○ Skin ulcerations

Treatment
○ Insulin replacement, meal planning, and exercise are recommended for the patient with type 1 diabetes. (Current forms of insulin replacement include single-dose, mixed-dose, split-mixed dose, and multiple-dose regimens by injection or insulin pump.)
○ Pancreas transplantation is a treatment option for type 1 diabetes and requires chronic immunosuppression.
○ Diet is specifically tailored to include the right amount and combination of foods with weight reduction (for the obese patient with type 2 diabetes) or high-calorie allotment, depending on growth stage and activity level (for type 2 diabetes).
○ Oral antidiabetic medication (including sulfonylureas, meglitinides, biguanides, alpha-glucosidase inhibitors, and thiazolidinediones) may be required in type 2 diabetes to stimulate endogenous insulin production, increase insulin sensitivity at the cellular level, and suppress hepatic gluconeogenesis.
○ Treatment of long-term diabetic complications includes transplantation or dialysis for renal failure, photocoagulation for retinopathy, and vascular surgery for large-vessel disease; meticulous blood glucose control is essential.

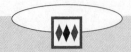

KEY TEACHING POINTS

Teaching about diabetes mellitus

Remember these key points when teaching your patient and his family about diabetes mellitus:

• Teach about the pathology underlying Type 1 or Type 2 diabetes.

• Discuss the prevention and treatment of acute and chronic complications of diabetes.

• Urge regular ophthalmologic examinations to detect diabetic retinopathy.

• Teach the patient about his individualized meal plan.

• Stress the importance of complying with the prescribed treatment program.

• Teach about prescribed antidiabetic medications, their names, indications, dosages, adverse effects, and special considerations.

• Stress the need for personal safety precautions because decreased sensation can mask injuries.

• Teach the patient how to care for his feet properly and urge him to report any changes to his primary health care provider. Advise the patient to have the podiatrist cut his toenails.

• Teach the patient how to manage his diabetes when he has a minor illness, such as a cold, flu, or upset stomach.

• To delay the clinical onset of diabetes, teach people at high risk to control modifiable risk factors. Advise genetic counseling for young adult diabetic patients who are planning families.

• Explain the importance of home blood glucose monitoring and demonstrate how to perform this procedure. Stress the effect of blood glucose control on long-term health.

• Teach the patient to keep a record of his glucose results.

○ Blood pressure control as well as smoking cessation in patients with type 2 diabetes reduces the onset and progression of complications, including cardiovascular disease.

 COLLABORATIVE MANAGEMENT
Care of the patient with DM involves several members of the interdisciplinary team. An interdisciplinary approach is vital to helping the patient normalize blood glucose levels and decrease complications through the use of insulin replacement, diet, and exercise. The primary health care provider monitors blood glucose levels and takes measures to prevent and treat complications. The nurse educates the patient about diabetes and self-care behaviors and monitors for complications. The dietitian helps the patient develop an individualized meal plan for his medical condition, weight, and lifestyle. The social worker assists with financial problems and obtaining supplies, and may provide counseling to help the patient and family cope with this chronic illness. The podiatrist provides foot examinations and care. The ophthalmologist monitors for retinopathy. The occupational therapist helps the patient with problems due to retinopathy, neuropathy, and peripheral vascular disease.

Special considerations

○ Watch for acute complications of diabetic therapy, especially hypoglycemia (vagueness, slow cerebration, dizziness, weakness, pallor, tachycardia, diaphoresis, seizures, and coma); immediately give carbohydrates, ideally in the form of fruit juice, glucose tablets, honey or, if the patient is unconscious, glucagon or dextrose I.V.

○ Be alert for signs of ketoacidosis (acetone breath, dehydration, weak and rapid pulse, and Kussmaul's respirations) and hyperosmolar coma (polyuria, thirst, neurologic abnormalities, and stupor). These hyperglycemic crises require I.V. fluids, insulin and, usually, potassium replacement.

○ Monitor diabetes control by obtaining blood glucose, glycohemoglobin, lipid levels, and blood pressure measurements regularly.

○ Minimize complications by maintaining strict blood glucose control.

○ Watch for diabetic effects on the cardiovascular system, such as cerebrovascular, coronary artery, and peripheral vascular impairment, and on the peripheral and autonomic nervous systems.

○ Treat all injuries, cuts, and blisters (particularly on the legs or feet) meticulously.

○ Be alert for signs of urinary tract infection and renal disease.

○ Assess for signs of diabetic neuropathy (numbness or pain in hands and feet, footdrop, neurogenic bladder).

○ Provide patient education. (See *Teaching about diabetes mellitus.*)

Applicable patient-teaching aids

○ Care and prevention of leg ulcers *
○ Coping with depression
○ Getting ready for an oral glucose tolerance test
○ Giving yourself a subcutaneous insulin injection *
○ Keeping a food diary *
○ Learning about daily food choices
○ Managing diabetes during illness
○ Mixing insulins in a syringe *
○ Preventing diabetic complications *
○ Taking care of your feet in diabetes *
○ Taking steps towards healthier legs
○ Testing your blood glucose level
○ Testing your urine for ketones
○ Travel tips for diabetic patients

Diverticular disease

In diverticular disease, bulging pouches (diverticula) in the GI wall push the mucosal lining through the surrounding muscle. The most common site for diverticula is in the sigmoid colon, but they may develop anywhere, from the proximal end of the pharynx to the anus. Other typical sites are the duodenum, near the pancreatic border or the ampulla of Vater, and the jejunum. Diverticular disease of the stomach is rare and is usually a precursor of peptic or neoplastic disease. Diverticular disease of the ileum (Meckel's diverticulum) is the most common congenital anomaly of the GI tract.

Diverticular disease has two clinical forms. In *diverticulosis,* diverticula are present but don't cause symptoms. In *diverticulitis,* diverticula are inflamed and may cause potentially fatal obstruction, infection, or hemorrhage.

The incidence of diverticular disease increases with age, but 20% of patients are younger than age 50. Right-sided diverticulitis is most common in Asians, accounting for 75% of cases in that ethnic group. Left-sided diverticulitis is more common in Western countries, where it accounts for 70% of cases.

Causes

Diverticula probably result from high intraluminal pressure on areas of weakness in the GI wall, where blood vessels enter. Diet may also be a contributing factor because insufficient fiber reduces fecal residue, narrows the bowel lumen, and leads to higher intra-abdominal pressure during defecation. The prevalence of diverticulosis in Western industrialized nations, where processing removes much of the roughage from foods, supports this theory.

Pathophysiology

In diverticulitis, retained undigested food mixed with bacteria accumulates in the diverticular sac, forming a hard mass (fecalith). This substance cuts off the blood supply to the thin walls of the sac, making them more susceptible to attack by colonic bacteria. Inflammation follows, possibly leading to perforation, abscess, peritonitis, obstruction, or hemorrhage. Occasionally, the inflamed colon segment may produce a fistula by adhering to the bladder or other organs. (See *How diverticular disease develops,* page 134.)

Assessment findings

Diverticulosis usually produces no symptoms, but it may cause recurrent left lower quadrant pain, which is commonly accompanied by alternating constipation and diarrhea and is relieved by defecation or the passage of flatus. Mild diverticulitis produces moderate left lower abdominal pain, mild nausea, gas, irregular bowel habits, low-grade fever, and leukocytosis. Severe diverticulitis produces signs and symptoms of rupture, such as abdominal rigidi-

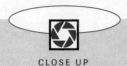

CLOSE UP

How diverticular disease develops

Diverticula probably result from high intraluminal pressure on an area of weakness in the GI wall, where blood vessels enter.

In diverticulitis, retained undigested food and bacteria accumulate in the diverticular sac. This hard mass cuts off the blood supply to the thin walls of the sac, making them more susceptible to attack by colonic bacteria. Inflammation follows and may lead to perforation, abscess, peritonitis, obstruction, or hemorrhage.

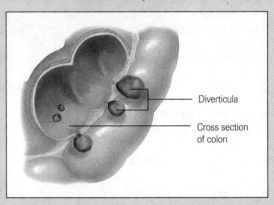

Diverticula

Cross section of colon

---

ty and left lower quadrant pain. The release of fecal material from the rupture site can lead to signs of sepsis and shock, such as high fever, chills, and hypotension. Rupture of diverticulum near a vessel may cause microscopic or massive hemorrhage. (See *Diverticulitis*.)

Chronic diverticulitis may cause fibrosis and adhesions that narrow the bowel's lumen and lead to bowel obstruction. Signs and symptoms of incomplete obstruction include constipation, ribbonlike stools, intermittent diarrhea, and abdominal distention. Increasing obstruction causes abdominal rigidity and pain, diminishing or absent bowel sounds, nausea, and vomiting.

Diagnosis
○ Upper GI series confirms or rules out diverticulosis of the esophagus and upper bowel.
○ Computed tomography reveals areas of inflammation.
○ Colonoscopy and sigmoidoscopy reveal diverticular disease.
○ Barium enema reveals filling of diverticula, which confirms the diagnosis.

○ Biopsy rules out cancer; however, a colonoscopic biopsy isn't recommended during acute diverticular disease because of the strenuous bowel preparation it requires.
○ Blood studies may show an elevated erythrocyte sedimentation rate in diverticulitis, especially if the diverticula are infected.

Complications
○ Fistula
○ Intestinal obstruction
○ Portal pyemia
○ Rectal hemorrhage
○ Ruptured diverticula that cause abdominal abscesses or peritonitis

Treatment
○ Diverticulosis that doesn't produce symptoms generally doesn't necessitate treatment.
○ Liquid or bland diet, stool softeners, and occasional doses of mineral oil may relieve symptoms, minimize irritation, and lessen the risk of progression to diverticulitis.
○ A high-residue diet and bulk medication, such as psyllium, may be given after pain sub-

sides to help decrease intra-abdominal pressure during defecation.

○ Bed rest, a liquid diet, stool softeners, and a broad-spectrum antibiotic (to prevent constipation and combat infection) may be used to treat mild diverticulitis without signs of perforation.

○ Colon resection is necessary to remove the involved segment if diverticulitis is refractory to medical treatment.

 COLLABORATIVE MANAGEMENT
Care of the patient with diverticular disease involves several members of the interdisciplinary team. The primary care provider recommends a treatment plan to reduce intestinal inflammation and prevent complications. If the patient requires surgery, the surgeon performs surgery based on the location and severity of the disease. The nurse educates the patient about the disease, preoperative and postoperative expectations and stoma care (if surgery is necessary), and helps the patient manage symptoms. The enterostomal therapist teaches about care of and adjustment to the stoma, if the patient requires a stoma. The social worker can help with financial issues and in obtaining supplies. The dietitian can assist with nutritional issues and management of GI symptoms.

Special considerations

○ Provide the patient with a diet high in digestible fiber.

○ Monitor the patient's stools carefully for frequency, color, and consistency, and keep accurate pulse and temperature charts because changes may signal developing inflammation or other complications.

After surgery to resect the colon:

○ Watch for signs of infection.

○ Provide meticulous wound care and change dressings as necessary.

○ Check drain sites frequently for signs of infection or fecal drainage.

○ Encourage coughing and deep breathing to prevent atelectasis.

○ Watch for signs of postoperative bleeding.

○ Document intake and output accurately.

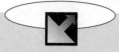

ACUTE EPISODE

Diverticulitis

If your patient presents with an acute episode of diverticulitis, take these steps:

● Administer I.V. fluids to prevent dehydration and replace electrolytes, as indicated; administer nothing by mouth.

● Monitor vital signs and intake and output.

● Observe for signs of shock, such as pallor, rapid pulse, and hypotension.

● To lessen pain, place the patient in semi-Fowler's position and medicate as ordered.

● Document the amount and color of nasogastric drainage, if a nasogastric tube was placed.

● If the patient has signs or symptoms of intestinal hemorrhage, prepare to administer blood component therapy.

● If diverticular bleeding occurs, prepare the patient for angiography and catheter placement for vasopressin infusion.

● Following angiography, inspect the insertion site frequently for bleeding, check pedal pulses often, and keep the patient from flexing his legs at the groin.

● Monitor the patient for vasopressin-induced fluid retention (apprehension, abdominal cramps, convulsions, oliguria, or anuria) and severe hyponatremia (hypotension; rapid, thready pulse; cold, clammy skin; and cyanosis).

● Monitor for signs and symptoms of perforation, peritonitis, obstruction, or fistula.

● Anticipate the need for a temporary colostomy to drain abscesses and rest the colon, followed by reanastomosis 6 weeks to 3 months after initial surgery.

○ Keep the nasogastric tube patent.

○ Arrange for a visit by an enterostomal therapist, who will provide ostomy care teaching and schedule a follow-up visit after the patient's discharge from the facility.

○ Provide patient education. (See *Teaching about diverticular disease,* page 136.)

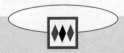

KEY TEACHING POINTS

Teaching about diverticular disease

Remember these key points when teaching your patient and his family about diverticular disease:

• Teach about the disease process and its treatments.

• Reinforce the importance of dietary fiber and the harmful effects of constipation and straining during defecation.

• Encourage increased intake of foods high in indigestible fiber, including fresh fruits and vegetables, whole grain bread, and wheat or bran cereals.

• Warn that a high-fiber diet may temporarily cause flatulence and discomfort.

• Advise the patient to relieve constipation with stool softeners or bulk-forming cathartics.

• Teach about prescribed medications, including their names, indications, dosages, adverse effects, and special considerations.

• Discuss warning signs of complications, such as obstruction, infection, and hemorrhage, and the need to seek immediate medical attention if they occur.

• If the patient is having surgery, explain surgical procedures and refer him to an enterostomal therapist.

Applicable patient-teaching aids

○ Adding fiber to your diet *
○ Learning about daily food choices
○ Preparing for a barium enema test
○ Preparing for a sigmoidoscopy or a colonoscopy *
○ Testing your stool for blood

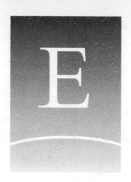

Emphysema

Emphysema, a form of chronic obstructive pulmonary disease, is the abnormal, permanent enlargement of the acini accompanied by destruction of alveolar walls. Its distinguishing characteristic is airflow limitation caused by lack of elastic recoil in the lungs. Obstruction results from tissue changes rather than mucus production, which occurs with asthma and chronic bronchitis.

Emphysema appears to be more prevalent in males than in females; about 65% of patients with well-defined emphysema are men and 35% are women.

Causes

Cigarette smoking is the primary cause of emphysema. However, it may also be caused by a deficiency of alpha$_1$-antitrypsin (AAT), a protein necessary for lung protection. In this autosomal recessive trait, homozygous individuals have up to an 80% chance of developing lung disease; people who smoke have a greater chance of developing emphysema.

Patients who develop emphysema before or during their early 40s and those who are nonsmokers are believed to have an AAT deficiency.

Pathophysiology

In emphysema, recurrent inflammation is associated with the release of proteolytic enzymes from lung cells. This causes irreversible enlargement of the air spaces distal to the terminal bronchioles. Enlargement of air spaces destroys the alveolar walls, which results in a breakdown of elasticity and loss of fibrous and muscle tissue, thus making the lungs less compliant.

In patients with emphysema, recurrent pulmonary inflammation damages and eventually destroys the alveolar walls, creating large air spaces. The alveolar septa are initially destroyed, eliminating a portion of the capillary bed and increasing air volume in the acinus. This breakdown leaves the alveoli unable to recoil normally after expanding and results in bronchiolar collapse on expiration. The damaged or destroyed alveolar walls can't support the airways to keep them open. The amount of air that can be expired passively is diminished, thus trapping air in the lungs and leading to overdistention.

Hyperinflation of the alveoli produces bullae (air spaces) adjacent to the pleura (blebs). Septal destruction also decreases airway calibration. Part of each inspiration is trapped because of increased residual volume and decreased calibration. Septal destruction may affect only the respiratory bronchioles and alveolar ducts, leaving alveolar sacs intact (centriacinar emphysema), or it can involve the entire acinus (panacinar emphysema), producing damage that's more random and involves the lower lobes of the lungs. (See *Understanding emphysema,* page 138.)

Associated pulmonary capillary destruction usually allows a patient with severe emphysema to match ventilation to perfusion. This process prevents the development of cyanosis. The lungs are usually enlarged; therefore, the total lung capacity and residual volume increase.

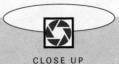

CLOSE UP

Understanding emphysema

In the patient with emphysema, recurrent pulmonary inflammation damages and eventually destroys the alveolar walls, creating large air spaces. The damaged alveoli can't recoil normally after expanding; therefore, bronchioles collapse.

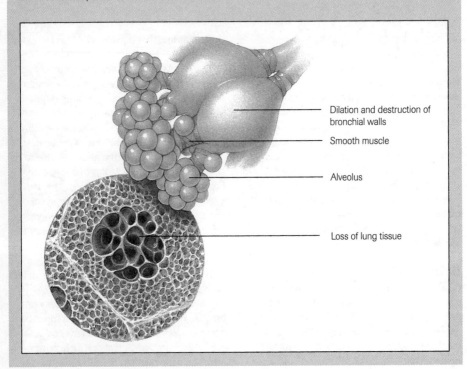

Dilation and destruction of bronchial walls

Smooth muscle

Alveolus

Loss of lung tissue

Assessment findings

Tachypnea and dyspnea on exertion are the most common findings in emphysema. Other findings include a barrel-shaped chest due to overdistention and overinflation of the lungs and prolonged expiration and grunting due to the use of accessory muscles for inspiration and abdominal muscles for expiration. The patient may also develop crackles, wheezing, decreased breath sounds, and decreased chest expansion. Palpation may reveal decreased tactile fremitus. Chest percussion may reveal hy-

perresonance. Chronic hypoxic changes may result in clubbed fingers and toes.

Diagnosis

○ Chest X-rays in advanced disease may show a flattened diaphragm, reduced vascular markings at the lung periphery, overaeration of the lungs, a vertical heart, enlarged anteroposterior chest diameter, and a large retrosternal air space.

○ Pulmonary function studies indicate increased residual volume and total lung capacity, reduced diffusing capacity, and increased inspiratory flow.

○ Arterial blood gas analysis usually reveals reduced partial pressure of arterial oxygen and a normal partial pressure of arterial carbon dioxide until late in the disease process, when carbon dioxide levels increase.

○ Electrocardiography may show tall, symmetrical P waves in leads II, III, and aV_F; a vertical QRS axis and signs of right ventricular hypertrophy are seen late in the disease.

○ Complete blood count usually reveals an increased hemoglobin level late in the disease when the patient has persistent, severe hypoxia.

Complications

○ Cor pulmonale
○ Peptic ulcer
○ Pneumomediastinum
○ Recurrent respiratory tract infections
○ Respiratory failure (see *Acute respiratory failure*, page 62)
○ Spontaneous pneumothorax

Treatment

○ Smoking cessation and avoiding air pollutants are the most effective treatments.

○ Antibiotics can be used to treat recurring infections.

○ Bronchodilators, such as beta-adrenergic blockers, albuterol, and ipratropium bromide, may reverse bronchospasms and promote mucociliary clearance.

○ Adequate hydration liquefies secretions and chest physiotherapy mobilizes secretions.

○ Ultrasonic or mechanical nebulizers loosen and mobilize secretions.

○ Aerosolized or systemic corticosteroids may be given to combat inflammation.

○ Diuretics may be used to reduce edema.

○ Oxygen at low settings may be necessary to treat hypoxia; transtracheal catheterization may be used to enable the patient to receive oxygen therapy at home.

○ Chest physiotherapy may help to mobilize secretions.

○ Mucolytics may help to thin secretions and aid in mucus expectoration.

○ Lung volume reduction surgery may be performed for selected patients to allow more functional lung tissue to expand and the diaphragm to return to its normally elevated position.

 COLLABORATIVE MANAGEMENT
Care of the patient with emphysema involves several members of the interdisciplinary team. The nurse typically coordinates the interdisciplinary team while providing education and therapeutic interventions. The physician diagnoses and directs the medical care, and the nurse practitioner may assist in care management. The physical therapist devises a program to promote muscle reconditioning and prevent further loss of muscle strength and tone. The occupational therapist teaches energy conservation techniques. The respiratory therapist performs pulmonary function tests, coordinates the use of oxygen, performs breathing treatments, and teaches the patient cough and breathing techniques. The dietitian assesses the patient's nutritional status and makes recommendations to maintain body weight and muscle mass. The social worker can aid in obtaining medical equipment and with financial difficulties.

Special considerations

○ Evaluate sputum quality and quantity, restlessness, increased tachypnea, and altered breath sounds. Report changes immediately.

○ Perform chest physiotherapy, including postural drainage and chest percussion and vibration for involved lobes, several times daily.

○ Weigh the patient three times weekly, and assess for edema.

○ Provide the patient with a high-calorie, protein-rich diet and offer small, frequent meals to conserve his energy and prevent fatigue.

○ Make sure the patient receives adequate fluids (at least 3 qt [3 L]/day) to loosen secretions.

○ Schedule respiratory therapy at least 1 hour before or after meals and provide mouth care after bronchodilator inhalation therapy.

○ Provide patient education. (See *Teaching about emphysema*, page 140.)

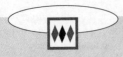

Applicable patient-teaching aids

○ Caring for aerosol equipment
○ Learning about immunization for the flu
○ Learning to do controlled coughing exercises *
○ Performing chest physiotherapy (for an adult)
○ Preparing for pulmonary function tests *
○ Preventing infection with proper hand washing *
○ Using an oral inhaler *

⭕ Endometriosis

Endometriosis is the presence of endometrial tissue outside the lining of the uterine cavity. Such ectopic tissue is generally confined to the pelvic area, most commonly around the ovaries, uterovesical peritoneum, uterosacral ligaments, and cul-de-sac, but it can appear anywhere in the body. This ectopic endometrial tissue responds to normal stimulation in the same way that the endometrium does. During menstruation, the ectopic tissue bleeds, which causes inflammation of the surrounding tissues. This inflammation causes fibrosis, leading to adhesions that produce pain and infertility.

Endometriosis may be classified in stages: Stage I, mild; Stage II, moderate; Stage III, severe; and Stage IV, extensive. Active endometriosis usually occurs between ages 20 and 40; it's uncommon before age 20. Severe symptoms of endometriosis may have an abrupt onset or may develop over many years. This disorder usually becomes progressively severe during the menstrual years; after menopause, it may subside.

Endometriosis occurs in 10% of women during the reproductive years. Prevalence may be as high as 25% to 35% among infertile women. A woman with a mother or sister with endometriosis is six times more likely to develop endometriosis than a woman without this familial history.

Causes

The cause of endometriosis remains unknown. The main theories to explain this disorder (one or more are perhaps true for certain populations of women) include:

○ retrograde menstruation with implantation at ectopic sites (retrograde menstruation alone may not be sufficient for endometriosis to occur because it occurs in women with no clinical evidence of endometriosis)

○ genetic predisposition and depressed immune system (may predispose to endometriosis)

○ coelomic metaplasia (repeated inflammation inducing metaplasia of mesothelial cells to the endometrial epithelium)

○ lymphatic or hematogenous spread (extraperitoneal disease).

Pathophysiology

The ectopic endometrial tissue responds to normal stimulation in the same way as the endometrium, but more unpredictably. The endometrial cells respond to estrogen and progesterone with proliferation and secretion. During menstruation, the ectopic tissue bleeds, which causes inflammation of the surrounding tissues. This inflammation causes fibrosis, leading to adhesions that produce pain and infertility.

Assessment findings

The classic symptom of endometriosis is acquired dysmenorrhea, which may produce constant pain in the lower abdomen and in the vagina, posterior pelvis, and back. This pain usually begins from 5 to 7 days before menses reaches its peak and lasts for 2 to 3 days.

Other clinical features depend on the location of the ectopic tissue:

○ *ovaries and oviducts* — infertility and profuse menses

○ *ovaries or cul-de-sac* — deep-thrust dyspareunia

○ *bladder* — suprapubic pain, dysuria, and hematuria

○ *small bowel and appendix* — nausea and vomiting, which worsen before menses, and abdominal cramps

○ *cervix, vagina, and perineum* — bleeding from endometrial deposits in these areas during menses.

Diagnosis

○ Palpation during pelvic examination may detect multiple tender nodules on uterosacral ligaments or in the rectovaginal septum in one-third of patients; these nodules enlarge and become more tender during menses. Ovarian enlargement in the presence of endometrial cysts on the ovaries or thickened, nodular adnexa (as in pelvic inflammatory disease) may also be noted.

○ Laparoscopy must confirm the diagnosis and determine the disease's stage before treatment is initiated.

Complications

○ Anemia secondary to excessive bleeding

○ Chronic pelvic pain

○ Infertility

○ Ovarian cyst

○ Pelvic adhesions

○ Severe dysmenorrhea

○ Spontaneous abortion

Treatment

Treatment varies according to the disease's stage and the patient's age and desire to have children. Conservative therapy for young women who want to have children includes:

○ androgens, such as danazol, which may produce a temporary remission in Stages I and II

○ progestins and hormonal contraceptives, which may also relieve symptoms

○ gonadotropin-releasing hormone agonists, which induce a pseudomenopause and, thus, a "medical oophorectomy," which may cause a remission of disease

○ surgery, which must rule out cancer when ovarian masses are present. (Conservative surgery includes laparoscopic removal of endometrial implants with conventional or laser techniques and presacral neurectomy for severe dysmenorrhea.)

Total abdominal hysterectomy with bilateral salpingo-oophorectomy is the treatment of choice for women who don't want to bear children or for extensive disease.

Special considerations

○ Because infertility is a possible complication, advise the patient who wants children not to postpone childbearing.

○ Recommend an annual pelvic examination and Papanicolaou test to all patients.

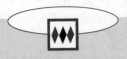

KEY TEACHING POINTS

Teaching about endometriosis

Remember these key points when teaching your patient and her family about endometriosis:
- Teach about the disease process, including its symptoms and treatments.
- Discuss warning signs of complications that require immediate medical attention.
- If the patient is having surgery, explain the surgical procedure and what to expect in the preoperative and postoperative periods.
- Teach about prescribed medications, including their names, indications, dosages, adverse effects, and special considerations.
- Tell the patient to avoid minor gynecological procedures immediately before and during menstruation.
- Caution the patient not to postpone childbearing due to potential for infertility.
- Reinforce the importance of having an annual pelvic examination and Papanicolaou test.

○ Provide patient education. (See *Teaching about endometriosis.*)

Applicable patient-teaching aids
○ Learning about laparoscopy *
○ Preparing for a pelvic exam

Epilepsy

Epilepsy, also called *seizure disorder,* is a condition of the brain marked by a susceptibility to recurrent seizures — paroxysmal events associated with abnormal electrical discharges of neurons in the brain.

Primary epilepsy is idiopathic without apparent structural changes in the brain. Secondary epilepsy, characterized by structural changes or metabolic alterations of the neuronal membranes, causes increased automaticity.

Epilepsy is believed to affect 1% to 2% of the population; approximately 2 million people have been diagnosed with epilepsy. The incidence is highest in childhood and old age. The prognosis is good if the patient adheres strictly to prescribed treatment.

Causes
In about one-half of epilepsy cases, the cause is unknown. However, some possible causes of epilepsy include:
○ anoxia (after respiratory or cardiac arrest)
○ birth trauma (inadequate oxygen supply to the brain, blood incompatibility, or hemorrhage)
○ head injury or trauma
○ infectious diseases (meningitis, encephalitis, or brain abscess)
○ ingestion of toxins (mercury, lead, or carbon monoxide)
○ inherited disorders or degenerative diseases, such as phenylketonuria or tuberous sclerosis
○ metabolic disorders, such as hypoglycemia or hypoparathyroidism
○ perinatal infection
○ stroke (hemorrhage, thrombosis, or embolism)
○ tumors of the brain.

Alcohol withdrawal can cause nonepileptic seizures.

Status epilepticus, a life-threatening, continuous seizure state that can occur in all seizure types, may result from abrupt withdrawal of anticonvulsant medications, hypoxic encephalopathy, acute head trauma, metabolic encephalopathy, or septicemia secondary to encephalitis or meningitis. (See *Status epilepticus.*)

Pathophysiology
Some neurons in the brain may depolarize easily or be hyperexcitable; this epileptogenic focus fires more readily than normal when stimulated. In these neurons, the membrane potential at rest is less negative or inhibitory connections are missing, possibly as a result of decreased gamma-aminobutyric acid activity or localized shifts in electrolytes.

On stimulation, the epileptogenic focus fires and spreads electric current to surrounding

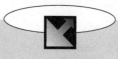

ACUTE EPISODE

Status epilepticus

When treating a patient for status epilepticus, follow these guidelines:

- Establish and maintain the patient's airway, using an oral airway; however, don't force it into the patient's mouth.
- Assist with endotracheal intubation or tracheostomy, if necessary. Administer oxygen and mechanical ventilation, as appropriate.
- Assess oxygen saturation via pulse oximetry and arterial blood gas analysis.
- Administer fast-acting anticonvulsants, such as diazepam or lorazepam I.V., and longer-acting anticonvulsants, such as phenytoin or fosphenytoin (if phenytoin can't be given).
- If phenobarbital is administered as the long-acting agent and it's given at the same time as the fast-acting agent, be alert for respiratory depression and hypotension. Have emergency intubation equipment readily available at the bedside, if it isn't already being used.
- Monitor the patient's response to anticonvulsant drugs.
- Anticipate general anesthesia using pentobarbital, propofol, or midazolam, if anticonvulsant therapy is ineffective. I.V. valproic acid, lidocaine, or neuromuscular blockers may also be used to stop seizure activity if initial treatment is unsuccessful.

- Assess neurological status to establish a baseline and then frequently reassess the patient, at least every 5 to 10 minutes initially, until stabilized.
- Assess respiratory status including rate, depth, and rhythm of respirations.
- Monitor the patient's vital signs every 2 to 3 minutes until stablized.
- Initiate continuous cardiac monitoring to evaluate for arrhythmias.
- Monitor blood glucose levels for hypoglycemia (a possible cause or effect of the patient's continued seizures) and administer glucose, as ordered.
- If alcohol withdrawal is determined to be the underlying cause, administer thiamine I.V. to prevent Wernicke's encephalopathy.
- Institute seizure precautions and ensure the patient's safety with raised, padded side rails, avoidance of restraints, and removal of dangerous objects.

cells. These cells fire in turn, and the impulse cascades to one side of the brain (a partial seizure), both sides of the brain (a generalized seizure), or to the cortical, subcortical, and brain stem areas.

The brain's metabolic demand for oxygen increases dramatically during a seizure. If this demand isn't met, hypoxia and brain damage ensue. Firing of inhibitory neurons causes the excitatory neurons to slow their firing and eventually stop. If this inhibitory action doesn't occur, the result is status epilepticus: one seizure occurring right after another and another; without treatment the anoxia is fatal.

Assessment findings

The hallmarks of epilepsy are recurring seizures, which can be classified as partial or generalized (some patients may be affected by more than one type). Other assessment findings vary with type of seizure. (See *Seizure types*, page 144.)

Diagnosis

○ Clinically, the diagnosis of epilepsy is based on the occurrence of one or more seizures and proof or the assumption that the condition that led to them is still present.

○ Computed tomography (CT) scan or magnetic resonance imaging may indicate abnormalities in internal structures.

○ EEG shows paroxysmal abnormalities and confirms the diagnosis by providing evidence of the continuing tendency to have seizures. A negative EEG doesn't rule out epilepsy because

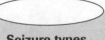

Seizure types

The various types of seizures – partial, generalized, status epilepticus, and unclassified – have distinct signs and symptoms.

Partial seizures

Arising from a localized area of the brain, partial seizures cause focal symptoms. These seizures are classified by their effect on consciousness and whether they spread throughout the motor pathway, causing a generalized seizure.

- A simple partial seizure begins locally and generally doesn't cause an alteration in consciousness. It may present with sensory symptoms (lights flashing, smells, hearing hallucinations), autonomic symptoms (sweating, flushing, pupil dilation), and psychic symptoms (dream states, anger, fear). The seizure lasts for a few seconds and occurs without preceding or provoking events. This type can be motor or sensory.
- A complex partial seizure alters consciousness. Amnesia for events that occur during and immediately after the seizure is a differentiating characteristic. During the seizure, the patient may follow simple commands. This seizure usually lasts for 1 to 3 minutes.

Generalized seizures

As the term suggests, generalized seizures cause a generalized electrical abnormality within the brain. They can be convulsive or nonconvulsive and include several types:

- Absence seizures occur most commonly in children, although they may affect adults. They usually begin with a brief change in level of consciousness, indicated by a blinking or rolling of the eyes, a blank stare, and slight mouth movements. The patient retains his posture and continues preseizure activity without difficulty. Typically, each seizure lasts from 1 to 10 seconds. If not properly treated, seizures can recur as often as 100 times per day. An absence seizure is a nonconvulsive seizure, but it may progress to a generalized tonic-clonic seizure.
- Myoclonic seizures are brief, involuntary muscular jerks of the body or extremities, typically occurring in early morning.
- Clonic seizures are characterized by bilateral rhythmic movements.

- Tonic seizures are characterized by a sudden stiffening of muscle tone, usually of the arms, but possibly including the legs.
- Generalized tonic-clonic seizures typically begin with a loud cry, precipitated by air rushing from the lungs through the vocal cords. The patient then loses consciousness and falls to the ground. The body stiffens (tonic phase) and then alternates between episodes of muscle spasm and relaxation (clonic phase). Tongue biting, incontinence, labored breathing, apnea, and subsequent cyanosis may occur. The seizure stops in 2 to 5 minutes, when abnormal electrical conduction ceases. When the patient regains consciousness, he's confused and may have difficulty talking. If he can talk, he may complain of drowsiness, fatigue, headache, muscle soreness, and arm or leg weakness. He may fall into a deep sleep after the seizure.
- Atonic seizures are characterized by a general loss of postural tone and a temporary loss of consciousness. They occur in young children and are sometimes called "drop attacks" because they cause the child to fall.

Status epilepticus

Status epilepticus is a continuous seizure state that can occur in all seizure types. The most life-threatening example is generalized tonic-clonic status epilepticus, a continuous generalized tonic-clonic seizure. Status epilepticus is accompanied by respiratory distress leading to hypoxia or anoxia. It can result from abrupt withdrawal of anticonvulsant medications, hypoxic encephalopathy, acute head trauma, metabolic encephalopathy, or septicemia secondary to encephalitis or meningitis.

Unclassified seizures

The category of unclassified seizures is reserved for seizures that don't fit the characteristics of partial or generalized seizures or status epilepticus. Included as unclassified are events that lack the data to make a more definitive diagnosis.

the paroxysmal abnormalities occur intermittently.

○ Serum glucose and calcium studies rule out other diagnoses.

○ Skull X-rays may show certain neoplasms within the brain substance or skull fractures.

○ Brain scan may show malignant lesions when X-ray findings are normal or questionable.

○ Cerebral angiography may show cerebrovascular abnormalities, such as aneurysm or tumor.

Complications
○ Anoxia
○ Traumatic injury

Treatment
○ Anticonvulsants, such as phenytoin, carbamazepine, phenobarbital, or primidone are given to treat generalized tonic-clonic seizures and complex partial seizures.

○ Valproic acid, clonazepam, and ethosuximide are commonly prescribed for absence seizures.

○ Surgery to remove a focal lesion may be performed to stop seizures if drug therapy fails.

○ Thiamine I.V. is administered for chronic alcoholism or withdrawal.

○ A vagus nerve stimulator implant may reduce the incidence of partial seizures in patients whose seizures aren't controlled with medication.

 COLLABORATIVE MANAGEMENT
Care of the patient with epilepsy involves several members of the interdisciplinary team. The neurologist diagnoses the problem and determines and monitors the treatment plan. The social worker promotes patient adherence to the drug regimen, assists with making lifestyle restrictions, and helps the patient cope with financial problems. The nurse educates the patient and his family about the disorder, monitors the effects of the therapeutic plan, and helps the patient to make lifestyle modifications.

KEY TEACHING POINTS

Teaching about epilepsy

Remember these key points when teaching your patient and his family about epilepsy:

● Teach about the disease process, including its signs and symptoms, complications, and treatments.

● Teach about prescribed medications, including their names, indications, dosages, frequencies, and special considerations.

● Stress the need for compliance with the prescribed drug schedule.

● Warn against possible adverse effects that should be reported immediately — drowsiness, lethargy, hyperactivity, confusion, and vision and sleep disturbances — all of which indicate the need for dosage adjustment. Instruct the patient to report adverse effects immediately.

● Emphasize the importance of having anticonvulsant blood levels checked at regular intervals, even if the seizures are under control.

● Warn the patient against drinking alcoholic beverages.

● Provide preoperative and postoperative teaching, if the patient will be having surgery.

● Discuss warning signs and symptoms of complications that require immediate medical attention.

● Review any activity restrictions, such as driving, if applicable.

● Discuss safety procedures with the patient if he feels a seizure is imminent.

● Teach the patient's family members how to protect the patient from injury and aspiration during a seizure and to observe and report the seizure activity.

● Stress the importance of wearing a medical identification bracelet.

Special considerations
○ Monitor the patient taking anticonvulsant drugs for toxic signs, including nystagmus, ataxia, lethargy, dizziness, drowsiness, slurred speech, irritability, nausea, and vomiting.

○ Encourage the patient and his family to express their feelings about the patient's condition.

○ When administering phenytoin I.V., use a large vein and monitor vital signs frequently. Avoid I.M. administration and mixing with dextrose solutions.

○ Refer the patient to the Epilepsy Foundation of America for general information and to the state motor vehicle department for information on how his disorder may affect his driving privileges.

○ After a seizure subsides, reassure the patient that he's all right, orient him to time and place, and inform him that he's had a seizure.

○ Provide patient education. (See *Teaching about epilepsy*, page 145.)

Applicable patient-teaching aids

○ Helping a seizure victim *
○ Preparing for a CT scan *
○ Taking phenytoin
○ Understanding seizures and your child *

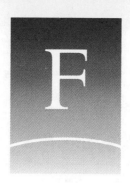

Fibromyalgia syndrome

Fibromyalgia syndrome (FMS), previously called *fibrositis,* is one of the most common causes of chronic musculoskeletal pain. A diffuse pain syndrome, its marked by multiple tender points in specific areas. (See *Tender points of fibromyalgia,* page 148.)

FMS is observed in up to 15% of patients seen in general rheumatology practice and 5% of patients seen in general medical clinics. Women are affected much more commonly than men, and although FMS can affect all age-groups, its peak incidence is between ages 20 and 60.

Causes

FMS may occur as a primary disorder or in association with an underlying disease, such as systemic lupus erythematosus, rheumatoid arthritis, osteoarthritis, sleep apnea syndrome, and neck trauma.

Pathophysiology

The exact pathophysiology of FMS isn't clear. Although the pain associated with FMS is located primarily in muscle areas, no distinct abnormalities have been documented on microscopic evaluation of biopsies of tender points when compared to normal muscle. Theories explaining FMS include decreased blood flow to muscle tissue (due to poor muscle aerobic conditioning versus other physiologic abnormalities); decreased blood flow in the thalamus and caudate nucleus, leading to a lowering of the pain threshold; endocrine dysfunction, such as ab-

normal pituitary-adrenal axis responses; and abnormal levels of the neurotransmitter serotonin in brain centers, affecting pain and sleep. Abnormal functioning of other pain-processing pathways may also be involved.

Considerable overlap of symptoms with other pain syndromes, such as chronic fatigue syndrome, raises the question of an association with an infection, such as with parvovirus B19. Human immunodeficiency virus infection and Lyme disease have also been associated with FMS.

It's possible that the development of FMS is multifactorial and is influenced by stress (physical and mental), physical conditioning, and quality of sleep as well as neuroendocrine, psychiatric and, possibly, hormonal factors (because of the female predominance).

Assessment findings

The primary symptom of fibromyalgia is diffuse, dull, aching pain that's typically concentrated across the neck, shoulders, lower back, and proximal limbs. It's typically worse in the morning and sometimes accompanied by stiffness, and it can vary from day to day and be exacerbated by stress, lack of sleep, weather changes, and inactivity. In patients who have an underlying illness, such as osteoarthritis and rheumatoid arthritis, sleep disturbances with frequent arousal and fragmented sleep or frequent waking throughout the night may develop secondary to pain. Other findings include irritable bowel syndrome, tension headaches, "puffy hands" (sensation of hand swelling, especially in the morning), and paresthesia.

147

Tender points of fibromyalgia

The patient with fibromyalgia syndrome may complain of specific areas of tenderness, which are shown in the illustrations below.

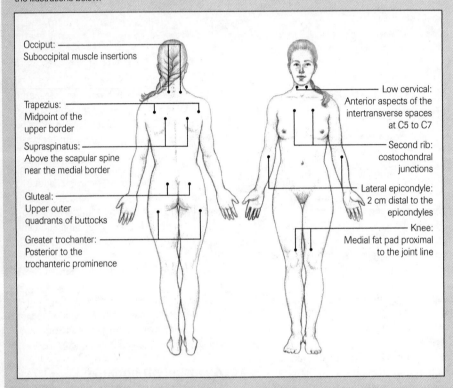

Occiput:
Suboccipital muscle insertions

Trapezius:
Midpoint of the
upper border

Supraspinatus:
Above the scapular spine
near the medial border

Gluteal:
Upper outer
quadrants of buttocks

Greater trochanter:
Posterior to the
trochanteric prominence

Low cervical:
Anterior aspects of the
intertransverse spaces
at C5 to C7

Second rib:
costochondral
junctions

Lateral epicondyle:
2 cm distal to the
epicondyles

Knee:
Medial fat pad proximal
to the joint line

Diagnosis

○ Diagnostic testing for FMS not associated with an underlying disease doesn't usually reveal significant abnormalities.
○ Pain that has lasted for at least 3 months and pain with palpation at 11 of 18 tender points indicates FMS.

Complications

○ Depression
○ Pain
○ Sleep deprivation

Treatments

○ Low-impact aerobic exercise can improve muscle conditioning, energy levels, and an overall sense of well-being. Exercise should be combined with preexercise and postexercise stretching to minimize injury.
○ Steroids or lidocaine, massage therapy, and ultrasound treatments may be helpful for problematic areas. Acupuncture, phototherapy, yoga, and tai chi may also be helpful.
○ Tricyclic antidepressants at bedtime may improve the patient's sleep patterns. A serotonin reuptake inhibitor taken during the day in con-

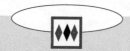

Teaching about fibromyalgia

Remember these key points when teaching your patient and her family about fibromyalgia:

● Teach about the disease process, including its symptoms, complications, and treatments.

● Teach about prescribed medications, including their names, indications, dosages, adverse effects, and special considerations.

● Advise the patient taking a tricyclic antidepressant to take the dose 1 to 2 hours before bedtime to improve sleep and reduce morning drowsiness.

● Tell the patient to avoid caffeine and decongestants before bedtime.

● Reassure the patient that although pain can be severe and chronic, it doesn't lead to deforming or life-threatening complications.

● Encourage a program of regular, low-impact aerobic exercise.

● Tell the patient she may feel increased muscle pain when starting a new exercise program and to decrease the duration or intensity if pain occurs.

Special considerations

○ Reassure the patient that FMS is common and, although chronic, can be treated.

○ Monitor the patient's pain level and response to treatment.

○ Provide emotional support and encourage the patient to express her feelings about FMS.

○ Provide patient education. (See *Teaching about fibromyalgia*.)

Applicable patient-teaching aids

○ Performing relaxation breathing exercises *

○ Relaxing your muscles

junction with a tricyclic antidepressant at bedtime may also be useful.

 COLLABORATIVE MANAGEMENT Care of the patient with FMS involves several members of the interdisciplinary team. The primary health care provider diagnoses and monitors the disorder. The nurse provides education, develops a therapeutic relationship, and assists with coping skills. The physical therapist can help the patient develop a low-impact aerobic exercise program with warm-up and cool-down stretches. The occupational therapist provides assistive devices to help the patient maintain independence with activities of daily living.

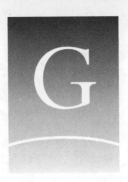

Gastroesophageal reflux disease

Gastroesophageal reflux disease (GERD) refers to the backflow of gastric or duodenal contents, or both, into the esophagus and past the lower esophageal sphincter (LES) without associated belching or vomiting. The reflux may cause symptoms or pathologic changes, and persistent reflux may cause reflux esophagitis (inflammation of the esophageal mucosa). Prognosis varies with the underlying cause.

About 25% to 40% of U.S. residents experience symptom-producing GERD at some point in their lives, while 7% to 10% experience symptoms daily. True incidence figures may be even higher, because many people with GERD take over-the-counter remedies without reporting their symptoms.

Causes

Several predisposing factors for GERD have been identified. Reflux of bile or pancreatic juice into the esophagus may occur following pyloric surgery and lead to the development of GERD. Nasogastric (NG) intubation that lasts for more than 4 days also puts a patient at risk for this disorder. Other risk factors for GERD include agents that lower LES pressure: food, alcohol, cigarettes, anticholinergics (atropine, belladonna, and propantheline), and other medications (morphine, diazepam, calcium channel blockers, and meperidine). An incompetent sphincter in a person with hiatal hernia and any condition or position that increases intra-abdominal pressure, such as straining, bending, coughing, pregnancy, obesity, and recurrent or persistent vomiting, also increases the risk of GERD.

Pathophysiology

The function of the LES—a high-pressure area in the lower esophagus, just above the stomach—is to prevent gastric contents from backing up into the esophagus. Normally, the LES creates pressure, closing the lower end of the esophagus, but relaxing after each swallow to allow food into the stomach. In GERD, the sphincter doesn't remain closed (usually due to deficient LES pressure or pressure within the stomach exceeding LES pressure) and the stomach pushes its contents into the esophagus. (See *How gastroesophageal reflux develops*.)

Assessment findings

The most common feature of GERD is heartburn, which may become more severe with vigorous exercise, bending, or lying down, and may be relieved by antacids or sitting upright. The pain of esophageal spasm resulting from reflux esophagitis tends to be chronic and may mimic angina pectoris, radiating to the neck, jaws, and arms.

Other symptoms include odynophagia, which may be followed by a dull substernal ache from severe, long-term reflux; dysphagia from esophageal spasm, stricture, or esophagitis; and bloody vomitus (bright red or dark brown). Nocturnal regurgitation may waken the patient with coughing, choking, and a mouthful of saliva. Reflux may be associated with hiatal hernia.

Pulmonary symptoms result from reflux of gastric contents into the throat; they include

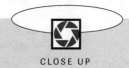

CLOSE UP

How gastroesophageal reflux develops

Hormonal fluctuations, mechanical stress, and the effects of certain foods and medications can decrease lower esophageal sphincter (LES) pressure. When LES pressure falls and intra-abdominal or intragastric pressure rises, the normally contracted LES relaxes inappropriately and allows reflux of gastric acid or bile secretions into the lower esophagus. There, the reflux irritates and inflames the esophageal mucosa, causing pyrosis (heartburn).

Persistent inflammation can cause LES pressure to decrease further, possibly triggering a recurrent cycle of reflux and pyrosis.

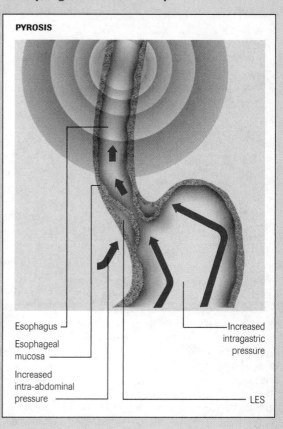

PYROSIS

Esophagus

Esophageal mucosa

Increased intra-abdominal pressure

Increased intragastric pressure

LES

---

chronic cough, hoarseness or nocturnal wheezing, and pulmonary diseases, such as bronchitis and asthma. In children, other signs consist of failure to thrive and forceful vomiting (which can lead to aspiration pneumonia) due to esophageal irritation.

Diagnosis

○ Esophageal acidity test evaluates the competence of the LES and provides objective measure of reflux.

○ Acid perfusion (Bernstein) test can show that reflux is the cause of symptoms.

○ Esophagoscopy allows visual examination of the lining of the esophagus to reveal the extent of the disease and confirm pathologic changes in the mucosa.

○ Barium swallow identifies hiatal hernia or motility problems.

○ Esophageal manometry evaluates resting pressure in the LES and determines sphincter competence.

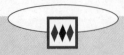

Teaching about GERD

Remember these key points when teaching your patient about gastroesophageal reflux disease (GERD):

● Explain the disease process and its treatments.

● Teach the patient what causes reflux, how to avoid reflux with an antireflux regimen (medication, diet, and positional therapy), and what symptoms to watch for and report.

● Tell the patient he shouldn't eat 2 hours before going to bed.

● Explain the need to elevate the head of the bed 6″ to 8″ (15 to 20 cm).

● Instruct the patient to avoid circumstances that increase intra-abdominal pressure (such as bending, coughing, vigorous exercise, tight clothing, constipation, and obesity) as well as substances that reduce sphincter control (cigarettes, alcohol, fatty foods, and caffeine).

● Advise the patient to sit upright, particularly after meals, and to eat small, frequent meals.

● Tell the patient to avoid highly seasoned food, acidic juices, alcoholic drinks, bedtime snacks, and foods high in fat or carbohydrates, which reduce LES pressure.

● Teach about prescribed medications, including their names, indications, dosages, adverse effects, and special considerations.

● Discuss warning signs and symptoms of complications that require immediate medical attention, such as coughing, choking, and difficulty breathing and swallowing.

● Tell the patient to take antacids, as ordered (usually 1 hour before or 3 hours after meals and at bedtime).

Complications

○ Anemia from esophageal bleeding
○ Barrett's esophagus
○ Esophageal stricture
○ Esophageal ulcer

○ Reflux aspiration leading to chronic pulmonary disease
○ Reflux esophagitis

Treatment

○ Diet therapy consists of a low-fat, high-fiber diet and avoidance of caffeine, alcohol, and carbonated beverages.

○ Position therapy consists of sitting up during and after meals and sleeping with the head of the bed elevated to reduce abdominal pressure and prevent reflux. Positioning is especially useful in infants and children who experience GERD without complications.

○ Proton pump inhibitors or histamine-2 (H$_2$) receptor antagonists help reduce gastric acidity.

○ Antacids neutralize acidic content of the stomach and minimize irritation.

○ Cholinergic agents increase the LES pressure.

○ Smoking cessation improves LES pressure and reduces symptoms of GERD.

○ Surgery, such as hiatal hernia repair, vagotomy or pyloroplasty, esophagectomy, and fundoplication, may be necessary to control severe and refractory symptoms, such as pulmonary aspiration, hemorrhage, obstruction, severe pain, perforation, an incompetent LES, or associated hiatal hernia.

 COLLABORATIVE MANAGEMENT
Care of the patient with GERD involves several members of the interdisciplinary team. The primary care provider diagnoses the disorder and develops the treatment plan. A surgeon may be consulted when symptoms are severe and fail to respond to drug, diet, and position therapy. The nurse educates the patient about the disorder and lifestyle modifications necessary to control symptoms. The dietitian provides the appropriate diet and reinforces the dietary modifications. The counselor or therapist can assist and support the patient in smoking cessation.

Special considerations

○ After surgery using a thoracic approach, carefully watch and record chest tube drainage and the patient's respiratory status. If needed, give chest physiotherapy and oxygen.

○ Position the patient with an NG tube in semi-Fowler's position to help prevent reflux.
○ Offer reassurance and emotional support.
○ Provide patient education. (See *Teaching about GERD*.)

Applicable patient-teaching aids
○ Relieving reflux and heartburn with diet *
○ Taking a proton-pump inhibitor

◯ Glaucoma

Glaucoma is a group of disorders characterized by an abnormally high intraocular pressure (IOP), which can damage the optic nerve. If untreated, it can lead to gradual peripheral vision loss and, ultimately, blindness. It occurs in several forms: chronic open-angle (primary), acute angle-closure, congenital (inherited as an autosomal recessive trait), and secondary to other causes. The prognosis for maintaining vision is good with early treatment.

In the United States, approximately 2.5 million people have been diagnosed with glaucoma; it's estimated that another 1 million people have the disorder but are undiagnosed. Glaucoma accounts for 12% of new cases of blindness in the United States.

Blacks have the highest incidence of glaucoma. It's the single most common cause of blindness in this group.

Causes
Chronic open-angle glaucoma is typically familial in origin and affects 90% of all patients with glaucoma. Diabetes and systemic hypertension have also been associated with this form of glaucoma.

Acute angle-closure (narrow-angle) glaucoma is four times more common in Blacks than Whites, and people with a family history of open-angle glaucoma are twice as likely to develop it as people without a family history of this disorder. The use of systemic anticholinergic medications, such as atropine or eye dilation drops, in a person who's already at high-risk for acute glaucoma increases the risk. Other risk factors include farsightedness and

ACUTE EPISODE

Acute angle-closure glaucoma

Acute angle-closure glaucoma is an ocular emergency requiring immediate treatment to lower high intraocular pressure (IOP). If your patient has acute angle-closure glaucoma, follow these guidelines:
● Administer prescribed medication, as ordered, to reduce IOP. I.V. mannitol (20%) or oral glycerin (50%) reduces IOP by creating an osmotic pressure gradient between the blood and intraocular fluid.
● Administer steroid drops (to reduce inflammation) in combination with latanoprost, a topical medication that helps drain the aqueous outflow from the eye and lower the IOP, as ordered.
● Administer I.V. acetazolamide to reduce IOP by decreasing the formation and secretion of aqueous humor, as ordered.
● Administer pilocarpine to constrict the pupil, thereby forcing the iris away from the trabeculae and allowing fluid to escape, as ordered.
● Administer timolol, a beta-adrenergic blocker, to decrease IOP, as ordered.
● Assess the patient for pain and administer opioid analgesics, as necessary.
● If drug therapy fails to reduce IOP, promptly prepare the patient for laser iridotomy or surgical peripheral iridectomy to release pressure and preserve vision by promoting outflow of aqueous humor. After laser peripheral iridectomy, administer cycloplegic drops, such as apraclonidine, in the affected eye, as ordered, to relax the ciliary muscle and reduce inflammation to prevent adhesions.

age-related changes that create an increase in IOP. (See *Acute angle-closure glaucoma*.)

Congenital glaucoma may be caused by congenital infections such as TORCH virus (*t*oxoplasmosis, *o*ther [varicella, mumps, parvovirus, human immunodeficiency virus], *r*ubella, *c*yto-

Congenital glaucoma

Congenital glaucoma, a rare disease, occurs when a congenital defect in the angle of the anterior chamber obstructs the outflow of aqueous humor. Congenital glaucoma is usually bilateral, with an enlarged cornea that may be cloudy and bulging. Symptoms in a neonate, although difficult to assess, may include tearing, pain, and photophobia.

Untreated, congenital glaucoma causes damage to the optic nerve and blindness. Surgical intervention (such as goniotomy, goniopuncture, trabeculotomy, or trabeculectomy) is necessary to reduce intraocular pressure and prevent vision loss.

megalovirus, and herpes), Sturge-Weber syndrome, or retinopathy of prematurity.

Secondary glaucoma can result from uveitis, trauma, or medications (such as steroids). Neovascularization in the angle can result from vein occlusion or diabetes.

Pathophysiology

Chronic open-angle glaucoma is bilateral, with an insidious onset and a slowly progressive course. It results from overproduction or obstruction of the outflow of aqueous humor through the trabecular meshwork or Schlemm's canal, causing increased IOP and damage to the optic nerve. In secondary glaucoma, conditions such as trauma and surgery increase the risk of obstruction of intraocular fluid outflow caused by edema or other abnormal processes.

Acute angle-closure (narrow-angle) glaucoma typically has a rapid onset, constituting an ophthalmic emergency. It results from obstruction to the outflow of aqueous humor due to anatomically narrow angles between the anterior iris and the posterior corneal surface, shallow anterior chambers, a thickened iris that causes angle closure on pupil dilation, or a bulging iris that presses on the trabeculae, closing the angle (peripheral anterior synechiae).

Any of these may cause IOP to increase suddenly. Unless treated promptly, acute-closure glaucoma produces blindness in 3 to 5 days.

Congenital glaucoma occurs when there is an abnormal fluid drainage angle of the eye. (See *Congenital glaucoma*.)

Assessment findings

Chronic open-angle glaucoma is usually bilateral, with insidious onset. Symptoms appear late in the disease and include halos around lights, loss of peripheral vision, mild aching in the eyes, and reduced visual acuity (especially at night) that isn't correctable with glasses.

Acute angle-closure glaucoma typically has a rapid onset. Symptoms include acute pain in a unilaterally inflamed eye, with pressure over the eye; blurring and decreased visual acuity; a cloudy cornea; halos around lights; moderate pupil dilation that's nonreactive to light; and photophobia. Increased IOP may induce nausea and vomiting, which may cause glaucoma to be misinterpreted as GI distress.

Diagnosis

○ Tonometry (using an applanation tonometer or air puff tonometer) and fingertip tension measure IOP.
○ Slit-lamp examination looks at the anterior structures of the eye: the cornea, iris, and lens.
○ Gonioscopy determines the angle of the anterior chamber of the eye to enable differentiation between chronic open-angle glaucoma and acute angle-closure glaucoma.
○ Ophthalmoscopy may show cupping of the optic disk in chronic open-angle glaucoma; a pale disk suggests acute angle-closure glaucoma.
○ Fundus photography shows optic disk changes.
○ Perimetry or visual field tests reveal the extent of damage to the optic neurons, signaled by an enlarged blind spot and loss of peripheral vision.

Complications

○ Total blindness
○ Varying degrees of vision loss

Treatment

○ Alpha antagonists, such as brimonidine tartrate or apraclonidine, reduce IOP.
○ Beta-adrenergic blockers, such as timolol or betaxolol, reduce aqueous humor production.
○ Anhydrase inhibitors, such as dorzolamide or acetazolamide, decrease the formation and secretion of aqueous humor.
○ Epinephrine reduces IOP by improving aqueous outflow.
○ Prostaglandins, such as latanoprost, reduce IOP.

Patients who are unresponsive to drug therapy may be candidates for surgical procedures:
○ Argon laser trabeculoplasty of the trabecular meshwork of an open angle produces a thermal burn that changes the surface of the meshwork and increases the outflow of aqueous humor.
○ Trabeculectomy (which removes scleral tissue) followed by peripheral iridectomy produces an opening for aqueous outflow under the conjunctiva, creating a filtering bleb.
○ A tuboplast or tube shunt or valve may be used to keep IOP within normal limits.

 COLLABORATIVE MANAGEMENT
Management of the patient with glaucoma requires several members of the interdisciplinary team. The ophthalmologist diagnoses and manages the care of the patient and consults the surgeon when medical therapy can't control IOP. The nurse educates the patient about medication therapy, provides preoperative and postoperative care, and encourages adherence to the treatment plan.

Special considerations

○ For the patient with acute angle-closure glaucoma, give medications as ordered, and prepare him physically and psychologically for laser iridotomy or surgery.
○ Postoperative care after peripheral iridectomy includes cycloplegic eyedrops to relax the ciliary muscle and to decrease inflammation, thus preventing adhesions.
○ Administer cycloplegic medications only in the affected eye. The use of these drops in the normal eye may precipitate an attack of acute

KEY TEACHING POINTS

Teaching about glaucoma

Remember these key points when teaching your patient and his family about glaucoma:
● Teach about the disease process, including its symptoms, complications, and treatments.
● Teach about prescribed medications, including their names, indications, dosages, adverse effects, and special considerations.
● Demonstrate how to administer eye drops properly.
● Stress the importance of meticulous compliance with prescribed drug therapy to prevent an increase in intraocular pressure and loss of vision.
● Reinforce the importance of glaucoma screening for early detection and prevention.
● Tell the patient what to expect before and after surgery, if applicable.
● Teach signs and symptoms that require immediate medical attention, such as sudden vision changes or eye pain.
● Explain that vision loss can't be restored but treatment can usually prevent further loss.

angle-closure glaucoma in this eye, threatening the patient's residual vision.
○ Encourage ambulation immediately after surgery.
○ Following surgical filtering, postoperative care includes dilation and topical steroids to rest the pupil.
○ Provide patient education. (See *Teaching about glaucoma.*)

Applicable patient-teaching aids

○ Administering eyedrops
○ Removing and applying an eye shield *

 # Gout

Gout, also called *gouty arthritis,* is a metabolic disease marked by urate deposits, which cause painfully arthritic joints. It can strike any joint but favors those in the feet and legs. Gout follows an intermittent course and typically leaves patients totally free from symptoms for years between attacks. In the chronic form, it can cause chronic disability or incapacitation, severe hypertension, and progressive renal disease. The prognosis is good with treatment.

Causes

Although the exact cause of primary gout remains unknown, it appears to be linked to a genetic defect in purine metabolism, which causes elevated blood levels of uric acid (hyperuricemia) due to overproduction of uric acid, retention of uric acid, or both. In secondary gout, which develops during the course of another disease (such as obesity, diabetes mellitus, hypertension, sickle cell anemia, and renal disease), hyperuricemia results from the breakdown of nucleic acids. Myeloproliferative and lymphoproliferative diseases, psoriasis, and hemolytic anemia are the most common causes.

Primary gout usually occurs in men and in postmenopausal women; secondary gout occurs in elderly people and can also follow drug therapy that interferes with uric acid excretion. Increased concentration of uric acid leads to urate deposits in joints or tissues and consequent local necrosis or fibrosis.

Pathophysiology

When uric acid becomes supersaturated in blood and other body fluids, it crystallizes and forms a precipitate of urate salts that accumulate in connective tissue throughout the body; these deposits are called *tophi*. The presence of the crystals triggers an acute inflammatory response when neutrophils begin to ingest the crystals. Tissue damage begins when the neutrophils release their lysosomes. The lysosomes not only damage the tissues, but also perpetuate the inflammation.

Assessment findings

Gout develops in four stages: asymptomatic, acute, intercritical, and chronic. Assessment findings vary with the stage. In *asymptomatic gout,* serum urate levels rise. The first attack of

acute gout is extremely painful, peaks quickly, and generally involves only one or a few joints that become hot, tender, inflamed, and appear dusky-red or cyanotic. The metatarsophalangeal joint of the great toe usually becomes inflamed first (podagra), followed by the instep, ankle, heel, knee, or wrist joints. Sometimes, a low-grade fever is present. If the attack is mild, symptoms may subside quickly but recur at regular intervals; if severe, symptoms may persist for days or weeks.

Intercritical periods are the symptom-free intervals between gout attacks. Most patients have a second attack within 6 months to 2 years, but in some the second attack doesn't occur for 5 to 10 years. Delayed attacks are more common in untreated patients and tend to be longer and more severe than initial attacks. Such attacks are also polyarticular, invariably affecting joints in the feet and legs and sometimes accompanied by fever. A migratory attack sequentially strikes various joints and the Achilles tendon and is associated with either subdeltoid or olecranon bursitis.

Chronic gout is marked by persistent, painful polyarthritis, with large, subcutaneous tophi in cartilage, synovial membranes, tendons, and soft tissue. Tophi form in fingers, hands, knees, feet, ulnar sides of the forearms, helix of the ear, Achilles tendons and, rarely, internal organs, such as the kidneys and myocardium. The skin over the tophus may ulcerate and release a chalky, white exudate or pus. (See *Gouty deposits.*)

Diagnosis

○ Monosodium urate monohydrate crystals in synovial fluid taken from an inflamed joint or tophus establishes the diagnosis.
○ Aspiration of synovial fluid (arthrocentesis) or of tophaceous material reveals needlelike intracellular crystals of sodium urate.
○ Serum uric acid is above normal, although hyperuricemia isn't specifically diagnostic of gout.
○ Urinary uric acid is usually higher in secondary gout than in primary gout.
○ Erythrocyte sedimentation rate and white blood cell (WBC) count may be elevated, and

the WBC count differential shows increased immature neutrophils (bands) in acute attacks.
❍ X-rays are normal initially; however, in chronic gout, X-rays show "punched out" erosions, sometimes with periosteal overgrowth. Outward displacement of the overhanging margin from the bone contour characterizes gout.

Complications
❍ Atherosclerotic disease
❍ Cardiovascular lesions
❍ Chronic renal dysfunction
❍ Coronary thrombosis
❍ Hypertension
❍ Infection (when tophi rupture)
❍ Nephrolithiasis
❍ Joint degeneration and deformity
❍ Stroke

Treatment
❍ Maintenance dosage of allopurinol may be given to suppress uric acid formation or control uric acid levels, preventing further attacks (use cautiously in the patient with renal failure).
❍ Colchicine is given to prevent recurrent acute attacks until uric acid returns to its normal level (doesn't affect uric acid level). It's effective in reducing pain, swelling, and inflammation in acute attacks. Other effective therapies include bed rest; immobilization and protection of the inflamed, painful joints; local application of heat or cold; and nonsteroidal anti-inflammatory drugs.
❍ Uricosuric agents (probenecid and sulfinpyrazone) promote uric acid excretion and inhibit accumulation of uric acid, but their value is limited in patients with renal impairment.
❍ Dietary restrictions include the avoidance of alcohol and purine-rich foods, such as organ meats, beer, wine, and certain types of fish.
❍ Obese patients should try to lose weight because obesity puts additional stress on painful joints.
❍ Surgery may be necessary in some cases to improve joint function or correct deformities and to excise and drain infected or ulcerated tophi.

Gouty deposits

The final stage of gout is marked by painful polyarthritis, with large, subcutaneous, tophaceous deposits in cartilage, synovial membranes, tendons, and soft tissue. The skin over the tophus is shiny, thin, and taut.

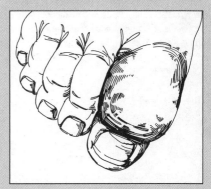

❍ Oral corticosteroids or an intra-articular corticosteroid injection may be ordered to relieve pain due to resistant inflammation.

COLLABORATIVE MANAGEMENT
Care of the patient with gout involves several members of the interdisciplinary team. The primary health care provider diagnoses the disorder and develops the treatment plan. The dietitian makes recommendations for dietary restrictions and weight loss (if the patient is obese). The nurse educates the patient, provides care during acute attacks, and helps identify and institute lifestyle modifications. The physical therapist helps the patient maintain joint function. The occupational therapist provides assistive devices to help the patient carry out activities of daily living.

Special considerations
❍ Encourage bed rest but use a bed cradle to keep bedcovers off extremely sensitive, inflamed joints.
❍ Give pain medication, as needed, especially during acute attacks.

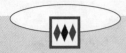

KEY TEACHING POINTS

Teaching about gout

Remember these key points when teaching your patient and his family about gout:

● Teach about the disease process, including its symptoms, complications, and treatments.

● Reinforce the importance of drinking plenty of fluids (up to 2 qt [2 L] per day).

● Discuss warning signs and symptoms of complications that require immediate medical attention.

● Teach relaxation techniques.

● Tell the patient to avoid high-purine foods, such as anchovies, liver, sardines, kidneys, sweetbreads, lentils, and alcoholic beverages — especially beer and wine — which raise the urate level.

● Explain the principles of a gradual weight-reduction diet to the patient who's obese.

● Teach about prescribed medications, including their names, indications, dosages, and special considerations.

● Advise the patient receiving allopurinol, probenecid, or other drugs to immediately report adverse effects, such as drowsiness, dizziness, nausea, vomiting, urinary frequency, and dermatitis.

○ Apply hot or cold packs to inflamed joints according to what the patient finds effective.

○ Administer anti-inflammatory medication and other medications, as ordered.

○ Monitor for adverse effects of medications. Be alert for GI disturbances with colchicine.

○ Watch for acute gout attacks 24 to 96 hours after surgery, because even minor surgery can precipitate an attack. Before and after surgery, administer colchicine as ordered, to help prevent gout attacks.

○ Provide patient education. (See *Teaching about gout*.)

Applicable patient-teaching aids

○ Protecting your joints *

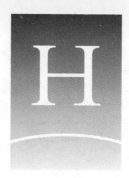

Headache, migraine

The most common patient complaint, headache usually occurs as a symptom of an underlying disorder. Ninety percent of all headaches are vascular, muscle contraction, or a combination; 10% are due to underlying intracranial, systemic, or psychological disorders.

Migraine headaches are throbbing, vascular headaches that usually begin to appear in childhood or adolescence and recur throughout adulthood. Affecting up to 10% of Americans, they're more common in females than in males and have a strong familial influence.

Causes

The exact cause of migraine headaches is unclear. Certain foods have been associated with migraine headache, including aged or processed cheese and meats, alcoholic beverages (particularly red wine), food additives (such as monosodium glutamate), and chocolate- and caffeine-containing foods. Changes in weather pattern, menstrual cycle fluctuations, sleep pattern changes, and too much or too little exercise as well as glaring lights and fatigue can also trigger a migraine headache. In addition, one of the more common causes of a recurring headache is the rebound effect that occurs when the original treatment used to get rid of the headache triggers the next episode.

Pathophysiology

Migraine headaches are believed to be associated with neuronal dysfunction of the trigeminal nerve pathway with secondary constriction and dilation of intracranial and extracranial arteries. During a migraine attack, certain bio-

chemical abnormalities, including local leakage of a vasodilator polypeptide called *neurokinin* through the dilated arteries and a decrease in the plasma level of serotonin, are thought to occur. (See *How migraine headache develops,* page 160.)

Assessment findings

Migraine headaches are commonly preceded by a scintillating scotoma, hemianopsia, unilateral paresthesia, or speech disorders. They initially produce unilateral, pulsating pain, which later becomes more generalized. As the headache progresses, it may produce irritability, anorexia, nausea, vomiting, and photophobia.

Diagnosis

○ History reveals recurrent headaches.
○ Physical examination of the head and neck reveals no other cause for headaches.
○ Skull X-rays, computed tomography, and magnetic resonance imaging are performed to rule out other causes of headaches.

Complications

○ Drug dependency
○ Emotional lability
○ Loss of work
○ Motor weakness
○ Photophobia
○ Worsening of existing hypertension

Treatment

○ 5-HT$_1$ receptor agonists, such as sumatriptan and zolmitriptan, are the abortive medications of choice for an acute migraine attack.

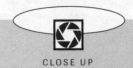

CLOSE UP

How migraine headache develops

Migraine headaches are thought to be associated with constriction and dilation of intracranial and extracranial arteries. Neurogenic inflammation can cause local vasoconstriction of innervated cerebral arteries and reduced cerebral blood flow. This causes compensatory vasodilation and biochemical abnormalities, including local leakage of neurokinin through dilated arteries and decreased plasma level of serotonin.

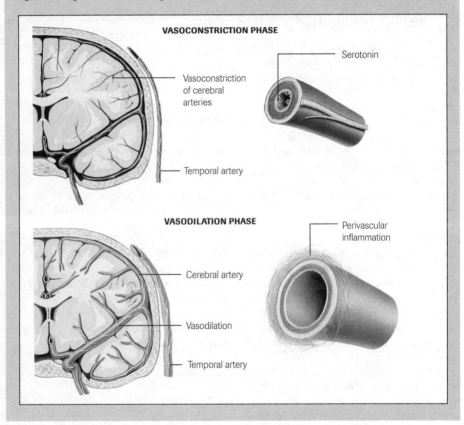

○ Ergotamine, alone or with caffeine, may be an effective treatment when taken early in the course of a migraine.
○ Nonsteroidal anti-inflammatory drugs, alone or in combination with drugs such as caffeine ergotamines, may be used for abortive measures.
○ Propranolol, atenolol, clonidine, and amitriptyline may also prevent migraines.

○ Antiemetics are given when nausea and vomiting accompany migraine headache.
○ Identification and elimination of causative factors may reduce or prevent migraine headaches.

 COLLABORATIVE MANAGEMENT
Care of the patient with migraine headaches involves several members of the interdisciplinary team. The primary care

KEY TEACHING POINTS

Teaching about migraine headache

Remember these key points when teaching your patient about migraine headache:

● Teach about the disease process, including its symptoms, complications, and treatments.

● Teach about prescribed medications, including their names, indications, dosages, adverse effects, and special considerations.

● Review possible triggers with the patient, including stress, hormonal changes, environmental factors, and dietary factors, and help her to develop a lifestyle modification plan to reduce these triggers.

● Encourage the patient to keep a headache log to help pinpoint individual triggers.

● Discuss nonpharmacologic strategies to prevent or abort migraines, such as relaxation techniques or biofeedback training.

provider or neurologist develops the care plan. The nurse educates the patient about preventing and managing migraine headaches. A cognitive-behavioral therapist teaches the patient relaxation techniques that may be useful in preventing migraines.

Special considerations

○ Help the patient identify exacerbating or triggering factors for migraine headaches and to develop a plan to reduce these triggers.

○ During a migraine headache, have the patient lie down in a dark, quiet room and place a cold pack or cloth on her forehead or over her eyes.

○ Avoid repeated use of opioids if possible.

○ Administer the prescribed preventative and abortive drugs, as indicated.

○ Refer the patient to the National Headache Foundation.

○ Provide patient education. (See *Teaching about migraine headache.*)

Applicable patient-teaching aids

○ Keeping a headache log *

○ Preventing vascular headaches through diet

◯ Heart failure

Heart failure is a syndrome characterized by myocardial dysfunction that leads to impaired pump performance (diminished cardiac output) or to frank heart failure and abnormal circulatory congestion. Congestion of systemic venous circulation may result in peripheral edema or hepatomegaly; congestion of pulmonary circulation may cause pulmonary edema. Pump failure usually occurs in a damaged left ventricle (left-sided heart failure) but may occur in the right ventricle (right-sided heart failure) either as a primary disorder or secondary to left-sided heart failure. Sometimes, left- and right-sided heart failure develop simultaneously.

Although heart failure may be acute (as a direct result of myocardial infarction [MI]), it's generally a chronic disorder associated with sodium and water retention by the kidneys. Advances in diagnostic and therapeutic techniques have greatly improved the outlook for patients with heart failure, but the prognosis still depends on the underlying cause and its response to treatment.

Heart failure affects approximately 2 of every 100 people between ages 27 and 74. It becomes more common with advancing age.

Causes

Causes of heart failure may be divided into four general categories: abnormal cardiac muscle function, abnormal left ventricular volume, abnormal left ventricular pressure, and abnormal left ventricular filling. (See *Causes of heart failure,* page 162.)

Pathophysiology

Heart failure may be classified according to the side of the heart affected (left- or right-sided heart failure) or by the cardiac cycle involved (systolic or diastolic dysfunction). (See *Understanding heart failure,* page 163.)

Left-sided heart failure occurs as a result of ineffective left ventricular contractile function.

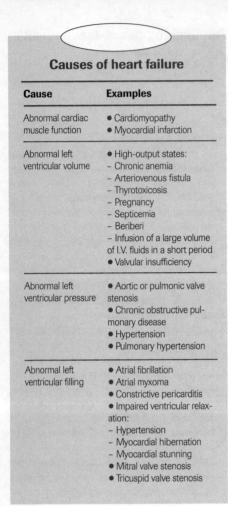

Causes of heart failure

Cause	Examples
Abnormal cardiac muscle function	• Cardiomyopathy • Myocardial infarction
Abnormal left ventricular volume	• High-output states: – Chronic anemia – Arteriovenous fistula – Thyrotoxicosis – Pregnancy – Septicemia – Beriberi – Infusion of a large volume of I.V. fluids in a short period • Valvular insufficiency
Abnormal left ventricular pressure	• Aortic or pulmonic valve stenosis • Chronic obstructive pulmonary disease • Hypertension • Pulmonary hypertension
Abnormal left ventricular filling	• Atrial fibrillation • Atrial myxoma • Constrictive pericarditis • Impaired ventricular relaxation: – Hypertension – Myocardial hibernation – Myocardial stunning • Mitral valve stenosis • Tricuspid valve stenosis

As the pumping ability of the left ventricle fails, cardiac output falls. Blood is no longer effectively pumped out into the body; it backs up into the left atrium and then into the lungs, causing pulmonary congestion, dyspnea, and activity intolerance. If the condition persists, pulmonary edema and right-sided heart failure may result. Common causes include left ventricular infarction, hypertension, and aortic and mitral valve stenosis.

Right-sided heart failure results from ineffective right ventricular contractile function. Consequently, blood isn't pumped effectively through the right ventricle to the lungs, causing

blood to back up into the right atrium and the peripheral circulation. The patient gains weight and develops peripheral edema and engorgement of the kidney and other organs. It may be due to an acute right ventricular infarction, pulmonary hypertension, or a pulmonary embolus. However, the most common cause is profound backward blood flow due to left-sided heart failure.

Systolic dysfunction occurs when the left ventricle can't pump enough blood out to the systemic circulation during systole and the ejection fraction falls. Consequently, blood backs up into the pulmonary circulation and pressure increases in the pulmonary venous system. Cardiac output falls; weakness, fatigue, and shortness of breath may occur. Causes of systolic dysfunction include MI and dilated cardiomyopathy.

Diastolic dysfunction occurs when the ability of the left ventricle to relax and fill during diastole is reduced and the stroke volume falls. Therefore, higher volumes are needed in the ventricles to maintain cardiac output. Consequently, pulmonary congestion and peripheral edema develop. Diastolic dysfunction may occur as a result of left ventricular hypertrophy, hypertension, or restrictive cardiomyopathy. This type of heart failure is less common than systolic dysfunction, and its treatment isn't as clear.

All causes of heart failure eventually lead to reduced cardiac output, which triggers compensatory mechanisms, such as increased sympathetic activity, activation of the renin-angiotensin-aldosterone system, ventricular dilation, and hypertrophy. These mechanisms improve cardiac output at the expense of increased ventricular work.

Increased sympathetic activity—a response to decreased cardiac output and blood pressure — enhances peripheral vascular resistance, contractility, heart rate, and venous return. Signs of increased sympathetic activity, such as cool extremities and clamminess, may indicate impending heart failure.

Increased sympathetic activity also restricts blood flow to the kidneys, causing them to secrete renin which, in turn, converts angioten-

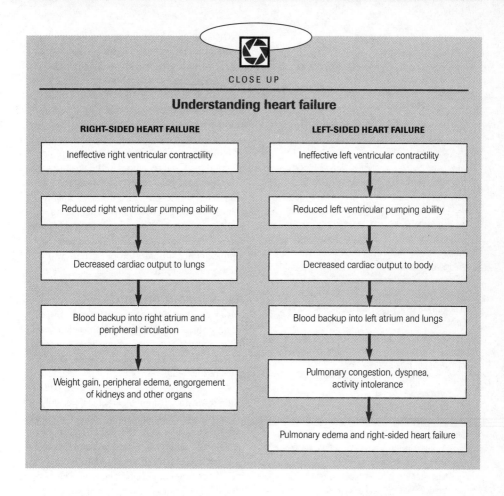

CLOSE UP

Understanding heart failure

RIGHT-SIDED HEART FAILURE

Ineffective right ventricular contractility

↓

Reduced right ventricular pumping ability

↓

Decreased cardiac output to lungs

↓

Blood backup into right atrium and peripheral circulation

↓

Weight gain, peripheral edema, engorgement of kidneys and other organs

LEFT-SIDED HEART FAILURE

Ineffective left ventricular contractility

↓

Reduced left ventricular pumping ability

↓

Decreased cardiac output to body

↓

Blood backup into left atrium and lungs

↓

Pulmonary congestion, dyspnea, activity intolerance

↓

Pulmonary edema and right-sided heart failure

sinogen to angiotensin I, which then becomes angiotensin II—a potent vasoconstrictor. Angiotensin causes the adrenal cortex to release aldosterone, leading to sodium and water retention and an increase in circulating blood volume. This renal mechanism is initially helpful; however, if it persists unchecked, it can aggravate heart failure as the heart struggles to pump against the increased volume.

In *ventricular dilation,* an increase in end-diastolic ventricular volume (preload) causes increased stroke work and stroke volume during contraction, stretching cardiac muscle fibers so that the ventricle can accept the increased intravascular volume. Eventually, the muscle becomes stretched beyond optimum limits and contractility declines.

In *ventricular hypertrophy,* an increase in ventricular muscle mass allows the heart to pump against increased resistance to the outflow of blood, improving cardiac output. However, this increased muscle mass also increases myocardial oxygen requirements. An increase in the ventricular diastolic pressure necessary to fill the enlarged ventricle may compromise diastolic coronary blood flow, limiting the oxygen supply to the ventricle, and causing ischemia and impaired muscle contractility.

In heart failure, counterregulatory substances—prostaglandins and atrial natriuretic factor—are produced in an attempt to reduce the negative effects of volume overload and vasoconstriction caused by the compensatory mechanisms.

Pulmonary edema

If your patient experiences pulmonary edema, follow these guidelines:

● Provide oxygen in high concentrations. Anticipate endotracheal intubation and mechanical ventilation if the patient fails to maintain an acceptable partial pressure of arterial oxygen.

● Monitor arterial blood gas levels, vital signs, oxygen saturation, breath sounds, intake and output and, in the patient with a pulmonary artery catheter, pulmonary end-diastolic and wedge pressures.

● Begin continuous cardiac monitoring.

● Administer diuretics, such as furosemide, to promote diuresis, which helps mobilize extravascular fluid.

● Administer positive inotropic agents, such as digoxin and inamrinone, to enhance contractility in myocardial dysfunction.

● Monitor for arrhythmias in the patient receiving a cardiac glycoside.

● Administer pressors to enhance contractility and promote vasoconstriction in peripheral blood vessels.

● Give antiarrhythmics for arrhythmias related to decreased cardiac output.

● Administer vasodilators, such as nitroprusside, to decrease peripheral vascular resistance, preload, and afterload.

● Monitor vital signs every 15 to 30 minutes while administering nitroprusside in dextrose 5% in water by I.V. drip. Protect the nitroprusside solution from light by wrapping the bottle or bag with aluminum foil, and discard unused solution after 4 hours.

● Give morphine to reduce anxiety and dyspnea and to dilate the systemic venous bed, promoting blood flow from pulmonary circulation to the periphery.

● Monitor for respiratory depression in the patient receiving morphine.

● Provide emotional support to the patient and his family and explain all procedures.

The kidneys release the prostaglandins, prostacyclin and prostaglandin E_2, which are potent vasodilators. These vasodilators also act to reduce volume overload produced by the renin-angiotensin-aldosterone system by inhibiting sodium and water reabsorption by the kidneys.

Atrial natriuretic factor is a hormone secreted mainly by the atria in response to stimulation of the stretch receptors in the atria caused by excess fluid volume. B-type natriuretic factor is secreted by the ventricles because of fluid volume overload. These natriuretic factors work to counteract the negative effects of sympathetic nervous system stimulation and the renin-angiotensin-aldosterone system by producing vasodilation and diuresis.

Assessment findings

Left-sided heart failure primarily produces pulmonary signs and symptoms; right-sided heart failure, primarily systemic signs and symptoms. However, heart failure usually affects both sides of the heart.

Clinical signs of left-sided heart failure include dyspnea, orthopnea, crackles, possibly wheezing, hypoxia, respiratory acidosis, cough, cyanosis or pallor, palpitations, arrhythmias, elevated blood pressure, and pulsus alternans.

Clinical signs of right-sided heart failure include dependent peripheral edema, hepatomegaly, splenomegaly, jugular vein distention, ascites, slow weight gain, arrhythmias, positive hepatojugular reflex, abdominal distention, nausea, vomiting, anorexia, weakness, fatigue, dizziness, and syncope.

Diagnosis

❍ Electrocardiography may reflect heart strain or enlargement, ischemia, old MI, atrial enlargement, tachycardia, and extrasystoles.

❍ Chest X-ray shows increased pulmonary vascular markings, interstitial edema, or pleural effusion and cardiomegaly.

❍ Pulmonary artery monitoring typically demonstrates elevated pulmonary artery and pulmonary artery wedge pressures, left ventricular end-diastolic pressure in left-sided heart failure, and elevated right atrial pressure or central venous pressure in right-sided heart failure.

○ Echocardiogram may demonstrate wall motion abnormalities and chamber dilation.

○ The plasma B-type natriuretic peptide assay is elevated.

○ Chest computed tomography scan, cardiac magnetic resonance imaging, or nuclear scans, such as multiple-gated acquisition and radionuclide ventriculography, may demonstrate enlargement of the heart or decreased functioning.

Complications

○ Activity intolerance
○ Arrhythmias
○ Cardiac cachexia
○ Cerebral insufficiency
○ Metabolic impairment
○ Pulmonary edema (may occur suddenly with left-sided heart failure and is marked by dyspnea, pleuritic chest pain, tachycardia, crackles on auscultation, neck vein distention and, early in its course, an S_3 heart sound) (see *Pulmonary edema*)
○ Renal impairment
○ Thromboembolism

Treatment

○ Angiotensin-converting enzyme (ACE) inhibitors are given to decrease peripheral vascular resistance.

○ Antiembolism stockings prevent venostasis and thromboembolus formation.

○ Carvedilol, a nonselective beta-adrenergic blocker with alpha-receptor blockade, reduces mortality and improves quality of life.

○ Digoxin or dopamine strengthens myocardial contractility and improves cardiac output.

○ Diuretics reduce total blood volume and circulatory congestion.

○ Inotropic agents, such as dobutamine and milrinone, given I.V. improve the heart's ability to pump.

○ Nesiritide, a recombinant form of endogenous human B-type natriuretic peptide, reduces sodium through its diuretic action.

○ Vasodilators increase cardiac output by reducing the impedance to ventricular outflow (afterload).

○ Dialysis may be used to remove excess fluid, if necessary.

○ Implanted devices, such as the intra-aortic balloon pump and the left ventricular assist device, may provide temporary assistance until the patient's condition stabilizes or surgery is performed.

○ Left ventricular remodeling surgery may be performed, resulting in a smaller organ that's able to pump blood more efficiently.

○ Heart transplantation may be an option for some people.

 COLLABORATIVE MANAGEMENT
Care of the patient with heart failure involves several members of the interdisciplinary team. The physician or cardiologist develops the treatment plan and monitors the patient. The nurse educates the patient, promotes compliance with the medical regimen, provides psychosocial support, and cares for the patient during acute exacerbations. The respiratory therapist provides oxygen therapy and breathing treatments to maximize pulmonary function. The dietitian assesses the patient's nutritional status, makes dietary recommendations, and reinforces dietary restrictions. The occupational therapist teaches energy conservation techniques and provides assistive devices, if needed. The social worker assists with financial difficulties and with obtaining medical equipment, such as home oxygen therapy. The interdisciplinary cardiac rehabilitation team (which may consist of cardiologists, exercise specialists, physical therapists, occupational therapists, dietitians, nurses, and social workers) provides supervised exercise, education, and cardiac risk modification.

Special considerations

○ Place the patient in Fowler's position and give him supplemental oxygen to help him breathe more easily.

○ Weigh the patient daily and check for peripheral edema. Carefully monitor intake and urine output, vital signs, and mental status.

Teaching about heart failure

Remember these key points when teaching your patient and his family about heart failure:

● Teach about the disease process, including its symptoms, complications, and treatments.

● Teach about prescribed medications, their names, indications, dosages, adverse effects, and special considerations.

● Explain to the patient that the potassium he loses through diuretic therapy may need to be replaced by taking a prescribed potassium supplement and eating high-potassium foods.

● Stress the importance of taking digoxin exactly as prescribed. Tell the patient to watch for and immediately report signs of toxicity, such as anorexia, vomiting, and yellow vision.

● Advise the patient to avoid foods high in sodium to curb fluid overload.

● Explain any fluid restrictions.

● Encourage participation in an outpatient cardiac rehabilitation program.

● Stress the need for regular checkups.

● Tell the patient to notify the physician promptly if his pulse is unusually irregular or measures less than 60 beats/minute; if he experiences dizziness, blurred vision, shortness of breath, a persistent dry cough, palpitations, increased fatigue, paroxysmal nocturnal dyspnea, swollen ankles, or decreased urine output; or if he notices rapid weight gain (3 to 5 lb [1.5 to 2.5 kg] in 1 week).

● Discuss the importance of smoking cessation.

○ Auscultate the heart for abnormal sounds (S_3 gallop) and the lungs for crackles or rhonchi.

○ Frequently monitor blood urea nitrogen, creatinine, and serum potassium, sodium, chloride, and magnesium levels.

○ Make sure the patient has continuous cardiac monitoring to identify and treat arrhythmias promptly.

○ To prevent deep vein thrombosis due to vascular congestion, assist the patient with range-of-motion exercises. Enforce bed rest and apply antiembolism stockings. Check regularly for calf pain and tenderness.

○ Allow adequate rest periods.

○ Provide patient education (See *Teaching about heart failure*.)

Applicable patient-teaching aids

○ Applying antiembolism stockings
○ Cutting down on salt *
○ How to measure fluid intake and output *
○ Learning about ACE inhibitors *
○ Learning about beta-adrenergic blockers *
○ Learning about digoxin *
○ Learning about potassium-rich foods *
○ Living with heart failure *
○ Overcoming shortness of breath
○ Preparing for cardiac catheterization *
○ Understanding your home oxygen equipment *
○ Using oxygen safely and effectively *

◯ Hemochromatosis

Hemochromatosis is an inherited disorder in which too much iron is absorbed and stored by the body. As iron levels rise, many organs are damaged, leading to cirrhosis, diabetes, cardiomegaly with heart failure, and arrhythmias.

Hemochromatosis is more common in whites than any other racial or ethnic group. The disorder affects both sexes, but men are approximately five times more likely to be diagnosed with it and more likely to develop complications at a younger age.

Causes

In some people, hemochromatosis is due to an autosomal recessive genetic defect in the HFE gene, which is involved in the regulation of iron absorption. A person who inherits the defective gene from both parents may develop the disorder, whereas a person who inherits the gene from only one parent is a carrier and may have a slight increase in iron absorption. The causes of juvenile hemochromatosis and neonatal hemochromatosis aren't clear.

Pathophysiology

Normally, the body absorbs approximately 10 percent of the iron that's ingested in food. Although most of the iron is stored in hemoglobin, a small portion is stored in the bone marrow, spleen, and liver. The body decreases the amount of iron absorbed when these iron stores are adequate. Patients with hemochromatosis absorb more iron than the body can use. Because this extra iron can't be eliminated from the body, it accumulates in organ tissue. Over time, high levels of iron damage the organs, leading to many chronic disorders including cirrhosis and diabetes.

Assessment findings

Common signs and symptoms of hemochromatosis include joint pain, fatigue, weight loss, abdominal pain, and a decreased libido. In advanced disease, the patient may develop bronze or gray-colored skin and signs and symptoms of other disorders, such as liver disease or cancer, diabetes, arthritis, and heart failure.

Diagnosis

○ Serum transferrin saturation test may reveal elevated amounts of iron bound to protein in the blood.
○ Serum ferritin may show elevated iron levels in the liver.
○ Deoxyribonucleic acid testing may reveal the HFE mutation.
○ Liver biopsy determines the amount of iron in the liver and whether liver damage is present.

Complications

○ Adrenal gland dysfunction
○ Arrhythmias
○ Arthritis
○ Bronze-colored skin
○ Diabetes
○ Heart failure
○ Hypopituitarism
○ Hypothyroidism

KEY TEACHING POINTS

Teaching about hemochromatosis

Remember these key points when teaching your patient and his family about hemochromatosis:
● Teach about the disease process, including its symptoms, complications, and treatments.
● Teach about prescribed medications, including their names, indications, dosages, adverse effects, and special considerations.
● Discuss warning signs and symptoms of complications that require immediate medical attention.
● Stress the importance of regular follow-up to assess for complications and to monitor serum ferritin levels.
● Advise the patient to refrain from taking iron supplements, drinking alcohol, and eating iron-rich foods.
● Explain that vitamin C supplements should also be avoided, especially with food, because it increases iron absorption.
● Discuss the need to avoid eating raw fish due to the increased susceptibility to infection.
● Advise parents, children, and siblings of the patient to consider testing for the disorder.

○ Liver disease, including hepatomegaly, cirrhosis, and liver failure
○ Premature menopause

Treatment

○ Phlebotomy is performed to remove excess iron from the body. Initially it's performed frequently until iron levels are lowered, then it's performed intermittently to maintain normal iron levels.

 COLLABORATIVE MANAGEMENT Care of the patient with hemochromatosis involves several members of the interdisciplinary team. Typically, a hepatologist, gastroenterologist, or hematologist will treat the disorder, but such specialists as the endocrinologist, cardiologist, or rheumatologist may also consult. The nurse educates the patient, monitors for complications, and cares for the patient during complications. The dietitian makes dietary recommendations and reinforces dietary restrictions.

Special considerations
○ Monitor serum ferritin levels regularly.
○ Assess the patient for associated disorders, such as liver disease, heart conditions, joint pain, and diabetes.
○ Provide patient education. (See *Teaching about hemochromatosis,* page 167.)

Applicable patient-teaching aids
○ Dietary do's and don'ts for cirrhosis *
○ Living with heart failure *
○ Preventing diabetic complications *

○ Hemophilia

Hemophilia is a hereditary bleeding disorder resulting from a deficiency of specific clotting factors. After a person with hemophilia forms a platelet plug at a bleeding site, the clotting factor deficiency impairs the blood's capacity to form a stable fibrin clot. Bleeding occurs primarily into large joints, especially after trauma or surgery. Spontaneous intracranial bleeding can occur and may be fatal.

There are two types: type A and type B. Type A, or *classic hemophilia,* is a deficiency of clotting factor VIII; it's more common than type B, affecting more than 80% of patients with hemophilia. Type B, or *Christmas disease,* affects 15% of patients with hemophilia and results from a deficiency of factor IX.

Advances in treatment have greatly improved the prognosis for patients with hemophilia, many of whom live normal life spans. Surgical procedures can be done safely at special treatment centers under the guidance of a hematologist.

Causes
Both hemophilia A and B are inherited as X-linked recessive traits. This means that female carriers have a 50% chance of transmitting the gene to each daughter, who would then be a carrier, and a 50% chance of transmitting the gene to each son, who would be born with hemophilia.

The factor VIII gene is located within the Xq28 region, and the factor IX gene is located within Xq27. Females with one defective factor VIII gene are carriers of hemophilia. A large number of disease-causing mutations have been identified in both genes. A specific inversion mutation in the noncoding region of the factor VIII gene is present in approximately 45% of families with severe hemophilia A.

Pathophysiology
Factors VIII and IX are components of the intrinsic clotting pathway; factor IX is an essential factor and factor VIII is a critical cofactor. Factor VIII accelerates the activation of factor X by several 1,000-fold. Excessive bleeding occurs when these clotting factors are reduced by more than 75%. A deficiency or nonfunction of factor VIII causes hemophilia A, and a deficiency or nonfunction of factor IX causes hemophilia B.

A person with hemophilia forms a platelet plug at a bleeding site, but clotting factor deficiency impairs the ability to form a stable fibrin clot. Delayed bleeding is more common than immediate hemorrhage. (See *Understanding hemophilia.*)

Hemophilia may be severe, moderate, or mild, depending on the degree of activation of clotting factors. Patients with severe disease have no detectable factor VIII or factor IX activity or less than 1% of normal. Moderately afflicted patients have 1% to 4% of normal clotting activity, and mildly afflicted patients have 5% to 25% of normal clotting activity.

Assessment findings
Hemophilia produces abnormal bleeding, which may be mild, moderate, or severe depending on the degree of factor deficiency.

Mild hemophilia commonly goes undiagnosed until adulthood because the patient doesn't bleed spontaneously or have prolonged bleeding after minor trauma. Severe hemophilia causes spontaneous bleeding. In many cases, the first sign of severe hemophilia is excessive bleeding after circumcision. Later, spontaneous bleeding or severe bleeding after minor trauma may produce large subcutaneous and deep intramuscular hematomas. Bleeding into joints and muscles causes pain, swelling, extreme tenderness and, possibly, permanent deformity.

Moderate hemophilia causes symptoms similar to severe hemophilia but produces only occasional spontaneous bleeding episodes.

Diagnosis

○ Characteristic findings in hemophilia A include:
– factor VIII-C assay, 0% to 30% of normal
– prolonged partial thromboplastin time (PTT)
– normal platelet count and function, bleeding time, and prothrombin time.
○ Characteristics of hemophilia B include:
– factor IX-C deficiency
– baseline coagulation results similar to hemophilia A, with normal factor VIII.
○ In both types of hemophilia, the degree of factor deficiency determines severity:
– mild hemophilia—factor levels 5% to 40% of normal
– moderate hemophilia—factor levels 1% to 5% of normal
– severe hemophilia—factor levels less than 1% of normal.

Complications

○ Death
○ Ischemia and gangrene
○ Pain, swelling, extreme tenderness, and permanent joint and muscle deformity
○ Peripheral neuropathies, pain, paresthesia, and muscle atrophy
○ Shock

Treatment

○ Prophylaxis with factor concentrates can prevent irreversible destructive arthritis that results from repeated hemarthrosis and synovial hypertrophy.
○ Replacement of the deficient factor before and after any surgery is required for the person with hemophilia; desmopressin may be given before dental extractions and surgery to pre-

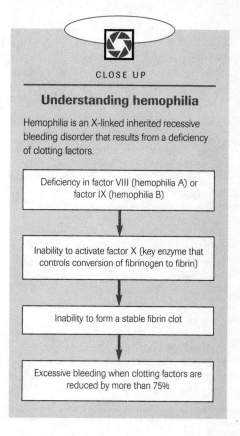

CLOSE UP

Understanding hemophilia

Hemophilia is an X-linked inherited recessive bleeding disorder that results from a deficiency of clotting factors.

> Deficiency in factor VIII (hemophilia A) or factor IX (hemophilia B)

> Inability to activate factor X (key enzyme that controls conversion of fibrinogen to fibrin)

> Inability to form a stable fibrin clot

> Excessive bleeding when clotting factors are reduced by more than 75%

vent bleeding; and epsilon-aminocaproic acid is commonly used for oral bleeding.

 COLLABORATIVE MANAGEMENT
Hemophilia isn't curable, but effective interdisciplinary treatment can prevent crippling deformities and prolong life expectancy. A hemophilia treatment center will devise a treatment plan for the patient's primary caregivers and is a resource for other health care providers, school personnel, dentists, and all others involved in the patient's care. A hematologist with expertise in hemophilia care carefully manages the patient with hemophilia. The nurse educates the patient and his family about hemophilia, monitors the chronic disorder, and provides care during acute episodes. The dietitian monitors the nutritional status and makes dietary recommendations. A therapist or social worker can help the patient and family cope with this disorder

Teaching about hemophilia

Remember these guidelines when teaching your patient and his family about hemophilia.

- Instruct parents to notify the physician immediately after a minor injury, but especially after an injury to the head, neck, or abdomen. Such injuries may require special blood factor replacement. Also, tell them to check with the physician before allowing dental extractions or any other surgery.
- Educate the patient and his parents on the early signs and symptoms of hemarthrosis: stiffness, tingling, or ache in joint, followed by decreased range of motion. If signs and symptoms are recognized early, treatment can begin earlier, potentially decreasing the possibility of long-term disability.
- Stress the importance of regular, careful toothbrushing with a soft-bristled toothbrush to prevent the need for dental surgery.
- Teach parents to be alert for signs of severe internal bleeding, such as severe pain or swelling in a joint or muscle, stiffness, decreased joint movement, severe abdominal pain, blood in urine, black tarry stools, and severe headache.
- Advise parents that the child is at risk for hepatitis from blood components. Early signs — headache, fever, decreased appetite, nausea, vomiting, abdominal tenderness, and pain over the liver — may appear 3 weeks to 6 months after treatment with blood components. Tell them to discuss with their physician the possibility of hepatitis vaccination.
- Urge parents to make sure their child wears a medical identification bracelet at all times.
- *Teach parents never to give their child aspirin,* which can aggravate the tendency to bleed. Advise them to give acetaminophen instead.
- Instruct parents to protect their child from injury, but to avoid unnecessary restrictions that impair his

normal development. For example, they can sew padded patches into the knees and elbows of a toddler's clothing to protect these joints during falls. They should forbid an older child to participate in contact sports such as football but can encourage him to swim or to play golf.

- Teach parents to elevate and apply cold compresses or ice bags to an injured area and to apply light pressure to a bleeding site. To prevent recurrence of bleeding, advise parents to restrict the child's activity for 48 hours after bleeding is under control.
- If parents have been trained to administer blood factor components at home to avoid frequent hospitalization, make sure they know proper venipuncture and infusion techniques and don't delay treatment during bleeding episodes.
- Instruct parents to keep blood factor concentrate and infusion equipment on hand at all times, even on vacation.
- Emphasize the importance of having the child keep routine medical appointments at the local hemophilia center.
- Instruct daughters of people with hemophilia to undergo genetic screening to determine if they're hemophilia carriers. Affected males should undergo counseling as well. If they produce offspring with a noncarrier, all of their daughters will be carriers; if they produce offspring with a carrier, each child has a 25% chance of being affected.
- For more information, refer parents to the National Hemophilia Foundation.

and with financial and vocational issues. Genetic counselors help people who carry hemophilia understand how this disease is transmitted.

Special considerations

○ Watch closely for signs of bleeding, such as increased pain and swelling, fever, or symptoms of shock.

○ Closely monitor PTT and other laboratory values.

○ Refer new patients to a hemophilia treatment center for evaluation.

○ Periodically assess the patient who has received blood products for hepatitis and human immunodeficiency virus. If he develops either of these disorders, provide appropriate support.

○ Refer patients and carriers for genetic counseling.

○ Provide patient education to reduce the risk of recurrent bleeding episodes. (See *Teaching about hemophilia*.)

Applicable patient-teaching aids

○ Avoiding excessive bleeding *
○ Caring for a child with hemophilia
○ Learning about blood transfusions
○ Learning self-infusion of clotting factors

○ Hepatitis B and C

Viral hepatitis is a fairly common systemic disease, marked by hepatic cell destruction, necrosis, and autolysis, leading to anorexia, jaundice, and hepatomegaly. In most patients, hepatic cells eventually regenerate with little or no residual damage. However, some people infected with the hepatitis B or hepatitis C virus develop chronic liver disease.

Approximately 90% of neonates infected at birth, 30% of children infected between ages 1 and 5, and 2% to 6% of infected older children and adults become chronically infected with hepatitis B. Over time, about 33% of these people develop chronic liver disease that may lead to liver fibrosis. Another 33% of people may develop cirrhosis or liver cancer, with about 15% to 25% of these people dying from liver complications.

In contrast to hepatitis B, about 75% to 85% of people with hepatitis C become chronically infected. Approximately 50% to 60% of these people develop mild to moderate chronic liver disease that may lead to fibrosis, 10% to 20% develop severe liver disease resulting in cirrhosis and liver cancer, and 1% to 5% die of chronic liver complications.

Causes

Hepatitis B (serum or long-incubation hepatitis), once thought to be transmitted only by the direct exchange of contaminated blood, is now known to be also transmitted by contact with human secretions and feces. As a result, nurses, physicians, laboratory technicians, and dentists are frequently exposed to type B hepatitis, in many cases as a result of wearing defective gloves. Transmission also occurs during intimate sexual contact as well as through perinatal transmission.

Incidence of hepatitis B is increasing among people with human immunodeficiency virus (HIV). Routine screening of donor blood for the hepatitis B surface antigen (HBsAg) has decreased the incidence of posttransfusion cases, but transmission through needles shared by drug abusers remains a major problem.

Although specific type C hepatitis viruses have been isolated, only a small percentage of patients have tested positive for them—perhaps reflecting the test's poor specificity. Usually, this type of hepatitis is transmitted through transfused blood from asymptomatic donors. Most exposures (60%) occur through the illicit use of I.V. drugs. However, sexual transmission is responsible for 20% of cases. More than 170 million people have the hepatitis C virus worldwide.

Pathophysiology

Hepatic damage is usually similar in all types of viral hepatitis. Varying degrees of cell injury and necrosis occur. On entering the body, the virus causes hepatocyte injury and death, either by directly killing the cells or by activating inflammatory and immune reactions. The inflammatory and immune reactions, in turn, injure or destroy hepatocytes by lysing the infected or neighboring cells. Later, direct antibody attack against the viral antigens causes further destruction of the infected cells. Edema and swelling of the interstitium lead to collapse of capillaries and decreased blood flow, tissue hypoxia, and scarring and fibrosis. Chronic hepatitis occurs in the patient whose liver has

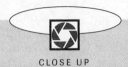

Effect of viral hepatitis on the liver

On entering the body, viral hepatitis either kills hepatocytes directly or activates inflammatory and immune reactions that injure or destroy the hepatocytes by lysing the infected or neighboring cells. Later, direct antibody attack against the viral antigens causes further destruction of the infected cells. Edema and swelling of the interstitium lead to collapse of capillaries and decreased blood flow, tissue hypoxia, and scarring and fibrosis.

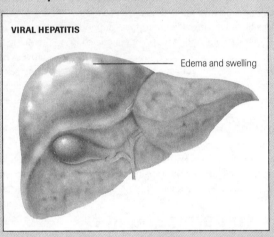

VIRAL HEPATITIS

Edema and swelling

been permanently damaged from the acute illness. (See *Effect of viral hepatitis on the liver*.)

Assessment findings

The patient with either hepatitis B or C may possibly present without any signs and symptoms. However, examination may reveal an enlarged liver and spleen, ascites, and pedal edema. If the patient also has cirrhosis, early findings may include abdominal pain, diarrhea or constipation, fatigue, nausea, vomiting, and muscle cramps; late findings, chronic dyspepsia, constipation, pruritus, weight loss, and bleeding tendencies.

Diagnosis

○ Chronic hepatitis B is diagnosed when the HBsAg test has been positive for at least 6 months.
○ Chronic hepatitis C is diagnosed when antibodies to anti-hepatitis C are present and serum aminotransferase levels remain elevated for more than 6 months.
○ Liver biopsy confirms the diagnosis of chronic hepatitis.

○ Liver function tests may indicate liver damage.
○ Prothrombin time may be prolonged.
○ Serum ammonia and serum bilirubin levels may be increased with cirrhosis.
○ Serum albumin levels may be decreased with cirrhosis.
○ Computed tomography, magnetic resonance imaging, and ultrasonography may be performed to assess liver size and density.

Complications

○ Cirrhosis
○ Death
○ Liver cancer
○ Liver failure

Treatment

○ Interferon alpha, adefovir dipivoxil, and lamivudine have been approved for the treatment of patients with chronic hepatitis B.
○ Interferon alpha and pegylated interferon in combination with ribavirin have been approved for the treatment of some patients with chronic hepatitis C.

◯ Antiemetics may be given 30 minutes before meals to relieve nausea and prevent vomiting.
◯ Treatment for cirrhosis may include paracentesis, restriction of fluids and sodium, diuretics, beta-adrenergic blockers and vasopressin, and an ammonia detoxicant. (See "Cirrhosis," page 97.)

 COLLABORATIVE MANAGEMENT Care of the patient with chronic hepatitis involves several members of the interdisciplinary team. The physician diagnoses the disorder and manages the treatment plan. The nurse provides psychosocial support and teaches the patient to reduce further liver damage and prevent the spread of infection. The social worker supports the patient and family, refers the patient to support groups for drug and alcohol abuse, and helps the patient manage financial concerns. The dietitian assesses nutritional status and devises an appropriate nutritional plan for the patient. The physical therapist may devise an activity program to maintain muscle strength and tone and prevent deconditioning while the occupational therapist teaches energy conservation skills. A drug and alcohol counselor can help the patient abstain from drinking and provide support.

Special considerations

◯ Practice standard precautions when providing nursing care.
◯ Provide the patient with rest periods throughout the day. Schedule treatments and tests so that he can rest between bouts of activity.
◯ Encourage the patient to eat. Don't overload his meal tray or overmedicate him because this will diminish his appetite.
◯ Administer supplemental vitamins and commercial feedings, as ordered. If symptoms are severe and the patient can't tolerate oral intake, provide I.V. therapy and parenteral nutrition, as ordered by the physician.
◯ Record the patient's weight daily, and document his intake and output. Observe stools for color, consistency, and amount and document the frequency of bowel movements.

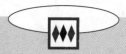

KEY TEACHING POINTS

Teaching about hepatitis B and C

Remember these key points when teaching your patient about hepatitis B and C:
● Explain the acute and chronic disease process to your patient.
● Reinforce the importance of regular follow-up appointments to monitor liver function and for early cancer detection.
● Teach about prescribed medications, including their names, indications, dosages, adverse effects, and special considerations.
● Discuss the importance of not taking any medications, even over-the-counter medications, without consulting a health care provider.
● Stress the importance of avoiding alcohol.
● Reinforce the need for yearly influenza vaccination.
● Reinforce the need to get vaccinated against hepatitis A (for patients with hepatitis B or C) and hepatitis B (for patients with hepatitis C).
● Review any dietary recommendations and caution against eating raw shellfish.
● Discuss the need to inform sex partners and household members about being infected with hepatitis and the importance of consulting with a health care provider for testing and vaccination.
● Discuss measures to prevent the spread of the hepatitis virus to others.
● Review signs and symptoms of complications that require immediate medical attention.

◯ Watch for signs of fluid shift, such as weight gain and orthostasis.
◯ Watch for signs of hepatic coma, dehydration, pneumonia, vascular problems, and pressure ulcers.
◯ Provide patient education. (See *Teaching about hepatitis B and C*.)

Applicable patient-teaching aids

◯ Avoiding excessive bleeding *
◯ Dietary do's and don'ts for cirrhosis *

○ How to detect — and prevent — infection *
○ Preparing for a liver biopsy
○ Preventing infection with proper hand washing *
○ Preventing the spread of hepatitis B, C, and D

○ Herpes simplex type 2

Herpes simplex is a recurrent viral infection. Herpes simplex type 2 primarily affects the genital area and is transmitted by sexual contact. Herpes simplex type 1, which is transmitted by oral and respiratory secretions, affects the skin and mucous membranes, commonly producing cold sores and fever blisters. However, cross-infection may result from orogenital sex or autoinoculation from one site to another. No cure for herpes exists; however, recurrences tend to be milder and of shorter duration than the primary infection. Herpes infection is equally common in males and females.

Causes

Herpes simplex type 2 is caused by *Herpesvirus hominis* (HVH), a widespread infectious agent. It's transmitted primarily by contact with genital secretions and mainly affects genital structures. Neonatal infection primarily occurs during delivery, but intrauterine transmission can occur.

Pathophysiology

The herpes simplex virus enters the mucosal surfaces or abraded skin sites in the genital area and initiates replication in the cells of the epidermis and dermis. This replication continues to permit the infection of sensory or autonomic nerve endings. The virus enters the neuronal cell and is transported intra-axonally to nerve cell bodies in the ganglia where the virus establishes latency and spreads by the peripheral nerve endings. (See *Understanding herpes simplex type 2*.)

The virus is spread through sexual contact with a person with active herpes. Lesions in the

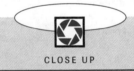

CLOSE UP

Understanding herpes simplex type 2

Herpes simplex type 2 is transmitted by contact with infectious lesions or secretions. The virus enters the skin, local replication of the virus occurs, and the virus enters cutaneous neurons. After the patient becomes infected, a latency period follows, although repeated outbreaks may develop at any time.

Initial infection
Highly infectious period, with manifestation of symptoms after incubation period (average period: 1 week)

↓

Latency
Intermittently infectious period, marked by viral dormancy or viral shedding and no disease symptoms

↓

Recurrent infection
Highly infectious period similar to initial infection, with milder symptoms that resolve faster than initial infection

genital area shed the virus, enabling further infection. Sometimes, the virus can be shed without any visible lesions. Although it isn't clear what causes the virus to become active again, outbreaks may occur following illness, stress, and heat or cold.

Assessment findings

Before an outbreak of herpes occurs, the patient may report tingling or itching in the genital area or pain in the buttocks or down the leg. Later, the patient may develop fluid-filled vesicles that ulcerate and heal in 1 to 3 weeks, fever, and regional lymphadenopathy. Future outbreaks are usually mild, only lasting for about a week.

Diagnosis

○ Tissue culture shows isolation of the virus.
○ Staining of scrapings from the base of the lesion may demonstrate characteristic giant cells or intranuclear inclusions of herpes virus infection.
○ Tissue analysis shows herpes simplex virus antigens or deoxyribonucleic acid in scrapings from lesions.

Complications

○ Cervical cancer
○ Erythema multiforme
○ Herpetic whitlow
○ Spontaneous abortion
○ Viral encephalitis
○ In patients who acquired the virus through congenital transmission, subclinical neonatal infection or severe infection with seizures, chorioretinitis, skin vesicles, and hepatosplenomegaly

Treatment

○ Analgesic-antipyretics reduce fever and relieve pain.
○ Drying agents, such as calamine lotion, ease the pain of labial or skin lesions. Avoid using petroleum-based ointments, which promote viral spread and slow healing.
○ Idoxuridine, trifluridine, and vidarabine are effective in reducing symptoms.

KEY TEACHING POINTS

Teaching about herpes simplex type 2

Remember these key points when teaching your patient and his family about herpes simplex type 2:
● Teach about the disease, including its symptoms, recurrences, complications, transmission, and treatments.
● Teach about prescribed medications, including their names, indications, dosages, adverse effects, and special considerations.
● Recommend that sexual partners be screened for sexually transmitted diseases.
● Teach the patient to use warm compresses or take sitz baths several times per day; to use a drying agent, such as povidone-iodine solution; to increase fluid intake; and to avoid all sexual contact during the active stage.
● Help the patient identify triggers for and to reduce the risk of recurrences.
● Discuss measures to prevent virus transmission.

○ Acyclovir, famciclovir, and valacyclovir may bring relief and may prevent future recurrences. Frequent prophylactic use of acyclovir in immunosuppressed transplant patients prevents disseminated disease.
○ Valacyclovir has been approved to prevent transmission of genital herpes.
○ Foscarnet can be used to treat a virus that's resistant to acyclovir.

 COLLABORATIVE MANAGEMENT Care of the patient with herpes simplex type 2 involves several members of the interdisciplinary team. The physician diagnoses the infection and recommends the treatment plan. The nurse provides support and educates the patient about the infection, reducing outbreaks, and preventing transmission. A therapist can help with issues related to self-esteem, relationships, and sexuality.

Special considerations

○ For pregnant women with active HVH infection at the time of delivery, a cesarean delivery is recommended to decrease the risk of infecting the neonate.

○ Use standard precautions, such as gloves, for contact with mucous membranes to prevent acquisition of herpetic whitlow.

○ Educate staff members and other susceptible people about the risk of contagion.

○ Encourage the patient to express concerns and provide support.

○ Provide patient education. (See *Teaching about herpes simplex type 2,* page 175.)

Applicable patient-teaching aids

○ Taking an antiviral medication

Human immunodeficiency virus infection

Human immunodeficiency virus (HIV) causes a serious secondary immunodeficiency disorder called acquired immunodeficiency syndrome (AIDS). Both diseases are characterized by the progressive destruction of cell-mediated (T-cell) immunity with subsequent effects on humoral (B-cell) immunity because of the pivotal role of the CD4+ helper T cells in immune reactions. The resultant immunodeficiency makes the patient susceptible to opportunistic infections, unusual cancers, and other abnormalities. (See *Common infections and neoplasms in HIV and AIDS.*)

The Centers for Disease Control and Prevention (CDC) first described AIDS in 1981. Since then, the CDC has declared a case surveillance definition for AIDS and modified it several times, most recently in January 2000.

Causes

HIV has two forms: HIV-1 and HIV-2. Both forms of HIV have the same modes of transmission and similar opportunistic infections associated with AIDS, but studies indicate that HIV-2 develops more slowly and presents with milder symptoms than HIV-1.

Transmission occurs through contact with infected blood or body fluids and is associated

Common infections and neoplasms in HIV and AIDS

This is a list of commonly seen disorders with human immunodeficiency virus (HIV) and acquired immunodeficiency syndrome (AIDS). AIDS is diagnosed when a patient diagnosed with HIV has a CD4+ T-cell count of less than 200 cells/mm³.

● Common infections in a patient with a CD4+ count less than 350 cells/mm³ include:
– herpes simplex virus
– herpes zoster
– *Mycobacterium tuberculosis*
– non-Hodgkin's lymphoma
– oral or vaginal thrush.
● Common infections in a patient with a CD4+ count less than 200 cells/mm³ include:
– *Candida* esophagitis
– *Pneumocystis carinii* pneumonia.
● Common infections in a patient with a CD4+ count less than 100 cells/mm³ include:
– AIDS dementia

– cryptococcal meningitis
– progressive multifocal leukoencephalopathy
– toxoplasmosis encephalitis
– wasting syndrome.
● Common infections in a patient with a CD4+ count less than 50 cells/mm³ include:
– cytomegalovirus infection
– *Mycobacterium avium.*
● Common neoplasms in patients with HIV and AIDS include:
– Hodgkin's disease
– Kaposi's sarcoma
– malignant lymphoma.

with identifiable high-risk behaviors. It's disproportionately represented in:
○ homosexual and bisexual men
○ persons who use illicit I.V. drugs
○ neonates of infected females
○ recipients of contaminated blood or blood products (incidence dramatically decreased since mid-1985)
○ heterosexual partners of persons in the former groups.

Pathophysiology

Infection with the HIV retrovirus, which is detectable only by laboratory tests, begins the natural history of AIDS. Twenty years of data strongly suggests that HIV isn't transmitted by casual household or social contact. The HIV virus may enter the body by any of several routes involving the transmission of blood or body fluids, for example:
○ direct inoculation during intimate sexual contact, especially associated with the mucosal trauma of receptive rectal intercourse
○ transfusion of contaminated blood or blood products (a risk diminished by routine testing of all blood products)
○ sharing contaminated needles
○ transplacental or postpartum transmission from infected mother to fetus (by cervical or blood contact at delivery and in breast milk).

HIV strikes helper T cells bearing the CD4+ antigen. Normally a receptor for major histocompatibility complex molecules, the antigen serves as a receptor for the retrovirus and allows it to enter the cell. Viral binding also requires the presence of a coreceptor (believed to be the chemokine receptor CCR5) on the cell surface. The virus also may infect CD4+ antigen–bearing cells of the GI tract, uterine cervix, and neuroglia. (See *HIV: How it progresses*, page 178.)

Like other retroviruses, HIV copies its genetic material in a reverse manner compared with other viruses and cells. Through the action of reverse transcriptase, HIV produces DNA from its viral RNA. Transcription is usually poor, leading to mutations, some of which make HIV resistant to antiviral drugs. The viral DNA enters the nucleus of the cell and is incorporated into the host cell's DNA, where it's transcribed into more viral RNA. If the host cell reproduces, it duplicates the HIV DNA along with its own and passes it on to the daughter cells. Thus, if activated, the host cell carries this information and, if activated, replicates the virus. Viral enzymes, proteases, arrange the structural components and RNA into viral particles that move out to the periphery of the host cell, where the virus buds and emerges from the host cell. Thus, the virus is now free to travel and infect other cells.

HIV replication may lead to cell death or it may become latent. HIV infection leads to profound disease, either directly through destruction of CD4+ cells, other immune cells, and neuroglial cells, or indirectly through the secondary effects of CD4+ T-cell dysfunction and resulting immunosuppression.

The HIV infectious process takes three forms:
○ immunodeficiency (opportunistic infections and unusual cancers)
○ autoimmunity (lymphoid interstitial pneumonitis, arthritis, hypergammaglobulinemia, and production of autoimmune antibodies)
○ neurologic dysfunction (AIDS dementia complex, HIV encephalopathy, and peripheral neuropathies).

Assessment findings

Initially, a person infected with HIV may remain asymptomatic for months or years. As the disease progresses, he may develop generalized adenopathy and nonspecific signs and symptoms, such as weight loss, fatigue, night sweats, and fevers. Neurologic symptoms, opportunistic infections, and certain normally rare cancers may develop as the patient's T-cell count lowers further. Eventually, lymph node and immunologic organ destruction can lead to major dysfunctions of the immunologic system.

Diagnosis

○ CD4+ T-cell count of at least 200 cells/mm³ confirms HIV infection.
○ Screening test enzyme-linked immunosorbent assay (ELISA) and confirmatory test

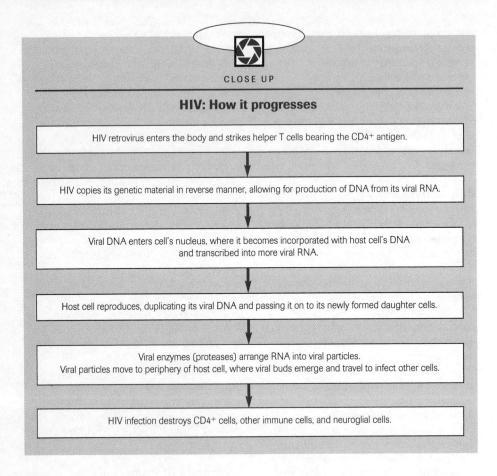

CLOSE UP

HIV: How it progresses

HIV retrovirus enters the body and strikes helper T cells bearing the CD4+ antigen.

HIV copies its genetic material in reverse manner, allowing for production of DNA from its viral RNA.

Viral DNA enters cell's nucleus, where it becomes incorporated with host cell's DNA and transcribed into more viral RNA.

Host cell reproduces, duplicating its viral DNA and passing it on to its newly formed daughter cells.

Viral enzymes (proteases) arrange RNA into viral particles.
Viral particles move to periphery of host cell, where viral buds emerge and travel to infect other cells.

HIV infection destroys CD4+ cells, other immune cells, and neuroglial cells.

(Western blot) detect the presence of HIV antibodies, which indicate HIV infection.
○ CD4+ and CD8+ T-lymphocyte subset counts, erythrocyte sedimentation rate, complete blood cell count, serum beta$_2$-microglobulin, p24 antigen, neopterin levels, and anergy testing are performed to support the diagnosis and help evaluate the severity of immunosuppression.

Complications
○ Neoplasms
○ Organ-specific syndrome
○ Premalignant diseases
○ Repeated opportunistic infections

Treatment
○ Highly active antiretroviral therapy (HAART) aims to reduce the number of HIV particles in the blood as measured by viral load, thus increasing T-cell counts and improving the immunologic system's functioning. Multiple combined antiviral drug therapies are used to suppress the replication of the HIV virus in the body. Initially, highly active antiviral therapy, consisting of a triple drug therapy regimen — a protease inhibitor and two non-nucleoside reverse transcriptase inhibitors — is recommended.
○ Nucleoside analogues (sometimes called *reverse transcriptase inhibitors*) have been the mainstay of AIDS therapy in recent years. These drugs interfere with viral reverse tran-

scriptase, which impairs HIV's ability to turn its RNA into DNA for insertion into the host cell.
○ Protease inhibitors (PIs) have greatly increased the life expectancy of patients with AIDS. They work by blocking the enzyme protease, which HIV needs to produce virions, the viral particles that spread the virus to other cells. The use of PIs dramatically reduces viral load while producing a corresponding increase in the CD4+ T-cell count.
○ Anti-infectives are used to combat opportunistic infections (some are used prophylactically to help patients resist opportunistic infections), and antineoplastic drugs are used to fight associated neoplasms.
○ Supportive treatments help maintain nutritional status and relieve pain and other distressing physical and psychological symptoms.

 COLLABORATIVE MANAGEMENT
Care of the patient with HIV involves several members of the interdisciplinary team. The physician manages the treatment plan. The nurse educates the patient and assists him in improving his quality of life. The dietitian assesses the patient's nutritional status and makes recommendations to optimize his condition. The respiratory therapist helps to optimize the patient's pulmonary status. The therapist recommends support groups and, if requested, spiritual counseling for the patient and his family. The physical therapist can help the patient maintain muscle strength and tone, and the occupational therapist can help the patient with peripheral neuropathy due to antiretroviral drugs to perform activities of daily living. Home health care agencies can help the patient maintain a satisfactory quality of life while maintaining as much independence as possible. The social worker can help with issues such as finances, housing, and social acceptance.

Special considerations
○ Advise health care workers and the public to use precautions in all situations that risk exposure to blood, body fluids, and secretions. Diligently practicing standard precautions can prevent the inadvertent transmission of HIV

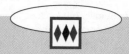

Teaching about HIV
Remember these key points when teaching your patient and his family about human immunodeficiency virus (HIV):
● Explain how HIV affects the immune response.
● Discuss the development of opportunistic infections, cancer, and neurologic effects associated with acquired immunodeficiency syndrome (AIDS).
● Explain diagnostic criteria for AIDS.
● Reinforce the importance of regular follow-up care.
● Talk about activity modifications, including adequate rest and moderate exercise.
● Reinforce the importance of adequate nutrition to prevent opportunistic infection.
● Teach about prescribed medications, including their names, indications, dosages, adverse effects, special considerations, and the importance of compliance.
● Discuss measures to prevent the transmission of the virus to sexual partners and household members. Explain safe sex practices, including how to use a condom. Reinforce the importance of informing potential sexual partners, caregivers, and health care workers of HIV infection.
● Review signs of impending infection and the importance of seeking immediate medical attention.
● Talk about the symptoms of AIDS dementia, including its stages and progression.

and other infectious diseases that are transmitted by similar routes.
○ Recognize that a diagnosis of HIV is profoundly distressing because of the disease's social impact and discouraging prognosis. The patient may lose his job and financial security as well as the support of family and friends. Do your best to help him cope with an altered body image, the emotional burden of serious illness, and the threat of death, and encourage and as-

sist the patient in learning about HIV and AIDS societies and support programs.

○ Provide patient education. (See *Teaching about HIV*, page 179.)

Applicable patient-teaching aids
○ Avoiding infection *
○ Caring for an AIDS patient at home
○ Preventing infection—and recognizing its symptoms *
○ Stimulating your appetite
○ Taking an antiviral medication
○ Using a condom correctly

○ Huntington's disease

Huntington's disease, also called *Huntington's chorea, hereditary chorea, chronic progressive chorea,* and *adult chorea,* is a hereditary disease in which degeneration in the cerebral cortex and basal ganglia causes chronic progressive chorea and mental deterioration, ending in dementia.

The disease usually strikes people between ages 35 and 55; however, 2% of cases occur in children, and 5% of cases occur as late as age 60. Death usually results 10 to 15 years after onset, from suicide, heart failure, or pneumonia. Genetic testing is available for persons with a family history of the disease.

Causes
Huntington's disease is inherited as a single faulty gene on chromosome #4, whereby part of the gene is repeated in multiple copies. It's transmitted as an autosomal dominant trait; either sex can transmit and inherit it. Each child of a parent with this disease has a 50% chance of inheriting it.

Pathophysiology
Huntington's disease involves a disturbance in neurotransmitter substances, primarily gamma-aminobutyric acid (GABA) and dopamine. In the basal ganglia, frontal cortex, and cerebellum, GABA neurons are destroyed and replaced by glial cells. The consequent deficiency of GABA (an inhibitory neurotransmitter) results in a relative excess of dopamine and abnormal neurotransmission along the affected pathways.

Assessment findings
Huntington's disease has an insidious onset. The patient eventually becomes totally dependent—emotionally and physically—through the loss of musculoskeletal control and the development of progressively severe choreic movements, which may be rapid, violent, and purposeless.

Ultimately, the patient with Huntington's diseases develops progressive dementia, which may progress at the same rate as the chorea. Personality changes include obstinacy, carelessness, untidiness, moodiness, apathy, inappropriate behavior, loss of memory and concentration and, occasionally, paranoia.

Diagnosis
○ Positron emission tomography and deoxyribonucleic acid analysis can detect the disease.
○ Diagnosis is based on a characteristic clinical history: progressive chorea and dementia, onset in early middle age (35 to 40), and confirmation of a genetic link.
○ Computed tomography scan and magnetic resonance imaging demonstrate brain atrophy.
○ Molecular genetics may detect the gene for Huntington's disease in people at risk while they're still asymptomatic.

Complications
○ Choking and aspiration
○ Heart failure
○ Infections
○ Pneumonia
○ Suicide

Treatment
○ Because Huntington's disease has no known cure, treatment is supportive, protective, and symptomatic.
○ Dopamine blockers, such as phenothiazine or haloperidol, help control choreic movements and reduce abnormal behaviors.
○ Reserpine and other drugs have been used with varying success.

○ Tetrabenazine and amantadine are used to control extra movements.

○ Some evidence suggests that co-enzyme Q10 may minimally decrease progression of the disease.

○ Institutionalization may be necessary because of mental deterioration, which can't be halted or managed by drugs.

 COLLABORATIVE MANAGEMENT
Care of the patient with Huntington's disease involves several members of the interdisciplinary team. The neurologist diagnoses and manages the disorder. The nurse educates the patient and his family about the disorder, helps the patient maintain the highest level of independent functioning for as long as possible, and provides support to the patient and his family. Speech therapy can help the patient with speech and swallowing issues. The social worker can facilitate the drafting of a living will and a power of attorney. During the later stages of the disease, the nurse and social worker can assist the patient and his family with end-of-life issues. Hospice nurses may provide care at the end of life.

Special considerations

○ Provide physical support by attending to the patient's basic needs, such as hygiene, skin care, bowel and bladder care, and nutrition. Increase this support as mental and physical deterioration make him increasingly immobile.

○ Offer emotional support to the patient and his family. Keep in mind the patient's dysarthria, and allow him extra time to express himself, thereby decreasing frustration.

○ Stay alert for possible suicide attempts. Control the patient's environment to protect him from suicide or other self-inflicted injury. Pad the side rails of the bed, but avoid restraints, which may cause the patient to injure himself with violent, uncontrolled movements.

○ If the patient has difficulty walking, provide a walker to help him maintain his balance.

○ Make sure affected families receive genetic counseling. All affected family members should realize that each of their offspring has a 50% chance of inheriting this disease.

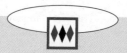

KEY TEACHING POINTS

Teaching about Huntington's disease

Remember these key points when teaching your patient and his family about Huntington's disease:

● Teach about the disease process, and listen to the patient's and his family's concerns and special problems.

● Teach the family to participate in the patient's care.

● Teach about prescribed medications, including their names, indications, dosages, adverse effects, and special considerations.

● Discuss warning signs of complications that require immediate medical attention.

● Discuss genetic testing with the family and refer those who desire genetic testing to centers specializing in Huntington's care, where psychosocial support is available.

● Refer the patient and his family to the Huntington's Disease Society of America.

● Demonstrate aspiration precautions to the patient and his family.

● Explain signs and symptoms of infection to report to the health care provider.

● Discuss alternate communication strategies.

○ Refer the patient and his family to the appropriate community organizations.

○ Provide patient education. (See *Teaching about Huntington's disease.*)

Applicable patient-teaching aids

○ Coping with depression
○ Learning to communicate without speech *
○ Repositioning a person in bed

○ Hypertension

Hypertension, an intermittent or sustained elevation in diastolic or systolic blood pressure, occurs as two major types: essential (idiopathic) hypertension, the most common, and secondary hypertension, which results from renal disease or another identifiable cause. Malignant hypertension is a severe, fulminant form of hypertension common to both types. Hypertension is a major cause of stroke, cardiac disease, and renal failure. The prognosis is good if this disorder is detected early and treatment begins before complications develop. Severely elevated blood pressure (hypertensive crisis) may be fatal.

Hypertension affects 25% of adults in the United States. If untreated, it carries a high mortality. The risk of hypertension increases with age and is higher for blacks than whites and in those with less education and lower income. Men have a higher incidence of hypertension in young and early middle adulthood; thereafter, women have a higher incidence.

Causes

Risk factors for hypertension include family history, race (most common in blacks), stress, obesity, a diet high in saturated fats or sodium, tobacco use, sedentary lifestyle, and aging.

Secondary hypertension may result from renal vascular disease; pheochromocytoma; primary hyperaldosteronism; Cushing's syndrome; thyroid, pituitary, or parathyroid dysfunction; coarctation of the aorta; pregnancy; neurologic disorders; and use of hormonal contraceptives or other drugs, such as cocaine, epoetin alfa (erythropoietin), and cyclosporine.

Pathophysiology

Arterial blood pressure is a product of total peripheral resistance and cardiac output. Cardiac output is increased by conditions that increase heart rate, stroke volume, or both. Peripheral resistance is increased by factors that increase blood viscosity or reduce the lumen size of vessels, especially the arterioles.

Several theories help to explain the development of hypertension, including:
○ changes in the arteriolar bed, causing increased peripheral vascular resistance
○ abnormally increased tone in the sympathetic nervous system that originates in the vaso-

motor system centers, causing increased peripheral vascular resistance
○ increased blood volume resulting from renal or hormonal dysfunction
○ an increase in arteriolar thickening caused by genetic factors, leading to increased peripheral vascular resistance
○ abnormal renin release, resulting in the formation of angiotensin II, which constricts the arteriole and increases blood volume.

Prolonged hypertension increases the heart's workload as resistance to left ventricular ejection increases. To increase contractile force, the left ventricle hypertrophies, raising the heart's oxygen demands and workload. Cardiac dilation and failure may occur when hypertrophy can no longer maintain sufficient cardiac output. Because hypertension promotes coronary atherosclerosis, the heart may be further compromised by reduced blood flow to the myocardium, resulting in angina or myocardial infarction (MI). Hypertension also causes vascular damage, leading to accelerated atherosclerosis and target organ damage, such as retinal injury, renal failure, stroke, and aortic aneurysm and dissection.

The pathophysiology of secondary hypertension is related to the underlying disease. For example:
○ The most common cause of secondary hypertension is chronic renal disease. Insult to the kidney from chronic glomerulonephritis or renal artery stenosis interferes with sodium excretion, the renin-angiotensin-aldosterone system, or renal perfusion, causing blood pressure to increase.
○ In Cushing's syndrome, increased cortisol levels raise blood pressure by increasing renal sodium retention, angiotensin II levels, and vascular response to norepinephrine.
○ In primary aldosteronism, increased intravascular volume, altered sodium concentrations in vessel walls, or very high aldosterone levels cause vasoconstriction and increased resistance.
○ Pheochromocytoma is a chromaffin cell tumor of the adrenal medulla that secretes epinephrine and norepinephrine. Epinephrine increases cardiac contractility and rate, whereas

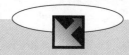

ACUTE EPISODE

Managing hypertensive crisis

If your patient experiences hypertensive crisis, follow these guidelines:

● Ensure a patent airway.

● Assess arterial blood gas levels and monitor oxygen saturation through pulse oximetry. Administer supplemental oxygen, as indicated.

● Institute continuous cardiac and arterial pressure monitoring.

● Administer I.V. sodium nitroprusside, as ordered, and titrate according to the patient's response. Take care not to reduce the patient's blood pressure too rapidly, because the patient's autoregulatory control is impaired. The current recommendation is to reduce the blood pressure by no more than 25% of the mean arterial pressure over the first 2 hours. Other agents that may be used include labetalol, nitroglycerin (the drug of choice for treating hypertensive crisis when myocardial ischemia, acute myocardial infarction, or pulmonary edema are present), and hydralazine (specifically indicated for treating hypertension in a pregnant woman with preeclampsia).

● Wrap the nitroprusside container in foil to protect it from light.

● Be alert for signs and symptoms of thiocyanate toxicity in the patient receiving nitroprusside, such as fatigue, nausea, tinnitus, blurred vision, and delirium. If the patient exhibits any of these, obtain a serum thiocyanate level. If the level is greater than 10 mg/dl, toxicity is present; notify the physician.

● Monitor blood pressure every 1 to 5 minutes while titrating drug therapy, then every 15 minutes to 1 hour as the patient's condition stabilizes.

● Continuously monitor the patient's electrocardiogram and institute treatment as indicated should arrhythmias occur.

● Auscultate for heart sounds, noting signs of heart failure such as the presence of an S_3 or S_4.

● Assess the patient's neurologic status every hour initially and then every 4 hours as the patient's condition stabilizes.

● Monitor urine output every hour. Notify the physician if output is less than 0.5 ml/kg/hour. Evaluate blood urea nitrogen and serum creatinine levels for changes, and monitor daily weight.

● As the patient's condition stabilizes, expect to begin oral antihypertensive therapy while gradually weaning I.V. agents to prevent hypotension.

● Administer diuretics as ordered if the patient is experiencing fluid overload.

● Assess the patient's vision and report such changes as increased blurred vision, diplopia, or loss of vision.

● Administer analgesics as ordered for headache; keep the environment quiet, with low lighting.

norepinephrine increases peripheral vascular resistance.

Assessment findings

Hypertension usually doesn't produce clinical effects until vascular changes in the heart, brain, or kidneys occur. However, when these changes do occur, the patient may present with elevated blood pressure readings on at least two consecutive occasions after the initial screening and an occipital headache, which may worsen in the morning. Other findings may include nausea and vomiting, epistaxis, dizzi-

ness, confusion, blurry vision, nocturia, edema, and fatigue. Auscultation may reveal bruits over the abdominal aorta or carotid, renal, and femoral arteries due to stenosis or aneurysm.

In hypertensive crisis, the patient may present with a severe, throbbing headache in the back of the head (most common complaint), nausea, vomiting, and anorexia. (See *Managing hypertensive crisis*.)

Diagnosis

○ Serial blood pressure measurements are obtained and compared to previous readings and

Classifying blood pressure readings

In 2003, the National Institutes of Health issued *The Seventh Report of the Joint National Committee on Prevention, Detection, Evaluation, and Treatment of High Blood Pressure (The JNC 7 Report)*. Updates since *The JNC 6* report include a new category, prehypertension, and the combining of stages 2 and 3 hypertension. Categories now are normal, prehypertension, and stages 1 and 2 hypertension.

The revised categories are based on the average of two or more readings taken on separate visits after an initial screening. They apply to adults ages 18 and older. (If the systolic and diastolic pressures fall into different categories, use the higher of the two pressures to classify the reading. For example, a reading of 160/92 mm Hg should be classified as stage 2.)

Normal blood pressure with respect to cardiovascular risk is a systolic reading below 120 mm Hg and a diastolic reading below 80 mm Hg. Patients with prehypertension are at increased risk for developing hypertension and should follow health-promoting lifestyle modifications to prevent cardiovascular disease.

In addition to classifying stages of hypertension based on average blood pressure readings, clinicians should also take note of target organ disease and additional risk factors, such as diabetes, left ventricular hypertrophy, and chronic renal disease. This additional information is important to obtain a true picture of the patient's cardiovascular health.

Category	Systolic		Diastolic
Normal	< 120 mm Hg	AND	< 80 mm Hg
Prehypertension	120 to 139 mm Hg	OR	80 to 89 mm Hg
Hypertension Stage 1	140 to 159 mm Hg	OR	90 to 99 mm Hg
Stage 2	≥ 160 mm Hg	OR	≥ 100 mm Hg

trends to reveal an increase in diastolic and systolic pressures. (See *Classifying blood pressure readings*.)

○ Ophthalmoscopy reveals arteriovenous nicking and, in hypertensive encephalopathy, papilledema.

○ Urinalysis may show protein, and red and white blood cell counts may indicate glomerulonephritis.

○ Excretory urography may reveal renal atrophy, indicating chronic renal disease; one kidney more than ⅝" (1.6 cm) shorter than the other suggests unilateral renal disease.

○ Serum potassium levels less than 3.5 mEq/L may indicate adrenal dysfunction (primary hyperaldosteronism).

○ Blood urea nitrogen levels that are elevated to more than 20 mg/dl and serum creatinine

levels that are elevated to more than 1.5 mg/dl suggest renal disease.

○ Electrocardiography may show left ventricular hypertrophy or ischemia.

○ Chest X-ray may show cardiomegaly.

○ Echocardiography may show left ventricular hypertrophy.

Complications
○ Blindness
○ Cardiac disease
○ Renal disease
○ Stroke

Treatment
The National Institutes of Health recommends the following approach for treating primary hypertension:

○ Lifestyle modifications should be made first, including weight reduction, moderation of alcohol intake, regular physical exercise, reduction of sodium intake, and smoking cessation.

○ Continue lifestyle modifications and begin drug therapy if the patient fails to achieve the desired blood pressure or make significant progress.

○ Thiazide-type diuretics are recommended for most patients for stage 1 hypertension in the absence of compelling indications, such as heart failure, post-MI, high coronary disease risk, diabetes, chronic kidney disease, or recurrent stroke prevention.

○ An angiotensin-converting enzyme inhibitor (ACEI), beta-adrenergic blocker, calcium channel blocker (CCB), angiotensin receptor blocker (ARB), or a combination may also be considered.

○ A two-drug combination (usually a thiazide-type diuretic and an ACEI, ARB, CCB, or beta-adrenergic blocker) may be ordered for stage 2 hypertension in the absence of compelling indications.

○ If the patient has one or more compelling indications, drug treatment is based on benefits from outcome studies or existing clinical guidelines.

– Chronic kidney disease—ACEI or ARB

– Diabetes—diuretic, beta-adrenergic blocker, ACEI, ARB, or CCB

– Heart failure—diuretic, beta-adrenergic blocker, ACEI, ARB, or aldosterone antagonist

– High coronary disease risk—diuretic, beta-adrenergic blocker, ACEI, or CCB

– Postmyocardial failure—beta-adrenergic blocker, ACEI, or aldosterone antagonist

– Recurrent stroke prevention—diuretic or ACEI.

○ If the patient fails to achieve the desired blood pressure, continue lifestyle modifications and optimize drug dosages until the goal blood pressure is achieved. Also, consider consultation with a hypertension specialist.

○ For the patient with secondary hypertension, correct the underlying cause of the disorder and control any hypertensive effects.

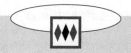

KEY TEACHING POINTS

Teaching about hypertension

Be sure to include the following points when teaching the patient with hypertension:

● Teach about the disease process, including its complications and treatment.

● Show the patient how to use a self-monitoring blood pressure cuff; instruct him to record the reading in a journal for review by the physician.

● Explain the importance of compliance with antihypertensive therapy and establishing a daily routine for taking prescribed drugs.

● Teach about prescribed medications, including their names, indications, and dosages, as well as the need to report adverse effects.

● Warn that uncontrolled hypertension may cause stroke and heart attack.

● Advise the patient to avoid high-sodium antacids and over-the-counter cold and sinus medications, which contain harmful vasoconstrictors.

● Encourage the patient to avoid high-sodium foods and to achieve and maintain a healthy weight.

● Help the patient examine and modify his lifestyle (for example, by reducing stress and exercising regularly).

● Stress the importance of follow-up care.

 COLLABORATIVE MANAGEMENT
Care of the patient with hypertension involves several members of the interdisciplinary team. Medical and nursing health care providers focus on administering medications to treat hypertension, preventing potential complications, and helping the patient make lifestyle modifications. The surgeon may be consulted to correct the underlying problem associated with secondary hypertension, such as removal of a tumor in pheochromocytoma. The dietitian can assist with dietary changes and weight loss.

Special considerations

○ If a patient is hospitalized with hypertension, find out if he was taking his prescribed medication. If he wasn't, ask why. If he can't afford the medication, refer him to appropriate social service agencies.

○ When routine blood pressure screening reveals elevated pressure, first make sure the cuff size is appropriate for the patient's upper arm circumference. Take the pressure in both arms in lying, sitting, and standing positions. Ask the patient if he smoked, drank a beverage containing caffeine, or was emotionally upset before the test. Advise him to return for blood pressure testing at frequent and regular intervals.

○ To help identify hypertension and prevent untreated hypertension, participate in public education programs dealing with hypertension and ways to reduce risk factors. Routinely screen all patients, especially those at risk (blacks and people with family histories of hypertension, stroke, or MI).

○ Provide patient education. (See *Teaching about hypertension*, page 185.)

Applicable patient-teaching aids

○ Cutting down on salt *
○ Exercising safely *
○ Learning about ACE inhibitors *
○ Learning about digoxin *
○ Learning about potassium-rich foods *
○ Performing relaxation breathing exercises *
○ Taking another person's blood pressure *
○ Taking your pulse *

○ Hyperthyroidism

Hyperthyroidism (also known as *Graves' disease, Basedow's disease,* and *thyrotoxicosis*) is a metabolic imbalance that results from thyroid hormone overproduction. The most common form of hyperthyroidism is Graves' disease, which increases thyroxine (T_4) production, enlarges the thyroid gland (goiter), and causes multiple system changes.

With treatment, most patients can lead normal lives. However, thyroid storm—an acute exacerbation of hyperthyroidism—is a medical emergency that may lead to life-threatening cardiac, hepatic, or renal failure.

Incidence of Graves' disease is highest between ages 30 and 40, especially in people with family histories of thyroid abnormalities; only 5% of hyperthyroid patients are younger than age 15.

Causes

Hyperthyroidism may result from both genetic and immunologic factors. An increased incidence of this disorder in monozygotic twins, for example, points to an inherited factor, probably an autosomal recessive gene. This disease occasionally coexists with abnormal iodine metabolism and other endocrine abnormalities, such as diabetes mellitus, thyroiditis, and hyperparathyroidism. Hyperthyroidism is also associated with the production of autoantibodies (thyroid-stimulating immunoglobulin and thyroid-stimulating hormone [TSH]-binding inhibitory immunoglobulin), possibly due to a defect in suppressor–T-lymphocyte function that allows the formation of autoantibodies.

In latent hyperthyroidism, excessive dietary intake of iodine and, possibly, stress can precipitate clinical hyperthyroidism. In a person with inadequately treated hyperthyroidism, stress—including surgery, infection, toxemia of pregnancy, and diabetic ketoacidosis—can precipitate thyroid storm.

Pathophysiology

The thyroid gland secretes the thyroid precursor, T_4, thyroid hormone or triiodothyronine (T_3), and calcitonin. T_4 and T_3 stimulate protein, lipid, and carbohydrate metabolism primarily through catabolic pathways. Calcitonin removes calcium from the blood and incorporates it into bone.

Biosynthesis, storage, and release of thyroid hormones are controlled by the hypothalamic-pituitary axis through a negative-feedback loop. Thyrotropin-releasing hormone (TRH) from the hypothalamus stimulates the release of TSH by the pituitary. Circulating T_3 levels provide negative feedback through the hypothalamus to decrease TRH levels, and through the pituitary to decrease TSH levels.

Graves' disease is an autoimmune disorder characterized by the production of autoantibodies that attach to and then stimulate TSH receptors on the thyroid gland. A goiter is an enlarged thyroid gland, either the result of increased stimulation or a response to increased metabolic demand. The latter occurs in iodine-deficient areas of the world, where the incidence of goiter increases during puberty (a time of increased metabolic demand). These goiters usually regress to normal size after puberty in males, but not in females. Sporadic goiter in non–iodine-deficient areas is of unknown origin. Endemic and sporadic goiters are nontoxic and may be diffuse or nodular. Toxic goiters may be uninodular or multinodular and may secrete excess thyroid hormone.

Pituitary tumors with TSH-producing cells are rare, as is hypothalamic disease causing TRH excess.

Assessment findings

The classic features of hyperthyroidism are an enlarged thyroid (goiter), nervousness, heat intolerance, weight loss despite increased appetite, sweating, diarrhea, tremor, and palpitations. Exophthalmos is considered most characteristic, but it's absent in many patients with hyperthyroidism. Many other symptoms are common because hyperthyroidism profoundly affects virtually every body system:

❍ *Central nervous system*—difficulty concentrating; excitability or nervousness; fine tremor, shaky handwriting, and clumsiness; and emotional instability and mood swings, ranging from occasional outbursts to overt psychosis

❍ *Skin, hair, and nails*—smooth, warm, flushed skin (patient sleeps with minimal covers and little clothing); fine, soft hair; premature graying and increased hair loss in both sexes; friable nails and onycholysis (distal nail separated from the bed); pretibial myxedema (dermopathy), producing thickened skin, accentuated hair follicles, raised red patches of skin that are itchy and sometimes painful, with occasional nodule formation.

❍ *Cardiovascular system*—tachycardia; full, bounding pulse; wide pulse pressure; cardiomegaly; increased cardiac output and blood volume; visible point of maximal impulse; paroxysmal supraventricular tachycardia and atrial fibrillation (especially in elderly patients); and, occasionally, systolic murmur at the left sternal border

❍ *Respiratory system*—dyspnea on exertion and at rest

❍ *GI system*—possible anorexia; nausea and vomiting; increased defecation; soft stools or, with severe disease, diarrhea; and liver enlargement

❍ *Musculoskeletal system*—weakness, fatigue, and muscle atrophy; rare coexistence with myasthenia gravis; generalized or localized paralysis associated with hypokalemia; and occasional acropachy—soft-tissue swelling, accompanied by underlying bone changes where new bone formation occurs

❍ *Reproductive system*—in females, oligomenorrhea or amenorrhea, decreased fertility, higher incidence of spontaneous abortions; in males, gynecomastia due to increased estrogen levels; in both sexes, diminished libido

❍ *Eyes*—exophthalmos; occasional inflammation of conjunctivae, corneas, or eye muscles; diplopia; and increased tearing.

When hyperthyroidism escalates to thyroid storm, these symptoms can be accompanied by extreme irritability, hypertension, tachycardia, vomiting, and temperature up to 106° F (41.1° C), delirium, and coma.

Diagnosis

❍ Radioimmunoassay shows increased serum T_4 and T_3 concentrations.

❍ Thyroid scan reveals increased uptake of radioactive iodine (^{131}I). This test is contraindicated if the patient is pregnant.

❍ TSH levels are decreased.

❍ Ultrasonography confirms subclinical ophthalmopathy.

❍ Antithyroglobulin antibody is positive in Graves' disease.

Complications

❍ Arrhythmias
❍ Corneal ulcers
❍ Decreased libido
❍ Gynecomastia

○ Heart failure
○ Hepatic or renal failure
○ Impaired fertility
○ Left ventricular hypertrophy
○ Muscle weakness and atrophy
○ Myasthenia gravis
○ Osteoporosis
○ Paralysis
○ Skin hyperpigmentation
○ Thyrotoxic crisis or thyroid storm
○ Vitiligo

Treatment

○ Thyroid hormone antagonists are given to block thyroid hormone synthesis. Antithyroid drug therapy is used for children, young adults, pregnant females, and patients who refuse surgery or ^{131}I treatment.
○ Beta-adrenergic blockers may be given concomitantly to manage tachycardia and other peripheral effects of excessive hypersympathetic activity.
○ [131]I in a single oral dose is the treatment of choice for patients not planning to have children.
○ Subtotal (partial) thyroidectomy, which decreases the thyroid gland's capacity for hormone production, is indicated for patients with a large goiter whose hyperthyroidism has repeatedly relapsed after drug therapy. It's also indicated for patients who refuse or aren't candidates for ^{131}I treatment.
○ Iodides (Lugol's solution or saturated solution of potassium iodide), antithyroid drugs, or high doses of propranolol may be given preoperatively, to help prevent thyroid storm. If euthyroidism isn't achieved, surgery should be delayed and propranolol administered to decrease hyperthyroidism's systemic effects (cardiac arrhythmias).
○ Long-term follow-up care is necessary after ablative treatment with ^{131}I or surgery, because the patient usually develops hypothyroidism, sometimes as long as several years after treatment.

○ Local applications of topical medications are used to treat hyperthyroid ophthalmopathy, but high doses of corticosteroids may be required.
○ External beam radiation therapy or surgical decompression to lessen pressure on the orbital contents may be needed in the patient with severe exophthalmos that causes pressure on the optic nerve.

 COLLABORATIVE MANAGEMENT
Care of the patient with hyperthyroidism involves several members of the interdisciplinary team. The endocrinologist can help manage the patient's hormonal status. A cardiologist manages arrhythmias, hypertension, and problems related to myocardial ischemia. The nurse educates the patient about the disorder, its treatments, and self-care issues and helps the patient to cope with the disorder. Because of the hypermetabolic state, the dietitian assesses the patient's nutritional status to ensure adequate nutrition and maintenance of body weight. The physical therapist can help develop a safe exercise program to overcome muscle deconditioning.

Special considerations

○ Document the patient's vital signs and weight.
○ Monitor serum electrolyte levels, and check periodically for hyperglycemia and glycosuria.
○ Carefully monitor cardiac function if the patient is elderly or has coronary artery disease. If the heart rate is more than 100 beats/minute, check blood pressure and pulse rate often.
○ Check level of consciousness and urine output.
○ Encourage bed rest, and keep the patient's room cool, quiet, and dark.
○ Place the patient with dyspnea in an upright or high Fowler's position.
○ Reassure the patient and his family that extreme nervousness may produce bizarre behavior that will probably subside with treatment. Provide sedatives as necessary.
○ To promote weight gain, provide a balanced diet, with six meals per day. If the patient has edema, suggest a low-sodium diet.
○ If iodide is part of the treatment, mix it with milk, juice, or water to prevent GI distress, and

administer it through a straw to prevent tooth discoloration.

○ Watch the patient taking propranolol for signs of hypotension (dizziness, decreased urine output).

○ Watch for signs of thyroid storm, such as tachycardia, hyperkinesis, fever, vomiting, and hypertension.

○ Check intake and output carefully to ensure adequate hydration and fluid balance.

○ Closely monitor blood pressure, cardiac rate and rhythm, and temperature. If the patient has a high fever, reduce it with appropriate hypothermic measures.

○ Maintain an I.V. line and give medications, as ordered.

○ Avoid excessive palpation of the thyroid to avoid precipitating thyroid storm.

○ If the patient has exophthalmos, moisten the conjunctivae often with isotonic eye drops

○ Provide meticulous postoperative care to prevent complications following thyroidectomy:

– Watch for evidence of hemorrhage into the neck, such as a tight dressing with no blood on it. Change dressings and perform wound care, as ordered; check the back of the dressing for drainage.

– Keep the patient in semi-Fowler's position, and support his head and neck with sandbags to ease tension on the incision.

– Check for dysphagia or hoarseness from possible laryngeal nerve injury.

– Watch for signs of hypoparathyroidism (tetany, numbness), a complication that results from accidental removal of the parathyroid glands during surgery.

– Check often for respiratory distress, and keep a tracheotomy tray at bedside.

– If the patient is taking propylthiouracil and methimazole, monitor complete blood count periodically to detect leukopenia, thrombocytopenia, and agranulocytosis.

○ Provide patient education. (See *Teaching about hyperthyroidism*.)

Applicable patient-teaching aids
○ Precautions after radioactive iodine therapy

Teaching about hyperthyroidism

Be sure to include the following points when teaching the patient about hyperthyroidism:

● Explain the disease process, including its signs and symptoms and treatments.

● If the patient has exophthalmos, suggest sunglasses or eye patches to protect his eyes from light.

● Warn the patient with severe lid retraction to avoid sudden physical movements that might cause the lid to slip behind the eyeball.

● Tell the patient who has received radioactive iodine (^{131}I) therapy not to expectorate or cough freely because his saliva will be radioactive for 24 hours. Stress the need for repeated measurement of serum thyroxine levels.

● Tell the patient taking propranolol to rise slowly after sitting or lying down to prevent orthostatic syncope.

● Instruct the patient receiving antithyroid drugs or ^{131}I therapy to report any symptoms of hypothyroidism.

● Instruct the patient to take propylthiouracil or methimazole with meals to minimize GI distress and to avoid over-the-counter cough preparations because many contain iodine.

● Tell the patient to report fever, enlarged cervical lymph nodes, sore throat, mouth sores, and other signs of blood dyscrasias and any rash or skin eruptions — signs of drug hypersensitivity.

● Stress the importance of regular medical follow-up for the patient who has had thyroidectomy because hypothyroidism may develop from 2 to 4 weeks postoperatively.

● Stress the importance of wearing medical identification.

● Explain complications that require immediate medical attention, such as thyroid storm.

● Reinforce the importance of adequate caloric intake.

⬭ Hypothyroidism

Hypothyroidism, a state of low serum thyroid hormone, results from hypothalamic, pituitary, or thyroid insufficiency. The disorder can progress to life-threatening myxedema coma.

Hypothyroidism is more prevalent in females than males, and frequency increases with age; in the United States, incidence is rising significantly in people ages 40 to 50.

Causes

Hypothyroidism results from inadequate production of thyroid hormone — usually because of dysfunction of the thyroid gland due to surgery (thyroidectomy), irradiation therapy (particularly with iodine 131 [^{131}I]), inflammation, chronic autoimmune thyroiditis (Hashimoto's disease) or, rarely, conditions such as amyloidosis and sarcoidosis. It may also result from pituitary failure to produce thyroid-stimulating hormone (TSH), hypothalamic failure to produce thyrotropin-releasing hormone, inborn errors of thyroid hormone synthesis, the inability to synthesize thyroid hormone because of iodine deficiency (usually dietary), or the use of antithyroid medications such as propylthiouracil. In patients with hypothyroidism, infection, exposure to cold, and sedatives may precipitate myxedema coma.

Pathophysiology

Hypothyroidism may reflect a malfunction of the hypothalamus, pituitary, or thyroid gland, all of which are part of the same negative-feedback mechanism. However, disorders of the hypothalamus and pituitary rarely cause hypothyroidism. Primary hypothyroidism, a disorder of the gland itself, is most common.

Chronic autoimmune thyroiditis, also called *chronic lymphocytic thyroiditis,* occurs when autoantibodies destroy thyroid gland tissue. Chronic autoimmune thyroiditis associated with goiter is called *Hashimoto's thyroiditis.* The cause of this autoimmune process is unknown, although heredity has a role, and specific human leukocyte antigen subtypes are associated with greater risk.

Outside the thyroid, antibodies can reduce the effect of thyroid hormone in two ways. First, antibodies can block the TSH receptor and prevent the production of TSH. Second, cytotoxic antithyroid antibodies may attack thyroid cells.

Subacute thyroiditis, painless thyroiditis, and postpartum thyroiditis are self-limited conditions that usually follow an episode of hyperthyroidism. Untreated subclinical hypothyroidism in adults is likely to become overt at a rate of 5% to 20% per year.

Assessment findings

Typically, the early clinical features of hypothyroidism are vague: fatigue, menstrual changes, hypercholesterolemia, forgetfulness, sensitivity to cold, unexplained weight gain, and constipation. As the disorder progresses, characteristic myxedematous signs and symptoms appear, such as decreasing mental stability; dry, flaky, inelastic skin; puffy face, hands, and feet; hoarseness; periorbital edema; upper eyelid droop; dry, sparse hair; and thick, brittle nails. (See *Facial signs of myxedema.*)

Cardiovascular involvement leads to decreased cardiac output, slow pulse rate, signs of poor peripheral circulation and, occasionally, an enlarged heart. Other common effects include anorexia, abdominal distention, menorrhagia, decreased libido, infertility, ataxia, intention tremor, nystagmus, and delayed relaxation time of reflexes (especially in the Achilles tendon).

Progression to myxedema coma is usually gradual but when stress (such as hip fracture, infection, or myocardial infarction) aggravates severe or prolonged hypothyroidism, coma may develop abruptly; clinical effects include progressive stupor, hypoventilation, hypoglycemia, hyponatremia, hypotension, and hypothermia.

Diagnosis

○ Radioimmunoassay confirms hypothyroidism with low triiodothyronine (T_3) and thyroxine (T_4) levels.
○ TSH level are increased when hypothyroidism is due to thyroid insufficiency; TSH levels

are decreased when hypothyroidism is due to hypothalamic or pituitary insufficiency.
○ Serum cholesterol, alkaline phosphatase, and triglyceride levels are elevated.
○ Complete blood cell count shows normocytic normochromic anemia.
○ Serum sodium levels and pH are reduced, and partial pressure of carbon dioxide is increased, indicating respiratory acidosis (myxedema coma).

Complications
○ Achlorhydria
○ Anemia
○ Arteriosclerosis
○ Benign intracranial hypertension
○ Bleeding tendencies
○ Cardiomegaly
○ Carpal tunnel syndrome
○ Conductive or sensorineural deafness
○ Dynamic colon
○ Heart failure
○ Hypercholesterolemia
○ Impaired fertility
○ Intestinal obstruction
○ Ischemic heart disease
○ Megacolon
○ Myxedema coma
○ Peripheral vascular disease
○ Pleural and pericardial effusion
○ Psychiatric disturbances

Treatment
○ Levothyroxine (for low T$_4$ levels) and, occasionally, liothyronine (for inadequate T$_3$ levels) may be ordered to gradually replace thyroid hormone.
○ Surgical excision, chemotherapy, or radiation may be ordered to treat hypothyroidism caused by tumors.

 COLLABORATIVE MANAGEMENT Care of the patient with hypothyroidism involves several members of the interdisciplinary team. The endocrinologist helps manage the patient's hormonal status. A cardiologist manages cardiovascular effects of hypothyroidism, such as heart failure and hypotension. The nurse educates the patient

Facial signs of myxedema

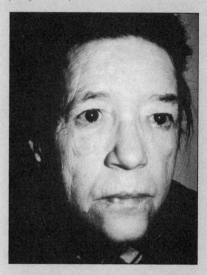

Characteristic myxedematous signs in adults include dry, flaky, inelastic skin; puffy face; and upper eyelid droop.

about the disorder, its treatments, and self-care issues, and helps the patient to cope. Because of the hypometabolic state, the dietitian assesses the patient's nutritional status and makes dietary recommendations. The physical therapist can help develop a safe exercise program to overcome muscle deconditioning. The social worker may assist with financial concerns and follow-up and long-term care planning, such as home care or referrals for community support.

Special considerations
○ Provide a high-bulk, low-calorie diet and encourage activity to combat constipation and promote weight loss. Administer cathartics and stool softeners, as needed.
○ After thyroid replacement therapy begins, watch for symptoms of hyperthyroidism, such

KEY TEACHING POINTS

Teaching about hypothyroidism

Remember these key points when teaching your patient about hypothyroidism:
● Teach about the disease process, including its signs and symptoms, complications, and treatments.
● Teach about prescribed medications, including their names, indications, dosages, adverse effects, and special considerations.
● Explain the signs and symptoms of myxedema that require immediate medical attention.
● To prevent myxedema coma, tell the patient to continue his course of thyroid medication even if his symptoms subside.
● Explain the need for lifelong hormone replacement therapy.
● Warn the patient to report infection immediately and to make sure any physician who prescribes medications for him knows about the underlying hypothyroidism.
● Discuss the need to adhere to a well-balanced, high-fiber, low-sodium diet.
● Talk about energy-conservation techniques and any activity restrictions.
● Reinforce the need to wear medical identification.
● Discuss the importance of keeping an accurate record of daily weight.

as restlessness, sweating, and excessive weight loss.
○ Tell the patient to report any signs of aggravated cardiovascular disease, such as chest pain and tachycardia.
○ Provide patient education. (See *Teaching about hypothyroidism*.)

Applicable patient-teaching aids
○ Learning about levothyroxine

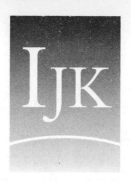

◯ Iron deficiency anemia

Iron deficiency anemia is a disorder of oxygen transport in which hemoglobin synthesis is deficient. A common disease worldwide, it affects 10% to 30% of the adult population of the United States. It occurs most commonly in premenopausal women, infants (particularly premature or low-birth-weight neonates), children, and adolescents (especially girls). Persons of low socioeconomic status who don't get a well-balanced diet that includes iron-rich foods are at increased risk.

Causes

Iron deficiency anemia may result from:
◯ inadequate dietary intake of iron (less than 1 to 2 mg/day), as in prolonged unsupplemented breast-feeding or bottle-feeding of infants or during periods of stress such as rapid growth in children and adolescents
◯ iron malabsorption, as in chronic diarrhea, partial or total gastrectomy, chronic diverticulosis, and malabsorption syndromes, such as celiac disease and pernicious anemia
◯ blood loss secondary to drug-induced GI bleeding (from anticoagulants, aspirin, and steroids) or due to heavy menses, hemorrhage from trauma, GI ulcers, esophageal varices, or cancer
◯ pregnancy, which diverts maternal iron to the fetus for erythropoiesis
◯ intravascular hemolysis-induced hemoglobinuria or paroxysmal nocturnal hemoglobinuria

◯ mechanical erythrocyte trauma caused by a prosthetic heart valve or vena cava filters.

Pathophysiology

Iron deficiency anemia occurs when the supply of iron is inadequate for optimal formation of red blood cells (RBCs), resulting in smaller (microcytic) cells with less color (hypochromic) on staining. Body stores of iron, including plasma iron, become depleted, and the concentration of serum transferrin, which binds with and transports iron, decreases. Insufficient iron stores lead to a depleted RBC mass with subnormal hemoglobin (Hb) concentration and, in turn, subnormal oxygen-carrying capacity of the blood.

Assessment findings

Because iron deficiency anemia progresses gradually, many patients are initially asymptomatic except for symptoms of any underlying condition. At advanced stages, decreased Hb levels and the consequent decrease in the blood's oxygen-carrying capacity cause the patient to develop dyspnea on exertion, fatigue, listlessness, pallor, inability to concentrate, irritability, headache, and a susceptibility to infection. Decreased oxygen perfusion causes the heart to compensate with increased cardiac output and tachycardia.

In chronic iron deficiency anemia, nails become spoon-shaped and brittle, the mouth's corners crack, the tongue turns smooth, and the patient complains of dysphagia or may develop pica. Associated neuromuscular effects include vasomotor disturbances, numbness and tingling of the extremities, and neuralgic pain.

193

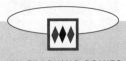

Teaching about iron deficiency anemia

Remember these key points when teaching your patient about iron deficiency anemia:

Nutritional needs
- If the patient is fatigued, urge her to eat small, frequent meals throughout the day.
- If the patient has oral lesions, suggest that she eat soft, cool, bland foods.
- If the patient has dyspepsia, advise her to eliminate spicy foods and to include dairy products in her diet.
- If the patient is anorexic and irritable, encourage her family to bring her favorite foods from home (unless her diet is restricted) and to keep her company during meals, if possible.

Activities
- If during physical activity the patient's pulse accelerates rapidly and she develops hypotension with hyperpnea, diaphoresis, light-headedness, palpitations, shortness of breath, or weakness, the activity is too strenuous.
- Tell the patient to pace her activities and allow for frequent rest periods.

Infection precautions
- Instruct the patient to avoid crowds and other sources of infection. Encourage her to practice good hand-washing technique. Stress the importance of receiving necessary immunizations and prompt medical treatment for any sign of infection.

Diagnostic tests
- Explain erythropoiesis, the function of blood, and the purpose of diagnostic and therapeutic procedures.

Complications
- Alert the patient to those sources of bleeding that may exacerbate anemia, including urine, stools, gums, and ecchymotic areas.
- If the patient is confined to strict bed rest, teach her and her family how to perform range-of-motion exercises. Stress the importance of frequent turning, coughing, and deep breathing.
- Warn the patient to move about and change positions slowly to minimize dizziness induced by cerebral hypoxia.

Diagnosis

○ Serum iron levels, total iron-binding capacity, serum ferritin levels, and iron stores in bone marrow may confirm iron deficiency anemia. Characteristic blood test results include:
– low Hb levels (in males, less than 12 g/dl; in females, less than 10 g/dl)
– low hematocrit (in males, less than 39%; in females, less than 35%)
– low serum iron levels, with high binding capacity
– low serum ferritin levels
– low RBC count, with microcytic and hypochromic cells (in early stages, RBC count may be normal, except in infants and children)
– decreased mean corpuscular Hb in severe anemia.

Bone marrow studies reveal depleted or absent iron stores (done by staining) and normoblastic hyperplasia. Other diagnostic tests must rule out other forms of anemia, such as those that result from thalassemia minor, cancer, and chronic inflammatory, hepatic, and renal disease.

Complications

○ Bleeding
○ Infection
○ Overdosage of oral or I.M. iron supplements
○ Pica (compulsive eating of nonfood materials, such as starch or dirt)
○ Pneumonia

Treatment

○ Identification and treatment of the underlying cause of anemia is the top priority. After that's determined, therapy can begin.

○ Treatment of choice is an oral iron preparation or a combination of iron and ascorbic acid (which enhances iron absorption).

○ Parenteral administration (I.V. or I.M.) of iron is necessary if the patient is noncompliant to the oral preparation, if he needs more iron than he can take orally, if malabsorption prevents adequate iron absorption, or if a maximum rate of Hb regeneration is desired.

 COLLABORATIVE MANAGEMENT
Care of the patient with iron deficiency anemia involves several members of the interdisciplinary team. The physician or hematologist typically diagnoses and treats the disorder. The nurse educates the patient and monitors for complications. The dietitian makes dietary recommendations and educates the patient about foods high in iron.

Special considerations

○ Monitor the patient's compliance with the prescribed iron supplement therapy.

○ If the patient receives I.V. iron, monitor the infusion rate carefully and observe for an allergic reaction. To minimize the risk of an allergic reaction to iron, an I.V. test dose of 0.5 ml should be given first. Stop the infusion and begin supportive treatment immediately if the patient shows signs of an adverse reaction. Also, watch for dizziness and headache and for thrombophlebitis around the I.V. site.

○ Use the Z-track injection method when administering iron I.M. to prevent skin discoloration, scarring, and irritating iron deposits in the skin.

○ Provide patient education. (See *Teaching about iron deficiency anemia*.)

Applicable patient-teaching aids

○ Choosing iron-rich foods *
○ Getting the most from oral iron supplements
○ Learning about daily food choices

○ Irritable bowel syndrome

Irritable bowel syndrome (IBS), also called *spastic colon* and *spastic colitis,* is a common condition marked by chronic or periodic diarrhea, alternating with constipation, and accompanied by straining and abdominal cramps. The prognosis is good. Supportive treatment or avoidance of a known irritant usually relieves symptoms.

IBS affects 10% to 20% of U.S. residents, with a yearly incidence rate of 1% to 2%. The condition occurs most frequently in women ages 20 to 30.

Causes

Mechanisms involved in IBS include visceral hypersensitivity and altered colonic motility. IBS is generally associated with psychological stress, which results in increased colonic contractions. It may result from physical factors, such as diverticular disease, ingestion of irritants (coffee, raw fruits, or vegetables), or lactose intolerance. Autonomic nervous system abnormalities, genetic and psychological factors, and a luminal component (impaired digestion and absorption of certain carbohydrates, such as artificial sweeteners and lactose) may also play a role. Secondary IBS can be caused by abuse of laxatives, food poisoning, or colon cancer.

Pathophysiology

IBS appears to reflect motor disturbances of the entire colon in response to stimuli. Some muscles of the small bowel are particularly sensitive to motor abnormalities and distention; others are particularly sensitive to certain foods and drugs. The patient may be hypersensitive to the hormones gastrin and cholecystokinin. The pain of IBS seems to be caused by abnormally strong contractions of the intestinal smooth muscle as it reacts to distention, irritants, or stress. (See *What happens in irritable bowel syndrome,* page 196.)

CLOSE UP

What happens in irritable bowel syndrome

Visceral hypersensitivity and altered colonic motility are the mechanisms involved in irritable bowel syndrome (IBS). Some muscles of the small bowel are particularly sensitive to motor abnormalities and distention; others are particularly sensitive to certain foods and drugs. Hypersensitivity to the hormones gastrin and cholecystokinin may also occur. In IBS, the entire colon appears to react to stimuli, causing abnormally strong contractions of the intestinal smooth muscle in response to distention, irritants, or stress.

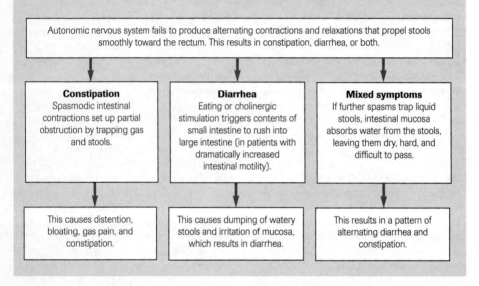

Autonomic nervous system fails to produce alternating contractions and relaxations that propel stools smoothly toward the rectum. This results in constipation, diarrhea, or both.

Constipation
Spasmodic intestinal contractions set up partial obstruction by trapping gas and stools.

Diarrhea
Eating or cholinergic stimulation triggers contents of small intestine to rush into large intestine (in patients with dramatically increased intestinal motility).

Mixed symptoms
If further spasms trap liquid stools, intestinal mucosa absorbs water from the stools, leaving them dry, hard, and difficult to pass.

This causes distention, bloating, gas pain, and constipation.

This causes dumping of watery stools and irritation of mucosa, which results in diarrhea.

This results in a pattern of alternating diarrhea and constipation.

Assessment findings

IBS characteristically produces lower abdominal pain (usually relieved by defecation or passage of gas) and diarrhea that typically occurs during the day. These symptoms alternate with constipation or normal bowel function. Stools are commonly small and contain visible mucus. Dyspepsia and abdominal distention may occur.

Diagnosis

○ History reveals contributing psychological factors such as a recent stressful life change.
○ Negative stool samples for ova, parasites, bacteria, and blood rule out infection.
○ Lactose intolerance test rules out lactose intolerance.

○ Barium enema may reveal colon spasm and tubular appearance of descending colon without evidence of cancers and diverticulosis.
○ Sigmoidoscopy and colonoscopy may reveal spastic contraction without evidence of colon cancer or inflammatory bowel disease.
○ Rectal biopsy rules out malignancy.

Complications

○ Chronic inflammatory bowel disease
○ Colon cancer
○ Diverticular disease
○ Malnutrition

Treatment

○ Treatment aims to relieve symptoms and includes counseling to help the patient understand the relationship between stress and the disorder.

○ Food irritants should be investigated and the patient should be instructed to avoid them.

○ Rest and heat applied to the abdomen are helpful, as is biofeedback.

○ Bowel training may help correct the condition if the cause is chronic laxative abuse.

○ Increased dietary fiber may be effective for both constipation and diarrhea.

○ Bulk laxatives (psyllium) help prevent constipation and diarrhea.

○ Antidiarrheal agents, such as loperamide, can be used to treat diarrhea.

○ 5-HT$_3$ receptor antagonist (alosetron) is a selective antagonist used for short-term treatment of women with IBS who have severe diarrhea. It's available through a restricted marketing program because of serious GI adverse effects, and only practitioners enrolled in the program can prescribe it.

○ 5-HT$_4$ receptor partial agonist (tegaserod) may be prescribed for short-term treatment of women with IBS whose primary symptom is constipation. It also relieves abdominal discomfort and bloating.

○ Antispasmodics may be used to relieve spasms and analgesics may be used for pain relief.

 COLLABORATIVE MANAGEMENT
Care of the patient with IBS involves several members of the interdisciplinary team. The physician or gastroenterologist diagnoses and manages the disorder. The nurse educates the patient, develops a therapeutic relationship, and cares for the patient during exacerbations. The dietitian can help the patient identify foods that may trigger a flare-up. A therapist can help the patient understand the relationship between stress and his illness and to develop coping strategies and lifestyle changes.

Special considerations

○ Monitor the patient's bowel elimination and provide medications (laxatives or antidiarrheals), as ordered.

○ Encourage increased fluid intake.

○ Provide a high-fiber diet.

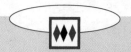

Teaching about irritable bowel syndrome

Remember these key points when teaching your patient and his family about irritable bowel syndrome (IBS):

● Teach about the disease process, including its symptoms, complications, and treatments.

● Teach about prescribed medications, including their names, indications, dosages, adverse effects, and special considerations.

● Tell the patient to avoid irritating foods and to drink 8 to 10 glasses of water each day.

● Encourage the patient to develop regular bowel habits.

● Help the patient deal with stress. Warn her against dependence on sedatives or antispasmodics.

● Encourage regular checkups because IBS is associated with a higher-than-normal incidence of diverticulitis and colon cancer. For patients older than age 40, emphasize the need for an annual sigmoidoscopy and rectal examination.

○ Because the patient with irritable bowel syndrome may not be hospitalized, nursing interventions focus on patient education. (See *Teaching about irritable bowel syndrome.*)

Applicable patient-teaching aids

○ Learning about daily food choices
○ Performing relaxation breathing exercises *
○ Preparing for a barium enema test
○ Preparing for a sigmoidoscopy or a colonoscopy *

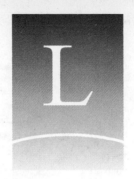

Leukemia, chronic granulocytic

Chronic granulocytic leukemia (CGL), also known as *chronic myelogenous leukemia* and *chronic myelocytic leukemia,* is characterized by the abnormal overgrowth of granulocytic precursors (myeloblasts, promyelocytes, metamyelocytes, and myelocytes) in bone marrow, peripheral blood, and body tissues.

CGL's clinical course proceeds in two distinct phases: the insidious chronic phase, with anemia and bleeding abnormalities and, eventually, the acute phase (blastic crisis), in which myeloblasts, the most primitive granulocytic precursors, proliferate rapidly. This disease is invariably fatal. Average survival time is 3 to 4 years after onset of the chronic phase and 3 to 6 months after onset of the acute phase.

CGL is most common in young and middle-age adults and is slightly more common in men than in women; it's rare in children. In the United States, approximately 4,300 cases of CGL develop annually, accounting for roughly 20% of all leukemias.

Causes

About 95% of patients with CGL have the Philadelphia, or Ph1, chromosome, an abnormality in which the long arm of chromosome 22 is translocated, usually to chromosome 9. Radiation and carcinogenic chemicals may induce this chromosome abnormality. Myeloproliferative diseases also seem to increase the incidence of CGL, and some clinicians suspect that an unidentified virus causes this disease.

Pathophysiology

CGL is a myeloproliferative disorder, originating in a progenitor stem cell. Malignant transformation is identified in erythroid, megakaryocytic, and macrophage cell lines. Malignant transformation arises from pluripotential stem cells or lymphoid stem cells.

Assessment findings

In patients with CGL, anemia may cause fatigue, weakness, decreased exercise tolerance, pallor, dyspnea, tachycardia, and headache. Thrombocytopenia is common, with resulting bleeding and clotting disorders, such as retinal hemorrhage, ecchymoses, hematuria, melena, bleeding gums, nosebleeds, and easy bruising. Hepatosplenomegaly may occur with abdominal discomfort and pain. Other signs and symptoms include sternal and rib tenderness from leukemic infiltrations of the periosteum; low-grade fever; weight loss; anorexia; renal calculi or gouty arthritis from increased uric acid excretion; occasionally, prolonged infection and ankle edema; and, rarely, priapism and vascular insufficiency.

Diagnosis

○ Chromosomal analysis of peripheral blood or bone marrow reveals the Philadelphia chromosome, and low leukocyte alkaline phosphatase levels confirm CGL.

○ White blood cell abnormalities include leukocytosis (leukocytes more than 50,000/mm³, ranging as high as 250,000/mm³), occasional leukopenia (leukocytes less than 5,000/mm³), neutropenia (neutrophils less than 1,500/mm³) despite high leukocyte count, and increased circulating myeloblasts.

○ Hemoglobin is commonly below 10 g/dl.

○ Hematocrit is low (less than 30%).

○ Platelet count reveals thrombocytosis (more than 1 million/mm³).

○ Serum uric acid may be more than 8 mg/dl.

○ Bone marrow aspirate or biopsy characteristically shows bone marrow infiltration by significantly increased number of myeloid elements (biopsy is done only if aspirate is dry); in the acute phase, myeloblasts predominate.

○ Computed tomography scan may identify the organs affected by leukemia.

Complications

○ Hemorrhage

○ Infection

○ Pain

Treatment

○ Aggressive chemotherapy has so far failed to produce remission in CGL. Consequently, the goal of treatment in the chronic phase is to control leukocytosis and thrombocytosis.

○ Imatinib mesylate, a tyrosine kinase inhibitor, has shown significant long-term effectiveness and has remarkably changed CGL treatment by normalizing blood counts.

○ Busulfan and hydroxyurea are the most commonly used oral agents to control leukocytosis and thrombocytosis.

○ Interferon-alpha–based therapy has been used to reduce leukemia cell division and boost the immune system's ability to fight the cancer.

○ Aspirin is commonly given to prevent stroke if the patient's platelet count is over 1 million/mm³.

○ Local splenic radiation or splenectomy may be necessary to increase the platelet count and decrease adverse effects related to splenomegaly.

○ Leukapheresis (selective leukocyte removal) may be performed to reduce leukocyte count.

○ Allopurinol may be given to prevent secondary hyperuricemia or colchicine to relieve gout caused by elevated serum uric acid levels.

○ Antibiotics and other anti-infectives are necessary for the prompt treatment of infections that may result from chemotherapy-induced bone marrow suppression.

○ Bone marrow transplant may produce long asymptomatic periods in the early phase of illness but has been less successful in the accelerated phase.

○ During the acute phase of CGL, lymphoblastic or myeloblastic leukemia may develop. Treatment is similar to that for acute lymphoblastic leukemia. Remission, if achieved, is commonly short lived. Despite vigorous treatment, CGL can progress after onset of the acute phase.

 COLLABORATIVE MANAGEMENT
Care of the patient with CGL involves several members of the interdisciplinary team. The oncologist recommends and manages chemotherapy and bone marrow transplantation. The nurse educates the patient about the disorder, provides measures to improve quality of life, plans interventions to minimize the adverse effects of therapy, and prepares the patient for bone marrow transplantation. The dietitian assesses the patient's nutritional status and makes dietary recommendations. The physical therapist develops an exercise program to help the patient maintain muscle strength and tone. The occupational therapist teaches the patient energy conservation techniques. The social worker helps the patient and family deal with end-of-life issues.

Special considerations

○ If the patient has persistent anemia, plan your care to help avoid exhausting the patient. Schedule laboratory tests and physical care with frequent rest periods in between, and assist the patient with walking, if necessary.

○ Regularly check the patient's skin and mucous membranes for pallor, petechiae, and bruising.

○ To minimize bleeding, suggest a soft-bristle toothbrush, an electric razor, and other safety precautions.

○ To minimize the abdominal discomfort of splenomegaly, provide small, frequent meals. For the same reason, prevent constipation with a stool softener or laxative, as needed. Ask the

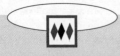

KEY TEACHING POINTS

Teaching about chronic granulocytic leukemia

Remember these key points when teaching your patient about chronic granulocytic leukemia:
• Teach about the disease process, including its symptoms, complications, and treatments.
• Teach about prescribed medications, including their names, indications, dosages, adverse effects, and special considerations.
• Discuss how to minimize bleeding and infection risks (such as by using a soft-bristled toothbrush, an electric razor, and other safety devices).
• Explain the importance of eating a high-calorie, high-protein diet.
• Reinforce the physician's explanation of the bone marrow procedure, possible outcomes, and potential adverse effects, if necessary.

If the patient is receiving chemotherapy, include these points:
• Explain expected adverse effects of chemotherapy. Pay particular attention to dangerous adverse effects such as bone marrow suppression.
• Tell the patient to watch for and immediately report signs and symptoms of infection: any fever over 100° F (37.8° C), chills, redness or swelling, sore throat, and cough.
• Instruct the patient to watch for signs of thrombocytopenia, to immediately apply ice and pressure to any external bleeding site, and to avoid aspirin and aspirin-containing compounds because of the risk of increased bleeding.
• Emphasize the importance of adequate rest to minimize the fatigue of anemia.
• Stress the importance of a high-calorie, high-protein diet to minimize the toxic effects of chemotherapy.

dietary department to provide a high-bulk diet, and maintain adequate fluid intake.
○ To prevent atelectasis, stress the need for coughing and deep-breathing exercises.

○ Provide patient education. (See *Teaching about chronic granulocytic leukemia*.)

Applicable patient-teaching aids
○ Avoiding infection *
○ Examining your lymph nodes
○ Learning about blood transfusions
○ Learning about bone marrow transplantation
○ Preparing for bone marrow aspiration and biopsy *

Leukemia, chronic lymphocytic

Chronic lymphocytic leukemia (CLL) is a generalized, progressive disease that's common in the elderly. It's the most benign and the most slowly progressive form of leukemia. Prognosis is poor if anemia, thrombocytopenia, neutropenia, bulky lymphadenopathy, and severe lymphocytosis are present.

According to the American Cancer Society, this disease accounts for about one-fourth of all new leukemia cases annually. Approximately 2 out of every 100,000 people develop CLL annually, with 90% of cases found in people older than age 50. Many cases go undetected by routine blood tests in people who are asymptomatic. The disease is common in Jewish people of Russian or Eastern European descent, and is uncommon in Asia.

Causes
Although the cause of CLL is unknown, researchers suspect hereditary factors (higher incidence has been recorded within families), still-undefined chromosome abnormalities, and certain immunologic defects (such as ataxia-telangiectasia or acquired agammaglobulinemia).

Pathophysiology
CLL is marked by an uncontrollable spread of abnormal, small lymphocytes in lymphoid tissue, blood, and bone marrow. After these cells infiltrate these areas, clinical signs begin to appear. Gross bone marrow replacement by abnormal lymphocytes is the most common cause

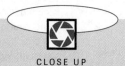

CLOSE UP

Understanding leukemia

Leukemias cause an abnormal proliferation of white blood cells (WBCs) and suppression of other blood components. A rapidly progressing disease, acute leukemia is characterized by the malignant proliferation of WBC precursors (blasts) in bone marrow or lymph tissue and by their accumulation in peripheral blood, bone marrow, and body tissues. In chronic forms of leukemia, disease onset occurs more insidiously, usually with no initial symptoms.

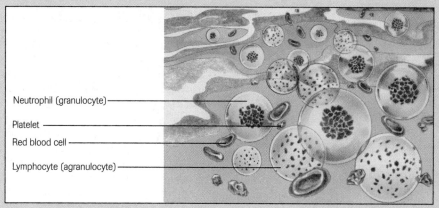

Neutrophil (granulocyte)

Platelet

Red blood cell

Lymphocyte (agranulocyte)

of death, usually within 4 to 5 years of diagnosis. (See *Understanding leukemia.*)

Assessment findings

In early stages, patients with CLL usually complain of fatigue, malaise, fever, and nodal enlargement and are particularly susceptible to infection. In advanced stages, patients may experience severe fatigue and weight loss, with liver or spleen enlargement, bone tenderness, and edema from lymph node obstruction. Pulmonary infiltrates may appear when lung parenchyma is involved. Skin infiltrations, manifested by macular to nodular eruptions, occur in about one-half of the cases of CLL.

As the disease progresses, bone marrow involvement may lead to anemia, pallor, weakness, dyspnea, tachycardia, palpitations, bleeding, and infection. Opportunistic fungal, viral, and bacterial infections commonly occur in late stages.

Diagnosis

○ Routine blood test reveals numerous abnormal lymphocytes (typically, CLL is an incidental finding during a routine complete blood count that reveals numerous abnormal lymphocytes).
○ White blood cell (WBC) count is mildly but persistently elevated in the early stages; granulocytopenia is the rule, but the WBC count climbs as the disease progresses.
○ Blood studies show hemoglobin levels under 11 g/dl, hypogammaglobulinemia, and depressed serum globulins; neutropenia (neutrophils less than 1,500/mm³); lymphocytosis (lymphocytes more than 10,000/mm³); and thrombocytopenia (platelets less than 150,000/mm³).
○ Bone marrow aspiration and biopsy show lymphocytic invasion.

Complications

○ Infection

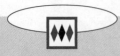

Teaching about chronic lymphocytic leukemia

Remember these key points when teaching your patient and his family about chronic lymphocytic leukemia:

● Teach about the disease process, including its symptoms, complications, and treatments.
● Teach about prescribed medications, including their names, indications, dosages, adverse effects, and special considerations.
● Advise the patient to avoid aspirin and aspirin-containing products because they thin the blood. Also tell him signs and symptoms of bleeding that he should report.
● Explain chemotherapy and radiation therapy and their possible adverse effects.
● Tell the patient to avoid coming in contact with obviously ill people, especially children with common contagious childhood diseases.
● Urge the patient to eat high-protein foods and drink high-calorie beverages.
● Stress the importance of follow-up care and frequent blood tests.
● Teach the patient the signs and symptoms of recurrence (swollen lymph nodes in the neck, axilla, and groin; increased abdominal size or discomfort), and tell him to notify his physician immediately if he detects any of these signs.
● Explain the need for activity restrictions and adequate rest.
● Prepare the patient and his family for bone marrow transplantation, if indicated.

○ In end-stage disease: anemia, progressive splenomegaly, leukemic cell replacement of the bone marrow, and profound hypogammaglobulinemia, which usually terminates with fatal septicemia

Treatment

○ Systemic chemotherapy includes alkylating agents—usually chlorambucil, cyclophosphamide, vincristine, or fludarabine (singly or in combination)—and steroids (prednisone) when autoimmune hemolytic anemia or thrombocytopenia occurs.
○ Humanized monoclonal antibodies, rituximab and alemtuzumab, which are recent advancements in the treatment of CLL, fight and suppress the disease.
○ Local radiation treatment can be used to reduce organ size when chronic lymphocytic leukemia causes obstruction or organ impairment or enlargement.
○ Allopurinol can be given to prevent hyperuricemia, a relatively uncommon finding in patients with CLL.

 COLLABORATIVE MANAGEMENT
Care of the patient with CLL involves several members of the interdisciplinary team. The oncologist makes recommendations for and manages chemotherapy. The radiation oncologist administers and supervises radiation therapy. The nurse educates the patient about the disorder, provides measures to improve quality of life, and plans interventions to minimize the adverse effects of chemotherapy and radiation therapy. The dietitian assesses the patient's nutritional status and makes dietary recommendations. The physical therapist develops an exercise program to help the patient maintain muscle strength and tone. The occupational therapist teaches the patient energy conservation techniques. The social worker helps the patient and family deal with end-of-life issues.

Special considerations

○ Plan patient care to relieve symptoms and prevent infection. Clean the patient's skin daily with mild soap and water. Frequent soaks may be ordered. Watch for signs or symptoms of infection: temperature over 100° F (37.8° C), chills, redness, or swelling of any body part.
○ Watch for signs and symptoms of thrombocytopenia (black tarry stools, easy bruising, nosebleeds, bleeding gums) and anemia (pale skin, weakness, fatigue, dizziness, palpitations).
○ Provide emotional support and be a good listener.

○ Provide patient education. (See *Teaching about chronic lymphocytic leukemia*.)

Applicable patient-teaching aids
○ Avoiding infection *
○ Examining your lymph nodes
○ Learning about blood transfusions
○ Learning about bone marrow transplantation
○ Preparing for bone marrow aspiration and biopsy *

◯ Lung cancer

Even though it's largely preventable, lung cancer has long been the most common cause of cancer death in men and is an increasing cause of cancer death in women. Lung cancer usually develops within the wall or epithelium of the bronchial tree. Its most common types are epidermoid (squamous cell) carcinoma, small-cell (oat cell) carcinoma, adenocarcinoma, and large-cell (anaplastic) carcinoma. Although the prognosis is usually poor, it varies with the extent of metastasis at the time of diagnosis and the cell type growth rate. Only about 14% of patients with lung cancer survive 5 years after diagnosis.

Causes

Most experts agree that lung cancer is attributable to inhalation of carcinogenic pollutants by a susceptible host. Who's most susceptible? Any smoker older than age 40, especially if he began to smoke before age 15, has smoked a whole pack or more per day for 20 years, or works with or near asbestos.

Pollutants in tobacco smoke cause progressive lung cell degeneration. Lung cancer is 10 times more common in smokers than in nonsmokers; 80% of patients with lung cancer are smokers. Cancer risk is determined by the number of cigarettes smoked daily, the depth of inhalation, how early in life smoking began, and the nicotine content of cigarettes. Other factors also increase susceptibility: exposure to second-hand smoke, carcinogenic industrial and air pollutants (asbestos, uranium, arsenic, nickel, iron oxides, chromium, radioactive dust, and coal dust) and familial susceptibility.

Pathophysiology

Lung cancer usually begins with the transformation of one epithelial cell within the patient's airway. Although the exact cause of such a change remains unclear, some lung cancers originating in the bronchi may be more vulnerable to injuries from carcinogens. As the tumor grows, it can partially or completely obstruct the airway, resulting in lobar collapse distal to the tumor. Early metastasis may occur to other thoracic structures as well.

In addition to their obvious interference with respiratory function, lung tumors may also alter the production of hormones that regulate body function or homeostasis. Clinical conditions that result from such changes are known as *hormonal paraneoplastic syndromes.* (See *How lung cancer develops,* page 204.)

Assessment findings

Because early-stage lung cancer usually produces no symptoms, this disease is usually in an advanced state at diagnosis. The following late-state symptoms commonly lead to diagnosis:
○ Epidermoid and small-cell carcinoma may result in smoker's cough, hoarseness, wheezing, dyspnea, hemoptysis, and chest pain.
○ Adenocarcinoma and large-cell carcinoma may produce fever, weakness, weight loss, anorexia, and shoulder pain.
○ Gynecomastia may result from large-cell carcinoma.
○ Hypertrophic pulmonary osteoarthropathy (bone and joint pain from cartilage erosion due to abnormal production of growth hormone) may occur with large-cell carcinoma and adenocarcinoma.
○ Cushing's and carcinoid syndromes may be caused by small-cell carcinoma.
○ Hypercalcemia may result from epidermoid tumors.

Metastatic signs and symptoms vary greatly, depending on the effect of tumors on intrathoracic and distant structures:

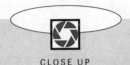

CLOSE UP

How lung cancer develops

Lung cancer usually begins with the transformation of one epithelial cell within the patient's airway. Although the exact cause of such change remains unclear, some lung cancers originating in the bronchi may be more vulnerable to injuries from carcinogens.

As the tumor grows, it can partially or completely obstruct the airway, resulting in lobar collapse distal to the tumor. Early metastasis may occur to other thoracic structures as well.

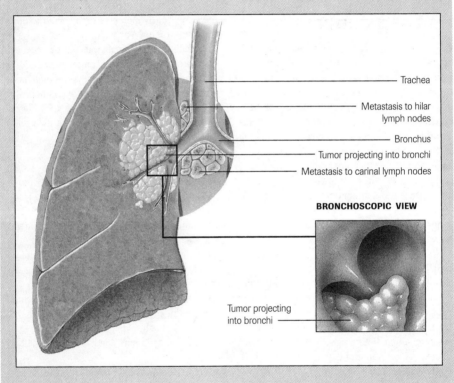

Trachea

Metastasis to hilar lymph nodes

Bronchus

Tumor projecting into bronchi

Metastasis to carinal lymph nodes

BRONCHOSCOPIC VIEW

Tumor projecting into bronchi

○ Bronchial obstruction may cause hemoptysis, atelectasis, pneumonitis, and dyspnea.
○ Cervical thoracic sympathetic nerve involvement produces miosis, ptosis, exophthalmos, and reduced sweating.
○ Chest wall invasion may result in piercing chest pain, increasing dyspnea, and severe shoulder pain, radiating down arm.
○ Esophageal compression leads to dysphagia.

○ Local lymphatic spread can produce cough, hemoptysis, stridor, and pleural effusion.
○ Pericardial involvement can result in pericardial effusion, tamponade, and arrhythmias.
○ Phrenic nerve involvement leads to dyspnea; shoulder pain; and unilateral paralyzed diaphragm, with paradoxical motion.
○ Recurrent nerve invasion produces hoarseness and vocal cord paralysis.

○ Vena caval obstruction causes venous distention and edema of the face, neck, chest, and back.

○ Distant metastasis may involve any part of the body, most commonly the central nervous system, liver, and bone.

Diagnosis

○ Chest X-ray usually shows an advanced lesion, but it can detect a lesion up to 2 years before symptoms appear. It also indicates tumor size and location.

○ Sputum cytology, which is 75% reliable, requires a specimen coughed up from the lungs and tracheobronchial tree, not postnasal secretions or saliva.

○ Computed tomography (CT) scan of the chest helps to delineate the tumor's size and its relationship to surrounding structures.

○ Bronchoscopy locates the tumor site. Bronchoscopic washings provide material for cytologic and histologic examination. The flexible fiber-optic bronchoscope increases the test's effectiveness.

○ Needle biopsy of the lungs allows firm diagnosis in 80% of patients.

○ Tissue biopsy of accessible metastatic sites includes supraclavicular and mediastinal node and pleural biopsy. Directed needle biopsy may be performed in conjunction with CT scan.

○ Thoracentesis allows chemical and cytologic examination of pleural fluid.

○ Mediastinoscopy or mediastinotomy rule out involvement of mediastinal lymph nodes (which would preclude curative pulmonary resection).

○ Bone scan, bone marrow biopsy (recommended in small-cell carcinoma), CT scan of the brain or abdomen, and positron emission tomography detect metastasis.

○ Staging determines the extent of the disease and helps in planning the treatment and predicting the prognosis.

Complications

○ Anorexia and weight loss
○ Esophageal compression with dysphagia
○ Hypoxemia

○ Lymphatic obstruction with pleural effusion
○ Neoplastic and paraneoplastic syndromes, including Pancoast's syndrome and syndrome of inappropriate secretion of antidiuretic hormone
○ Phrenic nerve paralysis with hemidiaphragm elevation and dyspnea
○ Spinal cord compression
○ Spread of primary tumor to intrathoracic structures
○ Sympathetic nerve paralysis with Horner's syndrome
○ Tracheal obstruction

Treatment

○ Surgery is the primary treatment for stage I, stage II, or selected stage III squamous cell cancer; adenocarcinoma; and large-cell carcinoma and may include partial removal of a lung (wedge resection, segmental resection, lobectomy, or radical lobectomy) or total removal (pneumonectomy or radical pneumonectomy).

○ Preoperative radiation therapy may reduce tumor bulk to allow for surgical resection. Preradiation chemotherapy helps improve response rates.

○ Radiation therapy is ordinarily recommended for stage I and stage II lesions, if surgery is contraindicated, and for stage III lesions when the disease is confined to the involved hemithorax and the ipsilateral supraclavicular lymph nodes.

○ High-dose radiation therapy or radiation implants may also be used.

○ Chemotherapy combinations of paclitaxel, gemcitabine, docetaxel, irinotecan, and vinorelbine are more active and better tolerated when combined with cisplatin or carboplatin. Many of these drugs are also used as single agents for the treatment of small-cell and non–small-cell lung cancers.

○ Laser therapy, directed through a bronchoscope, may destroy local tumors.

 COLLABORATIVE MANAGEMENT
Care of the patient with lung cancer involves several members of the interdisciplinary team. The surgeon resects the tumor and possibly removes a portion or all

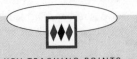

KEY TEACHING POINTS

Teaching about lung cancer

Remember these key points when teaching your patient about lung cancer:
- Teach about the disease process, including its symptoms, complications, and treatments.
- Teach about prescribed medications, including their names, indications, dosages, adverse effects, and special considerations.
- Explain what to expect during the preoperative and postoperative period, if applicable.
- Explain possible adverse effects of radiation and chemotherapy and ways to minimize their effects.
- Tell the patient receiving radiation therapy to avoid tight clothing, exposure to the sun, and harsh ointments on his chest.
- Teach exercises to help prevent shoulder stiffness.
- Encourage the patient to stop smoking and refer him to the American Cancer Society or a smoking-cessation program or suggest group therapy or individual counseling.
- Discuss pain management techniques, such as relaxation exercises.

of the lung. The radiation oncologist directs curative and palliative radiation therapy. The oncologist recommends and manages chemotherapy. The nurse educates the patient about the disorder and its treatments as well as manages problems, such as pain, dyspnea, weight loss, fatigue, adverse effects of chemotherapy and radiation therapy, and quality of life issues. The social worker assists with financial concerns, arranges for medical equipment, makes referrals for hospice, and addresses end-of-life issues. The dietitian teaches the patient and family about proper nutrition to prevent weight loss. The physical therapist works with the patient to prevent frozen shoulder syndrome.

Special considerations

○ If the patient is having surgery, tell him what to expect during the preoperative and postoperative periods.

After thoracic surgery:

○ Maintain a patent airway, and monitor chest tubes to reestablish normal intrathoracic pressure and prevent postoperative and pulmonary complications.

○ Check vital signs every 15 minutes during the 1st hour after surgery, every 30 minutes during the next 4 hours, and then every 2 hours.

○ Watch for and report abnormal respiration and other changes.

○ Suction the patient as needed, and encourage him to begin deep breathing and coughing as soon as possible. Monitor secretions, which may be thick and dark with blood, but should become thinner and grayish yellow within a day.

○ Monitor and document closed chest drainage. Keep chest tubes patent and watch for air leaks; if present, report them immediately.

○ Position the patient on the surgical side to promote drainage and lung reexpansion.

○ Watch for and report foul-smelling discharge and excessive drainage on dressing.

○ Monitor intake and output and maintain adequate hydration.

○ Watch for and treat infection, shock, hemorrhage, atelectasis, dyspnea, mediastinal shift, and pulmonary embolus.

○ To prevent pulmonary embolus, apply antiembolism stockings and encourage range-of-motion exercises.

If the patient is receiving chemotherapy and radiation:

○ Provide soft, nonirritating foods that are high in protein, and encourage the patient to eat high-calorie between-meal snacks.

○ Give antiemetics and antidiarrheals, as needed.

○ Schedule patient care activities in a way that helps the patient conserve his energy.

○ During radiation therapy, administer skin care to minimize skin breakdown.

○ Provide patient education. (See *Teaching about lung cancer*.)

Applicable patient-teaching aids
○ Caring for your hair and scalp during cancer treatment *
○ Controlling the side effects of chemotherapy *
○ Coping with depression
○ Performing exercises for healthier lungs and easier breathing
○ Preparing for bronchoscopy *
○ Taking morphine
○ Using an incentive spirometer
○ Using imagination to relieve pain

○ Lupus erythematosus, systemic

A chronic inflammatory disorder of the connective tissues, lupus erythematosus appears in two forms. *Discoid lupus erythematosus,* the less severe form, affects only the skin. *Systemic lupus erythematosus* (SLE) affects multiple organ systems as well as the skin and can be fatal. Like rheumatoid arthritis, SLE is characterized by recurring remissions and exacerbations, especially common during the spring and summer. The prognosis improves with early detection and treatment, but remains poor for patients who develop cardiovascular, renal, or neurologic complications or severe bacterial infections.

SLE strikes 8 times more women than men, increasing to 15 times more during childbearing years. It occurs worldwide but is most prevalent among Asians and Blacks.

Causes
The exact cause of SLE remains a mystery, but evidence points to interrelated immunologic, environmental, hormonal, and genetic factors. Autoimmunity is thought to be the prime causative mechanism.

Certain predisposing factors may make a person susceptible to SLE. Physical or mental stress, streptococcal or viral infections, exposure to sunlight or ultraviolet light, immunization, pregnancy, and abnormal estrogen metabolism may all affect this disease's development.

SLE may also be triggered or aggravated by treatment with certain drugs—for example, procainamide, hydralazine, anticonvulsants and, less commonly, penicillins, sulfa drugs, and hormonal contraceptives.

Pathophysiology
Autoimmunity is believed to be the prime mechanism involved with SLE. The body produces antibodies against components of its own cells, such as the antinuclear antibody (ANA), and immune complex disease follows. Patients with SLE may produce antibodies against many different tissue components, such as red blood cells (RBCs), neutrophils, platelets, lymphocytes, or almost any organ or tissue in the body. (See *Understanding systemic lupus erythematosus,* page 208.)

Assessment findings
The onset of SLE may be acute or insidious and produces no characteristic clinical pattern. However, its symptoms commonly include fever, weight loss, malaise, and fatigue as well as rashes and polyarthralgia. Most patients have joint involvement similar to that in rheumatoid arthritis. Skin lesions are most commonly erythematous rashes in areas exposed to light. The classic butterfly rash over the nose and cheeks occurs in fewer than 50% of the patients. Vasculitis can develop (especially in the digits), possibly leading to infarctive lesions, necrotic leg ulcers, or digital gangrene. Raynaud's phenomenon appears in about 20% of patients. Patchy alopecia and painless ulcers of the mucous membranes are common.

Constitutional symptoms of SLE include aching, malaise, fatigue, low-grade or spiking fever, chills, anorexia, and weight loss. Lymph node enlargement (diffuse or local, and nontender), abdominal pain, nausea, vomiting, diarrhea, and constipation may occur. Females may experience irregular menses or amenorrhea during the active phase of SLE. Headaches, irritability, and depression are common.

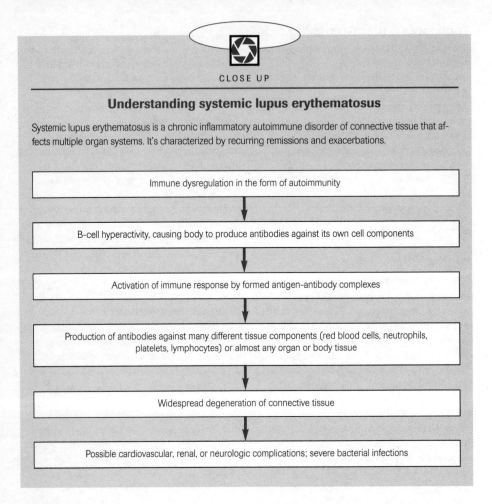

CLOSE UP

Understanding systemic lupus erythematosus

Systemic lupus erythematosus is a chronic inflammatory autoimmune disorder of connective tissue that affects multiple organ systems. It's characterized by recurring remissions and exacerbations.

Immune dysregulation in the form of autoimmunity

↓

B-cell hyperactivity, causing body to produce antibodies against its own cell components

↓

Activation of immune response by formed antigen-antibody complexes

↓

Production of antibodies against many different tissue components (red blood cells, neutrophils, platelets, lymphocytes) or almost any organ or body tissue

↓

Widespread degeneration of connective tissue

↓

Possible cardiovascular, renal, or neurologic complications; severe bacterial infections

Diagnosis

○ Diagnostic tests for patients with SLE include a complete blood count with differential (for signs of anemia and decreased white blood cell [WBC] count); platelet count (may be decreased); erythrocyte sedimentation rate (commonly elevated); and serum electrophoresis (may show hypergammaglobulinemia).

Specific tests for SLE include:

○ Antinuclear antibody panel, including anti-deoxyribonucleic acid (DNA) and anti-Smith antibodies are generally positive for lupus alone. (Because the anti-DNA test is rarely positive in other conditions, it's the most specific test for SLE. However, if the patient is in remission, anti-DNA may be reduced or absent [correlates with disease activity, especially renal involvement, and helps monitor response to therapy].

○ Urine studies may show RBCs and WBCs, urine casts and sediment, and significant protein loss (more than 0.5 g/24 hours).

○ Blood studies reveal decreased serum complement (C3 and C4) levels indicate active disease.

○ Chest X-ray may show pleurisy or lupus pneumonitis.

○ Electrocardiogram may show conduction defect with cardiac involvement or pericarditis.

○ Kidney biopsy determines disease stage and extent of renal involvement.

○ Lupus anticoagulant and anticardiolipin tests are possibly positive in some patients (usually in patients prone to antiphospholipid syndrome of thrombosis and thrombocytopenia).

Complications
○ Cardiopulmonary problems, such as pleuritis, pericarditis, dyspnea, myocarditis, endocarditis, tachycardia, parenchymal infiltrates, and pneumonitis
○ Central nervous system (CNS) involvement, producing emotional instability, psychosis, organic mental syndrome, and seizures
○ Concomitant infections
○ Osteonecrosis of hip from long-term steroid use
○ Renal failure
○ Urinary tract infections

Treatment
○ Nonsteroidal anti-inflammatory drugs, including aspirin, control arthritis symptoms in many patients.
○ Corticosteroid creams are recommended for acute skin lesions.
○ Intralesional corticosteroids or antimalarials such as hydroxychloroquine are used to treat refractory skin lesions.
○ Corticosteroids remain the treatment of choice for systemic symptoms of SLE, for acute generalized exacerbations, or for serious disease related to vital organ systems, such as pleuritis, pericarditis, lupus nephritis, vasculitis, and CNS involvement.
○ Dialysis or kidney transplant may be necessary if renal failure occurs.
○ Cytotoxic drugs may delay or prevent deteriorating renal status in some patients.
○ Antihypertensive drugs and dietary changes may also be warranted in renal disease.

 COLLABORATIVE MANAGEMENT
Care of the patient with lupus erythematosus involves several members of the health care team. The physician manages the disease and provides close follow-up care to prevent flare-ups. The nurse educates the patient about the disorder and plans interventions to prevent flare-ups, control pain, encourage self-care, and preserve self-esteem.

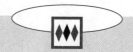

KEY TEACHING POINTS

Teaching about systemic lupus erythematosus

Remember these key points when teaching your patient and his family about systemic lupus erythematosus:
● Teach about the disease process, including its symptoms, complications, and treatments. Emphasize the unpredictable course of remissions and exacerbations.
● Teach about prescribed medications, including their names, indications, dosages, adverse effects, and special considerations.
● Explain measures to prevent infection and skin breakdown.
● Urge the patient to get plenty of rest.
● Encourage proper body alignment and regular exercise to maintain full range of motion and prevent contractures.
● Discuss pregnancy and family planning with patients of childbearing age.
● Offer cosmetic tips such as suggesting the use of hypoallergenic makeup and refer the patient to a hairdresser who specializes in scalp disorders.
● Tell the patient to wear protective clothing (hat, sunglasses, long sleeves, and slacks) and use a screening agent, with a sun protection factor of at least 15, when outdoors.

The social worker addresses financial and occupational concerns and makes referrals to community agencies.

Special considerations
○ Watch for constitutional symptoms: joint pain or stiffness, weakness, fever, fatigue, and chills. Observe for dyspnea, chest pain, and any edema of the extremities. Note the size, type, and location of skin lesions. Check urine for hematuria, scalp for hair loss, and skin and mucous membranes for petechiae, bleeding, ulceration, pallor, and bruising.

○ Provide a balanced diet. Renal involvement may mandate a low-sodium, low-protein diet.
○ Schedule diagnostic tests and procedures to allow adequate rest.
○ Apply heat packs to relieve joint pain and stiffness.
○ Watch for adverse effects, especially when the patient is taking high doses of corticosteroids.
○ Ensure that the patient receiving cyclophosphamide maintains adequate hydration. If prescribed, give mesna to prevent hemorrhagic cystitis and ondansetron to prevent nausea and vomiting.
○ Monitor vital signs, intake and output, weight, and laboratory reports. Check pulse rates and observe for orthopnea. Check stools and GI secretions for blood.
○ Observe for hypertension, weight gain, and other signs of renal involvement.
○ Assess for signs of neurologic damage: personality change, paranoid or psychotic behavior, ptosis, or diplopia. Take seizure precautions. If Raynaud's phenomenon is present, warm and protect the patient's hands and feet.
○ Refer the patient to the Lupus Foundation of America and the Arthritis Foundation as needed.
○ Provide patient education. (See *Teaching about systemic lupus erythematosus,* page 209.)

Applicable patient-teaching aids
○ Learning about corticosteroids
○ Protecting your joints *
○ Protecting your skin *

○ Lyme disease

Lyme disease is a multisystemic disorder that's caused by a tick-borne spirochete. It commonly begins in the summer with a papule that becomes red and warm but isn't painful. Weeks or months later, cardiac or neurologic abnormalities sometimes develop, possibly followed by arthritis of the large joints. This classic skin lesion is called erythema chronicum migrans (ECM), which may be confused with a similar rash caused by Southern tick-associated rash illness.

Initially, Lyme disease was identified in a group of children in Lyme, Connecticut. Now it's known to occur primarily in three parts of the United States: in the Northeast, from Massachusetts to Maryland; in the Midwest, in Wisconsin and Minnesota; and in the West, in California and Oregon. Although it's endemic to these areas, cases have been reported in all 50 states and in 20 other countries, including Germany, Switzerland, France, and Australia.

Causes
Lyme disease is caused by the spirochete *Borrelia burgdorferi,* carried by the minute tick *Ixodes dammini* (also called *I. scapularis*) or another tick in the Ixodidae family.

Pathophysiology
Lyme disease occurs when a tick injects spirochete-laden saliva into the bloodstream. After incubating for 3 to 32 days, the spirochetes migrate out to the skin, causing ECM. Then they disseminate to other skin sites or organs via the bloodstream or lymph system. They may survive for years in the joints, or they may trigger an inflammatory response in the host and then die. (See *Understanding Lyme disease.*)

Assessment findings
Typically, Lyme disease has three stages. ECM heralds stage one with a red macule or papule, commonly at the site of a tick bite, which feels hot and itchy, may grow to over 20″ (50.8 cm) in diameter, and resembles a bull's eye or target. Within a few days, more lesions may erupt, and a migratory, ringlike rash; conjunctivitis; or diffuse urticaria occurs. In 3 to 4 weeks, lesions are replaced by small red blotches, which persist for several more weeks. Malaise and fatigue are constant, but other findings are intermittent: headache, neck stiffness, fever, chills, achiness, and regional lymphadenopathy. Less common effects are meningeal irritation, mild encephalopathy, migrating musculoskeletal pain, hepatitis, and splenomegaly. A persistent

sore throat and dry cough may appear several days before ECM.

Weeks to months later, the second stage (disseminated infection) begins with neurologic abnormalities—fluctuating meningoencephalitis with peripheral and cranial neuropathy—that usually resolve after days or months. Facial palsy is especially noticeable. Cardiac abnormalities, such as a brief, fluctuating atrioventricular heart block, left ventricular dysfunction, or cardiomegaly may also develop.

Stage three (persistent infection) usually begins weeks or years later. Migrating musculoskeletal pain leads to frank arthritis with marked swelling, especially in the large joints. Recurrent attacks may precede chronic arthritis with severe cartilage and bone erosion.

Diagnosis

○ The characteristic ECM lesion and related clinical findings, especially in endemic areas, are used in the diagnosis of Lyme disease because isolation of *B. burgdorferi* is difficult in humans and serologic testing isn't standardized.

○ Immunofluorescence or enzyme-linked immunosorbent assay (ELISA) reveals antibodies to *B. burgdorferi*. Western blot analysis confirms ELISA findings.

○ Blood work may reveal mild anemia, an elevated erythrocyte sedimentation rate, and an elevated leukocyte count. It may also reveal elevated serum immunoglobulin M and aspartate aminotransferase levels.

Complications

○ Arrhythmias
○ Meningitis
○ Myocarditis
○ Pericarditis

   In untreated in acute phase:
○ Arthritis
○ Cranial or peripheral neuropathies
○ Encephalitis

Treatment

○ An antibiotic, such as doxycycline, is the treatment of choice for nonpregnant adults.

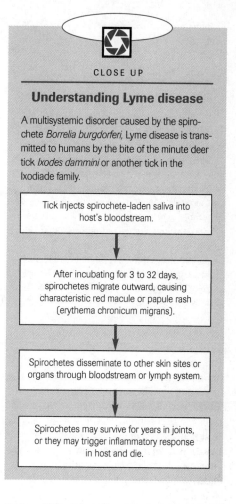

CLOSE UP

Understanding Lyme disease

A multisystemic disorder caused by the spirochete *Borrelia burgdorferi*, Lyme disease is transmitted to humans by the bite of the minute deer tick *Ixodes dammini* or another tick in the Ixodiade family.

> Tick injects spirochete-laden saliva into host's bloodstream.

> After incubating for 3 to 32 days, spirochetes migrate outward, causing characteristic red macule or papule rash (erythema chronicum migrans).

> Spirochetes disseminate to other skin sites or organs through bloodstream or lymph system.

> Spirochetes may survive for years in joints, or they may trigger inflammatory response in host and die.

Oral penicillin is usually prescribed for children. Alternatives include tetracycline, cefuroxime, and ceftriaxone.

○ I.V. ceftriaxone may be successful when given during the last stages.

 COLLABORATIVE MANAGEMENT Care of the patient with Lyme disease involves several members of the interdisciplinary team. Although the care of the patient may be managed by a primary physician, other specialists such as a cardiologist, neurologist, rheumatologist, or infection disease specialist may be involved. The nurse educates the patient and plans interventions to control symptoms and help the patient main-

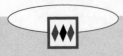

KEY TEACHING POINTS

Teaching about Lyme disease

Remember these key points when teaching your patient about Lyme disease:

- Teach about the disease process, including its symptoms, complications, and treatments.
- Teach about prescribed medications, including their names, indications, dosages, adverse effects, and special considerations.
- Emphasize the importance of follow-up care and reporting recurrent or new symptoms to the physician.
- Discuss the prevention of Lyme disease, such as avoiding tick-infested areas, covering the skin with clothing, using insect repellants, inspecting exposed skin for attached ticks at least every 4 hours, and removing found ticks promptly.

○ Check for cardiac abnormalities, such as arrhythmias and heart block.
○ Provide patient education. (See *Teaching about Lyme disease.*)

Applicable patient-teaching aids
○ Protecting your joints *
○ Restoring strength and relieving pain in arthritis *

tain an acceptable quality of life. The physical therapist helps the patient perform range-of-motion exercises to reduce joint stiffness and pain. The occupational therapist helps the patient perform activities of daily living at his highest level of functioning. The social worker addresses financial and occupational concerns.

Special considerations
○ Take a detailed patient history, asking about travel to endemic areas and exposure to ticks.
○ Check for drug allergies, and administer antibiotics carefully.
○ For a patient with arthritis, help with range-of-motion and strengthening exercises, but avoid overexertion. Ibuprofen helps relieve joint stiffness.
○ Assess the patient's neurologic function and level of consciousness frequently. Watch for signs of increased intracranial pressure and cranial nerve involvement, such as ptosis, strabismus, and diplopia.

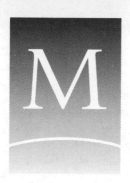

Macular degeneration, age-related

Macular degeneration is the atrophy or degeneration of the macular region of the retina. Two types of age-related macular degeneration occur. The dry or atrophic form is characterized by atrophic pigment epithelial changes and is most commonly associated with slow, progressive, mild vision loss. The wet, exudative form causes progressive visual distortion leading to vision loss. It's characterized by subretinal neovascularization that causes leakage, hemorrhage, and fibrovascular scar formation, which produce significant loss of central vision.

Macular degeneration is the most common cause of legal blindness in adults, accounting for about 12% of blindness cases in the United States and for about 17% of new blindness cases. It's also one of the causes of severe irreversible loss of central vision in elderly people; by age 75, almost 15% of people have this condition. Whites have the highest incidence. Other risk factors are family history and cigarette smoking.

Causes

Age-related macular degeneration results from underlying pathologic changes that occur primarily at the level of the retinal pigment epithelium, Bruch's membrane, and the choriocapillaris in the macular region. Drusen (bumps), which are common in elderly people, appear as yellow deposits beneath the pigment epithelium and may be prominent in the macula. No predisposing conditions have been identified; however, some forms of the disorder are hereditary.

Pathophysiology

Age-related macular degeneration results from hardening and obstruction of retinal arteries, which probably reflect normal degenerative changes. The formation of new blood vessels in the macular area obscures central vision. Underlying pathologic changes occur primarily in the retinal pigment epithelium, Bruch's membrane, and choriocapillaris in the macular region.

The dry form develops as yellow extracellular deposits, or *drusen*, accumulate beneath the pigment epithelium of the retina; they may be prominent in the macula. Drusen are common in elderly people. Over time, drusen grow and become more numerous. Vision loss occurs as the retinal pigment epithelium detaches and becomes atrophic.

Exudative macular degeneration develops as new blood vessels in the choroid project through abnormalities in Bruch's membrane and invade the potential space underneath the retinal pigment epithelium. As these vessels leak, fluid in the retinal pigment epithelium is increased, resulting in blurry vision.

Assessment findings

The patient notices a change in central vision. Initially, straight lines (for example, of buildings) become distorted; later, a blank area appears in the center of a printed page (central scotoma).

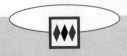

KEY TEACHING POINTS

Teaching about macular degeneration

Be sure to include the following points when teaching the patient with macular degeneration:
- Teach about the disease process, including its symptoms, complications, and treatments.
- Teach about prescribed medications, including their names, indications, dosages, adverse effects, and special considerations.
- Discuss the visual rehabilitation services that are available.
- Discuss special devices, such as low-vision optical aids, that are available to improve the quality of life in the patient with good peripheral vision.
- Assist the patient in identifying ways to modify his home to maintain safety.

Diagnosis
○ Indirect ophthalmoscopy may reveal gross macular changes.
○ I.V. fluorescein angiography may show leaking vessels as fluorescein dye flows into the tissues from the subretinal neovascular net.
○ Amsler's grid monitors visual field loss.

Complications
○ Nystagmus (if the macular degeneration is bilateral)
○ Vision impairment progressing to blindness

Treatment
○ Laser photocoagulation reduces the incidence of severe vision loss in patients with subretinal neovascularization, turning serous age-related macular degeneration to the dry form.
○ Photodynamic therapy is an option for patients with wet macular degeneration.

 COLLABORATIVE MANAGEMENT
Care of the patient with age-related macular degeneration involves sever-

al members of the interdisciplinary team. The ophthalmologist monitors the condition and makes recommendations for other treatments, such as laser surgery. A low-vision specialist can provide assistive devices to the patient with reduced vision to allow him to work and perform activities of daily living. The nurse provides education and support to the patient.

Special considerations
○ Ensure safety in the visually impaired patient.
○ Provide patient education. (See *Teaching about macular degeneration*.)

Applicable patient-teaching aids
○ Administering eyedrops

○ Malignant melanoma

A malignant neoplasm that arises from melanocytes, malignant melanoma is relatively rare, accounting for only 1% to 2% of all malignancies. However, incidence is increasing. The four types of melanomas are superficial spreading melanoma, nodular malignant melanoma, lentigo maligna, and acral lentiginous melanoma.

Melanoma spreads through the lymphatic and vascular systems and metastasizes to the regional lymph nodes, skin, liver, lungs, and central nervous system. Its course is unpredictable, however, and recurrence and metastasis may not appear for more than 5 years after resection of the primary lesion. The prognosis varies with tumor thickness. Generally, superficial lesions are curable, whereas deeper lesions tend to metastasize. The Breslow level method measures tumor depth from the granular level of the epidermis to the deepest melanoma cell. Melanoma lesions less than 0.76 mm deep have an excellent prognosis, whereas deeper lesions (more than 0.76 mm) are at risk for metastasis. The prognosis is better for a tumor on an extremity (which is drained by one lymphatic network) than for one on the head, neck, or trunk (drained by several networks).

Melanoma is slightly more common in women than in men and is rare in children. Peak incidence occurs between ages 50 and 70, although the incidence in younger age-groups is increasing.

Causes

Several factors seem to influence the development of melanoma. Excessive exposure to sunlight is a significant factor. Melanoma is most common in sunny, warm areas and typically develops on parts of the body that are exposed to the sun.

A person's skin type may also play a role. Most persons who develop melanoma have blond or red hair, fair skin, and blue eyes; are prone to sunburn; and are of Celtic or Scandinavian ancestry. Melanoma is rare among Blacks; when it does develop, it usually arises in lightly pigmented areas (the palms, plantar surface of the feet, or mucous membranes).

Hormones may be involved in the development of malignant melanoma because pregnancy may increase risk and exacerbate growth. Melanoma is also slightly more common within families. A past history of melanoma is also significant because a person who has had one melanoma is at greater risk for developing a second.

Pathophysiology

Malignant melanoma can arise on normal skin or from an existing mole. It arises from melanocytes, which produce the pigment melanin. These malignant cells can spread and invade nearby organs or may metastasize throughout the body through the lymphatic and vascular channels.

Assessment findings

Common sites for melanoma are on the head and neck in men, on the legs in women, and on the backs of persons exposed to excessive sunlight. Up to 70% arise from a preexisting nevus.

Suspect melanoma when any skin lesion or nevus enlarges, changes color, becomes inflamed or sore, itches, ulcerates, bleeds, undergoes textural changes, or shows signs of surrounding pigment regression (halo nevus or vitiligo). (See *Recognizing malignant melanoma,* page 216.)

Each type of melanoma has special characteristics:

○ *Superficial spreading melanoma,* the most common, usually arises on an area of chronic irritation. In women, it's most common between the knees and ankles; in Blacks and Asians, on the toe webs and soles (lightly pigmented areas subject to trauma). Characteristically, this melanoma has a red, white, and blue color over a brown or black background and an irregular, notched margin. Its surface is irregular, with small, elevated tumor nodules that may ulcerate and bleed.

○ *Nodular melanoma* grows vertically, invades the dermis, and metastasizes early. The lesion has a uniformly dark discoloration (it may be grayish), and looks like a blackberry. Occasionally, this melanoma is flesh-colored, with flecks of pigment around its base (possibly inflamed).

○ *Lentigo maligna melanoma* arises from a lentigo maligna on an exposed skin surface. This lesion looks like a large (3- to 6-cm) flat freckle of tan, brown, black, whitish, or slate color and has irregularly scattered black nodules on the surface. It develops slowly, usually over many years, and eventually may ulcerate. This melanoma commonly develops under the fingernails, on the face, and on the back of the hands.

○ *Acral lentiginous melanoma* develops in areas that are hard to see, such as the palms, soles, mucous membranes, and under fingernails. In its early stages, it looks like a bruise or a nail streak and is easily overlooked. As the cancer grows, it develops an irregular shape and color. The lesion may remain flat as the skin below is invaded. It's more common in Asian and Black people.

Diagnosis

○ Skin biopsy with histologic examination can distinguish malignant melanoma from a benign nevus, seborrheic keratosis, and pigmented basal cell epithelioma; it can also determine tumor thickness.

Recognizing malignant melanoma

Malignant melanoma arises from melanocytes in the dermis and epidermis. The lesions are asymmetrical with irregular borders that are ragged, uneven, or blurred, and they usually grow wider than 6 mm. The illustrations below show a cross-section of a malignant melanoma and its defining characteristics.

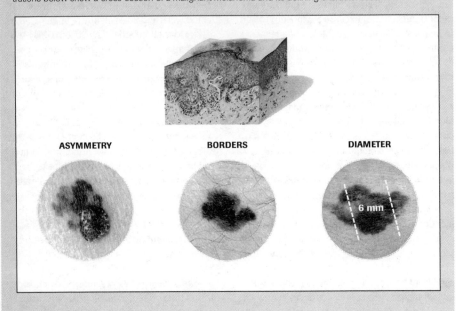

ASYMMETRY　　　　　BORDERS　　　　　DIAMETER

6 mm

○ Physical examination, paying particular attention to lymph nodes, can point to metastatic involvement.

○ Chest X-rays assist in staging.

○ Laboratory studies establish a baseline and include complete blood count with differential, erythrocyte sedimentation rate, platelet count, liver function studies, and urinalysis.

○ Computed tomography scan of the chest and abdomen and a bone scan may detect metastasis.

Complications

○ Metastasis to the lungs, liver, or brain

Treatment

○ Surgical resection is performed to remove the tumor. Closure of a wide resection may require a skin graft.

○ Regional lymphadenectomy may also be necessary.

○ Adjuvant chemotherapy and biotherapy may be used for deep primary lesions to eliminate or reduce the number of tumor cells.

○ Radiation therapy is usually reserved for metastatic disease because it doesn't prolong survival but may reduce tumor size and relieve pain.

COLLABORATIVE MANAGEMENT
Management of the melanoma patient requires careful physical, psychological, and social assessment by an interdisciplinary team. The lesions are removed by a surgeon. An oncologist makes recommendations for chemotherapy. The nurse educates the patient about the condition, reducing the risk of further lesions, and managing the effects of chemotherapy. With advanced disease,

KEY TEACHING POINTS

Teaching about malignant melanoma

Remember these key points when teaching your patient about malignant melanoma:
● Teach about the disease process, including its symptoms, complications, and treatments.
● Teach about prescribed medications, including their names, indications, dosages, adverse effects, and special considerations.
● Tell the patient what to expect before and after surgery and warn him that the donor site for a skin graft may be as painful as the tumor excision site, if not more so.
● Emphasize the need for close follow-up to detect recurrences early.
● Tell the patient how to recognize signs of recurrence.
● Stress the importance of regular use of a sunblock or a sunscreen and protective clothing and avoiding overexposure to solar radiation.

---

the social worker makes referrals for home care and assists with financial concerns.

Special considerations
○ Provide preoperative and postoperative teaching for the patient undergoing surgery.
○ After surgery, be careful to prevent infection. Check dressings often for excessive drainage, foul odor, redness, or swelling. If surgery included lymphadenectomy, minimize lymphedema by applying a compression stocking and instructing the patient to keep the extremity elevated.
○ During chemotherapy, monitor for adverse effects and take measures to minimize them. For instance, give an antiemetic, as ordered, to reduce nausea and vomiting.
○ Provide psychological support and encourage the patient to verbalize his fears.
○ Control and prevent pain in advanced metastatic disease with consistent, regularly scheduled administration of analgesics.

○ Make referrals for home care, social services, and spiritual and financial assistance, as needed.
○ If the patient is dying, identify the needs of the patient, his family, and friends, and provide appropriate support and care.
○ Provide patient education. (See *Teaching about malignant melanoma*.)

Applicable patient-teaching aids
○ Changing a dry dressing
○ Examining your skin *
○ Minimizing sun exposure *

○ Mitral insufficiency

Mitral insufficiency, also known as *mitral regurgitation,* allows the backflow of blood from the left ventricle to the left atrium. The condition may be acute (sudden volume overload of the left ventricle), chronic compensated (left ventricle compensates and left ventricular enlargement occurs), or chronic decompensated (left ventricle can't sustain forward cardiac output).

Causes
Mitral insufficiency results from rheumatic fever, hypertrophic cardiomyopathy, mitral valve prolapse, myocardial infarction, severe left-sided heart failure, or ruptured chordae tendineae. The condition is also associated with congenital anomalies, such as transposition of the great arteries. It's rare in children without other congenital anomalies.

Pathophysiology
In mitral insufficiency, blood from the left ventricle flows back into the left atrium during systole, causing the atrium to enlarge to accommodate the backflow. As a result, the left ventricle dilates to accommodate the increased volume of blood from the atrium and to compensate for diminishing cardiac output. Ventricular hypertrophy and increased end-diastolic pressure result in increased pulmonary artery pressure, eventually leading to left- and right-sided heart failure. (See *Understanding mitral insufficiency,* page 218.)

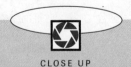

CLOSE UP

Understanding mitral insufficiency

An abnormality of the mitral leaflets, mitral annulus, chordae tendineae, papillary muscles, left atrium, or left ventricle can lead to mitral insufficiency. Blood from the left ventricle flows back into the left atrium during systole; the atrium enlarges to accommodate the backflow. As a result, the left ventricle also dilates to accommodate the increased blood volume from the atrium and to compensate for diminishing cardiac output. Ventricular hypertrophy and increased end-diastolic pressure result in increased pulmonary artery pressure, eventually leading to left-sided and right-sided heart failure.

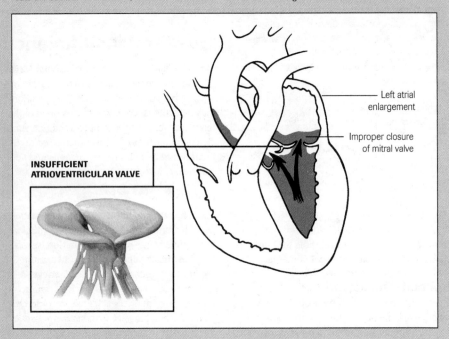

Left atrial enlargement

Improper closure of mitral valve

INSUFFICIENT ATRIOVENTRICULAR VALVE

Assessment findings

The patient with mitral insufficiency may report orthopnea, dyspnea, fatigue, angina, and palpitations. Examination may reveal peripheral edema, neck vein distention, and hepatomegaly (in right-sided heart failure). Auscultation may reveal crackles, tachycardia, a holosystolic murmur at the apex of the heart, a possible split S_2, and an S_3.

Diagnosis

○ Chest X-ray reveals left atrial and ventricular enlargement and pulmonary congestion.
○ Echocardiography shows abnormal valve leaflet motion and left atrial enlargement.
○ Cardiac catheterization reveals mitral insufficiency with increased left ventricular end-diastolic volume and pressure, increased atrial pressure and pulmonary artery wedge pressure, and decreased cardiac output.

○ Electrocardiography may show left atrial and ventricular hypertrophy, sinus tachycardia, or atrial fibrillation.

Complications
○ Arrhythmias
○ Endocarditis
○ Heart failure
○ Pulmonary edema
○ Thromboembolism

Treatment
○ Digoxin, a low-sodium diet, diuretics, vasodilators, and angiotensin-converting enzyme inhibitors are used to treat left left-sided heart failure.
○ Anticoagulants are administered to prevent thrombus formation around diseased or replaced valves.
○ Prophylactic antibiotics are necessary before and after surgery or dental care to prevent endocarditis.
○ Antiarrhythmics may be necessary to treat arrhythmias.
○ Valve replacement with a prosthetic valve or valve repair may be necessary to control symptoms.

 COLLABORATIVE MANAGEMENT
Care of the patient with mitral insufficiency involves several members of the interdisciplinary team. The cardiologist diagnoses the condition and determines the care plan. The surgeon may perform procedures such as annuloplasty or valve replacement. The nurse educates the patient about the condition and provides care to maximize cardiac function. The dietitian helps the patient to select low-sodium foods and prepare palatable low-sodium meals. Physical therapy may be needed in the postoperative period to assist the patient to regain maximum functioning. The interdisciplinary cardiac rehabilitation team (which may consist of cardiologists, exercise specialists, physical therapists, occupational therapists, dietitians, nurses, and social workers) provides supervised exercise, education, and cardiac risk modification.

Special considerations
○ Watch closely for signs of heart failure or pulmonary edema and for adverse effects of drug therapy.
○ If the patient has surgery, watch for hypotension, arrhythmias, and thrombus formation. Monitor vital signs, arterial blood gas values, intake and output, daily weight, blood chemistries, chest X-rays, and pulmonary artery catheter readings.
○ Place the patient in an upright position to relieve dyspnea, if indicated.
○ Provide patient education for valvular heart disease. (See *Teaching about valvular heart disease*, page 24.)

Applicable patient-teaching aids
○ Cutting down on salt *
○ Living with heart failure *
○ Preparing for echocardiography
○ Preventing infection with antibiotics *
○ Taking anticoagulants *
○ Taking warfarin

◯ Mitral stenosis

In mitral stenosis, narrowing of the mitral valve by valvular abnormalities, fibrosis, or calcification obstructs blood flow from the left atrium to the left ventricle. Consequently, left atrial volume and pressure rise and the left atrium dilates.

Mitral stenosis is most common in females. Typically, symptoms develop between ages 20 and 50 years in people who previously had rheumatic fever; as the incidence of rheumatic fever in the United States is declining, so is the incidence of mitral stenosis.

Causes
Mitral stenosis may be caused by rheumatic fever, congenital abnormalities, atrial myoma, and endocarditis. It may also be caused by an adverse effect of the fenfluramine-phentermine diet-drug combination (this drug combination has been removed from the U.S. drug market).

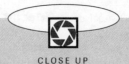

CLOSE UP

Understanding mitral stenosis

Mitral stenosis occurs when valve leaflets become thickened by fibrosis and calcification, resulting in narrowing of the valve orifice. The left atrium dilates as left atrial volume and pressure rise. Greater resistance to blood flow causes pulmonary hypertension, right ventricular hypertrophy, and right-sided heart failure. Inadequate filling of the left ventricle results in low cardiac output.

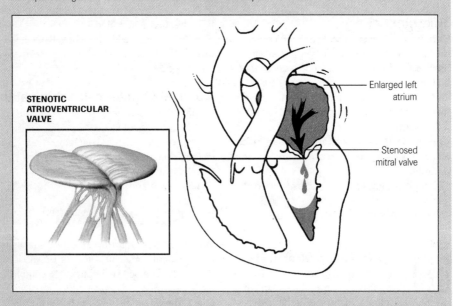

STENOTIC
ATRIOVENTRICULAR
VALVE

Enlarged left
atrium

Stenosed
mitral valve

Pathophysiology

In mitral stenosis, the valve leaflets become diffusely thickened by fibrosis and calcification. The mitral commissures and the chordae tendinae fuse and shorten, the valvular cusps become rigid, and the valve's apex becomes narrowed. This obstructs blood flow from the left atrium to the left ventricle, resulting in incomplete emptying. Left atrial volume and pressure increase, and the atrial chamber dilates. Increased resistance to blood flow causes pulmonary hypertension, right ventricular hypertrophy and, eventually, right-sided heart failure and reduced cardiac output. (See *Understanding mitral stenosis*.)

Assessment findings

The patient may report dyspnea on exertion, paroxysmal nocturnal dyspnea, fatigue, syncope, angina, and palpitations. Pulmonary congestion and left-sided heart failure may also be present. Examination may reveal diminished carotid pulses, pulsus alternans, and an irregular pulse. Auscultation may reveal a low-pitched diastolic murmur (heard best at the heart's apex), a loud S_1, and an opening diastolic snap heard at the left sternal border.

Diagnosis

○ Chest X-rays show left atrial and ventricular enlargement (in severe mitral stenosis), straightening of the left border of the cardiac silhouette, enlarged pulmonary arteries, dilation of the upper lobe pulmonary veins, and mitral valve calcification.

○ Echocardiography discloses thickened mitral valve leaflets and left atrial enlargement.

○ Cardiac catheterization shows a diastolic pressure gradient across the valve, elevated pulmonary artery wedge pressure (greater than 15 mm Hg), and pulmonary artery pressure in the left atrium with severe pulmonary hypertension.

○ Electrocardiography reveals left atrial enlargement, right ventricular hypertrophy, right axis deviation, and (in 40% to 50% of cases) atrial fibrillation.

Complications
○ Arrhythmias, especially atrial fibrillation
○ Endocarditis
○ Thromboembolism

Treatments
○ Digoxin, a low-sodium diet, diuretics, vasodilators, and angiotensin-converting enzyme inhibitors are given to treat left-sided heart failure.

○ Nitroglycerin relieves angina.

○ Anticoagulants prevent thrombus formation around diseased or replaced valves.

○ Prophylactic antibiotics must be administered before and after surgery or dental care to prevent endocarditis.

○ Antiarrhythmics may be necessary to treat arrhythmias.

○ Valve replacement with a prosthetic valve or balloon valvuloplasty enlarges the orifice of the stenotic valve.

 COLLABORATIVE MANAGEMENT
Care of the patient with mitral stenosis involves several members of the interdisciplinary team. The cardiologist diagnoses the disorder and determines the treatment plan. The nurse plays a crucial role in educating the patient about the disease and its treatments. The dietitian reinforces the need for a low-sodium diet and helps the patient with making proper food choices. The interdisciplinary cardiac rehabilitation team (which may consist of cardiologists, exercise specialists, physical therapists, occupational therapists, dietitians, nurses, and social workers) provides supervised exercise, education, and cardiac risk modification.

Special considerations
○ Watch closely for signs of heart failure or pulmonary edema and for adverse effects of drug therapy.

○ If the patient has surgery, watch for hypotension, arrhythmias, and thrombus formation. Monitor vital signs, arterial blood gas values, intake and output, daily weight, blood chemistries, chest X-rays, and pulmonary artery catheter readings.

○ Place the patient in an upright position to relieve dyspnea, if indicated.

○ Provide patient education for valvular heart disease. (See *Teaching about valvular heart disease,* page 24.)

Applicable patient-teaching aids
○ Cutting down on salt *
○ Living with heart failure *
○ Preparing for cardiac catheterization *
○ Preventing infection with antibiotics *
○ Taking anticoagulants *

◯ Multiple sclerosis

Multiple sclerosis (MS) is a progressive disease caused by demyelination of the white matter of the brain and spinal cord. In this disease, sporadic patches of demyelination throughout the central nervous system (CNS) induce widely disseminated and varied neurologic dysfunction. Characterized by exacerbations and remissions, MS is a major cause of chronic disability in young adults.

The prognosis varies; MS may progress rapidly, disabling some patients by early adulthood or causing death within months of onset. However, 70% of patients lead active, productive lives with prolonged remissions.

MS usually begins between ages 20 and 40. It affects more women than men. A family history of MS and living in a geographical area with higher incidence of MS (northern Europe,

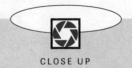

CLOSE UP

How myelin breaks down

Myelin speeds electrical impulses to the brain for interpretation. This lipoprotein complex (formed of glial cells or oligodendrocytes) protects the neuron's axon much like the insulation on an electrical wire. Its high electrical resistance and low capacitance allow the myelin to conduct nerve impulses from one node of Ranvier to the next.

Myelin is susceptible to injury (for example, by hypoxemia, toxic chemicals, vascular insufficiencies, or autoimmune responses). The sheath becomes inflamed, and the membrane layers break down into smaller components that become well-circumscribed plaques (filled with microglial elements, macroglia, and lymphocytes). This process is called *demyelination*.

The damaged myelin sheath can't conduct normally. The partial loss or dispersion of the action potential causes neurologic dysfunction.

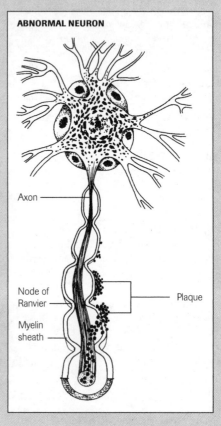

ABNORMAL NEURON

Axon

Node of Ranvier

Myelin sheath

Plaque

---

northern United States, southern Australia, and New Zealand) increase the risk.

Causes

The exact cause of MS is unknown, but current theories suggest a slow-acting or latent viral infection and an autoimmune response. Other theories suggest that environmental and genetic factors may also be linked to MS. Emotional stress, overwork, fatigue, pregnancy, and acute respiratory tract infections have been known to precede the onset of this illness.

Pathophysiology

In MS, sporadic patches of axon demyelination and nerve fiber loss occur throughout the CNS, inducing widely disseminated and varied neurologic dysfunction. (See *How myelin breaks down*.)

New evidence of nerve fiber loss may provide an explanation for the invisible neurologic deficits experienced by many patients with MS. The axons determine the presence or absence of function; loss of myelin doesn't correlate with loss of function. Clinical findings in MS depend on the extent and site of myelin destruction, the extent of remyelination, and the adequacy of subsequent restored synaptic transmission.

Assessment findings

Signs and symptoms in MS may be transient, last for hours or weeks, wax and wane with no predictable pattern, vary from day to day, and be bizarre and difficult for the patient to describe. In most patients, vision problems and sensory impairment, such as numbness and tingling sensations (paresthesia), are the first signs that something may be wrong. Other characteristic changes include the following:

○ Ocular disturbances include optic neuritis, diplopia, ophthalmoplegia, blurred vision, and nystagmus.

○ Muscle dysfunction leads to weakness, paralysis ranging from monoplegia to quadriplegia, spasticity, hyperreflexia, intention tremor, and gait ataxia.

○ Urinary incontinence, frequency, urgency, and frequent infections may also occur.

○ The person with MS may have characteristic mood swings, irritability, euphoria, and depression.

○ Associated signs and symptoms include poorly articulated or scanning speech and dysphagia.

○ Clinical effects may be so mild that the patient is unaware of them or so bizarre that he appears hysterical.

Diagnosis

○ Magnetic resonance imaging may detect MS lesions.

○ EEG findings are abnormal in one-third of patients.

○ Lumbar puncture shows elevated gamma globulin fraction of immunoglobulin G but normal total cerebrospinal fluid (CSF) protein levels. Elevated CSF gamma globulin is significant only when serum gamma globulin levels are normal because it reflects hyperactivity of the immune system due to chronic demyelination. Oligoclonal bands of immunoglobulin can be detected when gamma globulin in CSF is examined by electrophoresis, and these bands are

present in most patients, even when the percentage of gamma globulin in CSF is normal. In addition, the white blood cell count in CSF may rise.

○ Evoked potential studies show slowed conduction of nerve impulses.

Complications

○ Constipation
○ Contractures
○ Depression
○ Injuries from falls
○ Pneumonia
○ Pressure ulcers
○ Urinary tract infections

Treatment

○ Immune modulating therapy, with interferon or glatiramer acetate, is used in those patients with relapsing-remitting courses.

○ Steroids are used to reduce the associated edema of the myelin sheath during exacerbations.

○ Baclofen, tizanidine, or diazepam may relieve spasticity.

○ Cholinergic agents relieve urine retention and minimize frequency and urgency.

○ Amantadine relieves fatigue.

○ Antidepressants help with mood or behavioral symptoms.

○ Supportive care is given during acute exacerbations and includes bed rest, comfort measures such as massages, prevention of fatigue, prevention of pressure ulcers, bowel and bladder training (if necessary), administration of antibiotics for bladder infections, physical therapy, and counseling.

 COLLABORATIVE MANAGEMENT An interdisciplinary approach is necessary to maximize patient functioning and reduce the risk of complications in the patient with MS. The neurologist diagnoses and manages the disorder. The nurse provides support, education, and cares for the patient during acute exacerbations. The nurse also helps the patient maintain the highest level of independent functioning for as long as possible, and provides support to the patient and his family. If the patient is depressed, a med-

Teaching about multiple sclerosis

Remember these key points when teaching your patient about multiple sclerosis (MS):
- Teach about the disease process, including its symptoms, complications, and treatments.
- Teach about prescribed medications, including their names, indications, dosages, adverse effects, and special considerations.
- Discuss the chronic course of MS and that exacerbations are unpredictable, requiring physical and emotional adjustments in lifestyle.
- Emphasize the need to avoid temperature extremes, stress, fatigue, and infections and other illnesses, all of which can trigger an MS attack.
- Advise the patient to maintain independence by developing new ways of performing daily activities.
- Stress the importance of eating a nutritious, well-balanced diet that contains sufficient roughage and adequate fluids to prevent constipation.
- Teach the correct use of suppositories to help establish a regular bowel schedule.
- Discuss methods to relieve urinary incontinence and retention, including Credé's maneuver and self-catheterization.
- Encourage daily physical exercise and regular rest periods to prevent fatigue.
- Discuss sexual dysfunction and childbearing concerns.

ical social worker or therapist can help provide counseling for this progressive, fatal illness. The physical therapist and occupational therapist assist in promoting the highest level of independent functioning and recommend the use of appliances and assistive devices. The speech therapist can help the patient with speech and swallowing issues. The dietitian provides nutritional counseling. The social worker can facilitate the drafting of a living will and power of attorney.

Special considerations

○ Assist with active, resistive, and stretching exercises to maintain muscle tone and joint mobility, decrease spasticity, improve coordination, and boost morale.

○ Evaluate the need for bowel and bladder training during hospitalization. Encourage adequate fluid intake and regular urination. Eventually, the patient may require urinary drainage by self-catheterization or, in men, condom drainage.

○ Promote emotional stability.

○ Help the patient establish a daily routine to maintain optimal functioning.

○ Refer the patient to the National Multiple Sclerosis Society.

○ Provide patient education. (See *Teaching about multiple sclerosis*.)

Applicable patient-teaching aids

○ Caring for an indwelling catheter
○ Caring for your urinary catheter *
○ Catheterizing yourself: For men *
○ Catheterizing yourself: For women *
○ Choosing the right wheelchair *
○ Coping with falls
○ Dealing with a blocked indwelling catheter
○ Helping a person into or out of a wheelchair
○ Irrigating a blocked indwelling catheter
○ Learning about wheelchair transfers
○ Performing active range-of-motion exercises *
○ Performing chest physiotherapy (for an adult)
○ Performing self-massage
○ Performing stretching exercises
○ Preventing infection from an indwelling catheter
○ Recording pressure ulcers
○ Repositioning a person in bed
○ What is autogenic training?

⃝ Muscular dystrophy

Muscular dystrophy is actually a group of congenital disorders characterized by progressive symmetrical wasting of skeletal muscles without neural or sensory defects. Paradoxically, these wasted muscles tend to enlarge because of connective tissue and fat deposits, giving an erroneous impression of muscle strength. The main types of muscular dystrophy are Duchenne's (pseudohypertrophic), Becker's (benign pseudohypertrophic), facioscapulohumeral (Landouzy-Dejerine), and limb-girdle dystrophy.

The prognosis varies. Duchenne's muscular dystrophy generally strikes during early childhood and usually results in death by age 20. Patients with Becker's muscular dystrophy typically live into their 40s. Facioscapulohumeral and limb-girdle dystrophies usually don't shorten life.

Causes

Muscular dystrophy is caused by various genetic mechanisms. Duchenne's and Becker's muscular dystrophies are X-linked recessive disorders. Both result from defects in the gene coding for the muscle protein dystrophin; the gene has been mapped to the Xp21 locus. Both affect males almost exclusively.

Facioscapulohumeral dystrophy is an autosomal dominant disorder. Limb-girdle dystrophy is usually autosomal recessive. These two types affect both sexes about equally.

Pathophysiology

Abnormally permeable cell membranes allow leakage of various muscle enzymes, particularly creatine kinase. This metabolic defect, which causes the muscle cells to die, is present from fetal life onward. The absence of progressive muscle wasting at birth suggests that other factors compound the effect of dystrophin deficiency. The specific trigger is unknown, but phagocytosis of the muscle cells by inflammatory cells causes scarring and loss of muscle function.

As the disease progresses, skeletal muscle becomes almost totally replaced by fat and connective tissue. The skeleton eventually becomes deformed, causing progressive immobility. Cardiac and smooth muscle of the GI tract typically become fibrotic. No consistent structural abnormalities are seen in the brain.

Assessment findings

Duchenne's muscular dystrophy begins insidiously. It initially affects leg and pelvic muscles but eventually spreads to the involuntary muscles. Muscle weakness produces a waddling gait, toe walking, and lordosis. Children have difficulty climbing stairs, fall down often, can't run properly, and their scapulae flare out (or "wing") when they raise their arms. Calf muscles especially become enlarged and firm. Muscle deterioration progresses rapidly, and contractures develop. Some have abrupt intermittent oscillations of the irises in response to light (Gowers' sign). Usually, these children are confined to wheelchairs by ages 9 to 12. Late in the disease, progressive weakening of cardiac muscle causes tachycardia, electrocardiogram abnormalities, and pulmonary complications. Death commonly results from sudden heart failure, respiratory failure, or infection.

Signs and symptoms of Becker's muscular dystrophy resemble those of Duchenne's muscular dystrophy, but they progress more slowly. Although symptoms start around age 5, the patient can still walk well beyond age 15 — sometimes into his 40s.

Facioscapulohumeral dystrophy is a slowly progressive and relatively benign form of muscular dystrophy that commonly occurs before age 10 but may develop during early adolescence. Initially, it weakens the muscles of the face, shoulders, and upper arms but eventually spreads to all voluntary muscles, producing a pendulous lower lip and absence of the nasolabial fold. Early symptoms include the inability to pucker the mouth or whistle, abnormal facial movements, and the absence of facial movements when laughing or crying. Other signs consist of diffuse facial flattening that leads to a masklike expression, winging of the scapulae, the inability to raise the arms above the head and, in infants, the inability to suckle.

Limb-girdle dystrophy follows a similarly slow course and commonly causes only slight disability. Usually, it begins between ages 6 and 10; less commonly, in early adulthood. Muscle weakness first appears in the upper arm and pelvic muscles. Other symptoms include winging of the scapulae, lordosis with abdominal

protrusion, waddling gait, poor balance, and the inability to raise the arms.

Diagnosis

○ Electromyography typically demonstrates short, weak bursts of electrical activity or high-frequency, repetitive waxing and waning discharges in affected muscles.
○ Muscle biopsy shows variations in the size of muscle fibers and, in later stages, shows fat and connective tissue deposits; dystrophin is absent in Duchenne's dystrophy and diminished in Becker's dystrophy.
○ Serum creatine kinase is markedly elevated in Duchenne's, but only moderately elevated in Becker's and facioscapulohumeral dystrophies.

○ Immunologic and molecular biological assays available in specialized medical centers facilitate accurate prenatal and postnatal diagnosis of Duchenne's and Becker's muscular dystrophies and are replacing muscle biopsy and elevated serum creatine kinase levels in diagnosing these dystrophies. These assays can also help to identify carriers.

Complications

○ Arrhythmias
○ Cardiac hypertrophy
○ Contractures
○ Crippling disability
○ Dysphagia
○ Pneumonia

Treatment

○ No treatment stops the progressive muscle impairment of muscular dystrophy.
○ Orthopedic appliances, exercise, physical therapy, and surgery to correct contractures can help preserve the patient's mobility and independence.
○ Prednisone improves muscle strength in patients with Duchenne's muscular dystrophy.

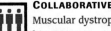 **COLLABORATIVE MANAGEMENT**
Muscular dystrophy can't be cured, but proper treatment by an interdisciplinary team can help affected children reach and maintain their fullest potential. Such treatment requires a comprehensive and cooperative effort involving physicians, nurses, teachers, psychologists, and the child's family. Rehabilitation includes physical, occupational, and speech therapy to maintain or improve functional abilities. Splints, braces, surgery to correct contractures, trapeze bars, overhead slings, and a wheelchair can help preserve mobility. Home care is usually possible. Children with milder forms of muscular dystrophy should attend a regular school; severely afflicted children may need special classes. Psychological counseling can help the parents deal with unreasonable guilt about their child's disability and the stress that comes with caring for a child with a chronic illness.

Special considerations

◯ When respiratory involvement occurs in Duchenne's muscular dystrophy, encourage coughing, deep-breathing exercises, and diaphragmatic breathing.

◯ Encourage and assist with active and passive range-of-motion exercises to preserve joint mobility and prevent muscle atrophy.

◯ Refer the patient for physical therapy. A footboard or high-topped sneakers and a foot cradle increase comfort and prevent footdrop.

◯ Because inactivity may cause constipation, encourage adequate fluid intake, increase dietary bulk, and obtain an order for a stool softener.

◯ Always allow the patient plenty of time to perform even simple physical tasks because he's likely to be slow and awkward.

◯ Encourage communication between the patient's family members to help them deal with the emotional strain this disorder produces. Provide emotional support to help the patient cope with continual changes in body image.

◯ Help the child with Duchenne's muscular dystrophy maintain peer relationships and realize his intellectual potential by encouraging his parents to keep him in a regular school as long as possible.

◯ If necessary, refer adult patients for counseling. Refer those who must acquire new job skills for vocational rehabilitation. (Contact the Department of Labor and Industry in your state for more information.) For information on social services and financial assistance, refer these patients and their families to the Muscular Dystrophy Association.

◯ Refer the patient's family members for genetic counseling.

◯ Provide patient education. (See *Teaching about muscular dystrophy.*)

Applicable patient-teaching aids

◯ Adding fiber to your diet *
◯ Avoiding burnout: Aid for the caregiver *
◯ Choosing the right wheelchair *
◯ Performing active range-of-motion exercises *

◯ Myasthenia gravis

Myasthenia gravis produces sporadic but progressive weakness and abnormal fatigability of striated (skeletal) muscles, exacerbated by exercise and repeated movement, but improved by anticholinesterase drugs. Usually, this disorder affects muscles innervated by the cranial nerves (face, lips, tongue, neck, and throat), but it can affect any muscle group. Myasthenia gravis follows an unpredictable course of recurring exacerbations and periodic remissions. There's no known cure. Drug treatment has improved prognosis and allows patients to lead relatively normal lives except during exacerbations. When the disease involves the respiratory system, it may be life-threatening.

Myasthenia gravis affects 3 of every 10,000 people. It's most common in young women and older men.

Causes

The exact cause of myasthenia gravis is unknown. However, it's believed to be the result of an autoimmune response, ineffective acetylcholine (ACh) release, or inadequate muscle fiber response to ACh. About 20% of neonates born to mothers with myasthenia gravis have transient (or occasionally persistent) myasthenia. This disease may coexist with immunologic and thyroid disorders; about 15% of patients with myasthenia gravis have thymomas.

Pathophysiology

Myasthenia gravis causes a failure in transmission of nerve impulses at the neuromuscular junction. The site of action is the postsynaptic membrane. Theoretically, antireceptor antibodies block, weaken, or reduce the number of ACh receptors available at each neuromuscular junction and thereby impair muscle depolarization necessary for movement. (See *Impaired transmission in myasthenia gravis,* page 228.)

Assessment findings

Onset of symptoms in myasthenia gravis may be sudden or insidious. In many patients, weak eye closure, ptosis, and diplopia are the first signs that something is wrong.

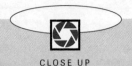

CLOSE UP

Impaired transmission in myasthenia gravis

During normal neuromuscular transmission, a motor nerve impulse travels to a motor nerve terminal, stimulating release of a chemical neurotransmitter called *acetylcholine* (ACh). When ACh diffuses across the synapse, receptor sites in the motor end plate react and depolarize the muscle fiber. Depolarization spreads through the muscle fiber, causing muscle contraction.

In myasthenia gravis, antibodies attach to the ACh receptor sites. They block, destroy, and weaken these sites, leaving them insensitive to ACh, thereby blocking neuromuscular transmission.

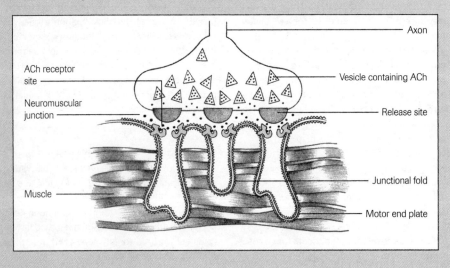

The dominant symptoms of myasthenia gravis are skeletal muscle weakness and fatigability. In the early stages, easy fatigability of certain muscles may appear with no other findings; later, it may be severe enough to cause paralysis. Typically, myasthenic muscles are strongest in the morning but weaken throughout the day, especially after exercise; short rest periods temporarily restore muscle function. Muscle weakness is progressive and eventually some muscles may lose function entirely.

Patients with myasthenia gravis usually have blank, expressionless faces, nasal vocal tones, frequent nasal regurgitation of fluids, and difficulty chewing and swallowing. Their eyelids droop (ptosis), and they may have to tilt their heads back to see. Neck muscles may become too weak to support their heads without bobbing.

In patients with weakened respiratory muscles, decreased tidal volume and vital capacity make breathing difficult and predispose to pneumonia and other respiratory tract infections. Respiratory muscle weakness (myasthenic crisis) may be severe enough to require an emergency airway and mechanical ventilation. (See *Myasthenic crisis and cholinergic crisis*.)

Diagnosis
○ The classic proof of myasthenia gravis is improved muscle function after an I.V. injection of edrophonium or neostigmine (anticholinesterase drugs).

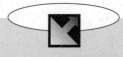

ACUTE EPISODE

Myasthenic crisis and cholinergic crisis

Myasthenic crisis is an acute exacerbation of the muscular weakness that occurs in myasthenia gravis. It can be triggered by infection, surgery, emotional stress, drug interaction, alcohol ingestion, temperature extremes, or pregnancy. Insufficient anticholinesterase medication can also cause myasthenic crisis. Signs and symptoms of myasthenic crisis include:
- anxiety, restlessness, irritability
- respiratory distress progressing to apnea
- dysarthria
- dysphagia
- extreme fatigue
- fever
- inability to move jaw or raise one or both eyelids
- increased muscular weakness.

Cholinergic crisis results from an overdose of, or toxicity to, anticholinesterase agents that block the acetylcholine receptors, ultimately leading to a neuromuscular blockage. Typical signs and symptoms of cholinergic crisis include:
- increasing anxiety and apprehension
- anorexia, nausea, vomiting, abdominal cramps
- excessive salivation

- sweating
- fasciculation (twitching) around the eyes
- muscle cramps and spasms
- increasing muscle weakness
- dysarthria
- increasing dysphagia
- respiratory distress.

Both myasthenic and cholinergic crises are emergency situations that require immediate intervention. When caring for a patient who experiences one of these crises, follow these guidelines:
- Notify the physician immediately.
- Maintain a patent airway; provide respiratory support as needed, including oxygen therapy or assisted ventilation.
- Assist with the administration of edrophonium (Tensilon) I.V.
- Provide supportive care, including parenteral fluids, antibiotics (if the crisis was due to infection), enteral feedings, or the insertion of an indwelling urinary catheter.
- Provide emotional support and be sure to explain all the events as they're happening to help allay some of the patient's fears and anxieties.

○ Repeated muscle use over a very short time that fatigues and then improves with rest suggests myasthenia gravis. Electromyography, with repeated neural stimulation, may help confirm this diagnosis.

○ ACh receptor antibodies may be present in the blood.

○ ACh receptor antibody titer may be elevated in generalized myasthenia.

Complications
○ Aspiration
○ Myasthenic crisis
○ Pneumonia
○ Respiratory distress

Treatment
○ Anticholinesterase drugs, such as neostigmine and pyridostigmine, counteract fatigue and muscle weakness and allow about 80% of normal muscle function.

○ Immunosuppressants, such as corticosteroids, azathioprine, cyclosporine, and cyclophosphamide are used to relieve symptoms.

○ Plasmapheresis is used in severe myasthenic exacerbation.

○ Patients with thymomas require thymectomy, which may cause remission in some cases of adult-onset myasthenia.

○ Emergency treatment is necessary for acute exacerbations of myasthenia gravis that cause severe respiratory distress.

Teaching about myasthenia gravis

Remember these key points when teaching your patient about myasthenia gravis:

● Teach about the disease process, including its symptoms, complications, and treatments.
● Teach about prescribed medications, including their names, indications, dosages, adverse effects, and special considerations.
● Help the patient plan daily activities to coincide with energy peaks.
● Stress the need for frequent rest periods throughout the day.
● Emphasize that periodic remissions, exacerbations, and day-to-day fluctuations are common.
● Teach the patient how to recognize adverse effects and signs and symptoms of toxicity of anticholinesterase drugs (headaches, weakness, sweating, abdominal cramps, nausea, vomiting, diarrhea, excessive salivation, and bronchospasm) and corticosteroids (euphoria, insomnia, edema, and increased appetite).
● Warn the patient to avoid strenuous exercise, stress, infection, and needless exposure to the sun or cold, which can worsen signs and symptoms.
● Teach the patient about thymectomy, if indicated.

○ Immediate hospitalization and vigorous respiratory support is necessary for myasthenic crisis.

COLLABORATIVE MANAGEMENT
Care of the patient with myasthenia gravis requires an interdisciplinary approach because this disease can affect muscle functioning in any body system. The nurse educates the patient, develops a therapeutic relationship, and cares for the patient during exacerbations. The respiratory therapist provides measures to improve respiratory muscle function and ventilation. The physical therapist provides exercises to strength muscles and assistive devices to aid ambulation. The occupational therapist provides adaptations needed for activities of daily living. The speech therapist provides guidance with swallowing difficulties. Social services may be necessary to assist the patient with referrals to community support groups, financial concerns, and home care issues because the disease involves remissions and exacerbations.

Special considerations

○ Establish an accurate neurologic and respiratory baseline.
○ Assess the patient's respiratory function, monitor his need for ventilatory support, and perform frequent suctioning to remove accumulated secretions.
○ Be alert for signs of an impending crisis (increased muscle weakness, respiratory distress, and difficulty in talking or chewing).
○ To prevent relapses, adhere closely to the ordered drug administration schedule. Be prepared to give atropine for anticholinesterase overdose or toxicity.
○ Plan exercise, meals, patient care, and activities to make the most of energy peaks. For example, give medication 20 to 30 minutes before meals to facilitate chewing or swallowing.
○ When swallowing is difficult, give soft, solid foods instead of liquids to lessen the risk of choking.
○ Refer the patient to the Myasthenia Gravis Foundation to give him an opportunity to obtain more information and meet other people with myasthenia gravis who lead full, productive lives.
○ Provide patient education. (See *Teaching about myasthenia gravis*.)

Applicable patient-teaching aids

○ Avoiding infection *
○ Calling for help during a myasthenic crisis *
○ Learning about plasmapheresis

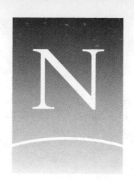

Neurogenic bladder

Neurogenic bladder (also known as *neuromuscular dysfunction of the lower urinary tract, neurologic bladder dysfunction,* and *neuropathic bladder*) refers to all types of bladder dysfunction caused by an interruption of normal bladder innervation. Subsequent complications include incontinence, residual urine retention, urinary infection, stone formation, and renal failure. A neurogenic bladder can be spastic (hypertonic, reflex, or automatic) or flaccid (hypotonic, atonic, nonreflex, or autonomous).

Causes

At one time, neurogenic bladder was thought to result primarily from spinal cord injury; now, it appears to stem from a host of underlying conditions. Cerebral disorders that may result in neurogenic bladder include stroke, brain tumor (meningioma and glioma), Parkinson's disease, multiple sclerosis, dementia, and incontinence caused by aging.

Conditions that lead to spinal cord disease or trauma may also cause neurogenic bladder, such as herniated vertebral disks, spina bifida, myelomeningocele, spinal stenosis (causing cord compression) or arachnoiditis (causing adhesions between the membranes covering the cord), cervical spondylosis, myelopathies from hereditary or nutritional deficiencies and, rarely, tabes dorsalis.

Disorders of peripheral innervation, including autonomic neuropathies resulting from endocrine disturbances such as diabetes mellitus (most common), can also result in neurogenic bladder. Metabolic disturbances, such as hypothyroidism, porphyria, or uremia (infrequent) are yet another cause.

Other conditions that may lead to neurogenic bladder include acute infectious diseases, such as transverse myelitis; heavy metal toxicity; chronic alcoholism; collagen diseases, such as systemic lupus erythematosus; vascular diseases, such as atherosclerosis; distant effects of cancer, such as primary oat cell carcinoma of the lung; herpes zoster; and sacral agenesis.

Pathophysiology

An upper motor neuron lesion (at or above T12) causes spastic neurogenic bladder, with spontaneous contractions of detrusor muscles, increased intravesical voiding pressure, bladder wall hypertrophy with trabeculation, and urinary sphincter spasms. The patient may experience small urine volume, incomplete emptying, and loss of voluntary control of voiding. Urinary retention also sets the stage for infection.

A lower motor neuron lesion (at or below S2 to S4) affects the spinal reflex that controls micturition. The result is a flaccid neurogenic bladder with decreased intravesical pressure, and increased bladder capacity, residual urine retention, and poor detrusor contraction. The bladder may not empty spontaneously. The patient experiences loss of voluntary and involuntary control of urination. Lower motor neuron lesions lead to overflow incontinence. When sensory neurons are interrupted, the patient can't perceive the need to void.

Interruption of the efferent nerves at the cortical, or upper motor neuron, level results in loss of voluntary control. Higher centers also control micturition, and voiding may be incomplete. Sensory neuron interruption leads to

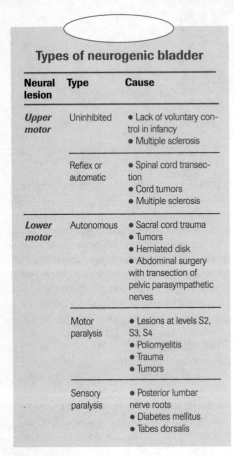

Types of neurogenic bladder

Neural lesion	Type	Cause
Upper motor	Uninhibited	• Lack of voluntary control in infancy • Multiple sclerosis
	Reflex or automatic	• Spinal cord transection • Cord tumors • Multiple sclerosis
Lower motor	Autonomous	• Sacral cord trauma • Tumors • Herniated disk • Abdominal surgery with transection of pelvic parasympathetic nerves
	Motor paralysis	• Lesions at levels S2, S3, S4 • Poliomyelitis • Trauma • Tumors
	Sensory paralysis	• Posterior lumbar nerve roots • Diabetes mellitus • Tabes dorsalis

dribbling and overflow incontinence. Altered bladder sensation often makes symptoms difficult to discern. (See *Types of neurogenic bladder*.)

Retention of urine contributes to renal calculi as well as infection. Neurogenic bladder can lead to deterioration of renal function if not promptly diagnosed and treated.

Assessment findings

Usually, neurogenic bladder causes some degree of incontinence, changes in initiation or interruption of micturition, and the inability to empty the bladder completely. Other effects include vesicoureteral reflux, deterioration or infection in the upper urinary tract, and hydroureteral nephrosis.

Depending on the site and extent of the spinal cord lesion, spastic neurogenic bladder may produce involuntary or frequent scanty

urination, without a feeling of bladder fullness, and possibly spontaneous spasms of the arms and legs. Anal sphincter tone may be increased. Tactile stimulation of the abdomen, thighs, or genitalia may precipitate voiding and spontaneous contractions of the arms and legs. With cord lesions in the upper thoracic (cervical) level, bladder distention can trigger hyperactive autonomic reflexes, resulting in severe hypertension, bradycardia, and headaches.

Flaccid neurogenic bladder may be associated with overflow incontinence, diminished anal sphincter tone, fecal impaction, and a greatly distended bladder (evident on percussion or palpation), but without the accompanying feeling of bladder fullness due to sensory impairment.

Diagnosis

○ Voiding cystourethrography evaluates bladder neck function, vesicoureteral reflux, and continence.
○ Urine flow study (uroflow) shows diminished or impaired urine flow.
○ Cystometry evaluates bladder nerve supply, detrusor muscle tone, and intravesical pressures during bladder filling and contraction.
○ Urethral pressure profile determines urethral function with respect to the length of the urethra and the outlet pressure resistance.
○ Sphincter electromyelography correlates the neuromuscular function of the external sphincter with bladder muscle function during bladder filling and contraction. This evaluates how well the bladder and urinary sphincter muscles work together.
○ Retrograde urethrography reveals the presence of strictures and diverticula. This test may not be performed on a routine basis.

Complications

○ Calculus formation
○ Incontinence
○ Renal failure
○ Residual urine retention
○ Urinary tract infection

Treatment

○ Valsalva's maneuver promotes evacuation of the bladder.

○ Credé's method — application of manual pressure over the lower abdomen — promotes complete emptying of the bladder.

○ Intermittent self-catheterization allows complete emptying of the bladder without the risks that an indwelling catheter poses and, when used in conjunction with a bladder-retraining program, is especially useful for patients with flaccid neurogenic bladder.

○ Bethanechol and phenoxybenzamine may be given to facilitate bladder emptying.

○ Propantheline, methantheline, flavoxate, dicyclomine, and imipramine may be given to facilitate urine storage.

○ Surgery may correct the structural impairment through transurethral resection of the bladder neck, urethral dilatation, external sphincterotomy, or urinary diversion procedures.

○ Implantation of an artificial urinary sphincter may be necessary if permanent incontinence follows surgery for neurogenic bladder.

 COLLABORATIVE MANAGEMENT
Care of the patient with neurogenic bladder involves many members of the interdisciplinary team. The physician or urologist develops the treatment plan and monitors patient progress. A surgeon may be consulted if conservative treatment fails. If urinary diversion procedure is to be performed, an enterostomal therapist meets with the patient to provide instruction on care of the skin and stoma. The nurse educates the patient about the condition and its treatments and provides emotional support.

Special considerations

○ Use strict sterile technique during insertion of an indwelling catheter. Don't interrupt the closed drainage system for any reason. Obtain urine specimens with a syringe and small-bore needle inserted through the aspirating port of the catheter itself. Irrigate in the same manner if ordered.

○ Provide meticulous catheter care.

○ Watch for signs of infection (fever, cloudy or foul-smelling urine).

○ Encourage the patient to drink plenty of fluids to prevent calculus formation and infection from urinary stasis.

KEY TEACHING POINTS

Teaching about neurogenic bladder

Remember these key points when teaching your patient about neurogenic bladder:
● Teach about the disease process, including its symptoms and treatments.
● Teach about prescribed medications, including their names, indications, dosages, adverse effects, and special considerations.
● Encourage the patient to drink plenty of fluids.
● If the patient is having surgery, explain the surgical procedure and refer him to an enterostomal therapist.
● Teach the patient and his family evacuation techniques, such as Credé's method, Valsalva's maneuver, and intermittent catheterization, as necessary.
● Teach catheter care, if the patient has an indwelling urinary catheter.
● Counsel the patient regarding sexual activities.
● Discuss complications that may occur, such as urinary tract infection and hydronephrosis, and when to seek medical attention for them.

○ Keep the patient as mobile as possible. Perform passive range-of-motion exercises if needed.

○ If urinary diversion procedure is ordered, arrange for consultation with an enterostomal therapist and coordinate the care plans.

○ Provide emotional support.

○ Provide patient education. (See *Teaching about neurogenic bladder.*)

Applicable patient-teaching aids

○ Caring for an indwelling catheter
○ Catheterizing yourself: For men *
○ Catheterizing yourself: For women *
○ Dealing with a blocked indwelling catheter
○ Preventing infection from an indwelling catheter
○ Treating and preventing urinary tract infections *

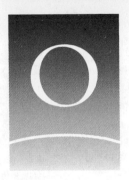

Obesity

Obesity is an excess of body fat, generally 20% above ideal body weight. The prognosis for correction of obesity is poor: Fewer than 30% of patients succeed in losing 20 lb (9 kg), and only half of these maintain the loss over a prolonged period. Rates of obesity are climbing, and the percentage of children and adolescents who are obese has doubled in the last 30 years.

Causes

Obesity results from excessive calorie intake and inadequate expenditure of energy. Theories to explain this condition include hypothalamic dysfunction of hunger and satiety centers, genetic predisposition, abnormal absorption of nutrients, and impaired action of GI and growth hormones and of hormonal regulators such as insulin. An inverse relationship between socioeconomic status and the prevalence of obesity has been documented, especially in women. Obesity in parents increases the probability of obesity in children from genetic or environmental factors such as activity levels and learned patterns of eating. Psychological factors, such as stress or emotional eating, may also contribute to obesity.

Pathophysiology

Unused or excess dietary fats leave the capillary circulation and enter fat cells (adipocytes). When the body needs fuel, it can draw on this stored energy. Fat, in the form of triglycerides, is the major component of the adipocyte.

Adipocytes increase in size in response to dietary intake. When the cells can no longer expand, they increase in number. With weight loss, the size of the fat cells decreases, but the number of cells doesn't.

Assessment findings

The patient may report such associated signs and symptoms as snoring and sleep apnea, gastroesophageal reflux, and arthritis. He may also show signs of poor body image, poor self-esteem, and depression.

Diagnosis

○ Height and weight comparison to a standard table indicates obesity.
○ Body mass index calculations are 30 or greater. (See *BMI measurements.*)
○ Measurement of the thickness of subcutaneous fat folds with calipers provides an approximation of total body fat. (See *Taking anthropometric arm measurements.*)

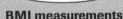

BMI measurements

Use these steps to calculate body mass index (BMI):
● Multiply weight in pounds by 705.
● Divide this number by height in inches.
● Then divide it by height in inches again.
● Compare results to these standards:
  – 18.5 to 24.9: normal
  – 25 to 29.9: overweight
  – 30 to 39.9: obese
  – 40 or greater: morbidly obese.

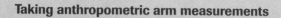

Taking anthropometric arm measurements

Follow these steps to determine triceps skinfold thickness, midarm circumference, and midarm muscle circumference.

Triceps skinfold thickness
● Find the midpoint circumference of the arm by placing the tape measure halfway between the axilla and the elbow. Grasp the patient's skin with your thumb and forefinger, about ⅜" (1 cm) above the midpoint, as shown below.
● Place calipers at the midpoint, and squeeze for 3 seconds.
● Record the measurement to the nearest millimeter.
● Take two more readings, and use the average.

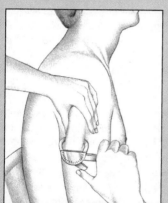

Remember, a measurement less than 90% of the standard indicates caloric deprivation. A measurement over 90% indicates adequate or more-than-adequate energy reserves.

Midarm circumference and midarm muscle circumference
● At the midpoint, measure the midarm circumference, as shown below. Record the measurement in centimeters.
● Calculate the midarm muscle circumference by multiplying the triceps' skinfold thickness — measured in millimeters — by 3.14.
● Subtract this number from the midarm circumference.

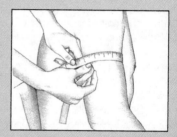

Recording the measurements
Record all three measurements as a percentage of the standard measurements (see table below), using this formula:

$$\frac{\text{Actual measurement}}{\text{Standard measurement}} \times 100\%$$

Measurement	Standard	90%
Triceps skinfold thickness	Men: 12.5 mm Women: 16.5 mm	Men: 11.3 mm Women: 14.9 mm
Midarm circumference	Men: 29.3 cm Women: 28.5 cm	Men: 26.4 cm Women: 25.7 cm
Midarm muscle circumference	Men: 25.3 cm Women: 23.3 cm	Men: 22.8 cm Women: 20.9 cm

Complications
○ Cardiovascular disease
○ Diabetes mellitus
○ Gallbladder disease
○ Hypertension
○ Menstrual irregularities
○ Premature death
○ Psychosocial difficulties
○ Renal disease
○ Respiratory difficulties

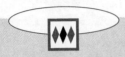

KEY TEACHING POINTS

Teaching about obesity

Remember these key points when teaching your patient about obesity:

● Explain the principles of energy balance and their relationship to obesity and weight loss.

● Talk about the assessment of obesity with height-weight charts, body mass index, and skin-fold measurements.

● Explain complications, such as diabetes, coronary artery disease, and respiratory problems.

● Discuss the prescribed diet as well as dietary tips to reduce food consumption.

● Teach about prescribed medications, their names, indications, dosages, adverse effects, and special considerations.

● Teach the importance of good skin care to prevent breakdown in moist skin folds.

● To help prevent obesity in children, teach parents to avoid overfeeding their infants and to familiarize themselves with actual nutritional needs and optimum growth rates.

● Discourage parents from using food to reward or console their children, from emphasizing the importance of "clean plates," and from allowing eating to prevent hunger rather than to satisfy it.

● Encourage physical activity and exercise, especially in children and young adults, to establish lifelong patterns.

● Review procedures and surgery to treat morbid obesity, as indicated.

● Explain how to keep a food diary.

● Discuss behavior modification techniques.

Treatment

○ Total fasting is an effective method of rapid weight reduction but requires close monitoring and supervision to minimize risks of ketonemia, electrolyte imbalance, hypotension, and loss of lean body mass.

○ Prolonged fasting and very-low-calorie diets have been associated with sudden death, possibly resulting from cardiac arrhythmias caused by electrolyte abnormalities.

○ Hypnosis and behavior modification techniques, which promote fundamental changes in eating habits and activity patterns, may work in some patients.

○ Psychotherapy may be beneficial for some patients, because weight reduction may lead to depression or even psychosis. Antidepressants are also helpful in weight loss.

○ Amphetamines and amphetamine congeners have been used to enhance compliance with a prescribed diet by temporarily suppressing the appetite and creating a feeling of well-being. However, their value in long-term weight control is questionable, and they have significant potential for dependence.

○ Surgery may be performed as a last resort for morbid obesity (body weight that's 50% to 100% higher than ideal), body weight that's 100 pounds higher than ideal, or a body mass index greater than 39, using bariatric procedures such as vertical banded gastroplasty and gastric bypass surgery.

COLLABORATIVE MANAGEMENT
An interdisciplinary approach is needed to help the obese individual achieve lifelong maintenance of healthy eating and exercise patterns. Regular follow-up care with a primary physician is necessary to help the obese patient lose weight and maintain an acceptable body weight. The nurse establishes a trusting and ongoing relationship with the patient, allowing more effective education, encouragement, and guidance. The surgeon can help the patient achieve and maintain weight loss when more conservative methods have failed. The dietitian educates the patient about healthy eating patterns and discourages fad diets. The physical therapist can help the patient develop an exercise program that's safe and takes into account concurrent medical problems, such as diabetes or hypertension. A therapist can help the patient address issues such as body image and self-esteem. Weight loss support groups may help some individuals.

Special considerations

○ Obtain an accurate diet history to identify the patient's eating patterns and the importance of food to his lifestyle. Ask the patient to keep a careful record of what, where, and when he eats to help identify situations that normally provoke overeating.

○ To increase calorie expenditure, promote increased physical activity, including an exercise program. Recommend varying activity levels according to the patient's general condition and cardiovascular status.

○ If the patient is taking appetite-suppressing drugs, watch carefully for signs of dependence or abuse and for adverse effects, such as insomnia, excitability, dry mouth, and GI disturbances.

○ Provide patient education. (See *Teaching about obesity.*)

Applicable patient-teaching aids

○ Diet-consciousness tips for dining out *
○ Keeping a food diary *
○ Learning about daily food choices
○ Personalizing your exercise program *

○ Obsessive-compulsive disorder

Obsessive thoughts and compulsive behaviors represent recurring efforts to control overwhelming anxiety, guilt, or unacceptable impulses that persistently enter the consciousness. The word *obsession* refers to a recurrent idea, thought, impulse, or image that's intrusive and inappropriate, causing marked anxiety or distress. A *compulsion* is a ritualistic, repetitive, and involuntary defensive behavior. Performing a compulsive behavior reduces the patient's anxiety, thereby increasing the probability that the behavior will recur. Compulsions are commonly associated with obsessions.

Patients with obsessive-compulsive disorder (OCD) are prone to abuse psychoactive substances, such as alcohol and anxiolytics, in an attempt to relieve their anxiety. In addition, other anxiety disorders and major depression commonly coexist with OCD.

OCD is typically a chronic condition with remissions and flare-ups. Mild forms of the disorder are relatively common in the population at large. OCD affects 2% to 3% of Americans—about 7 million people. Symptoms are usually noticed between ages 20 and 30, with 75% of patients displaying symptoms before age 30.

Causes

The cause of OCD is unknown. Some studies suggest the possibility of brain lesions, but the most useful research and clinical studies base an explanation on psychological theories. In addition, major depression, organic brain syndrome, and schizophrenia may contribute to the onset of OCD. Some authorities think OCD is closely related to some eating disorders.

Pathophysiology

OCD is an anatomic-physiologic disturbance that's thought to involve an alteration in the frontal-subcortical neural circuitry of the brain. Several studies on patients with OCD have shown brain abnormalities, such as decreased caudal size and decreased white matter, but results have been inconsistent.

Assessment findings

The patient's psychiatric history may reveal the presence of obsessive thoughts, words, or mental images such as thoughts of violence (such as stabbing, shooting, maiming, or hitting), thoughts of contamination (images of dirt, germs, or excrement), repetitive doubts and worries about a tragic event, and repeating or counting images, words, or objects in the environment. The patient recognizes that the obsessions are a product of his own mind and that they interfere with normal daily activities.

The patient may also have compulsions, including repetitive touching, sometimes combined with counting; doing and undoing (for instance, opening and closing doors or rearranging things); washing (especially hands); and checking (to be sure no tragedy has occurred since the last time he checked). In many cases, the patient's anxiety is so strong that he will avoid the situation or the object that evokes the impulse.

Diagnosing obsessive-compulsive disorder

Obsessive-compulsive disorder is diagnosed when the patient's signs and symptoms meet the established criteria put forth in the *Diagnostic and Statistical Manual,* Fourth Edition, Text Revision.

Either obsessions or compulsions
Obsessions are defined as all of the following:
- Recurrent and persistent thoughts, impulses, or images perceived to be intrusive and inappropriate by the patient, causing anxiety or distress at some point in time during the disturbance.
- The thoughts, impulses, or images aren't simply excessive worries about real-life problems.
- The person attempts to ignore or suppress such thoughts or impulses, or to neutralize them with some other thought or action.
- The person recognizes that the obsessions are the products of his mind and not externally imposed.
Compulsions are defined as all of the following:
- Repetitive behaviors or mental acts performed by the patient, who feels driven to perform them in response to an obsession, or according to rules that must be applied rigidly.
- The behavior or mental acts are aimed at preventing or reducing distress or preventing some dreaded event or situation. However, either the activity isn't connected in a realistic way with what it's designed to neutralize or prevent, or it's clearly excessive.

- The patient recognizes that his behavior is excessive or unreasonable. (This may not be true for young children or for patients whose obsessions have evolved into overvalued ideas.)

Additional criteria
- At some point, the patient recognizes that the obsessions or compulsions are excessive or unreasonable.
- The obsessions or compulsions cause marked distress, are time-consuming (take more than 1 hour a day), or significantly interfere with the patient's normal routine, occupational functioning, or usual social activities or relationships.
- If another axis I disorder is present, the content of the obsession is unrelated to it; for example, the ideas, thoughts, or images aren't about food in the presence of an eating disorder, about drugs in the presence of a psychoactive substance abuse disorder, or about guilt in a major depressive disorder.
- The disturbance isn't due to the direct physiologic effects of a substance or a general medical condition.

Reprinted with permission from *the Diagnostic and Statistical manual of mental Disorders,* copyright 2000. American Psychiatric Association.

Feelings of shame, nervousness, or embarrassment may prompt the patient to try limiting compulsive acts to his own private time. The patient typically reports moderate to severe impairment of social and occupational functioning.

Diagnosis
For characteristic findings in patients with this condition, see *Diagnosing obsessive-compulsive disorder.*

Complications
○ Endangerment of health and safety
○ Impairment of occupational and social functioning

Treatment
○ Clomipramine, a tricyclic antidepressant; selective serotonin reuptake inhibitors, such as fluoxetine, paroxetine, sertraline, and fluvoxamine; and the benzodiazepine, clonazepam, may be effective in treating this disorder.
○ Behavioral therapies—aversion therapy, thought-stopping, thought-switching, flooding, implosion therapy, and response prevention—have also been effective in treating OCD. (See *Behavioral therapies.*)

 COLLABORATIVE MANAGEMENT
Care of the patient with OCD involves many members of the interdisciplinary team. The psychiatrist or neurologist diagnoses and treats the disorder. The therapist

can help the patient reduce anxiety, learn stress reduction techniques, and decrease obsessive thoughts and compulsions. The nurse develops a therapeutic relationship and reinforces coping strategies and relaxation techniques.

Special considerations

○ Approach the patient unhurriedly.

○ Provide an accepting atmosphere; don't appear shocked, amused, or critical of the ritualistic behavior.

○ Provide for basic needs, such as rest, nutrition, and grooming, if the patient becomes involved in ritualistic thoughts and behaviors to the point of self-neglect.

○ Let the patient know you're aware of his behavior and help him explore feelings associated with the behavior.

○ Make reasonable demands and set reasonable limits.

○ Avoid creating situations that increase frustration and provoke anger, which may interfere with treatment.

○ Explore patterns leading to the behavior or recurring problems.

○ Listen attentively, offering feedback.

○ Encourage the use of appropriate defenses to relieve loneliness and isolation.

○ Engage the patient in activities to create positive accomplishments and raise his self-esteem and confidence.

○ Encourage active diversionary activities, such as whistling or humming a tune, to divert attention from the unwanted thoughts and to promote a pleasurable experience.

○ Help the patient develop new ways to solve problems, and cultivate more effective coping skills by setting limits on unacceptable behavior.

○ Identify insight and improved behavior (reduced compulsive behavior and fewer obsessive thoughts).

○ Identify disturbing topics of conversation that reflect underlying anxiety or terror.

○ Help the patient identify progress and set realistic expectations.

○ Work with the patient and other interdisciplinary team members to establish behavioral

Behavioral therapies

The following behavioral therapies are used to treat the patient with obsessive-compulsive disorder.

Aversion therapy
Application of a painful stimulus creates an aversion to the obsession that leads to undesirable behavior (compulsion).

Flooding
Flooding is frequent, full-intensity exposure (through the use of imagery) to an object that triggers a symptom. It must be used with caution because it produces extreme discomfort.

Implosion therapy
A form of desensitization, implosion therapy calls for repeated exposure to a highly feared object.

Response prevention
Preventing compulsive behavior by distraction, persuasion, or redirection of activity, response prevention may require hospitalization or involvement of the patient's family to be effective.

Thought-stopping
Thought-stopping breaks the habit of fear-inducing anticipatory thoughts. The patient learns to stop unwanted thoughts by saying the word "stop" and then focusing his attention on achieving calmness and muscle relaxation.

Thought-switching
To replace fear-inducing self-instructions with competent self-instructions, the patient learns to replace negative thoughts with positive ones until the positive thoughts become strong enough to overcome the anxiety-provoking ones.

goals and to help the patient tolerate anxiety in pursuing these goals.

○ Provide patient education. (See *Teaching about obsessive-compulsive disorder,* page 240.)

Applicable patient-teaching aids

○ Performing relaxation breathing exercises *
○ Taking your medication correctly

○ Osteoarthritis

Osteoarthritis, the most common form of arthritis, is a chronic disease that causes deterioration of the joint cartilage and formation of reactive new bone at the margins and subchondral areas of the joints. This degeneration results from a breakdown of chondrocytes, most commonly in the distal interphalangeal and proximal interphalangeal joints, but also in the hip and knee joints.

Osteoarthritis is widespread, occurring equally in both sexes. Its earliest symptoms typically begin after age 40 and may progress with advancing age. Disability depends on the site and severity of involvement and can range from minor limitation of the dexterity of the fingers to severe disability in persons with hip or knee involvement. The rate of progression varies, and joints may remain stable for years in an early stage of deterioration.

Osteoarthritis may first appear between ages 30 and 40, and is present in almost everyone by age 70. Before age 55, it affects men and women equally, but after age 55 the incidence is higher in women.

Causes

Studies indicate that osteoarthritis is acquired and probably results from a combination of metabolic, genetic, chemical, and mechanical factors. Secondary osteoarthritis usually follows an identifiable predisposing event—most commonly trauma, congenital deformity, or obesity—and leads to degenerative changes.

Pathophysiology

Osteoarthritis occurs in synovial joints. The joint cartilage deteriorates, and reactive new bone forms at the margins and subchondral areas of the joints. (See *Digital joint deformities*.) The degeneration results from damage to the chondrocytes. Cartilage softens with age, narrowing the joint space. Mechanical injury erodes articular cartilage, leaving the underlying bone unprotected. This causes sclerosis, or thickening and hardening of the bone underneath the cartilage. (See *What happens in osteoarthritis.*)

Cartilage flakes irritate the synovial lining, which becomes fibrotic and limits joint movement. Synovial fluid may be forced into defects in the bone, causing cysts. New bone, called *osteophyte* (bone spur), forms at joint margins as the articular cartilage erodes, causing gross alteration of the bony contours and enlargement of the joint.

Assessment findings

The most common symptom of osteoarthritis is a deep, aching joint pain, particularly after exercise or weight bearing, usually relieved by rest. Other symptoms include stiffness in the morning and after exercise (relieved by rest), aching during changes in weather, "grating" of the joint during motion, and altered gait contractures. These symptoms increase with poor posture, obesity, and stress to the affected joint.

Osteoarthritis of the interphalangeal joints produces irreversible joint changes and forma-

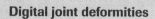

Digital joint deformities

Osteoarthritis of the interphalangeal joints produces irreversible changes in the distal joints (Heberden's nodes, left) and the proximal joints (Bouchard's nodes, right). Initially painless, these nodes gradually progress to or suddenly flare up as redness, swelling, tenderness, and impaired sensation and dexterity.

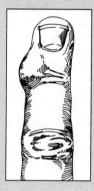
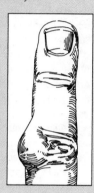

tion of nodes that eventually become red, swollen, and tender, causing numbness and loss of dexterity.

Diagnosis
○ X-rays of the affected joint help confirm diagnosis of osteoarthritis but may be normal in the early stages. X-rays may require many views and typically show:
– narrowing of joint space or margin
– cystlike bony deposits in joint space and margins and sclerosis of the subchondral space
– joint deformity due to degeneration or articular damage
– bony growths at weight-bearing areas
– fusion of joints.

Complications
○ Ankylosis
○ Bony cysts
○ Cauda equine syndrome
○ Central cord syndrome
○ Deformity

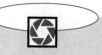

CLOSE UP

What happens in osteoarthritis

The characteristic breakdown of articular cartilage is a gradual response to aging or to predisposing factors, such as joint abnormalities or traumatic injury.

Chondrocytes break down.

Cartilage degenerates.

Degeneration of cartilage

Osteophytes (bony spurs) form.

Fragments of bone float freely in joint.

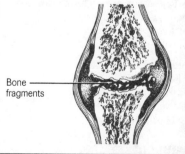

Bone fragments

Stiffness and decreased movement result.

Teaching about osteoarthritis

Remember these key points when teaching your patient about osteoarthritis:

● Teach about the disease process, including its symptoms, complications, and treatments.

● Teach about prescribed medications, including their names, indications, dosages, adverse effects, and special considerations.

● Teach the patient to pace daily activities and plan for adequate rest during the day, after exertion, and at night.

● Caution the patient to avoid overexertion, take care to stand and walk correctly, minimize weight-bearing activities, and be especially careful when stooping or picking up objects.

● Emphasize the importance of wearing well-fitting, supportive shoes and not letting heels become too worn down.

● Advise the patient to install safety devices at home such as guard rails in the bathrooms.

● Recommend maintaining a proper body weight to lessen strain on the joints.

● Discuss nonpharmacologic measures to reduce pain, including heat and cold therapy and massage.

● Explain preoperative and postoperative expectations, if the patient is having surgery.

● Teach how to properly use protective and assistive devices to avoid joint fatigue.

● Demonstrate range-of-motion, extension, flexion, and isometric exercises.

○ Flexion contractures
○ Gross bony overgrowth
○ Nerve root compression
○ Subluxation

Treatment

○ Medications include nonsteroidal anti-inflammatory drugs and in some cases, intra-articular injections of corticosteroids.

○ Glucosamine and chondroitin may be useful in controlling symptoms and reducing functional impairment.

○ Artificial joint fluid injections into the knee can provide pain relief for up to 6 months.

○ Crutches, braces, canes, walkers, cervical collars, or traction are effective treatments that reduce stress and support or stabilize the joint.

○ Exercise, such as through physical therapy, is important to maintaining or improving joint mobility.

○ Other supportive measures include massage, moist heat, paraffin dips for hands, protective techniques to prevent undue stress on the joints, and adequate rest (particularly after activity).

○ Surgical treatment is reserved for patients who have severe disability or uncontrollable pain and may include:

– Arthroplasty (partial or total): replacement of deteriorated part of joint with prosthetic appliance

– Arthrodesis: surgical fusion of bones, used primarily in spine (laminectomy)

– Osteoplasty: scraping and lavage of deteriorated bone from joint

– Osteotomy: change in alignment of bone to relieve stress by excision of wedge of bone or cutting of bone.

COLLABORATIVE MANAGEMENT
Care of the patient with osteoarthritis involves many members of the interdisciplinary team. The primary care provider diagnoses and manages the disorder. The surgeon is consulted when medical treatment can no longer provide acceptable pain relief. The nurse educates the patient and helps him to maintain mobility and minimize disability. The physical therapist works with the patient to maintain range of motion and muscle strength and tone. The occupational therapist helps the patient perform activities of daily living and teaches the use of assistive devices.

Special considerations

○ Promote adequate rest, particularly after activity. Plan rest periods during the day, and provide for adequate sleep at night.

○ Assist with physical therapy, and encourage the patient to perform gentle, isometric range-of-motion exercises.

○ Provide emotional support and reassurance to help the patient cope with limited mobility.

Specific patient care depends on the affected joint:

○ *Hand:* Apply hot soaks and paraffin dips to relieve pain, as ordered.

○ *Spine (lumbar* and *sacral):* Recommend a firm mattress (or bed board) to decrease morning pain.

○ *Spine (cervical):* Check cervical collar for constriction; watch for redness with prolonged use.

○ *Hip:* Use moist heat pads to relieve pain and administer antispasmodic drugs, as ordered. Assist with range-of-motion and strengthening exercises, always making sure the patient gets the proper rest afterward. Check crutches, canes, braces, and walkers for proper fit, and teach the patient to use them correctly. Recommend the use of cushions when sitting as well as the use of an elevated toilet seat.

○ *Knee:* Assist with range-of-motion exercises, exercises to maintain muscle tone, and progressive resistance exercises to increase muscle strength. Provide elastic supports or braces if needed.

○ Provide patient education. (See *Teaching about osteoarthritis.*)

Applicable patient-teaching aids

○ Adjusting to a total hip replacement *
○ Exercising for a stronger back
○ Learning about canes *
○ Performing active range-of-motion exercises *
○ Protecting your joints *
○ Recognizing warning signs of ulcer complications *
○ Restoring strength and relieving pain in arthritis *
○ Taking naproxen *
○ Using good posture to protect your back
○ Using special kitchen helpers in arthritis
○ Walking with a cane

○ Osteoporosis

Osteoporosis is a metabolic bone disorder in which the rate of bone resorption accelerates while the rate of bone formation slows down, causing a loss of bone mass. Bones affected by this disease lose calcium and phosphate salts and thus become porous, brittle, and abnormally vulnerable to fractures. Osteoporosis may be primary or secondary to an underlying disease. Primary osteoporosis is commonly called *postmenopausal osteoporosis* because it typically develops in postmenopausal women.

The incidence of osteoporosis is high, with an estimated 10 million Americans suffering from osteoporosis and another 18 million Americans suffering from low bone mass, or *osteopenia.* Incidence is higher in women than in men, with women accounting for 80% of cases.

Causes

The cause of primary osteoporosis is unknown; however, a mild but prolonged negative calcium balance, resulting from an inadequate dietary intake of calcium, may be an important contributing factor—as may declining gonadal or adrenal function, faulty protein metabolism due to estrogen deficiency, and sedentary lifestyle. Causes of secondary osteoporosis are many: prolonged therapy with steroids or heparin, total immobilization or disuse of a bone (as with hemiplegia, for example), alcoholism, malnutrition, malabsorption, scurvy, lactose intolerance, osteogenesis imperfecta, Sudeck's atrophy (localized to hands and feet, with recurring attacks), and endocrine disorders (hypopituitarism, acromegaly, thyrotoxicosis, long-standing diabetes mellitus, and hyperthyroidism).

Pathophysiology

In normal bone, the rates of bone formation and resorption are constant; replacement follows resorption immediately, and the amount of bone replaced equals the amount of bone resorbed. Osteoporosis develops when the remodeling cycle is interrupted, and new bone formation falls behind resorption.

When bone is resorbed faster than it forms, the bone becomes less dense. Men have approximately 30% greater bone mass than women, which may explain why osteoporosis develops later in men. (See *How osteoporosis develops,* page 244.)

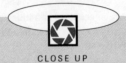

CLOSE UP

How osteoporosis develops

A metabolic bone disorder, osteoporosis develops as the rate of bone
resorption accelerates while the rate
of bone formation slows, causing a
loss of bone mass. Bones weaken
as local cells reabsorb bone tissue.
Trabecular bone at the core becomes less dense, and cortical bone
on the perimeter loses thickness.
Bones affected by this disease lose
calcium and phosphate salts and
become porous, brittle, and abnormally vulnerable to fractures.

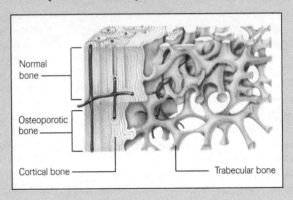

Assessment findings

Vertebral collapse, causing a backache with
pain that radiates around the trunk, is the most
common presenting feature of osteoporosis;
movement or jarring aggravates the backache.

Osteoporosis can develop insidiously, with
increasing deformity, kyphosis, loss of height
and, possibly, a dowager hump. As bones
weaken, spontaneous wedge fractures, pathologic fractures of the neck or femur, Colles'
fractures after a minor fall, and hip fractures
become increasingly common.

Diagnosis

○ Bone mineral density testing, the gold standard for evaluating osteoporosis, is performed
in dual-energy X-ray absorptiometry (DEXA)
and measures the mineralization of bones.
○ A computed tomography scan of the spine
shows demineralization; quantitative computed
tomography can evaluate bone density but is
less available and more expensive than DEXA.
○ X-rays show fracture or vertebral collapse in
severe cases.
○ Urine calcium can provide evidence of bone
turnover but is limited in value.

○ Urinary N-telopeptide is a newer test to help
diagnose osteoporosis.

Complications

○ Bone fractures (vertebra, femoral neck, and
distal radius)
○ Shock, hemorrhage, or fat embolism

Treatment

○ Bisphosphonates, such as alendronate and
risedronate, are given to prevent bone loss and
reduce the risk of fractures.
○ Calcium and vitamin D supplements are giv-
en to support normal bone metabolism.
○ Raloxifene and calcitonin have also been
used effectively to prevent and treat osteoporosis.
○ A back brace may be needed to support
weakened vertebrae.
○ Surgery can correct pathologic fractures of
the femur by open reduction and internal fixa-
tion. Colles' fracture requires reduction with
plaster immobilization for 4 to 10 weeks.
○ An adequate intake of dietary calcium and
regular exercise is necessary to reduce the incidence of primary osteoporosis. Fluoride treatments may also offer some preventive benefit.

○ Hormone replacement therapy with estrogen and progesterone may retard bone loss and prevent the occurrence of fractures; however, this therapy remains controversial.

○ Correction of the underlying disease as well as corticosteroid therapy, early mobilization after surgery or trauma, careful observation for signs of malabsorption, and prompt treatment of hyperthyroidism can prevent secondary osteoporosis.

○ Decreased alcohol consumption and caffeine use, as well as smoking cessation, are also helpful preventive measures.

 COLLABORATIVE MANAGEMENT
Care of the patient with osteoporosis involves many members of the interdisciplinary team. The primary care provider diagnoses and develops a treatment plan to slow down or prevent bone loss, prevent additional fractures, and control pain. The nurse educates the patient about the disorder and helps the patient make the appropriate lifestyle modifications. The physical therapist provides a program of gentle weight-bearing exercise. The occupational therapist prescribes assistive devices, as appropriate, to perform activities of daily living at the highest level of independence. The dietitian teaches the patient to follow a diet rich in calcium and makes recommendations for calcium and vitamin D supplementation.

Special considerations

○ Check the patient's skin daily for redness, warmth, and new sites of pain, which may indicate new fractures.

○ Administer analgesics and heat to relieve pain.

○ Encourage activity and help the patient walk several times daily.

○ As appropriate, perform passive range-of-motion exercises or encourage the patient to perform active exercises.

○ Institute safety measures: Move the patient gently and carefully at all times, and have him call for assistance when getting out of bed or a chair.

Teaching about osteoporosis

Remember these key points when teaching your patient about osteoporosis:

● Explain how an imbalance between bone formation and resorption leads to osteoporosis.

● Discuss risk factors for osteoporosis and how lifestyle modifications can reduce the risk.

● Encourage a weight-bearing exercise program.

● Advise the patient to report any new pain immediately, especially after trauma.

● Recommend that the patient sleep on a firm mattress and avoid excessive bed rest.

● Demonstrate how to correctly apply a back brace, if appropriate.

● Teach the patient good body mechanics — to stoop before lifting anything and to avoid twisting movements and prolonged bending.

● Teach about prescribed medications, including their names, indications, dosages, adverse effects, and special considerations.

● Review foods high in calcium and vitamin D.

● Teach female patients receiving estrogen therapy to perform monthly breast self-examinations.

● Teach the female patient to report vaginal bleeding promptly.

○ Provide a balanced diet, high in nutrients that support skeletal metabolism: vitamin D, calcium, and protein.

○ Provide patient education. (See *Teaching about osteoporosis.*)

Applicable patient-teaching aids

○ Caring for your cast *
○ Exercising casted limbs
○ Exercising for a stronger back
○ Learning about canes *
○ Learning about how broken bones heal
○ Performing active range-of-motion exercises *
○ Performing stretching exercises
○ Planning a calcium-rich diet *

○ Troubleshooting your casted limb
○ Using good posture to protect your back
○ Walking with a cane

Ovarian cancer

Ovarian cancer is one of the leading causes of gynecological deaths in the United States. In women with previously treated breast cancer, metastatic ovarian cancer is more common than cancer at any other site and may be linked to mutations in the BRCA1 or BRCA2 gene.

The prognosis varies with the histologic type and stage of the disease but is generally poor because ovarian tumors produce few early signs and are usually advanced at diagnosis. About 46% of women with ovarian cancer survive for 5 years.

Three main types of ovarian cancer exist:
○ *Primary epithelial tumors* account for 90% of all ovarian cancers and include serous cystadenocarcinoma, mucinous cystadenocarcinoma, and endometrioid and mesonephric malignancies. Serous cystadenocarcinoma is the most common type and accounts for 50% of all cases.
○ *Germ cell tumors* include endodermal sinus malignancies, embryonal carcinoma (a rare ovarian cancer that appears in children), immature teratomas, and dysgerminoma.
○ *Sex cord (stromal) tumors* include granulosa cell tumors (which produce estrogen and may have feminizing effects), granulosa-theca cell tumors, and the rare arrhenoblastomas (which produce androgen and have virilizing effects).

Causes

Exactly what causes ovarian cancer isn't known, but the greatest number of cases occurs in the fifth decade of life. However, it can occur during childhood. Other contributing factors include infertility; nulliparity; familial tendency; ovarian dysfunction; irregular menses; and possible exposure to asbestos, talc, and industrial pollutants.

Pathophysiology

Primary epithelial tumors arise in the müllerian epithelium; germ cell tumors, in the ovum itself; and sex cord tumors, in the ovarian stroma. Ovarian tumors spread rapidly intraperitoneally by local extension or surface seeding and, occasionally, through the lymphatics and the bloodstream. Generally, extraperitoneal spread is through the diaphragm into the chest cavity, which may cause pleural effusions. Other metastasis is rare.

Assessment findings

In the early stages, ovarian cancer may be asymptomatic or cause vague abdominal discomfort, dyspepsia, and other mild GI disturbances. As the cancer progresses, it causes urinary frequency, constipation, pelvic discomfort, distention, and weight loss. Tumor rupture, torsion, or infection may cause pain, which, in young patients, may mimic appendicitis.

Granulosa cell tumors have feminizing effects (such as bleeding between periods in premenopausal women); conversely, arrhenoblastomas have virilizing effects.

Advanced ovarian cancer causes ascites, postmenopausal bleeding and pain (rare), and symptoms relating to metastatic sites (most commonly pleural effusions).

Diagnosis

○ Abdominal ultrasonography, computed tomography scan, or X-ray may delineate tumor size.
○ Excretory urography provides information on renal function and possible urinary tract anomalies or obstruction.
○ Chest X-ray checks for distant metastasis and pleural effusions.
○ Barium enema (especially in patients with GI symptoms) may reveal obstruction and size of tumor.
○ Lymphangiography shows lymph node involvement.
○ Mammography is performed to rule out primary breast cancer.
○ Laboratory tumor marker studies, such as Ca-125, carcinoembryonic antigen, and human chorionic gonadotropin may show abnormalities that indicate complications.
○ Aspiration of ascetic fluid can reveal atypical cells.

Staging ovarian cancer

The International Federation of Gynecology and Obstetrics uses this staging system for ovarian cancer.

Stage I
Growth limited to the ovaries; T1, N0, M0
STAGE IA — growth limited to one ovary; no ascites; no tumor on the external surface; capsule intact
STAGE IB — growth limited to both ovaries; no ascites; no tumor on the external surfaces; capsules intact
STAGE IC — tumor either stage IA or IB but on surface of one or both ovaries; or with capsule ruptured; or with ascites containing malignant cells or with positive peritoneal washings

Stage II
Growth involving one or both ovaries with pelvic extension; T2, N0, M0
STAGE IIA — extension or metastasis, or both, to the uterus or tubes (or both)
STAGE IIB — extension to pelvic tissues
STAGE IIC — tumor either stage IIA or IIB, but with tumor on surface of one or both ovaries; with capsule (or capsules) ruptured; or with ascites present containing malignant cells or with positive peritoneal washings

Stage III
Tumor involving one or both ovaries with peritoneal implants outside the pelvis or positive retroperitoneal or inguinal nodes; superficial liver metastasis equals stage III; tumor limited to the true pelvis but with confirmed extension to small bowel or omentum; T3, N0, M0
STAGE IIIA — tumor grossly limited to the true pelvis with negative nodes but with confirmed microscopic seeding of abdominal peritoneal surfaces
STAGE IIIB — tumor of one or both ovaries with confirmed implants of abdominal peritoneal surfaces none exceeding 2 cm in dimension; nodes are negative
STAGE IIIC — abdominal implants greater than 2 cm or positive retroperitoneal or inguinal nodes or both

Stage IV
Growth involving one or both ovaries with distant metastasis (such as pleural effusion and abnormal cells or parenchymal liver metastasis)

○ Exploratory laparotomy, including lymph node evaluation and tumor resection, is required for accurate diagnosis and staging. (See *Staging ovarian cancer.*)

Complications
○ Ascites
○ Fluid and electrolyte imbalance
○ Intestinal obstruction
○ Leg edema
○ Profound cachexia
○ Recurrent malignant effusions

Treatment
○ Total abdominal hysterectomy and bilateral salpingo-oophorectomy with tumor resection are performed.
○ Omentectomy, appendectomy, lymph node biopsies with lymphadenectomy, tissue biopsies, and peritoneal washings may also be required.
○ Bilateral salpingo-oophorectomy in a prepubertal girl necessitates hormone replacement therapy, beginning at puberty, to induce the development of secondary sex characteristics.
○ Chemotherapeutic drugs useful in ovarian cancer include carboplatin, cisplatin, cyclophosphamide, docetaxel, doxorubicin, paclitaxel, and topotecan. These drugs are usually given in combination and they may be administered intraperitoneally.
○ Radiation therapy generally isn't used for ovarian cancer because the resulting myelosuppression would limit the effectiveness of chemotherapy.
○ Radioisotopes have been used as adjuvant therapy, but they cause small-bowel obstructions and stenosis.

Teaching about ovarian cancer

Remember these key points when teaching your patient about ovarian cancer:

- Teach about the disease process, including its symptoms, complications, and treatments.
- Teach about prescribed medications, including their names, indications, dosages, adverse effects, and special considerations.
- Explain all preoperative tests, the expected course of treatment, and surgical and postoperative procedures.
- Reinforce what the surgeon has told the patient about the surgical procedures listed in the surgical consent form. Explain that this form lists multiple procedures because the extent of the surgery can only be determined after the surgery itself has begun.
- Explain to the premenopausal woman that bilateral salpingo-oophorectomy artificially induces early menopause.
- Teach the patient relaxation techniques.
- Discuss the importance of preventing infection, emphasizing proper hand washing.
- Discuss self-care techniques following chemotherapy and radiation.

COLLABORATIVE MANAGEMENT
Care of the patient with ovarian cancer involves many members of the interdisciplinary team. The primary health care provider and the oncologist recommend and carry out the treatment regimen, assisted by the surgeon and radiation oncologist, as needed. The nurse educates the patient about the disease process, treatments, and self-care following surgery, radiation therapy, or chemotherapy. The therapist can help with issues, such as relationships and sexuality. The social worker can provide additional supportive care.

Special considerations

○ Tell the patient what to expect in the preoperative and postoperative periods.

After surgery:

○ Monitor vital signs frequently, and check I.V. fluids often. Monitor intake and output. Check the dressing regularly for excessive drainage or bleeding, and watch for signs of infection.

○ Provide abdominal support, and watch for abdominal distention.

○ Encourage coughing and deep breathing. Reposition the patient often, and encourage her to walk shortly after surgery.

○ Monitor and treat adverse effects of radiation and chemotherapy.

○ Provide psychological support for the patient and her family.

○ Provide patient education. (See *Teaching about ovarian cancer.*)

Applicable patient-teaching aids

○ Controlling the side effects of chemotherapy *

○ How to reduce incisional pain

○ Minimizing hair loss from chemotherapy

○ Using imagination to relieve pain

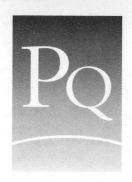

Paget's disease

Paget's disease, also called *osteitis deformans,* is a slowly progressive metabolic bone disease characterized by an initial phase of excessive bone resorption (osteoclastic phase), followed by a reactive phase of excessive abnormal bone formation (osteoblastic phase). The new bone structure, which is chaotic, fragile, and weak, causes painful deformities of both external contour and internal structure.

Paget's disease usually localizes in one or more areas of the skeleton (most frequently the lower torso), but occasionally skeletal deformity is widely distributed. It can be fatal, particularly when it's associated with heart failure (widespread disease creates a continuous need for high cardiac output), bone sarcoma, or giant-cell tumors.

Paget's disease occurs worldwide, but is more common in Europe, Australia, and New Zealand, where it's seen in up to 5% of the elderly population.

Causes

Although the exact cause of Paget's disease is unknown, one theory holds that early viral infection causes a dormant skeletal infection that erupts many years later as Paget's disease. Genetic factors are also suspected. Other possible causes include benign or malignant bone tumors, vitamin D deficiency during the bone-developing years of childhood, autoimmune disease, and estrogen deficiency.

Pathophysiology

Repeated episodes of accelerated osteoclastic resorption of spongy bone occur. The trabeculae diminish, and vascular fibrous tissue replaces marrow. This is followed by short periods of rapid, abnormal bone formation. The collagen fibers in this new bone are disorganized, and glycoprotein levels in the matrix decrease. The partially resorbed trabeculae thicken and enlarge because of excessive bone formation, and the bone becomes soft and weak.

Assessment findings

Clinical signs of Paget's disease vary. Early stages may be asymptomatic, but when pain does develop, it's usually severe and persistent and may coexist with impaired movement resulting from impingement of abnormal bone on the spinal cord or sensory nerve root. Such pain intensifies with weight bearing.

The patient with skull involvement shows characteristic cranial enlargement over frontal and occipital areas (hat size may increase) and may complain of headaches. Other deformities include kyphosis (spinal curvature due to compression fractures of pagetic vertebrae), accompanied by a barrel-shaped chest and asymmetrical bowing of the tibia and femur, which commonly reduces height. Pagetic sites are warm and tender and are susceptible to pathologic fractures (which heal slowly and usually incompletely) after minor trauma.

Bony impingement on the cranial nerves may cause blindness and hearing loss with tinnitus and vertigo.

Diagnosis

○ X-rays taken before overt symptoms develop show increased bone expansion and density.

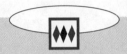

○ Bone scan clearly shows early pagetic lesions (radioisotope collects around areas of active disease).

○ Computed tomography scan or magnetic resonance imaging shows extra bony extension if sarcomatous degeneration occurs.

○ Bone biopsy reveals characteristic mosaic pattern.

○ Serum alkaline phosphatase levels (an index of osteoblastic activity and bone formation) and serum calcium levels are elevated.

○ 24-hour urine levels for hydroxyproline are elevated (amino acid excreted by kidneys and an index of osteoclastic hyperactivity).

○ Red blood cell count shows signs of anemia.

○ Serum osteocalcin and N-telopeptide are usually increased.

Complications

○ Blindness and hearing loss with tinnitus and vertigo
○ Fractures
○ Gout
○ Heart failure
○ Hypercalcemia
○ Hypertension
○ Osteoarthritis
○ Paraplegia
○ Renal calculi
○ Sarcoma

Treatment

○ Calcitonin (subcutaneously or intranasally) is used to retard bone resorption (which relieves bone lesions) and reduce levels of serum alkaline phosphate and urinary hydroxyproline secretion.

○ Bisphosphonates, such as alendronate, etidronate, pamidronate, risedronate, and tiludronate produce rapid reduction in bone turnover, relieve pain, and reduce serum alkaline phosphate and urinary hydroxyproline secretion.

○ Plicamycin, a cytotoxic antibiotic, is used to decrease calcium, urinary hydroxyproline, and serum alkaline phosphatase and is reserved for severe cases with neurologic compromise and for those resistant to other therapies.

○ Orthopedic surgery is used to correct specific deformities in severe cases, reduce or prevent pathologic fractures, correct secondary deformities, or relieve neurologic impairment.

○ Analgesics or nonsteroidal anti-inflammatory drugs may be given to control pain.

 COLLABORATIVE MANAGEMENT
Care of the patient with Paget's disease involves several members of the interdisciplinary team. The primary care provider diagnoses and manages the disorder. The surgeon is consulted to correct deformities, reduce fractures, and relieve pain. The nurse educates the patient to improve his level of functioning and to help him slow the progress of the disease and reduce the risk of com-

plications. The dietitian helps the patient plan a diet that's high in calcium and vitamin D and to achieve and maintain a healthy body weight. The physical therapist helps the patient develop an exercise program that reduces stress on pagetic bones. The occupational therapist teaches the patient to use assistive devices that will improve his functional abilities. The social worker counsels the patient about financial and occupational concerns.

Special considerations
○ To evaluate the effectiveness of analgesics, assess the patient's level of pain daily.
○ Watch the patient for new areas of pain or restricted movements, which may indicate new fracture sites.
○ Monitor the patient for sensory or motor disturbances, such as difficulty in hearing, seeing, or walking.
○ Monitor serum calcium and alkaline phosphatase levels.
○ If the patient is confined to prolonged bed rest, prevent pressure ulcers by providing good skin care. Reposition the patient frequently, and use a flotation mattress. Provide high-topped sneakers to prevent footdrop.
○ Monitor intake and output. Encourage adequate fluid intake to minimize renal calculi formation.
○ Help the patient and his family make use of community support resources such as a visiting nurse or home health agency. For more information, refer them to the Paget's Disease Foundation.
○ Provide patient education. (See *Teaching about Paget's disease*.)

Applicable patient-teaching aids
○ Caring for your cast *
○ Exercising casted limbs
○ Exercising for a stronger back
○ Learning about canes *
○ Learning about how broken bones heal
○ Performing active range-of-motion exercises *
○ Performing stretching exercises
○ Planning a calcium-rich diet *

○ Troubleshooting your casted limb
○ Using good posture to protect your back
○ Walking with a cane

○ Pancreatitis, chronic

Pancreatitis, inflammation of the pancreas, occurs in acute and chronic forms and may be due to edema, necrosis, or hemorrhage. In men, this disease is commonly associated with alcoholism, trauma, or peptic ulcer; in women, it's linked to biliary tract disease. Patients with acquired immunodeficiency syndrome have a higher incidence of pancreatitis.

The prognosis is good when pancreatitis follows biliary tract disease, but poor when it follows alcoholism. Mortality rises as high as 60% when pancreatitis is associated with necrosis and hemorrhage.

Causes
Chronic pancreatitis is usually associated with alcoholism (in over half of all patients) but can also follow hyperparathyroidism (causing hypercalcemia), hyperlipidemia or, infrequently, gallstones, trauma, prolonged fasting, or peptic ulcer. Inflammation and fibrosis cause progressive pancreatic insufficiency and eventually destroy the pancreas.

Other causes of pancreatitis are biliary tract disease, pancreatic cancer, trauma, or use of certain drugs, such as glucocorticoids, sulfonamides, chlorothiazide, and azathioprine. This disease also may develop as a complication of peptic ulcer, mumps, or hypothermia. Rarer causes are stenosis or obstruction of the sphincter of Oddi, hemochromatosis, vasculitis or vascular disease, viral infections, mycoplasmal pneumonia, and pregnancy.

Pathophysiology
In chronic pancreatitis, persistent inflammation produces irreversible changes in the structure and function of the pancreas. It sometimes follows an episode of acute pancreatitis. Protein precipitates block the pancreatic duct and eventually harden or calcify. Structural changes lead to fibrosis and atrophy of the glands.

Growths called *pseudocysts* contain pancreatic enzymes and tissue debris. An abscess results if pseudocysts become infected.

If pancreatitis damages the islets of Langerhans, diabetes mellitus may result. Sudden severe pancreatitis causes massive hemorrhage and total destruction of the pancreas, manifested as diabetic acidosis, shock, or coma.

Assessment findings

Symptoms of chronic pancreatitis include constant dull pain in the midepigastrium, left chest, and back that may be constant with acute episodes aggravated by meals and relieved by bending forward. Other findings include anorexia, severe weight loss, and hyperglycemia (leading to diabetic symptoms). The patient may report bulky, foul-smelling stools

and nausea and vomiting. The area around the navel may appear bluish with bruising of the loin skin. Vital signs may reveal tachycardia, hypotension, and a low-grade fever. The patient's abdomen may be tender and swollen.

Diagnosis

○ Serum amylase, trypsin, and lipase levels may be elevated during acute attacks but may be normal at other times.

○ Pancreatic polypeptide levels may be reduced following a high protein meal in advanced chronic pancreatitis.

○ Erythrocyte sedimentation rate may be elevated.

○ Serum glucose levels may be elevated, indicating the development of diabetes.

○ Serum calcium, potassium, and magnesium levels may be decreased.

○ Abdominal X-rays or computed tomography scans show dilation of the small or large bowel or calcification of the pancreas.

○ Endoscopic retrograde cholangiopancreatography identifies ductal system abnormalities, such as calcification or strictures, and helps differentiate pancreatitis from other disorders such as pancreatic cancer.

Complications

○ Diabetes mellitus
○ Fluid and electrolyte imbalance
○ Gallbladder disease
○ GI bleeding, from peptic ulcers or variceal bleeding
○ Hypovolemia
○ Malabsorption and steatorrhea
○ Opioid addiction
○ Pancreatic cancer
○ Pseudocyst and fistula formation
○ Splenic and portal vein obstruction
○ Stenosis of the common bile duct
○ Weight loss

Treatment

○ Analgesics are administered to control severe pain.

○ Pancreatic enzymes taken at meal times decrease pancreatic enzyme secretion and reduce steatorrhea.

○ Insulin or oral hypoglycemics may be needed to control hyperglycemia.

○ A low-fat, high-carbohydrate diet may help control steatorrhea.

○ Surgical repair of biliary or pancreatic ducts or the sphincter of Oddi may be required to reduce pressure and promote the flow of pancreatic juice.

○ Alcohol cessation is important to improve prognosis.

 COLLABORATIVE MANAGEMENT
Care of the patient with chronic pancreatitis involves several members of the interdisciplinary team. The primary health care provider, gastroenterologist, or pancreatic specialist diagnoses or manages the disorder. The nurse educates the patient about the disorder, guides him in making necessary lifestyle modifications, and works with him to control pain. The social worker refers the patient to support groups for alcohol counseling and explores financial concerns. The dietitian assesses the patient's nutritional status and recommends a nutritional plan, such as a low-fat, high-carbohydrate diet with pancreatic enzyme replacement. The physical therapist plans an activity program to maintain the patient's muscle strength and tone and prevent deconditioning while the occupational therapist teaches energy conservation skills. An alcohol counselor can help the patient abstain from drinking and provide support.

Special considerations

○ Administer analgesics as needed to relieve the patient's pain.

○ Monitor glucose levels and administer insulin or oral hypoglycemics, as ordered.

○ Plan for frequent rest periods to help the patient conserve energy.

○ Consult with the dietitian to provide the patient with a low-fat, high-carbohydrate diet.

○ Administer pancreatic enzymes with meals.

○ Provide perineal care to the patient with steatorrhea.

○ Prepare the patient for surgery, if appropriate.

○ Provide patient education. (See *Teaching about chronic pancreatitis*.)

Applicable patient-teaching aids

○ Combating pancreatitis with a low-fat diet

○ Giving yourself a subcutaneous insulin injection *

○ Performing chest physiotherapy (for an adult)

○ Preventing diabetic complications *

○ Testing your blood glucose level

○ Using imagination to relieve pain

◯ Panic disorder

Characterized by recurrent episodes of intense apprehension, terror, and impending doom, panic disorder represents anxiety in its most severe form. Initially unpredictable, panic attacks may become associated with specific situations or tasks. The disorder often exists concurrently with agoraphobia. Equal numbers of men and women are affected by panic disorder alone, whereas panic disorder with agoraphobia occurs in about twice as many women.

Panic disorder typically has an onset in late adolescence or early adulthood, often in response to a sudden loss. It may also be triggered by severe separation anxiety experienced during early childhood. Without treatment, panic disorder can persist for years, with alternating exacerbations and remissions. The patient with panic disorder is at high risk for a psychoactive substance abuse disorder: He may resort to alcohol or anxiolytics in an attempt to relieve his extreme anxiety.

Panic disorder affects about 2% of the population. Symptoms usually develop between ages 24 and 44. Panic disorder is more common in women, and people who are separated or divorced.

Causes

Like other anxiety disorders, panic disorder may stem from a combination of physical and psychological factors. For example, some theorists emphasize the role of stressful events or unconscious conflicts that occur early in childhood. Panic disorder may develop as a persistent pattern of maladaptive behavior acquired by learning. It may also have a hereditary component.

Pathophysiology

Although the exact cause of panic attacks isn't clear, one theory is that increased sensitivity to adrenergic central nervous system discharges, with hypersensitivity of presynaptic alpha-2 receptors may occur. Alterations in brain biochemistry, especially in norepinephrine, serotonin, and gamma-aminobutyric acid activity, may also contribute to panic disorder.

Assessment findings

The patient with panic disorder typically complains of repeated episodes of unexpected apprehension, fear, and, rarely, intense discomfort. These panic attacks may last for minutes or hours and leave the patient shaken, fearful, and exhausted. They occur several times a week, sometimes even daily. Because the attacks occur spontaneously, without exposure to a known anxiety-producing situation, the patient generally worries between attacks about when the next episode will occur.

Physical examination of the patient during a panic attack may reveal signs of intense anxiety, such as hyperventilation, tachycardia, trembling, and profuse sweating. The patient may also complain of difficulty breathing, digestive disturbances, chest pain, and feelings of unreality or being detached from self.

Diagnosis

○ Urine and serum toxicology tests may reveal the presence of psychoactive substances that can precipitate panic attacks, including barbiturates, caffeine, and amphetamines.
○ Various tests may be ordered to rule out an organic basis for the symptoms, for example, tests for serum glucose levels rule out hypoglycemia; studies of urine catecholamines and vanillylmandelic acid rule out pheochromocytoma; and thyroid function tests rule out hyperthyroidism. (See *Diagnosing panic disorder*.)

Complications

○ Psychoactive substance use disorder

Treatment

○ Cognitive-behavioral therapy works best when agoraphobia accompanies panic disorder because the identification of anxiety-inducing situations is easier. The patient learns to recognize panic symptoms as a misinterpretation of essentially harmless physical sensations.
○ Psychotherapy allows patients time to explore social or personal difficulties.
○ Progressive relaxation using visual imaging and systematic desensitization to reduce panic attacks.
○ Drug therapy includes antianxiety drugs, such as diazepam, alprazolam, and clonazepam; and beta-adrenergic blockers, such as propranolol, to provide symptomatic relief.
○ Antidepressants, including tricyclic antidepressants, selective serotonin reuptake inhibitors, and monoamine oxidase inhibitors, are also effective.

COLLABORATIVE MANAGEMENT
Care of the patient with panic disorder involves several members of the interdisciplinary team. The primary care provider or psychiatrist diagnoses the disorder and develops the care plan. A therapist can help the patient reduce anxiety and learn stress reduction techniques. The nurse educates the patient and reinforces coping strategies and relaxation techniques.

Special considerations

○ Provide emotional support by staying with the patient until the attack subsides. If left alone, he may become even more anxious.
○ Maintain a calm, serene approach. Statements such as, "I won't let anything here hurt you," and "I'll stay with you," can assure the patient that you're in control of the immediate situation. Avoid giving him insincere expressions of reassurance.
○ The patient's perceptual field may be narrowed, and excessive stimuli may cause him to feel overwhelmed. Dim bright lights or raise dim lights as necessary.
○ If the patient loses control, move him to a smaller, quieter space.
○ The patient may be so overwhelmed that he can't follow lengthy or complicated instructions. Speak in short, simple sentences, and slowly give one direction at a time. Avoid giving lengthy explanations and asking too many questions.

Diagnosing panic disorder

The diagnosis of panic disorder is confirmed when the patient meets the criteria put forth in the *Diagnostic and Statistical Manual of Mental Disorders,* Fourth Edition, Text Revision.

Panic attack

A discrete period of intense fear or discomfort in which at least four of the following symptoms develop abruptly and reach a peak within 10 minutes:
- chest pain or discomfort
- depersonalization or derealization
- dizziness or faintness
- fear of dying
- fear of losing control or going crazy
- feeling of choking
- hot flashes or chills
- nausea or abdominal distress
- numbness or tingling sensations (paresthesia)
- palpitations, pounding heart, or tachycardia
- shortness of breath or smothering sensations
- sweating
- trembling or shaking.

Panic disorder without agoraphobia

- The person experiences recurrent unexpected panic attacks and at least one of the attacks has been followed by 1 month (or more) or one (or more) of the following:
– persistent concern about having additional attacks
– worry about the implications of the attack or its consequences
– a significant change in behavior related to the attacks.

- The panic attacks aren't due to the direct physiologic effects of a substance or a general medical condition.
- The panic attacks aren't better accounted for by another mental disorder, such as social phobia, specific phobia, obsessive-compulsive disorder, post-traumatic stress disorder, or separation anxiety disorder.

Panic disorder with agoraphobia

- The person experiences recurrent unexpected panic attacks and at least one of the attacks has been followed by 1 month (or more) or one (or more) of the following:
– persistent concern about having additional attacks
– worry about the implications of the attack or its consequences
– a significant change in behavior related to the attacks.
- The person exhibits agoraphobia (the fear of being alone or of open space).
- The panic attacks aren't due to the direct physiologic effects of a substance or a general medical condition.
- The panic attacks aren't better accounted for by another mental disorder, such as social phobia, specific phobia, obsessive-compulsive disorder, post-traumatic stress disorder, or separation anxiety disorder.

○ Allow the patient to pace around the room (provided he isn't belligerent) to help expend energy.

○ Show him how to take slow, deep breaths if he's hyperventilating.

○ Avoid touching the patient until you've established rapport. Unless he trusts you, he may be too stimulated or frightened to find touch reassuring.

○ Administer medication as prescribed.

○ During and after a panic attack, encourage the patient to express his feelings. Discuss his fears and help him identify situations or events that trigger the attacks.

○ Encourage the patient and his family to use community resources such as the Anxiety Disorders Association of America.

○ Provide patient education. (See *Teaching about panic disorder,* page 256.)

Teaching about panic disorder

Remember these key points when teaching your patient and his family about panic disorder:
● Teach about the disease process, including its symptoms, complications, and treatments.
● Teach about prescribed medications, including their names, indications, dosages, adverse effects, and special considerations.
● Caution the patient to notify the physician before discontinuing any medication because abrupt withdrawal could cause severe symptoms.
● Teach the patient relaxation techniques, and explain how he can use them to relieve stress or avoid a panic attack.
● Help the patient recognize situations that trigger an attack and how these situations can be changed.
● Discuss how the use of alcohol, cocaine, amphetamines, caffeine, and nicotine can trigger panic attacks and should be avoided.

Applicable patient-teaching aids
○ Performing relaxation breathing exercises *
○ Taking your medication correctly

Parkinson's disease

Parkinson's disease, also called *parkinsonism, paralysis agitans,* and *shaking palsy,* is one of the most common crippling diseases in the United States. Parkinson's disease characteristically produces progressive muscle rigidity, akinesia, involuntary tremor, and dementia. Death may result from aspiration pneumonia or an infection.

Parkinson's disease strikes 2 in every 1,000 people, most often developing in those older than age 50; however, it also occurs in children and young adults. Because of increased longevity, this amounts to roughly 60,000 new cases diagnosed annually in the United States alone. Incidence increases in persons with repeated brain injury, including professional athletes, and persons using psychoactive substances, whether prescribed or illicit.

Causes
Although the cause of Parkinson's disease is unknown, study of the extrapyramidal brain nuclei (corpus striatum, globus pallidus, and substantia nigra) has established that a dopamine deficiency prevents affected brain cells from performing their normal inhibitory function within the central nervous system. Parkinson's disease is hereditary in some cases; in others, it's secondary to external factors such as medications used to treat schizophrenia.

Pathophysiology
Parkinson's disease is a degenerative process involving the dopaminergic neurons in the substantia nigra (the area of the basal ganglia that produces and stores the neurotransmitter dopamine). This area plays an important role in the extrapyramidal system, which controls posture and coordination of voluntary motor movements. (See *Neurotransmitter action in Parkinson's disease.*)

Normally, stimulation of the basal ganglia results in refined motor movement because acetylcholine (excitatory) and dopamine (inhibitory) release are balanced. Degeneration of the dopaminergic neurons and loss of available dopamine leads to an excess of excitatory acetylcholine at the synapse and consequent rigidity, tremors, and bradykinesia.

Other nondopaminergic neurons may be affected, possibly contributing to depression and the other nonmotor symptoms associated with this disease. Moreover, the basal ganglia is interconnected to the hypothalamus, potentially affecting autonomic and endocrine function as well.

Current research on the pathogenesis of Parkinson's disease focuses on damage to the substantia nigra from oxidative stress. Oxidative stress is believed to diminish brain iron content, impair mitochondrial function, inhibit antioxidant and protective systems, reduce glutathione secretion, and damage lipids, proteins, and deoxyribonucleic acid. Brain cells are less capable of repairing oxidative damage than are other tissues.

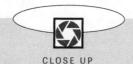

CLOSE UP

Neurotransmitter action in Parkinson's disease

Parkinson's disease is a degenerative process involving the dopaminergic neurons in the substantia nigra (the area of the basal ganglia that produces and stores the neurotransmitter dopamine). Dopamine deficiency prevents affected brain cells from performing their normal inhibitory function. Other nondopaminergic receptors may be affected, possibly contributing to depression and other nonmotor symptoms.

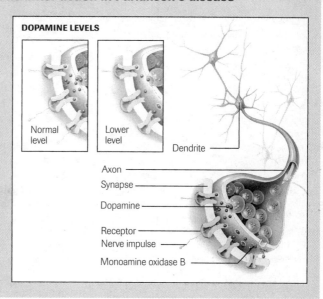

DOPAMINE LEVELS

Normal level

Lower level

Dendrite

Axon

Synapse

Dopamine

Receptor

Nerve impulse

Monoamine oxidase B

Assessment findings

The cardinal symptoms of Parkinson's disease are muscle rigidity; bradykinesia; akinesia; and an insidious resting tremor that begins in the fingers (unilateral pill-roll tremor), increases during stress or anxiety, and decreases with purposeful movement and sleep. Muscle rigidity results in resistance to passive muscle stretching, which may be uniform (lead-pipe rigidity) or jerky (cogwheel rigidity). Bradykinesia causes the patient to walk with difficulty (gait is festinant). Akinesia produces a high-pitched, monotone voice; drooling; a masklike facial expression; stooped posture; and freezing movement, dysarthria, dysphagia, or both. Occasionally, akinesia may also cause oculogyric crises (eyes are fixed upward, with involuntary tonic movements) or blepharospasm (eyelids are completely closed). Other findings include excessive sweating, decreased motility of GI and genitourinary smooth muscle, orthostatic hypotension, and oily skin.

Diagnosis

○ Conclusive diagnosis is possible only after ruling out other causes of tremor, involutional depression, cerebral arteriosclerosis and, in patients younger than age 30, intracranial tumors, Wilson's disease, or phenothiazine or other drug toxicity.

Complications

○ Food aspiration
○ Injury from falls
○ Skin breakdown
○ Urinary tract infections

Treatment

○ Levodopa, a dopamine replacement, is most effective during early stages and is given in increasing doses until symptoms are relieved or adverse effects appear.
○ Carbidopa may be given in combination with levodopa to halt peripheral dopamine synthesis and reduce serious adverse effects of levodopa.

Teaching about Parkinson's disease

Remember these key points when teaching your patient and his family about Parkinson's disease:

- Teach about the disorder, including its progressive symptoms, complications, and treatments.
- Discuss warning signs of complications that require immediate medical attention.
- If the patient is having surgery, explain surgical procedures and what to expect preoperatively and postoperatively.
- Teach about prescribed medications, including their names, indications, dosages, adverse effects, and special considerations (such as dietary restrictions and the need to stand up slowly for the patient on levodopa).
- Reinforce the importance of range-of-motion exercises, routine daily activities, walking, and baths and massage to help relax muscles.
- Explain to the patient and family how to prevent pressure ulcers and contractures by proper positioning.
- Explain household safety measures to prevent accidents.
- Reinforce a swallowing therapy regimen to prevent food aspiration.

○ Alternative drug therapy is used when levodopa is ineffective and includes anticholinergics such as trihexyphenidyl, antihistamines such as diphenhydramine, and amantadine, an antiviral agent.

○ Entacapone may be given to potentiate the effects of levodopa-carbidopa treatment so that less frequent doses are required (levodopa-carbidopa has been associated with an acceleration of disease process).

○ Selegiline, an enzyme-inhibiting agent, allows conservation of dopamine and enhances the therapeutic effect of levodopa; selegiline used with tocopherols delays the time when the patient with Parkinson's disease becomes disabled.

○ Catechol-O-methyltransferase inhibitors given with levodopa-carbidopa increases available dopamine in the brain.

○ Stereotactic neurosurgery, such as subthalamotomy and pallidotomy, may be an alternative to relieve symptoms when drug therapy fails and is most effective in young, otherwise healthy people with unilateral tremor or muscle rigidity.

○ Brain stimulator implantation alters the activity of the area where Parkinson's disease symptoms originate, reducing the need for medication, thus reducing the medication-related adverse effects experienced by the patient.

○ Fetal cell transplantation, in which fetal cells are injected into brain tissue, may allow the brain to process dopamine, thereby either halting or reversing disease progression.

○ Neurotransplantation techniques, including the use of nerve cells from other parts of the patient's body, have been attempted with varying results.

○ Individually planned physical therapy complements drug treatment and neurosurgery to maintain normal muscle tone and function and includes both active and passive range-of-motion exercises, routine daily activities, walking, and baths and massage to help relax muscles.

COLLABORATIVE MANAGEMENT
Because Parkinson's disease has no cure, the primary aim of treatment is to relieve symptoms and keep the patient functional as long as possible. The neurologist diagnoses and manages the disorder. The nurse educates the patient and family about the disorder and helps the patient maintain the highest level of independent functioning. The speech therapist helps the patient with swallowing issues. The physical therapist works with the patient to develop an exercise program to maintain muscle tone and function. The social worker can facilitate the drafting of a living will and power of attorney.

Special considerations

○ Monitor drug treatment and adjust dosage, if necessary, to minimize adverse effects.

○ If the patient has surgery, watch for signs of hemorrhage and increased intracranial pressure by frequently checking level of consciousness and vital signs.

○ Encourage the patient to be as independent as possible.

○ Help the patient overcome problems related to eating. For example, if he has difficulty eating, offer supplementary or small, frequent meals to increase caloric intake.

○ Take measures to prevent aspiration.

○ Stress the importance of rest periods between activities.

○ Provide frequent warm baths and massage.

○ Assist with ambulation and range-of-motion exercises.

○ Help establish a regular bowel routine by encouraging the patient to drink at least 2 qt (2 L) of liquids daily and eat high-fiber foods. He may need an elevated toilet seat to assist him from a standing to a sitting position.

○ Give the patient and his family emotional support and help them express their feelings and frustrations about the progressively debilitating effects of the disease.

○ Refer the patient and his family to the National Parkinson Foundation or the United Parkinson Foundation for more information.

○ Provide patient education. (See *Teaching about Parkinson's disease*.)

Applicable patient-teaching aids
○ Performing stretching exercises
○ Using dressing aids *
○ Walking with a wide-based gait *

○ Pernicious anemia

Pernicious anemia, also known as *Addison's anemia,* is a megaloblastic anemia characterized by decreased gastric production of hydrochloric acid and deficiency of intrinsic factor, a substance normally secreted by the parietal cells of the gastric mucosa that's essential for vitamin B_{12} absorption in the ileum. The resulting deficiency of vitamin B_{12} causes serious neurologic, gastric, and intestinal abnormalities. Untreated pernicious anemia may lead to permanent neurologic disability and death.

Pernicious anemia primarily affects people of northern European ancestry. It's rare in children and infants. Onset typically occurs after age 35, and incidence increases with age. It affects about 2% of people older than age 60.

Causes
Familial incidence of pernicious anemia suggests a genetic predisposition. The disease is associated with human leucocyte antigen types A2, A3, and B7 and type A blood group. Significantly higher incidence in patients with immunologically related diseases, such as thyroiditis, myxedema, and Graves' disease, seems to support a widely held theory that an inherited autoimmune response causes gastric mucosal atrophy and, therefore, deficiency of hydrochloric acid and intrinsic factor. Iatrogenic induction can follow partial gastrectomy.

Juvenile pernicious anemia, occurring in children younger than age 10, stems from a congenital stomach disorder that causes secretion of abnormal intrinsic factor. With age, vitamin B_{12} absorption may also diminish, resulting in reduced erythrocyte mass and decreased hemoglobin levels and hematocrit.

Pathophysiology
Pernicious anemia is characterized by decreased production of hydrochloric acid in the stomach and a deficiency of intrinsic factor, which is normally secreted by the parietal cells of the gastric mucosa and is essential for vitamin B_{12} absorption in the ileum. The resulting vitamin B_{12} deficiency inhibits deoxyribonucleic acid synthesis and cell replication, particularly of red blood cells (RBCs), leading to production of fewer, deformed RBCs with poor oxygen-carrying capacity. It also causes neurologic damage by impairing myelin formation. (See *Understanding pernicious anemia*, page 260.)

Assessment findings
Characteristically, pernicious anemia has an insidious onset but eventually causes an unmistakable triad of symptoms: weakness, sore tongue, and numbness and tingling in the extremities. The lips, gums, and tongue appear markedly bloodless. Hemolysis-induced hyperbilirubinemia may cause faintly jaundiced scle-

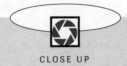

CLOSE UP

Understanding pernicious anemia

Pernicious anemia is characterized by decreased production of hydrochloric acid in the stomach and a deficiency of intrinsic factor, which is normally secreted by the parietal cells of the gastric mucosa and essential for vitamin B_{12} absorption in the ileum. The resulting vitamin B_{12} deficiency inhibits cell growth, particularly of red blood cells (RBCs), leading to production of scant, deformed RBCs with poor oxygen-carrying capacity. RBCs are abnormally large due to excess ribonucleic acid production of the hemoglobin. Pernicious anemia also causes neurologic damage by impairing myelin formation.

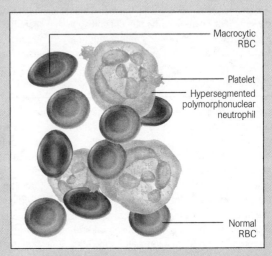

ra and pale to bright-yellow skin. In addition, the patient may become highly susceptible to infection, especially of the genitourinary tract.

Other systemic symptoms of pernicious anemia include the following:

○ *GI:* nausea, vomiting, anorexia, weight loss, flatulence, diarrhea, steatorrhea, constipation, and gingival bleeding and tongue inflammation that may hinder eating and intensify anorexia

○ *Central nervous system (CNS):* neuritis; weakness in extremities; peripheral numbness and paresthesia; disturbed position sense; lack of coordination; ataxia; impaired fine finger movement; positive Babinski's and Romberg's signs; light-headedness; diplopia and blurred vision, altered taste, and tinnitus; optic muscle atrophy; loss of bowel and bladder control; irritability, poor memory, headache, depression, and delirium; and, in males, impotence

○ *Cardiovascular:* weakness, fatigue, light-headedness, palpitations, wide pulse pressure, dyspnea, orthopnea, tachycardia, premature beats and, eventually, heart failure

○ *Musculoskeletal:* scissors gait (can also occur as a late sign of untreated anemia).

Diagnosis

○ Hemoglobin level is decreased (4 to 5 g/dl) and RBC count is low.

○ Mean corpuscular volume (greater than 120/μl) is increased; because larger-than-normal RBCs *each* contain increased amounts of hemoglobin, mean corpuscular hemoglobin concentration is also increased.

○ White blood cell and platelet counts may be low; platelets may be large and malformed.

○ Serum vitamin B_{12} assay levels are less than 0.1 mcg/ml.

○ Serum lactate dehydrogenase levels are elevated.

○ Bone marrow aspiration reveals erythroid hyperplasia (crowded red bone marrow), with increased numbers of megaloblasts, but few normally developing RBCs.

○ Gastric analysis shows absence of free hydrochloric acid after histamine or pentagastrin injection.

○ Schilling test, the definitive test for pernicious anemia, may reveal a urinary excretion of less than 3% in the first 24 hours in patients with pernicious anemia; it may reveal normal excretion of vitamin B_{12} when repeated with intrinsic factor added.

○ Serologic findings may include intrinsic factor antibodies and antiparietal cell antibodies.

Complications

○ Heart failure (with severe anemia)
○ Loss of sphincter control of bowel and bladder
○ Myocardial ischemia
○ Paralysis
○ Peptic ulcer disease
○ Permanent CNS symptoms (if patient isn't treated within 6 months of appearance of symptoms)
○ Psychotic behavior

Treatment

○ Parenteral vitamin B_{12} replacement can reverse pernicious anemia, minimize complications and, possibly, prevent permanent neurologic damage.
○ Concomitant iron and folic acid replacement is necessary to prevent iron deficiency anemia (rapid cell regeneration increases the patient's iron and folate requirements).
○ Maintenance vitamin B_{12} injections are given monthly after the patient's condition improves and must be continued for life.
○ Bed rest is required for extreme fatigue until hemoglobin levels rise.
○ Blood transfusions may be needed if hemoglobin levels are dangerously low.
○ Digoxin, a diuretic, and a low-sodium diet may be necessary for a patient with heart failure.
○ Antibiotics help combat accompanying infections.

COLLABORATIVE MANAGEMENT
Care of the patient with pernicious anemia involves several members of the interdisciplinary team. The primary care provider or hematologist typically diagnose and treat the disorder. Other specialists, such as a cardiologist or neurologist, may consult based on complications that develop. The nurse educates the patient about the disorder, teaches how to give vitamin B_{12} injections, and monitors for complications. The dietitian makes dietary recommendations and educates

Teaching about pernicious anemia

Remember these key points when teaching your patient about pernicious anemia:
● Teach about the disease process, including its symptoms, complications, and treatments.
● Teach about prescribed medications, including their names, indications, dosages, adverse effects, and special considerations.
● Warn the patient to guard against infections and tell him to report signs of infection promptly.
● Discuss warning signs of complications that require immediate medical attention.
● Teach the patient to eat foods high in vitamin B_{12}, folic acid, iron, and vitamin C.
● Discuss safety measures to avoid falls in the home.
● Demonstrate proper B_{12} injection technique.
● Stress that vitamin B_{12} replacement isn't a permanent cure and that these injections *must* be continued for life, even after symptoms subside.
● Reinforce the importance of avoiding exposure to extreme heat or cold on the extremities.
● Discuss the importance of pacing activities and planning for rest periods.

the patient about eating a well-balanced diet high in vitamin B_{12}. The dietitian also counsels the patient on following a low-sodium diet, if heart failure is a problem. The physical therapist plans an activity and exercise program to help the patient safely regain strength, while the occupational therapist teaches energy conservation techniques.

Special considerations

○ If the patient has severe anemia, plan activities, rest periods, and necessary diagnostic tests to conserve his energy. Monitor his pulse rate; tachycardia means his activities are too strenuous.
○ To ensure accurate Schilling test results, make sure that all urine over a 24-hour period

is collected and that the specimens are uncontaminated.

○ Provide a well-balanced diet, including foods high in vitamin B_{12} (meat, liver, fish, eggs, and milk).

○ Because a sore mouth and tongue make eating painful, avoid giving the patient irritating foods. Provide diluted mouthwash or, with severe conditions, swab the patient's mouth with tap water or warm saline solution.

○ If the patient is incontinent, establish a regular bowel and bladder routine.

○ If neurologic damage causes behavioral problems, assess mental and neurologic status often and provide appropriate safety measures.

○ To prevent pernicious anemia, emphasize the importance of vitamin B_{12} supplements for patients who have had extensive gastric resections or who follow strict vegetarian or vegan diets.

○ Provide patient education. (See *Teaching about pernicious anemia,* page 261.)

Applicable patient-teaching aids
○ Learning about blood transfusions
○ Learning about daily food choices
○ Preventing infection with proper hand washing *

○ Polycystic ovarian syndrome

Polycystic ovarian syndrome is a metabolic disorder characterized by varying degrees of hirsutism, obesity, and infertility. It's often associated with hyperinsulinemia, or insulin resistance, dyslipidemia, and hypertension. About 22% of the women in the United States have the disorder, and obesity is present in 50% to 80% of these women. Among those who seek treatment for infertility, more than 75% have some degree of polycystic ovarian syndrome, usually manifested by anovulation alone. Prognosis is good for ovulation and fertility with appropriate treatment.

Causes
The precise cause of polycystic ovarian syndrome is unknown. A possible genetic basis has been suggested with an autosomal dominant mode of inheritance. Hyperinsulinemia plays a key role in androgen excess, anovulation, and pathogenesis of polycystic ovarian syndrome.

Pathophysiology
A general feature of all anovulation syndromes is a lack of pulsatile release of gonadotropin-releasing hormone. Initial ovarian follicle development is normal. Many small follicles begin to accumulate because there's no selection of a dominant follicle. These follicles may respond abnormally to the hormonal stimulation, causing an abnormal pattern of estrogen secretion during the menstrual cycle. Endocrine abnormalities may be the cause of polycystic ovarian syndrome or cystic abnormalities; muscle and adipose tissue are resistant to the effects of insulin, and lipid metabolism is abnormal.

Assessment findings
The woman with polycystic ovarian syndrome may report mild pelvic discomfort, lower back pain, dyspareunia, and menstrual disturbance, usually dating back to menarche. Abnormal uterine bleeding may occur secondary to a disturbed ovulatory pattern. Other findings include hirsutism, acne, male-pattern hair loss, and bilaterally enlarged polycystic ovaries.

Diagnosis
○ Ultrasound permits visualization of the ovaries.
○ Urinary 17-ketosteroid levels are slightly elevated.
○ Basal body temperature graphs and endometrial biopsy may reveal anovulation.
○ Ratio of luteinizing hormone to follicle-stimulating hormone (usually 3:1 or greater) is elevated.
○ Testosterone and androstenedione levels may be elevated.
○ Unopposed estrogen action occurs during the menstrual cycle due to anovulation.
○ Laparoscopy permits direct visualization of the ovaries to rule out paraovarian cysts of the broad ligament, salpingitis, endometriosis, and neoplastic cysts.
○ Surgery may confirm the diagnosis.

Complications

○ Addison's disease
○ Cardiovascular disease
○ Endometrial carcinoma
○ Infertility
○ Oligomenorrhea
○ Ovarian atrophy
○ Secondary amenorrhea
○ Type 2 diabetes mellitus

Treatment

○ Clomiphene may be given to induce ovulation.
○ Metformin may be used before or concurrent with clomiphene.
○ Medroxyprogesterone may be administered for 10 days each month for a patient wanting to become pregnant.
○ Low-dose hormonal contraceptives treat abnormal bleeding for the patient needing reliable contraception.
○ Weight loss, diet, and exercise reduce obesity.
○ Surgery, in the form of laparoscopy or exploratory laparotomy with possible ovarian cystectomy or oophorectomy, may be necessary if an ovarian cyst is found to be persistent or suspicious.

 COLLABORATIVE MANAGEMENT
Care of the patient with polycystic ovarian syndrome includes several members of the interdisciplinary team. The primary care provider diagnoses the disorder and develops the care plan. Referrals to specialists, such as a surgeon, cardiologist, endocrinologist, may be necessary. The nurse educates the patient, provides care following surgery, and helps the patient identify necessary lifestyle modifications. The dietitian assesses the patient's nutritional status and makes dietary recommendations for losing weight, controlling blood glucose levels, and reducing cardiovascular risk. The physical therapist helps the patient develop a regular exercise program.

Special considerations

○ Preoperatively, watch for signs of cyst rupture, such as increasing abdominal pain, distention, and rigidity; monitor vital signs for

Teaching about polycystic ovarian syndrome

Remember these key points when teaching your patient about polycystic ovarian syndrome:
● Teach about the disease process, including its symptoms, complications, and treatments.
● Discuss warning signs and symptoms of complications that require immediate medical attention.
● If the patient is having surgery, explain the surgical procedure and what to expect in the preoperative and postoperative periods.
● Teach about prescribed medications, including their names, indications, dosages, adverse effects, and special considerations.
● Discuss dietary recommendations for weight loss and diabetic control, as necessary.
● Reinforce the importance of regular follow-up care.
● Discuss concerns related to fertility issues.

fever, tachypnea, or hypotension (possibly indicating peritonitis or intraperitoneal hemorrhage).
○ Postoperatively, encourage frequent movement in bed and early ambulation as ordered to prevent pulmonary embolism.
○ Provide emotional support, offering appropriate reassurance if the patient fears cancer or infertility.
○ Provide patient education. (See *Teaching about polycystic ovarian syndrome.*)

Applicable patient-teaching aids

○ How to take your basal body temperature
○ Learning about daily food choices
○ Learning about laparoscopy *
○ Understanding the menstrual cycle *

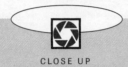

CLOSE UP

How prostate cancer develops

Prostate cancer (commonly a form of adeno-carcinoma) grows slowly. When primary lesions metastasize beyond the prostate, they invade the prostate capsule and spread along the ejaculatory ducts in the space between the seminal vesicles.

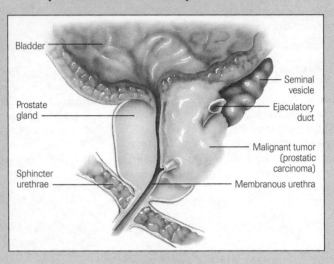

⬭ Prostate cancer

Prostate cancer is the most common cancer in men older than age 50. Adenocarcinoma is its most common form; sarcoma occurs only rarely. Most prostate carcinomas originate in the posterior prostate gland; the rest originate near the urethra. Malignant prostate tumors seldom result from the benign hyperplastic enlargement that commonly develops around the prostatic urethra in elderly men. Prostate cancer seldom produces symptoms until it's advanced, and its treatment depends on clinical assessment, the patient's tolerance of therapy and his expected lifespan, and the disease's stage.

Incidence of prostate cancer is highest in Blacks and lowest in Asians. In fact, Blacks have the highest prostate cancer incidence in the world and are considered at high risk for the disease. Incidence also increases with age more rapidly than any other cancer.

Causes

Four factors have been suspected in the development of prostatic cancer: family or racial predisposition, exposure to environmental elements, co-existing sexually transmitted diseases, and endogenous hormonal influence. Eating fat-containing animal products has also been implicated. Although androgens regulate prostate growth and function and may also speed tumor growth, no definite link between increased androgen levels and prostatic cancer has been found.

Pathophysiology

Prostate cancer is slow-growing and seldom causes signs and symptoms until it's well advanced. Typically, when a primary prostatic lesion spreads beyond the prostate gland, it invades the prostatic capsule and spreads along ejaculatory ducts in the space between the seminal vesicles or perivascular fascia. Endocrine factors may play a role, leading researchers to suspect that androgens speed tumor growth. Malignant prostatic tumors sel-

Staging prostate cancer

The American Joint Committee on Cancer recognizes the TNM (tumor, node, metastasis) cancer staging system for assessing prostate cancer.

Primary tumor
TX — primary tumor can't be assessed
T0 — no evidence of primary tumor
T1 — tumor an incidental histologic finding
T1a — three or fewer microscopic foci of cancer
T1b — more than three microscopic foci of cancer
T2 — tumor limited to the prostate gland
T2a — tumor involves one-half of 1 lobe or less
T2b — tumor involves more than one-half of 1 lobe but not both lobes
T2c — tumor involves both lobes
T3 — unfixed tumor extends into the prostatic apex or into or beyond the prostatic capsule, bladder neck, or seminal vesicle
T4 — tumor fixed or invades adjacent structures not listed in T3

Regional lymph nodes
NX — regional lymph nodes can't be assessed
N0 — no evidence of regional lymph-node metastasis
N1 — metastasis in a single lymph node, 2 cm or less in greatest dimension

N2 — metastasis in a single lymph node, between 2 and 5 cm in greatest dimension, or metastasis to several lymph nodes, none more than 5 cm in greatest dimension
N3 — metastasis in a lymph node more than 5 cm in greatest dimension

Distant metastasis
MX — distant metastasis can't be assessed
M0 — no known distant metastasis
M1 — distant metastasis

Staging categories
Prostatic cancer progresses from mild to severe as follows:
STAGE 0 or STAGE I — T1a, N0, M0; T2a, N0, M0
STAGE II — T1b, N0, M0; T2b, N0, M0
STAGE III — T3, N0, M0
STAGE IV — T4, N0, M0; any T, N1, M0; any T, N2, M0; any T, N3, M0; any T, any N, M1

---

dom result for the benign hyperplastic enlargement that commonly develops around the prostatic urethra in older men. (See *How prostate cancer develops*.)

Assessment findings
Signs and symptoms of prostate cancer appear only in the advanced stages and include difficulty initiating a urine stream, dribbling, urine retention, unexplained cystitis, back pain and, rarely, hematuria. Pain may be present with urination, ejaculation, and bowel movement. (See *Staging prostate cancer*.)

Diagnosis
○ Digital rectal examination (DRE) reveals a small, hard nodule.
○ Biopsy confirms the diagnosis of prostate cancer.

○ Prostate-specific antigen (PSA) levels are elevated in all men with metastatic prostate cancer.
○ Serum acid phosphatase levels are elevated in two-thirds of men with metastatic prostate cancer.
○ Magnetic resonance imaging, computed tomography scan, and excretory urography may also aid diagnosis.
○ Elevated alkaline phosphatase levels and a positive bone scan point to bone metastasis.

Complications
○ Death
○ Deep vein thrombosis
○ Myelophthisis
○ Pulmonary emboli
○ Spinal cord compression

Teaching about prostate cancer

Remember these key points when teaching your patient about prostate cancer:

● Teach about the disease process, including its symptoms, complications, and treatments.

● Teach about prescribed medications, including their names, indications, dosages, adverse effects, and special considerations.

● Discuss warning signs of complications that require immediate medical attention.

● Before radiation therapy, explain possible adverse effects.

● If the patient is having surgery, explain the surgical procedure and what to expect in the preoperative and postoperative periods.

● Before prostatectomy, explain the expected aftereffects of surgery (such as erectile dysfunction and incontinence) and radiation and discuss tube placement and dressing changes.

● After prostatectomy or suprapubic prostatectomy, teach the patient to do perineal exercises.

● After perineal and retropubic prostatectomy, explain that urine leakage after catheter removal is normal and will subside.

● Reinforce the importance of follow-up care.

● Discuss self-care measures for the patient undergoing chemotherapy or radiation therapy.

● Reinforce any activity restrictions.

Treatment

○ Expectant management (watchful waiting) is used to closely monitor the cancer without active treatment for slow-growing tumors.

○ Radical prostatectomy is usually effective for localized lesions.

○ Transurethral resection of the prostate or cryosurgery may also be performed.

○ Orchiectomy may be performed to reduce androgen production.

○ Radiation therapy is used to cure some locally invasive lesions and to relieve pain from metastatic bone involvement.

○ Radionuclide strontium-89, given as a single injection, is also used to treat pain caused by bone metastasis.

○ Luteinizing hormone–releasing hormone (LHRH) agonists or LHRH antagonists are used to lower testosterone levels.

○ Hormone therapy with synthetic estrogen (diethylstilbestrol [DES]) and antiandrogens, such as cyproterone, megestrol, and flutamide, may also be administered in some patients.

○ Chemotherapy (using combinations of mitoxantrone with prednisone, estramustine, docetaxel, and paclitaxel) may be tried if hormone therapy, surgery, and radiation therapy aren't feasible or successful.

COLLABORATIVE MANAGEMENT
Because prostate cancer usually affects older men, who commonly have such coexisting disorders as hypertension, diabetes, and cardiac disease, care of the patient with prostate cancer involves several members of the interdisciplinary team. The primary health care provider provides screening through DRE and PSA levels. If cancer is detected, the surgeon is consulted. The radiation oncologist makes recommendations for and monitors the use of radiation therapy. The oncologist makes recommendations for and monitors the use of chemotherapy. The nurse educates the patient and provides care to the patient undergoing surgery, radiation therapy, and chemotherapy. The therapist can help the patient deal with issues such as anxiety, uncertainty, and sexuality.

Special considerations

○ Explain to the patient what he can expect in the preoperative and postoperative periods.

○ After prostatectomy or suprapubic prostatectomy, regularly check the dressing, incision, and drainage systems for excessive bleeding; watch the patient for signs of bleeding (pallor, falling blood pressure, rising pulse rate) and infection.

○ Maintain adequate fluid intake.

○ Give antispasmodics, as ordered, to control postoperative bladder spasms.

○ Assess for pain and give analgesics as needed.

○ Keep the patient's skin clean, dry, and free from drainage and urine.

○ Encourage perineal exercises within 24 to 48 hours after surgery after prostatectomy or suprapubic prostatectomy.

○ Provide meticulous catheter care—especially if a three-way catheter with a continuous irrigation system is in place. Check the tubing for kinks and blockages, especially if the patient reports pain.

○ After transurethral prostate resection, watch for signs of urethral stricture (dysuria, decreased force and caliber of urine stream, and straining to urinate) and for abdominal distention (from urethral stricture or catheter blockage). Irrigate the catheter as ordered.

○ After perineal prostatectomy, avoid taking a rectal temperature or inserting any kind of rectal tube. Provide pads to absorb urine leakage and sitz baths for pain and inflammation.

○ After perineal and retropubic prostatectomy, explain that urine leakage after catheter removal is normal and will subside.

○ When a patient receives hormonal therapy, watch for adverse effects. Gynecomastia, fluid retention, nausea, vomiting, erectile dysfunction, and thrombophlebitis may occur with DES.

○ After radiation therapy, watch for these common adverse effects: proctitis, diarrhea, bladder spasms, and urinary frequency. Internal radiation usually results in cystitis in the first 2 to 3 weeks. Urge the patient to drink at least 67.5 oz (2,000 ml) of fluid daily.

○ Provide analgesics and antispasmodics, as ordered.

○ Provide patient education. (See *Teaching about prostate cancer*.)

Applicable patient-teaching aids

○ Caring for your urinary catheter *
○ Controlling the side effects of chemotherapy *
○ Speeding your recovery after prostate surgery *

○ Psoriasis

Psoriasis is a chronic, recurrent disease marked by epidermal proliferation. Its lesions, which appear as erythematous papules and plaques covered with silvery scales, vary widely in severity and distribution. Psoriasis is characterized by recurring partial remissions and exacerbations. Flare-ups are usually related to specific systemic and environmental factors but may be unpredictable; they can usually be controlled with therapy.

Psoriasis affects approximately 2% of the population in the United States, and incidence is higher in whites than other races. Although this disorder is most common in young adults, it may strike at any age, including infancy.

Causes

The tendency to develop psoriasis is genetically determined. Researchers have discovered a significantly higher-than-normal incidence of certain human leukocyte antigens (HLAs) in families with psoriasis, suggesting a possible immune disorder. Onset of the disease is also influenced by environmental factors. Trauma can trigger the isomorphic effect or Koebner's phenomenon, in which lesions develop at sites of injury. Infections, especially those resulting from beta-hemolytic streptococci, may cause a flare of guttate (drop-shaped) lesions. Other contributing factors include pregnancy, endocrine changes, climate (cold weather tends to exacerbate psoriasis), and emotional stress.

Pathophysiology

A skin cell normally takes 14 days to move from the basal layer to the stratum corneum, where it's sloughed off after 14 days of normal wear and tear. Thus, the life cycle of a normal skin cell is 28 days compared with only 4 days for a psoriatic skin cell. This markedly shortened cycle doesn't allow time for the cell to mature. Consequently, the stratum corneum becomes thick and flaky, producing the cardinal manifestations of psoriasis. (See *Understanding psoriasis*, page 268.)

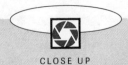

CLOSE UP

Understanding psoriasis

Psoriasis is a chronic, nonconta-
gious inflammatory skin disease
marked by reddish papules (solid
elevations) and plaques covered
with silvery scales. Psoriatic skin
cells have a shortened maturation
time as they migrate from the
basal membrane to the surface or
stratum corneum. As a result, the
stratum corneum develops thick,
scaly plaques, the chief sign of
psoriasis.

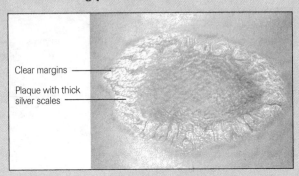

Clear margins

Plaque with thick
silver scales

Assessment findings

The most common complaint of the patient
with psoriasis is itching and, occasionally, pain
from dry, cracked, encrusted lesions. (See
Psoriatic plaques.) Psoriatic lesions are erythematous and usually form well-defined plaques,
sometimes covering large areas of the body,
most commonly the face, scalp, chest, elbows,
knees, shins, back, and buttocks. The plaques
consist of characteristic silvery white scales
that either flake off easily or can thicken, covering the lesion. Removal of psoriatic scales frequently produces fine bleeding points (Auspitz
sign). Occasionally, small guttate lesions appear, either alone or with plaques; these lesions
are typically thin and erythematous, with few
scales.

Widespread shedding of scales is common in
exfoliative or erythrodermic psoriasis and may
also develop in chronic psoriasis.

In localized pustular (Barber's) psoriasis,
pustules appear on the palms and soles and remain sterile until opened. In generalized pustular (*von Zumbusch's*) psoriasis, which often
occurs with fever, leukocytosis, and malaise,
groups of pustules coalesce to form lakes of
pus on red skin and commonly involve the
tongue and oral mucosa.

In about 30% of patients, psoriasis spreads to
the fingernails, producing small indentations

and yellow or brown discoloration. In severe
cases, the accumulation of thick, crumbly debris under the nail causes it to separate from
the nail bed.

Some patients with psoriasis develop arthritic symptoms (psoriatic arthritis), usually in one
or more joints of the fingers or toes, or sometimes in the sacroiliac joints, which may
progress to spondylitis. Such patients may
complain of morning stiffness.

Diagnosis

○ Serum uric acid level is elevated as a result
of accelerated nucleic acid degradation, but indications of gout are absent.
○ HLA-Cw6, B-13, and B-w57 may be present
in early-onset psoriasis.
○ Skin biopsy rules out other diseases.

Complications

○ Altered self-image
○ Depression
○ Infection
○ Social isolation

Treatment

○ Appropriate treatment depends on the type
of psoriasis, the extent of the disease, the patient's response to it, and what effect the disease has on the patient's lifestyle. No perma-

nent cure exists, and all methods of treatment are palliative. No effective treatment exists for psoriasis of the nails.

○ Occlusive ointment bases, such as petroleum jelly, salicylic acid preparations, or preparations containing urea are used to remove psoriatic scales.

○ Baker P & S liquid (phenol, sodium chloride, and liquid paraffin), applied to the scalp at bedtime, or liquid carbonis detergens in Nivea oil is also effective.

○ Ultraviolet light (UVB or natural sunlight) exposure to the point of minimal erythema retards rapid cell production.

○ Tar preparations or crude coal tar itself may be applied to affected areas about 15 minutes before exposure to UVB or may be left on overnight and wiped off the next morning.

○ Petroleum jelly may be applied in a thin layer before UVB exposure (the most common treatment for generalized psoriasis).

○ Steroid creams and ointments are useful to control symptoms of psoriasis and require application twice daily, preferably after bathing to facilitate absorption, and overnight use of occlusive dressings, such as plastic wrap, plastic gloves or booties, or a vinyl exercise suit (under direct medical or nursing supervision).

○ Intralesional steroid injections may be used for small, stubborn plaques.

○ Anthralin, combined with a paste mixture, may be used for well-defined plaques but must not be applied to unaffected areas because it causes injury and stains normal skin; petroleum jelly is applied around the affected skin before applying anthralin.

○ Anthralin and steroids may be used with anthralin application at night and steroid use during the day.

○ Goeckerman regimen — which combines tar baths and UVB treatments — may help achieve the longest remission and clear the skin in 3 to 5 weeks in the patient with severe chronic psoriasis.

○ Ingram technique is a variation of the Goeckerman regimen, using anthralin instead of tar.

○ PUVA therapy combines administration of psoralens (accelerates exfoliation) with exposure to high-intensity UVA.

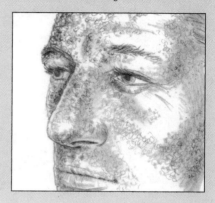

Psoriatic plaques

In this patient with psoriasis, plaques consisting of silver scales cover a large area of the face.

○ Cytotoxin, usually methotrexate, or cyclosporine, an immunosuppressant, may help severe, refractory psoriasis.

○ Etretinate, a retinoid compound, is effective in treating extensive cases of psoriasis; however, it's a strong teratogen and has numerous adverse effects that many patients find intolerable.

○ Low-dose antihistamines, oatmeal baths, emollients, and open wet dressings may help relieve pruritus.

○ Aspirin and local heat help alleviate the pain of psoriatic arthritis; severe cases may require nonsteroidal anti-inflammatory drugs.

○ Tar shampoo followed by application of a steroid lotion is used to treat psoriasis of the scalp; ketoconazole and anthralin may also be effective.

○ Tazarotene, a newer topical retinoid, combined with a medium-strength topical corticosteroid is also effective in treating mild to moderate plaques.

○ Alefacept, the first biological therapy for psoriasis, works by simultaneously blocking and reducing the cellular component (activated T cells) of the immune system that play a role in the psoriasis disease process.

Teaching about psoriasis

Remember these key points when teaching your patient and his family about psoriasis:

- Explain the disease process, including its course of alternating remissions and recurrences.
- Reinforce that there's no cure for psoriasis.
- Assure the patient that psoriasis isn't contagious.
- Discuss factors that can trigger flare-ups, such as stress, sunburn, and skin injury, and help the patient learn to cope with these situations.
- Explain the patient's prescribed therapy and provide written instructions to avoid confusion.
- Teach correct application of prescribed ointments, creams, and lotions.
- Discuss proper skin care, including cleaning, dressings, and measures to relieve itching.
- Reinforce the importance of avoiding sun exposure.
- Explain how to prevent flare-ups.
- Talk about ways to cope with the psychosocial effects of psoriasis.
- Discuss warning signs and symptoms of complications that require immediate medical attention.
- Caution the patient receiving psoralen plus ultraviolet light A therapy to stay out of the sun on the day of treatment, to protect his eyes with sunglasses that screen ultraviolet light A for 24 hours after treatment, and to wear goggles during exposure to this light.
- Explain the relationship between psoriasis and arthritis, but point out that psoriasis causes no other systemic disturbances.

COLLABORATIVE MANAGEMENT
Care of the patient with psoriasis involves several members of the interdisciplinary team. The primary care provider or dermatologist diagnoses and manages the disorder. The nurse educates the patient and family, administers treatments, and provides emotional support. The psoriasis day-care center can provide intensive treatment along with psychosocial support. The social worker helps with financial and occupational concerns. The therapist helps with self-esteem, coping, and psychosocial concerns. The physical therapist may provide whirlpool treatments to soften and remove scales over widespread areas of the body.

Special considerations

○ Apply topical medications, especially those containing anthralin and tar, with a downward motion to avoid rubbing them into the follicles.

○ Apply a steroid cream in a thin film and rub it gently into the skin until the cream disappears.

○ Wear gloves when applying anthralin because it stains and injures the skin. After application, suggest that the patient dust himself with powder to prevent anthralin from rubbing off on his clothes. Use mineral oil, then soap and water, to remove anthralin.

○ Caution the patient to avoid scrubbing his skin vigorously, to prevent Koebner's phenomenon.

○ Watch for adverse effects, especially allergic reactions to anthralin, atrophy and acne from steroids, and burning, itching, nausea, and squamous cell epitheliomas from PUVA.

○ Evaluate the patient on methotrexate weekly, then monthly for red blood cell, white blood cell, and platelet counts because cytotoxins may cause hepatic or bone marrow toxicity.

○ Provide care to the patient following liver biopsy to assess the effects of methotrexate.

○ Refer all patients to the National Psoriasis Foundation, which provides information and directs patients to local chapters.

○ Provide patient education. (See *Teaching about psoriasis.*)

Applicable patient-teaching aids

○ Learning about anthralin
○ Performing daily skin care for psoriasis
○ Preventing infection with proper hand washing *

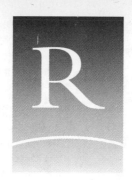

Renal failure, chronic

Chronic renal failure is usually the end result of a gradually progressive loss of renal function; occasionally, it's the result of a rapidly progressive disease of sudden onset. Few symptoms develop until after more than 75% of glomerular filtration is lost; then the remaining normal parenchyma deteriorates progressively, and symptoms worsen as renal function decreases.

If this condition continues unchecked, uremic toxins accumulate and produce potentially fatal physiologic changes in all major organ systems. If the patient can tolerate it, maintenance dialysis or kidney transplantation can sustain life.

Chronic renal failure and end-stage renal disease affect about 2 out of every 1,000 people in the United States.

Causes

Diabetes and hypertension are the primary causes of chronic renal failure, accounting for about 66% of cases. Other causes of chronic renal failure include:
○ chronic glomerular disease such as glomerulonephritis
○ chronic infections, such as chronic pyelonephritis or tuberculosis
○ congenital anomalies such as polycystic kidneys
○ vascular diseases such as renal nephrosclerosis
○ obstructive processes such as calculi
○ collagen diseases such as systemic lupus erythematosus

○ nephrotoxic agents such as long-term aminoglycoside therapy.

These conditions gradually destroy the nephrons and eventually cause irreversible renal failure. Similarly, acute renal failure that fails to respond to treatment becomes chronic renal failure.

Pathophysiology

Chronic renal failure often progresses through four stages:
○ reduced renal reserve (creatinine clearance glomerular filtration rate [GFR] is 40 to 70 ml/minute)
○ renal insufficiency (GFR 20 to 40 ml/minute)
○ renal failure (GFR 10 to 20 ml/minute)
○ end-stage renal disease (GFR less than 10 ml/minute).

Nephron damage is progressive; damaged nephrons can't function and don't recover. (See *Understanding chronic renal failure,* page 272.) The kidneys can maintain relatively normal function until about 75% of the nephrons are nonfunctional. Surviving nephrons hypertrophy and increase their rate of filtration, reabsorption, and secretion. Compensatory excretion continues as GFR diminishes.

Urine may contain abnormal amounts of protein, red blood cells (RBCs), and white blood cells or casts. The major end products of excretion remain essentially normal, and nephron loss becomes significant. As GFR decreases, plasma creatinine levels increase proportionately without regulatory adjustment. As sodium delivery to the nephron increases, less is reabsorbed, and sodium deficits and volume deple-

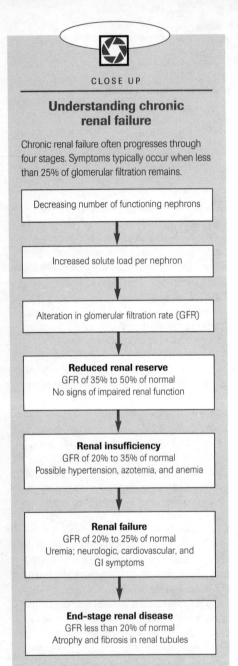

CLOSE UP

Understanding chronic renal failure

Chronic renal failure often progresses through four stages. Symptoms typically occur when less than 25% of glomerular filtration remains.

Decreasing number of functioning nephrons

⬇

Increased solute load per nephron

⬇

Alteration in glomerular filtration rate (GFR)

⬇

Reduced renal reserve
GFR of 35% to 50% of normal
No signs of impaired renal function

⬇

Renal insufficiency
GFR of 20% to 35% of normal
Possible hypertension, azotemia, and anemia

⬇

Renal failure
GFR of 20% to 25% of normal
Uremia; neurologic, cardiovascular, and GI symptoms

⬇

End-stage renal disease
GFR less than 20% of normal
Atrophy and fibrosis in renal tubules

nephron—precedes failure, as do such problems as renal tubular acidosis, salt-wasting, and difficulty diluting and concentrating urine. If vascular or glomerular damage is the primary cause, proteinuria, hematuria, and nephrotic syndrome are more prominent.

Changes in acid-base balance affect phosphorus and calcium balance. Renal phosphate excretion and $1,25(OH)_2$ vitamin D_3 synthesis are diminished. Hypocalcemia results in secondary hypoparathyroidism, diminished GFR, and progressive hyperphosphatemia, hypocalcemia, and dissolution of bone. In early renal insufficiency, acid excretion and phosphate reabsorption increase to maintain normal pH. When GFR decreases by 30% to 40%, progressive metabolic acidosis ensues and tubular secretion of potassium increases. Total-body potassium levels may increase to life-threatening levels requiring dialysis.

In glomerulosclerosis, distortion of filtration slits and erosion of the glomerular epithelial cells lead to increased fluid transport across the glomerular wall. Large proteins traverse the slits but become trapped in glomerular basement membranes, obstructing the glomerular capillaries. Epithelial and endothelial injuries cause proteinuria. Mesangial-cell proliferation, increased production of extracellular matrix, and intraglomerular coagulation cause the sclerosis.

Tubulointerstitial injury occurs from toxic or ischemic tubular damage, as with acute tubular necrosis. Debris and calcium deposits obstruct the tubules. The resulting defective tubular transport is associated with interstitial edema, leukocyte infiltration, and tubular necrosis. Vascular injury causes diffuse or focal ischemia of renal parenchyma, associated with thickening, fibrosis, or focal lesions of renal blood vessels. Decreased blood flow then leads to tubular atrophy, interstitial fibrosis, and functional disruption of glomerular filtration, medullary gradients, and concentration.

The structural changes trigger an inflammatory response. Fibrin deposits begin to form around the interstitium. Microaneurysms result from vascular wall damage and increased pressure secondary to obstruction or hypertension. Eventual loss of the nephron triggers compen-

tion follow. The kidney becomes incapable of concentrating and diluting urine.

If tubular interstitial disease is the cause of chronic renal failure, primary damage to the tubules—the medullary portion of the satory hyperfunction of uninjured nephrons, which initiates a positive-feedback loop of increasing vulnerability.

Eventually, the healthy glomeruli are so overburdened that they become sclerotic, stiff, and necrotic. Toxins accumulate and potentially fatal changes ensue in all major organ systems.

Assessment findings

Chronic renal failure produces major changes in all body systems. The presence and severity of manifestations depend on the duration of renal failure and its response to treatment. (See *Chronic renal failure: A multisystem disorder,* page 274.)

Diagnosis

○ Blood studies show elevated blood urea nitrogen, serum creatinine, and potassium levels; decreased arterial pH and bicarbonate; low hemoglobin (Hb) level and hematocrit (HCT); and decreased red blood cell (RBC) survival time, mild thrombocytopenia, and platelet defects.
○ Urine specific gravity becomes fixed at 1.010; urinalysis may show proteinuria, glycosuria, erythrocytes, leukocytes, and casts, depending on the etiology.
○ X-ray studies include kidney-ureter-bladder films, excretory urography, nephrotomography, renal scan, and renal arteriography and may reveal reduced kidney size.
○ Renal or abdominal computed tomography scan, magnetic resonance imaging, or ultrasound indicate changes associated with chronic renal failure, including abnormally small size in both kidneys.
○ Kidney biopsy allows histologic identification of the underlying pathology.

Complications

○ Anemia
○ Cardiopulmonary dysfunction
○ Electrolyte imbalances
○ GI disturbances
○ Infection
○ Lipid disorders
○ Peripheral neuropathy
○ Platelet dysfunction
○ Pulmonary edema

○ Sexual dysfunction
○ Skeletal defects

Treatment

○ Treatment aims to control associated diseases that cause or result from chronic renal failure, such as hypertension.
○ A low-protein diet reduces the production of end products of protein metabolism that the kidneys can't excrete.
○ A high-protein diet is recommended for patients receiving continuous peritoneal dialysis.
○ A high-calorie diet prevents ketoacidosis and the negative nitrogen balance that results in catabolism and tissue atrophy.
○ Sodium and potassium restrictions prevent elevated levels.
○ Fluid restrictions help maintain fluid balance.
○ Loop diuretics, such as furosemide, reduce fluid retention.
○ Cardiac glycosides may be used to mobilize edema fluids.
○ Antihypertensives control blood pressure and associated edema.
○ Antiemetics taken before meals may relieve nausea and vomiting; cimetidine or ranitidine may decrease gastric irritation.
○ Methylcellulose or docusate helps prevent constipation.
○ Iron and folate supplements treat anemia; severe anemia requires infusion of fresh frozen packed cells or washed packed cells.
○ Epoetin alpha increases RBC production.
○ Antipruritics, such as trimeprazine or diphenhydramine, relieve itching.
○ Aluminum hydroxide gel or calcium acetate lowers serum phosphate levels.
○ Supplementary vitamins (particularly B vitamins and vitamin D) and essential amino acids are also needed to meet nutritional requirements.
○ Hemodialysis or peritoneal dialysis (particularly continuous ambulatory peritoneal dialysis and continuous cyclic peritoneal dialysis) controls most manifestations of end-stage renal disease; altering dialyzing bath fluids can correct fluid and electrolyte disturbances. (See *Comparing peritoneal dialysis and hemodialysis,* page 275, and *Continuous ambulatory peritoneal dialysis,* page 276.)

Chronic renal failure: A multisystem disorder

The clinical manifestations caused by chronic renal failure affect many body systems:

- *Renal and urologic:* Initially, salt-wasting and consequent hyponatremia produce hypotension, dry mouth, loss of skin turgor, listlessness, fatigue, and nausea; later, somnolence and confusion develop. As the number of functioning nephrons decreases, so does the kidneys' capacity to excrete sodium, resulting in salt retention and overload. Accumulation of potassium causes muscle irritability, then muscle weakness as the potassium level continues to rise. Fluid overload and metabolic acidosis also occur. Urinary output decreases; urine is very dilute and contains casts and crystals.
- *Cardiovascular:* Renal failure leads to hypertension, arrhythmias (including life-threatening ventricular tachycardia or fibrillation), cardiomyopathy, uremic pericarditis, pericardial effusion with possible cardiac tamponade, heart failure, and periorbital and peripheral edema.
- *Respiratory:* Pulmonary changes include reduced pulmonary macrophage activity with increased susceptibility to infection, pulmonary edema, pleuritic pain, pleural friction rub and effusions, crackles, thick sputum, uremic pleuritis and uremic lung (or *uremic pneumonitis*), dyspnea due to heart failure, and Kussmaul's respirations as a result of acidosis.
- *GI:* Inflammation and ulceration of GI mucosa cause stomatitis, gum ulceration and bleeding and, possibly, parotitis, esophagitis, gastritis, duodenal ulcers, lesions on the small and large bowel, uremic colitis, pancreatitis, and proctitis. Other GI symptoms include a metallic taste in the mouth, uremic fetor (ammonia smell to breath), anorexia, nausea, and vomiting.
- *Cutaneous:* Typically, the skin is pallid, yellowish bronze, dry, and scaly. Other cutaneous symptoms include severe itching; purpura; ecchymoses; petechiae; uremic frost (most often in critically ill or terminal patients); thin, brittle fingernails with characteristic lines; and dry, brittle hair that may change color and fall out easily.
- *Neurologic:* Restless leg syndrome, one of the first signs of peripheral neuropathy, causes pain, burning, and itching in the legs and feet, which may be relieved by voluntarily shaking, moving, or rocking them. Eventually, this condition progresses to paresthesia and motor nerve dysfunction (usually bilateral footdrop) unless dialysis is initiated. Other signs and symptoms include muscle cramping and twitching, shortened memory and attention span, apathy, drowsiness, irritability, confusion, coma, and seizures. EEG changes indicate metabolic encephalopathy.
- *Endocrine:* Common endocrine abnormalities include stunted growth patterns in children (even with elevated growth hormone levels), infertility and decreased libido in both sexes, amenorrhea and cessation of menses in females, and impotence, decreased sperm production, and testicular atrophy in males. Increased aldosterone secretion (related to increased renin production) and impaired carbohydrate metabolism (increased blood glucose levels similar to diabetes mellitus) may also occur.
- *Hematopoietic:* Anemia, decreased red blood cell survival time, blood loss from dialysis and GI bleeding, mild thrombocytopenia, and platelet defects occur. Other problems include increased bleeding and clotting disorders, demonstrated by purpura, hemorrhage from body orifices, easy bruising, ecchymoses, and petechiae.
- *Skeletal:* Calcium-phosphorus imbalance and consequent parathyroid hormone imbalances cause muscle and bone pain, skeletal demineralization, pathologic fractures, and calcifications in the brain, eyes, gums, joints, myocardium, and blood vessels. Arterial calcification may produce coronary artery disease. In children, renal osteodystrophy (renal rickets) may develop.

○ Kidney transplantation may be the treatment of choice for some patients with end-stage renal disease.

COLLABORATIVE MANAGEMENT
Care of the patient with chronic renal failure requires an interdisciplinary approach to control symptoms, minimize com-

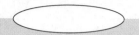

Comparing peritoneal dialysis and hemodialysis

Advantages, disadvantages, and complications of peritoneal dialysis and hemodialysis are described below.

Type	Advantages	Disadvantages	Possible complications
Peritoneal dialysis	• Can be performed immediately • Requires less complex equipment and less specialized personnel than hemodialysis does • Requires small amounts of heparin or none at all • No blood loss; minimal cardiovascular stress • Can be performed by patient anywhere (continuous ambulatory peritoneal dialysis), without assistance and with minimal patient teaching • Allows patient independence without long interruptions in daily activities because exchange may be done at night while he sleeps • Lower infection rate • Lower cost	• Contraindicated within 72 hours of abdominal surgery • Requires 48 to 72 hours for significant response to treatment • Severe protein loss necessitates high-protein diet (up to 100 g/day) • High risk of peritonitis; repeated bouts may cause scarring, preventing further treatments with peritoneal dialysis • Urea clearance less than with hemodialysis (60%)	• Abdominal hernias • Anorexia • Atelectasis and pneumonia • Bacterial or chemical peritonitis • Catheter displacement or obstruction • Catheter site inflammation, infection, or leakage • Constipation • Excessive fluid loss • Fluid overload • Hypertriglyceridemia • Hypotension • Pain (abdominal, low back, shoulder) • Severe loss of protein into the dialysis solution in the abdominal cavity (10 to 20 g/day) • Shortness of breath, or dyspnea
Hemodialysis	• Takes only 3 to 5 hours per treatment • Faster results in an acute situation • Total number of hours of maintenance treatment that's only half that of peritoneal dialysis • In an acute situation, can use an I.V. route without a surgical access route	• Requires surgical creation of a vascular access between circulation and dialysis machine • Requires complex water treatment, dialysis equipment, and highly trained personnel • Requires administration of larger amounts of heparin • Confines patient to special treatment unit	• Air emboli • Arrhythmias • Headache • Hemolytic anemia • Heparin overdose, possibly causing hemorrhage • Hypotension or hypertension • Increased risk of hepatitis • Itching • Leg cramps • Metastatic calcification • Nausea and vomiting • Pain (generalized or in chest) • Rapid fluid and electrolyte imbalance (disequilibrium syndrome) • Septicemia

plications, and slow the progression of the disease. The renal specialist or nephrologist evaluates, treats, and manages the patient's kidney function. Other specialists, such as the cardiologist or pulmonologist, may be consulted, depending on the patient's history and complications. The nurse educates the patient, promotes self-care, and implements measures to minimize symptoms and prevent complications. The dietitian recommends necessary food and fluid restrictions or supplementations. The physical therapist helps the patient maintain muscle strength and tone while the occupational therapist teaches energy conser-

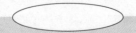

Continuous ambulatory peritoneal dialysis

Continuous ambulatory peritoneal dialysis is a useful alternative to hemodialysis in patients with renal failure. Using the peritoneum as a dialysis membrane, it allows almost uninterrupted exchange of dialysis solution. With this method, four to six exchanges of fresh dialysis solution are infused each day. The approximate dwell-time for daytime exchanges is 5 hours; for overnight exchanges, the dwell-time is 8 to 10 hours. After each dwell-time, the patient removes the dialyzing solution by gravity drainage. This form of dialysis offers the unique advantages of being a simple, easily taught procedure and provides patient independence from a special treatment center.

In this procedure, a Tenckhoff catheter, Gore-Tex catheter, or column-disk catheter is surgically implanted in the patient's abdomen, just below the umbilicus. A bag of dialysis solution is aseptically attached to the tube, and the fluid is allowed to flow into the peritoneal cavity (this takes about 10 minutes).

The fluid is then drained out of the peritoneal cavity through gravity flow by unrolling the bag and suspending it below the pelvis (drainage takes about 20 minutes). After the fluid drains, the patient aseptically connects a new bag of dialyzing solution and fills the peritoneal cavity again. He repeats this procedure four to six times per day.

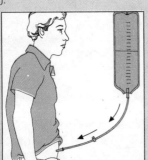

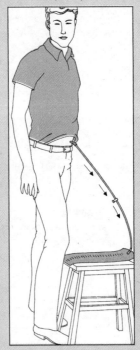

The dialyzing fluid remains in the peritoneal cavity for 4 to 6 hours. During this time, the bag may be rolled up and placed under a shirt or blouse, and the patient can go about normal activities while dialysis takes place.

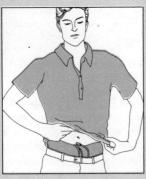

vation techniques. The social worker can help with financial and occupational concerns, obtaining equipment, coordinating home care, and dealing with end-of-life issues.

Special considerations

○ Bathe the patient using superfatted soaps, oatmeal baths, and skin lotion without alcohol to ease pruritus. Don't use glycerin-containing soaps because they'll cause skin drying. Give good perineal care, using mild soap and water.
○ Pad the side rails to guard against ecchymoses.
○ Turn the patient often, and use a convoluted foam mattress to prevent skin breakdown.
○ Provide good oral hygiene using a soft brush or sponge tip. Sugarless hard candy and mouthwash minimize bad taste in the mouth and alleviate thirst.
○ Offer small, palatable, nutritious meals; try to provide favorite foods within dietary restrictions. Encourage intake of high-calorie foods.
○ Watch for hyperkalemia. Monitor for cramping of the legs and abdomen, diarrhea, muscle irritability, and a weak pulse rate. Monitor the electrocardiogram for tall, peaked T waves, widening QRS segment, prolonged PR interval, and disappearance of P waves, indicating hyperkalemia.
○ Check for jugular vein distention and peripheral edema, and auscultate the lungs for crackles. Measure daily intake and output, including all drainage, emesis, diarrhea, and blood loss. Record daily weight.
○ Prevent pathologic fractures by turning the patient carefully and ensuring his safety.
○ Provide passive range-of-motion exercises for the bedridden patient.
○ Encourage deep breathing and coughing to prevent pulmonary congestion. Listen for crackles, rhonchi, and decreased breath sounds. Be alert for pulmonary edema, such as dyspnea, restlessness, and crackles. Administer diuretics and other medications, as ordered.
○ Maintain strict sterile technique. Watch for signs of infection (listlessness, high fever, and leukocytosis).
○ Carefully observe and document seizure activity. Infuse sodium bicarbonate for acidosis, and sedatives or anticonvulsants for seizures, as ordered. Keep an oral airway and suction setup at bedside.
○ Assess neurologic status, and check for Chvostek's and Trousseau's signs, indicators of low serum calcium levels.
○ Watch for prolonged bleeding at puncture sites and at the vascular access site used for hemodialysis. Monitor Hb levels and HCT, and check stool, urine, and vomitus for blood.
○ Report signs of pericarditis, such as a pericardial friction rub and chest pain.
○ Schedule medications carefully. Give iron before meals, aluminum hydroxide gels after meals, and antiemetics, as necessary, a half hour before meals. Administer antihypertensives at appropriate intervals.
○ If the patient requires a rectal infusion of sodium polystyrene sulfonate for dangerously high potassium levels, apply an emollient to soothe the perianal area. Be sure the sodium polystyrene sulfonate enema is expelled; otherwise, it will cause constipation and won't lower potassium levels.

If the patient requires dialysis:
○ Check the vascular access site for patency and the extremity for adequate blood supply and nerve function (temperature, pulse rate, capillary refill, and sensation). If a fistula is present, lightly feel for a thrill and listen for a bruit. Report signs of possible clotting.
○ Don't use the arm with the vascular access site to take blood pressure readings, draw blood, or give injections as these procedures may rupture the fistula or occlude blood flow.
○ Withhold antihypertensives on the morning of dialysis.
○ Use standard precautions when handling body fluids and needles.
○ Monitor Hb levels and HCT and assess the patient's tolerance of his levels.
○ After dialysis, check for disequilibrium syndrome, a result of sudden correction of blood chemistry abnormalities. Symptoms range from a headache to seizures. Also, check for excessive bleeding from the dialysis site. Apply pressure dressing or absorbable gelatin sponge, as indicated. Monitor blood pressure carefully after dialysis.

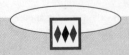

○ Refer the patient and his family to the National Kidney Foundation and appropriate counseling agencies for assistance in coping with chronic renal failure.

○ Provide patient education. (See *Teaching about chronic renal failure*.)

Applicable patient-teaching aids

○ Coping with depression
○ How to measure fluid intake and output *
○ Learning about hemodialysis
○ Learning about peritoneal dialysis
○ Performing a solution exchange
○ Preventing peritonitis *

○ Rheumatoid arthritis

A chronic, systemic, autoimmune, inflammatory disease, rheumatoid arthritis (RA) primarily attacks peripheral joints and surrounding muscles, tendons, ligaments, and blood vessels. Spontaneous remissions and unpredictable exacerbations mark the course of this potentially crippling disease. RA usually requires lifelong treatment and, sometimes, surgery. In most patients, the disease follows an intermittent course and allows normal activity, although 10% suffer total disability from severe articular deformity, associated extra-articular symptoms, or both. The prognosis worsens with the development of nodules, vasculitis, and high titers of rheumatoid factor (RF).

RA occurs worldwide, striking three times more females than males. Although it can occur at any age, it begins most often between ages 25 and 55. This disease affects more than 7 million people in the United States alone.

Causes

What causes the chronic inflammation characteristic of RA isn't known, but various theories point to infectious, genetic, and endocrine factors. Currently, it's believed that a genetically susceptible individual develops abnormal or altered immunoglobulin (Ig) G antibodies when exposed to an antigen. This altered IgG antibody isn't recognized as "self," and the individual forms an antibody against it—an antibody known as *RF*. By aggregating into complexes, RF generates inflammation. Eventually, cartilage damage by inflammation triggers additional immune responses, including activation of complement. This process, in turn, attracts polymorphonuclear leukocytes and stimulates release of inflammatory mediators, which enhance joint destruction.

Pathophysiology

Much more is known about the pathogenesis of RA than about its causes. If unarrested, the inflammatory process within the joints occurs in four stages. First, *synovitis* develops from congestion and edema of the synovial membrane and joint capsule. Infiltration by T-lymphocytes,

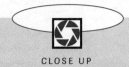

CLOSE UP

Understanding rheumatoid arthritis

A potentially crippling disease, rheumatoid arthritis primarily attacks peripheral joints and surrounding tissues through chronic inflammation. If not arrested, the inflammatory process occurs in four stages:

● Synovitis develops from congestion and edema of the synovial membrane and joint capsule. Infiltration by lymphocytes, macrophages, and neutrophils continues the local inflammatory response. These cells, as well as fibroblast-like synovial cells, produce enzymes that help degrade bone and cartilage.

● Pannus (thickened layers of granulation tissue) covers and invades cartilage, eventually destroying the joint capsule and bone.

● Fibrous ankylosis (fibrous invasion of the pannus and scar formation) occludes the joint space. Bone atrophy and misalignment cause visible deformities and disrupt the articulation of opposing bones, resulting in muscle atrophy and imbalance and, possibly, partial dislocations (subluxations).

● Fibrous tissue calcifies, resulting in bony ankylosis and total immobility.

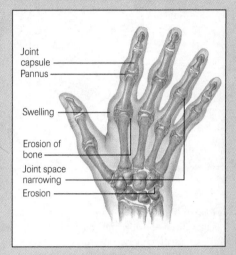

(particularly CD4+ cells and cytotoxic CD8 varieties), interleukin-1, and tumor necrosis factor continues the local inflammatory response. These cells and factors, as well as fibroblast-like synovial cells, produce enzymes that help to degrade bone and cartilage. (See *Understanding rheumatoid arthritis*.)

Formation of *pannus*—thickened layers of granulation tissue—marks the second stage's onset. Pannus covers and invades cartilage and eventually destroys the joint capsule and bone.

Progression to the third stage is characterized by *fibrous ankylosis*—fibrous invasion of the pannus and scar formation that occludes the joint space. Bone atrophy and misalignment cause visible deformities and disrupt the articulation of opposing bones, causing muscle atrophy and imbalance and, possibly, partial dislocations or *subluxations*.

In the fourth stage, *fibrous tissue calcifies*, resulting in bony ankylosis and total immobility.

Assessment findings

RA usually develops insidiously and initially produces nonspecific signs and symptoms, such as fatigue, malaise, anorexia, persistent low-grade fever, weight loss, lymphadenopathy, and vague articular symptoms. Later, more specific localized articular symptoms develop, commonly in the fingers at the proximal interphalangeal, metacarpophalangeal, and metatarsophalangeal joints; symptoms usually occur bilaterally and symmetrically and may extend to the wrists, knees, elbows, and ankles. The affected joints stiffen after inactivity, especially upon rising in the morning. The fingers may assume a spindle shape from marked edema and joint congestion.

The joints become tender and painful, at first only when the patient moves them, but eventually even at rest. They commonly feel hot to the touch. Ultimately, joint function is diminished.

Proximal interphalangeal joints may develop flexion deformities or become hyperextended.

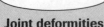

Joint deformities

In advanced rheumatoid arthritis, marked edema and congestion cause spindle-shaped interphalangeal joints and severe flexion deformities.

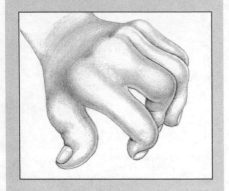

(See *Joint deformities.*) Metacarpophalangeal joints may swell dorsally, and volar subluxation and stretching of tendons may pull the fingers to the ulnar side ("ulnar drift"). The fingers may become fixed in a characteristic "swan's neck" appearance, or "boutonnière" deformity. The hands appear foreshortened, the wrists boggy; carpal tunnel syndrome from synovial pressure on the median nerve causes tingling paresthesia in the fingers.

The most common extra-articular finding is the gradual appearance of rheumatoid nodules—subcutaneous, round or oval, nontender masses—usually on pressure areas such as the elbows. Vasculitis can lead to skin lesions, leg ulcers, and multiple systemic complications.

Diagnosis

○ X-rays in the early stages show bone demineralization and soft-tissue swelling; later, loss of cartilage and narrowing of joint spaces; finally, cartilage and bone destruction and erosion, subluxations, and deformities.
○ Rheumatoid factor test is positive in 75% to 80% of patients as indicated by a titer of 1:160 or higher.
○ Synovial fluid analysis reveals increased volume and turbidity but decreased viscosity and

complement (C3 and C4) levels; and increased white blood cell count.
○ Erythrocyte sedimentation rate is elevated in 85% to 90% of patients (may be useful to monitor response to therapy because elevation commonly parallels disease activity).
○ Complete blood count usually reveals moderate anemia and slight leukocytosis.
○ C-reactive protein test can help monitor response to therapy.

Complications
○ Cardiopulmonary lesions
○ Carpal tunnel syndrome
○ Fibrous or bony ankylosis
○ Hip joint necrosis
○ Joint deformities
○ Lymphadenopathy
○ Myositis
○ Osteoporosis
○ Pericarditis
○ Peripheral neuropathy
○ Pleuritis
○ Recurrent infections
○ Scleritis and episcleritis
○ Sjögren's syndrome
○ Soft-tissue contractures
○ Spinal cord compression
○ Temporomandibular joint disease
○ Upper-motor-neuron signs and symptoms

Treatment
○ Salicylates, particularly aspirin, are the mainstay of RA therapy because they decrease inflammation and relieve joint pain. Other useful medications include nonsteroidal anti-inflammatory drugs (such as indomethacin, fenoprofen, and ibuprofen), antimalarials (hydroxychloroquine), gold salts, penicillamine, and corticosteroids (prednisone). Biologic response modifiers, such as infliximab, adalimumab, and etanercept, often work in patients in whom other therapies have failed. Immunosuppressants, such as cyclophosphamide, methotrexate, and azathioprine, are also therapeutic and are being used more commonly in early disease. (See *Drug therapy for arthritis.*)
○ Supportive measures include 8 to 10 hours of sleep every night, frequent rest periods be-

Drug therapy for arthritis

Drug and adverse effects	Clinical considerations
ASPIRIN	
Prolonged bleeding time; GI disturbances, including nausea, dyspepsia, anorexia, ulcers, and hemorrhage; hypersensitivity reactions ranging from urticaria to anaphylaxis; salicylism (mild toxicity: tinnitus, dizziness; moderate toxicity: restlessness, hyperpnea, delirium, marked lethargy; and severe toxicity: coma, seizures, severe hyperpnea)	• Don't use in patients with GI ulcers, bleeding, or hypersensitivity or in neonates. • Tell the patient to take the drug with food, milk, antacid, or large glass of water to reduce GI adverse effects. • Monitor the patient's salicylate level. Remember that toxicity can develop rapidly in febrile, dehydrated children. • Teach the patient to reduce the dose, one tablet at a time, if tinnitus occurs. • Teach the patient to watch for signs of bleeding, such as bruising, melena, and petechiae.
FENOPROFEN, IBUPROFEN, NAPROXEN, PIROXICAM, SULINDAC, AND TOLMETIN	
Prolonged bleeding time; central nervous system abnormalities (headache, drowsiness, restlessness, dizziness, and tremor); GI disturbances, including hemorrhage and peptic ulcer; increased blood urea nitrogen and liver enzyme levels	• Don't use in patients with renal disease, in patients with asthma who have nasal polyps, or in children. • Use cautiously in patients with GI and cardiac disease or if a patient is allergic to other nonsteroidal anti-inflammatory drugs (NSAIDs). • Tell the patient to take the drug with milk or meals to reduce GI adverse effects. • Tell the patient that the drug effect may be delayed for 2 to 3 weeks. • Monitor kidney, liver, and auditory functions in long-term therapy. Stop the drug if abnormalities develop. • Use cautiously in elderly patients; they may experience severe GI bleeding without warning.
GOLD (ORAL AND PARENTERAL)	
Dermatitis, pruritus, rash, stomatitis, nephrotoxicity, blood dyscrasias and, with oral form, GI distress and diarrhea	• Watch for and report adverse effects. Observe for nitritoid reaction (flushing, fainting, and sweating). • Check the patient's urine for blood and albumin before giving each dose. If positive, hold the drug and notify the physician. Stress to the patient the need for regular follow-up, including blood and urine testing. • To avoid local nerve irritation, mix the drug well and give it via a deep I.M. injection in the buttock. • Advise the patient not to expect improvement for 3 to 6 months. • Tell the patient to report rash, bruising, bleeding, hematuria, or oral ulcers.
HYDROXYCHLOROQUINE AND SULFASALAZINE	
Blood dyscrasias, GI irritation, corneal opacities, and keratopathy or retinopathy	• Don't use in patients with retinal or visual field changes. • Use cautiously in patients with hepatic disease, alcoholism, glucose-6-phosphate dehydrogenase deficiency, or psoriasis. • Perform complete blood count (CBC) and liver function tests before therapy and during chronic therapy. The patient should also have regular ophthalmologic examinations. • Tell the patient to take the drug with food or milk to minimize GI adverse effects. • Warn the patient that dizziness may occur.

(continued)

Drug therapy for arthritis *(continued)*

Drug and adverse effects	Clinical considerations
INFLIXIMAB, ADALIMUMAB, ETANERCEPT	
Headache, rhinitis, nausea, and upper respiratory tract infection	• Watch for infusion-related reactions, such as fever, chills, pruritus, uticaria, dyspnea, hypotension, hypertension, and chest pain. • Instruct the patient to report signs of infection. • Tell the patient that injection site reactions generally occur within the first month of therapy.
METHOTREXATE	
Tubular necrosis, bone marrow depression, leukopenia, thrombocytopenia, pulmonary interstitial infiltrates, hyperuricemia, stomatitis, rash, pruritus, dermatitis, alopecia, diarrhea, dizziness, cirrhosis, and hepatic fibrosis	• Don't give to women who are pregnant or breast-feeding or to patients who are alcoholic. • Monitor the patient's uric acid levels, CBC, and intake and output. • Warn the patient to promptly report any unusual bleeding (especially GI) or bruising. • Warn the patient to avoid alcohol, aspirin, and NSAIDs. • Advise the patient to follow the prescribed regimen.

Note: Other drugs that may be used in resistant cases include prednisone, chloroquine, azathioprine, and cyclophosphamide.

tween daily activities, and splinting to rest inflamed joints.

○ Physical therapy, including range-of-motion exercises and carefully individualized therapeutic exercises, forestalls joint function loss.

○ Heat application relaxes muscles and relieves pain.

○ Ice packs are effective during acute episodes.

○ Synovectomy, joint reconstruction, or total joint arthroplasty may be performed in advanced disease.

○ Surgical procedures in RA include metatarsal head and distal ulnar resectional arthroplasty, insertion of a Silastic prosthesis between the metacarpophalangeal and proximal interphalangeal joints, and arthrodesis (joint fusion).

○ Arthrodesis sacrifices joint mobility for stability and pain relief.

○ Synovectomy (removal of destructive, proliferating synovium, usually in the wrists, knees, and fingers) may halt or delay the course of this disease.

○ Osteotomy (the cutting of bone or excision of a wedge of bone) can realign joint surfaces and redistribute stresses.

○ Tendon transfers may prevent deformities or relieve contractures. Tendons may rupture spontaneously, requiring surgical repair. (See *When arthritis requires surgery.*)

 COLLABORATIVE MANAGEMENT
Care of the patient with RA involves several members of the interdisciplinary team. The rheumatologist manages the patient care. The nurse educates the patient and plans interventions to reduce pain and help the patient attain the highest degree of mobility possible. The physical therapist teaches the patient exercises to maintain joint mobility and body alignment and provides treatments such as heat and whirlpool. The occupational therapist helps the patient maintain independence with activities of daily of living through the use of assistive devices and grooming aids. The social worker addresses financial and occupational concerns.

Special considerations

○ Assess all joints carefully. Look for deformities, contractures, immobility, and inability to perform everyday activities.

When arthritis requires surgery

Arthritis severe enough to necessitate total knee or total hip arthroplasty calls for comprehensive preoperative teaching and postoperative care.

Before surgery

● Explain preoperative and surgical procedures. Show the patient the prosthesis to be used if available.

● Teach the patient postoperative exercises, such as isometrics, and supervise his practice. Also, teach deep-breathing and coughing exercises that will be necessary after surgery.

● Explain that total hip or knee arthroplasty requires frequent range-of-motion exercises of the leg after surgery; total knee arthroplasty requires frequent leg-lift exercises.

● Show the patient how to use a trapeze to move himself about in bed after surgery, and make sure he has a fracture bedpan handy.

● Tell the patient what kind of dressings to expect after surgery. After total knee arthroplasty, the patient's knee may be placed in a constant-passive-motion device to increase postoperative mobility and prevent emboli. After total hip arthroplasty, he'll have an abduction pillow between the legs to help keep the hip prosthesis in place.

After surgery

● Closely monitor and record vital signs. Watch for complications, such as steroid crisis and shock in patients receiving steroids. Monitor distal leg pulses often, marking them with a waterproof marker to make them easier to find.

● As soon as the patient awakens, have him do active dorsiflexion; if he can't, report this immediately. Supervise isometric exercises every 2 hours. After total hip arthroplasty, check traction for pressure areas and keep the bed's head raised between 30 and 45 degrees.

● Change or reinforce dressings, as needed, using sterile technique. Check wounds for hematoma, excessive drainage, color changes, or foul odor – all possible signs of hemorrhage or infection. (Wounds on patients with rheumatoid arthritis may heal slowly.) Avoid contaminating dressings while helping the patient use the urinal or bedpan.

● Administer blood replacement products, antibiotics, and pain medication, as ordered.

● Monitor serum electrolyte and hemoglobin levels and hematocrit.

● Have the patient turn, cough, and deep-breathe every 2 hours; then percuss his chest.

● After total knee arthroplasty, keep the patient's leg extended and slightly elevated.

● After total hip arthroplasty, keep the patient's hip in abduction to prevent dislocation by using such measures as a wedge pillow. Prevent external and internal rotation and avoid hip flexion greater than 90 degrees. Watch for and immediately report any inability to rotate the hip or bear weight on it, increased pain, or a leg that appears shorter than the other leg – all may indicate dislocation.

● As soon as allowed, help the patient get out of bed and sit in a chair, keeping his weight on the unaffected side. When he's ready to walk, consult with the physical therapist for walking instruction and aids.

○ Monitor the patient's vital signs, and note weight changes and sensory disturbances.

○ Assess the patient's pain level; administer analgesics, as ordered, and watch for adverse effects.

○ Provide meticulous skin care. Check for rheumatoid nodules as well as pressure ulcers and breakdowns due to immobility, vascular impairment, corticosteroid treatment, or improper splinting. Use lotion or cleansing oil, not soap, for dry skin.

○ Monitor the duration, not the intensity, of morning stiffness because duration more accurately reflects the disease's severity. Encourage the patient to take hot showers or baths at bedtime or in the morning to reduce the need for pain medication.

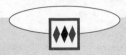

Teaching about rheumatoid arthritis

Remember these key points when teaching your patient about rheumatoid arthritis:
● Teach about the disease process, including its symptoms, complications, and treatments.
● Explain the prescribed medications, including their names, indications, dosages, adverse effects, and special considerations.
● Discuss warning signs and symptoms of complications that require immediate medical attention.
● Discuss the chronic nature of rheumatoid arthritis and the need for major changes in lifestyle.
– Stress the need for a balanced diet and weight control.
– Encourage the use of daily living aids, such as a long-handled shoehorn; elastic shoelaces; zipper-pulls; button hooks; easy-to-handle cups, plates, and silverware; elevated toilet seats; and battery-operated toothbrushes.
– Discuss sexual aids: alternative positions, pain medication, and moist heat to increase mobility.
– Encourage the patient to follow the recommended exercise routine when he's able to tolerate it.
– Recommend mobility aids that promote self-care, including an overhead grasping trapeze to get out of bed, easy-to-open drawers, handheld shower nozzles, handrails, and grab bars.
– Instruct the patient to pace daily activities and alternate sitting and standing tasks.
– Advise the patient to sleep on his back on a firm mattress and avoid placing a pillow under his knees, which encourages flexion deformity.
– Teach the use of good body mechanics.
● Discuss surgical options, when appropriate.

○ Apply splints carefully and correctly. Observe for pressure ulcers if the patient is in traction or wearing splints.
○ Activities of daily living that can be done in a sitting position should be encouraged. Allow the patient enough time to calmly perform these tasks.
○ Provide emotional support. Encourage the patient to discuss his fears concerning dependency, sexuality, body image, and self-esteem. Refer him to an appropriate social service agency as needed.
○ Refer the patient to the Arthritis Foundation for more information on coping with the disease.
○ Provide patient education. (See *Teaching about rheumatoid arthritis*.)

Applicable patient-teaching aids
○ Protecting your joints *
○ Recognizing warning signs of ulcer complications *
○ Restoring strength and relieving pain in arthritis *
○ Taking naproxen *
○ Using special kitchen helpers in arthritis

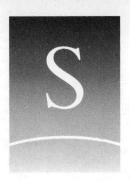

Sarcoidosis

Sarcoidosis is a multisystem, granulomatous disorder that characteristically produces lymphadenopathy, pulmonary infiltration, and skeletal, liver, eye, or skin lesions. Acute sarcoidosis usually resolves within 2 years. Chronic, progressive sarcoidosis, which is uncommon, is associated with pulmonary fibrosis and progressive pulmonary disability.

Sarcoidosis occurs most commonly in adults ages 30 to 50. In the United States, sarcoidosis affects twice as many women as men and occurs predominantly among blacks.

Causes

The cause of sarcoidosis is unknown, but several factors may play a role. It may occur as a hypersensitivity response (possibly from T-cell imbalance) to such agents as atypical mycobacteria, fungi, and pine pollen. Sarcoidosis may also occur in those individuals with a genetic predisposition (suggested by a slightly higher incidence of sarcoidosis within the same family). It's also thought that the disorder may also result from an extreme immune response to infection.

Pathophysiology

In sarcoidosis, organ dysfunction results from accumulation of T lymphocytes, mononuclear phagocytes, and nonsecreting epithelial granulomas, which distort normal tissue architecture in tissues and organs, such as the lungs, skin, eyes, mouth, salivary glands, liver, spleen, or lymph nodes. As these granulomas grow larger, they impair organ function.

Granulomas form and enlarge during the active stage of the disease, causing the development of scar tissue. In the nonactive stage of the disease, the granulomas remain stable, shrink, or become scars.

Assessment findings

Initial symptoms of sarcoidosis include arthralgia (in the wrists, ankles, and elbows), fatigue, malaise, and weight loss. Other clinical features vary according to the extent and location of the fibrosis:

○ Respiratory involvement may cause breathlessness, cough (usually nonproductive), and substernal pain. Complications in advanced pulmonary disease include pulmonary hypertension and cor pulmonale.

○ Cutaneous findings include erythema nodosum, subcutaneous skin nodules with maculopapular eruptions, and extensive nasal mucosal lesions.

○ Ophthalmic involvement may lead to anterior uveitis (common), glaucoma, and blindness (rare).

○ Lymphatic affects may produce bilateral hilar and right paratracheal lymphadenopathy and splenomegaly.

○ Musculoskeletal signs and symptoms may consist of muscle weakness, polyarthralgia, pain, and punched-out lesions on phalanges.

○ Hepatic effects include granulomatous hepatitis, which is usually asymptomatic.

○ Genitourinary findings may produce hypercalciuria.

○ Cardiovascular involvement leads to arrhythmias (premature beats, bundle-branch or complete heart block) and, rarely, cardiomyopathy.

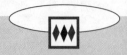

○ Central nervous system effects may produce cranial or peripheral nerve palsies, basilar meningitis, seizures, and pituitary and hypothalamic lesions producing diabetes insipidus.

Diagnosis

○ Skin lesion biopsy supports the diagnosis.
○ Chest X-ray may reveal bilateral hilar and right paratracheal adenopathy with or without diffuse interstitial infiltrates; occasionally large nodular lesions are present in lung parenchyma.
○ Lymph node or lung biopsy shows noncaseating granulomas with negative cultures for mycobacteria and fungi.
○ Pulmonary function tests show decreased total lung capacity and compliance, and decreased diffusing capacity.
○ Arterial blood gas (ABG) analysis shows a decreased arterial oxygen tension and increased carbon dioxide levels.

○ Negative tuberculin skin test, fungal serologies, and sputum cultures for mycobacteria and fungi, as well as negative biopsy cultures, help rule out infection.

Complications

○ Cor pulmonale
○ Pulmonary fibrosis
○ Pulmonary hypertension

Treatment

○ Corticosteroids are required by patients severely affected by the disorder and is usually continued for 1 to 2 years, but some patients may need lifelong therapy.
○ Immunosuppressive agents, such as methotrexate, azathioprine, and cyclophosphamide, may also be used.
○ Transplantation may be required if organ failure occurs.
○ Other measures include a low-calcium diet and avoidance of direct exposure to sunlight in patients with hypercalcemia.

COLLABORATIVE MANAGEMENT
Care of the patient with sarcoidosis involves several members of the interdisciplinary team. Depending on the organs affected by the disorder, specialists such as a cardiologist, neurologist, or pulmonologist may be involved in the patient's care. The nurse educates the patient and helps the patient cope with the disorder. The dietitian assesses the patient's nutritional status and makes dietary recommendations, such as a nutritious, high-calorie diet or a low-calcium diet for the patient with hypercalcemia. The respiratory therapist provides breathing treatments, monitors pulmonary function, and assists the patient with pulmonary exercises and hygiene. A low-vision specialist may be consulted if the patient has reduced vision.

Special considerations

○ Watch for and report any complications. Monitor laboratory results and report any abnormalities (anemia, for example).
○ For the patient with arthralgia, administer analgesics as ordered. Record signs of progressive muscle weakness.

○ Provide a nutritious, high-calorie diet and plenty of fluids. If the patient has hypercalcemia, suggest a low-calcium diet. Weigh the patient regularly to detect weight loss.

○ Monitor respiratory function. Note and record any bloody sputum or increase in sputum. If the patient has pulmonary hypertension or end-stage cor pulmonale, check ABG levels, observe for arrhythmias, and administer oxygen, as needed.

○ Because steroids may induce or worsen diabetes mellitus, perform fingerstick glucose tests at least every 12 hours at the beginning of steroid therapy. Also, watch for other steroid adverse effects, such as fluid retention, electrolyte imbalance (especially hypokalemia), moon face, hypertension, and personality change. During or after steroid withdrawal (particularly in association with infection or other types of stress), watch for and report vomiting, orthostatic hypotension, hypoglycemia, restlessness, anorexia, malaise, and fatigue. Remember that the patient on long-term or high-dose steroid therapy is vulnerable to infection.

○ Refer the patient with failing vision to community support and resource groups, and the American Foundation for the Blind, if necessary.

○ Provide patient education. (See *Teaching about sarcoidosis.*)

Applicable patient-teaching aids
○ Avoiding infection *
○ Learning about corticosteroids
○ Preventing infection with proper hand washing *

○ Schizophrenia

Schizophrenia is characterized by disturbances (for at least 6 months) in thought content and form, perception, affect, sense of self, volition, interpersonal relationships, and psychomotor behavior. The *Diagnostic and Statistical Manual of Mental Disorders*, Fourth Edition, Text Revision (*DSM-IV-TR*), recognizes paranoid, disorganized, catatonic, undifferentiated, and residual schizophrenia. Onset of symptoms usually occurs during adolescence or early adulthood. The disorder produces varying degrees of impairment. Up to one-third of patients with schizophrenia have just one psychotic episode and no more. Some patients have no disability between periods of exacerbation; others need continuous institutional care. The prognosis worsens with each episode.

Schizophrenia affects 1% to 2% of the population in the United States and is equally prevalent in both sexes.

Causes
Schizophrenia may result from a combination of genetic, biological, cultural, and psychological factors. Some evidence supports a genetic predisposition. Close relatives of people with schizophrenia have a greater likelihood of developing schizophrenia; the closer the degree of biological relatedness, the higher the risk.

The most widely accepted biochemical theory holds that schizophrenia results from excessive activity at dopaminergic synapses. Other neurotransmitters may also be involved.

Numerous psychological and sociocultural causes, such as disturbed family and interpersonal patterns, also have been proposed. Schizophrenia is more common in lower socioeconomic groups, possibly due to downward social drift, lack of upward socioeconomic mobility, and high stress levels that may stem from poverty, social failure, illness, and inadequate social resources. Higher incidence is also linked to low birth weight and congenital deafness.

Pathophysiology
Schizophrenia may result from too much activity at dopaminergic synapses. Other neurotransmitter alterations, such as serotonin increases, may also contribute to schizophrenic symptoms. In addition, patients with schizophrenia have structural abnormalities of the frontal and temporolimbic systems. Computed tomography scan and magnetic resonance imaging studies show a variety of structural brain abnormalities, including frontal lobe atrophy and increased lateral and third ventricles. Positron-emission tomography scans substantiate frontal lobe hypometabolism.

Assessment findings

Schizophrenia is associated with a variety of abnormal behaviors. Watch for these signs and symptoms:

○ ambivalence—coexisting strong positive and negative feelings, leading to emotional conflict

○ apathy and other affective abnormalities

○ clang associations—words that rhyme or sound alike used in an illogical, nonsensical manner—for instance, "It's the rain, train, pain"

○ concrete associations—inability to form or understand abstract thoughts

○ delusions—false ideas or beliefs accepted as real by the patient; delusions of grandeur, persecution, and reference (distorted belief regarding the relation between events and one's self—or example, a belief that television programs address the patient on a personal level); feelings of being controlled, somatic illness, and depersonalization

○ echolalia—automatic and meaningless repetition of another's words or phrases

○ echopraxia—involuntary repetition of movements observed in others

○ flight of ideas—rapid succession of incomplete and loosely connected ideas

○ hallucinations—false sensory perceptions with no basis in reality; usually visual or auditory, but may also be olfactory (smell), gustatory (taste), or tactile (touch)

○ illusions—false sensory perceptions with some basis in reality, for example, a car backfiring mistaken for a gunshot

○ loose associations—rapid shifts among unrelated ideas

○ magical thinking—belief that thoughts or wishes can control others or events

○ neologisms—bizarre words that have meaning only for the patient

○ poor interpersonal relationships

○ regression—return to an earlier developmental stage

○ thought blocking—sudden interruption in the patient's train of thought

○ withdrawal—disinterest in objects, people, or surroundings

○ word salad—illogical word groupings, such as "She had a star, barn, plant."

Diagnosis

○ A diagnosis of schizophrenia is made if the patient's symptoms match those in the *DSM-IV-TR*. (See *Diagnosing schizophrenia*.)

Complications

○ Impaired health
○ Impaired social functioning
○ Suicide

Treatment

○ Antipsychotic drugs (also called *neuroleptic drugs*) reduce the incidence of psychotic symptoms. Other psychiatric drugs, such as antidepressants and anxiolytics, may control associated signs and symptoms. (See *Reviewing adverse effects of antipsychotic drugs,* page 290.)

○ Psychotherapy may be an effective adjunct to drug therapy.

○ Psychosocial rehabilitation, education, and social skills training may be effective in treating chronic schizophrenia.

○ Family therapy may be helpful to reduce family guilt and disappointment as well as improve acceptance of the patient and his bizarre behavior.

 COLLABORATIVE MANAGEMENT
Care of the patient with schizophrenia requires a multidisciplinary approach to meet the physical and psychosocial needs of the patient. The psychiatrist diagnoses and manages schizophrenia. The nurse educates the patient and family, maintains a safe environment for the patient who is hospitalized, develops a therapeutic relationship with the patient, and monitors for adverse effects of drug therapy. Treatment may combine drug therapy, long-term psychotherapy for the patient and his family, psychosocial rehabilitation, vocational counseling, and the use of community resources.

Special considerations

○ Assess the patient's ability to carry out activities of daily living.

Diagnosing schizophrenia

The following criteria described in the *Diagnostic and Statistical Manual of Mental Disorders,* Fourth Edition, Text Revision, are used to diagnose a person with schizophrenia.

Characteristic symptoms

A person with schizophrenia has two or more of the following symptoms (each present for a significant time during a 1-month period — or less if successfully treated):
- delusions
- hallucinations
- disorganized speech
- grossly disorganized or catatonic behavior
- negative symptoms (affective flattening, alagia, anhedonia, attention impairment, apathy, and avolition).

The diagnosis requires only one of these characteristic symptoms if the person's delusions are bizarre, or if hallucinations consist of a voice issuing a running commentary on the person's behavior or thoughts, or two or more voices conversing.

Social and occupational dysfunction

For a significant period since the onset of the disturbance, one or more major areas of functioning (such as work, interpersonal relations, or self-care) are markedly below the level achieved before the onset.

When the disturbance begins in childhood or adolescence, the dysfunction takes the form of failure to achieve the expected level of interpersonal, academic, or occupational development.

Duration

Continuous signs of the disturbance persist for at least 6 months. The 6-month period must include at least 1 month of symptoms (or less if signs and symptoms have been successfully treated) that match the characteristic symptoms and may include periods of prodromal or residual symptoms.

During the prodromal or residual period, signs of the disturbance may be manifested by only negative symptoms or by two or more characteristic symptoms in a less severe form.

Schizoaffective and mood disorder exclusion

Schizoaffective disorder and mood disorder with psychotic features have been ruled out for these reasons: Either no major depressive, manic, or mixed episodes have occurred concurrently with the active-phase symptoms, *or,* if mood disorder episodes have occurred during active-phase symptoms, their total duration has been brief relative to the duration of the active and residual periods.

Substance and general medical condition exclusion

The disturbance isn't due to the direct physiologic effects of a substance or a general medical condition.

Relationship to a pervasive developmental disorder

If the person has a history of autistic disorder or another pervasive developmental disorder, the additional diagnosis of schizophrenia is appropriate only if prominent delusions or hallucinations are also present for at least 1 month (or less if successfully treated).

❍ Monitor the patient's nutritional status and monitor his weight. If he thinks that his food is poisoned, let him fix his own food when possible, or offer foods in closed containers that he can open. If you give liquid medication in a unit-dose container, allow the patient to open the container.
❍ Maintain a safe environment, minimizing stimuli.
❍ Administer prescribed medications to decrease symptoms and anxiety.

Reviewing adverse effects of antipsychotic drugs

The newer atypical agents such as olanzapine, quetiapine, risperidone, sertindole, and ziprasidone produce fewer extrapyramidal symptoms than the first, older class of antipsychotics. Risperidone is associated with increases in serum prolactin. Olanzapine, in moderate doses, induces little extrapyramidal symptoms, but has been associated with weight gain and blood glucose abnormalities. Quetiapine can cause weight gain, hypotension, and sedation.

Older classes of antipsychotic drugs (sometimes known as *neuroleptic drugs*) can cause sedative, anticholinergic, or extrapyramidal effects; orthostatic hypotension; and, rarely, neuroleptic malignant syndrome.

Sedative, anticholinergic, and extrapyramidal effects

High-potency drugs (such as haloperidol) are minimally sedative and anticholinergic but cause a high incidence of extrapyramidal adverse effects. Intermediate-potency agents (such as molindone) are associated with a moderate incidence of adverse effects, whereas low-potency drugs (such as chlorpromazine) are highly sedative and anticholinergic but produce few extrapyramidal adverse effects.

The most common extrapyramidal effects are dystonia, parkinsonism, and akathisia. Dystonia usually occurs in young male patients within the first few days of treatment. Characterized by severe tonic contractions of the muscles in the neck, mouth, and tongue, dystonia may be misdiagnosed as a psychotic symptom. Diphenhydramine or benztropine administered I.M. or I.V. provides rapid relief of this symptom.

Drug-induced parkinsonism results in bradykinesia, muscle rigidity, shuffling or propulsive gait, stooped posture, flat facial affect, tremors, and drooling. Parkinsonism may occur from 1 week to several months after the initiation of drug treatment. Drugs prescribed to reverse or prevent this syndrome include benztropine, trihexyphenidyl, and amantadine.

Tardive dyskinesia can occur after only 6 months of continuous therapy and is usually irreversible. No effective treatment is available for this disorder, which is characterized by various involuntary movements of the mouth and jaw; flapping or writhing; purposeless, rapid, and jerky movements of the arms and legs; and dystonic posture of the neck and trunk.

Signs and symptoms of akathisia include restlessness, pacing, and an inability to rest or sit still. Propranolol relieves this adverse effect.

Orthostatic hypotension

Low-potency neuroleptics can cause orthostatic hypotension because they block alpha-adrenergic receptors. If hypotension is severe, the patient is placed in the supine position and given I.V. fluids for hypovolemia. If further treatment is necessary, an alpha-adrenergic agonist, such as norepinephrine or metaraminol, may be ordered to relieve hypotension. Mixed alpha- and beta-adrenergic drugs (such as epinephrine) or beta-adrenergic drugs (such as isoproterenol) shouldn't be given because they can further reduce blood pressure.

Neuroleptic malignant syndrome

Neuroleptic malignant syndrome is a life-threatening syndrome that occurs in up to 1% of patients taking antipsychotic drugs. Signs and symptoms include fever, muscle rigidity, and altered level of consciousness occurring hours to months after initiating drug therapy or increasing the dose. Treatment is symptomatic, largely consisting of dantrolene and other measures to counter muscle rigidity associated with hyperthermia. You'll need to monitor the patient's vital signs and mental status continuously.

○ Adopt an accepting and consistent approach with the patient. Short, repeated contacts are best until trust has been established.

○ Avoid promoting dependence. Reward positive behavior to help the patient improve his level of functioning.

○ Engage the patient in reality-oriented activities that involve human contact, such as inpatient social skills training groups, outpatient day care, and sheltered workshops.

○ Provide reality-based explanations for distorted body images or hypochondriacal complaints. Explain to the patient that his private language, autistic inventions, or neologisms aren't understood. Set limits on inappropriate behavior.

○ If the patient is hallucinating, explore the content of the hallucinations. If he hears voices, find out if he believes that he must do what they command. Explore the emotions connected with the hallucinations, but don't argue about them. If possible, change the subject.

○ Assist the patient to recognize the nonreality of his hallucinatory experience.

○ Don't tease or joke with a schizophrenic patient. Choose words and phrases that are unambiguous and clearly understood.

○ If the patient expresses suicidal thoughts, institute suicide precautions. Document his behavior and your actions.

○ If he's expressing homicidal thoughts (for example, "I have to kill my mother"), institute homicidal precautions. Notify the physician and the potential victim. Document the patient's comments and the names of those you notified.

○ Don't touch the patient without telling him first what you're going to do.

○ Postpone procedures that require physical contact with hospital personnel until the patient is less suspicious or agitated.

○ Mobilize community resources to provide a support system for the patient. Ongoing support is essential to his mastery of social skills.

○ Monitor the patient for adverse reactions to drug therapy, including acute dystonia, drug-induced parkinsonism, akathisia, tardive dyskinesia, and malignant neuroleptic syndrome. Document and report such reactions promptly.

○ Help the patient explore possible connections between anxiety and stress and the exacerbation of symptoms.

For catatonic schizophrenia:

○ Assess for physical illness because the patient who's mute won't complain of pain or physical symptoms; if he's in a bizarre posture,
he's at risk for pressure ulcers or decreased circulation to a body area.

○ Meet the patient's physical needs for adequate food, fluid, exercise, and elimination.

○ Provide range-of-motion exercises for the patient or help him ambulate.

○ Prevent physical exhaustion and injury during periods of hyperactivity.

○ Tell the patient specifically which procedures need to be done. Don't offer the patient who is negativistic a choice.

○ Spend some time with the patient even if he's mute and unresponsive. The patient is acutely aware of his environment even though he seems not to be. Your presence can be reassuring and supportive.

○ Verbalize for the patient the message that his nonverbal behavior seems to convey; encourage him to do so as well.

○ Offer reality orientation. Emphasize reality in all contacts to reduce distorted perceptions.

○ Stay alert for violent outbursts; if they occur, get help promptly to ensure the patient's safety and your own.

For paranoid schizophrenia:

○ When the patient is newly admitted, minimize his contact with the hospital staff.

○ Don't crowd the patient physically or psychologically; he may strike out to protect himself.

○ Be flexible; allow the patient some control. Approach him in a calm and unhurried manner. Initially, keep the conversation light and social and avoid entering into power struggles.

○ Respond to the patient's condescending attitudes (arrogance, put-downs, sarcasm, or open hostility) with neutral remarks.

○ Don't let the patient put you on the defensive, and don't take his remarks personally. If he tells you to leave him alone, do leave but return soon. Brief contacts with the patient may be most useful at first.

○ Don't make attempts to combat the patient's delusions with logic. Instead, respond to feelings, themes, or underlying needs.

○ Be honest and dependable. Don't threaten the patient or make promises that you can't fulfill.

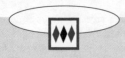

○ Provide patient education. (See *Teaching about schizophrenia.*)

Applicable patient-teaching aids
○ Taking your medication correctly

○ Scleroderma

Scleroderma, a systemic sclerosis that's also known as *progressive systemic sclerosis,* is a diffuse connective tissue disease characterized by fibrotic, degenerative, and occasionally inflammatory changes in skin, blood vessels, synovial membranes, skeletal muscles, and internal organs (especially the esophagus, intestinal tract, thyroid, heart, lungs, and kidneys). (See *Forms of scleroderma.*)

Scleroderma affects more women than men, especially between ages 30 and 50. Approximately 30% of patients with scleroderma die within 5 years of onset.

Causes
The cause of scleroderma is unknown. Known risk factors include exposure to silica dust and polyvinyl chloride. Anticancer agents, such as bleomycin, or nonopioid analgesics, such as pentazocine, may also result in scleroderma. Fibrosis may also occur due to an abnormal immune system response. There may be an underlying vascular cause with tissue changes initiated by inconsistent perfusion. Asymptomatic or common viral infections may also be involved.

Pathophysiology
Scleroderma usually begins in the fingers and extends proximally to the upper arms, shoulders, neck, and face. The skin atrophies, edema and infiltrates containing CD4+ T cells surround the blood vessels, and inflamed collagen fibers become degenerative and edematous, losing strength and elasticity. The dermis becomes tightly bound to the underlying structures, resulting in atrophy of the affected dermal appendages and destruction of the distal phalanges by osteoporosis. As the disease progresses, this atrophy can affect other areas. For example, in some patients, muscles and joints become fibrotic. (See *Scleroderma: How it happens,* page 294.)

Assessment findings
Scleroderma typically begins with Raynaud's phenomenon—blanching, cyanosis, and erythema of the fingers and toes in response to stress or exposure to cold. Progressive phalangeal resorption may shorten the fingers. Later symptoms include pain, stiffness, and finger and joint swelling. Skin thickening produces taut, shiny skin over the entire hand and forearm. Facial skin also becomes tight and in-

Forms of scleroderma

Scleroderma occurs in distinctive forms:

- *CREST syndrome* — a benign form of scleroderma characterized by calcinosis, Raynaud's phenomenon, esophageal dysfunction, sclerodactyly, and telangiectasia
- *diffuse systemic sclerosis* — characterized by generalized skin thickening and invasion of internal organ systems
- *localized scleroderma* — characterized by patchy skin changes with a droplike appearance known as *morphea*

- *linear scleroderma* — characterized by a band of thickened skin on the face or extremities that severely damages underlying tissues, causing atrophy and deformity (most common in childhood).

Other forms of scleroderma include *chemically induced localized scleroderma, eosinophilia myalgia syndrome* (recently associated with ingestion of L-tryptophan), *toxic oil syndrome* (associated with contaminated oil), and *graft-versus-host disease.*

---

elastic, causing a masklike appearance and "pinching" of the mouth.

GI dysfunction causes frequent reflux, heartburn, dysphagia, and bloating after meals; abdominal distention; diarrhea; constipation; and malodorous floating stools.

Diagnosis

○ Blood studies show slightly elevated erythrocyte sedimentation rate, positive rheumatoid factor in 25% to 35% of patients, and a positive antinuclear antibody test.

○ Chest X-rays reveal bilateral basilar pulmonary fibrosis.

○ Electrocardiogram shows possible nonspecific abnormalities related to myocardial fibrosis.

○ GI X-rays reveal distal esophageal hypomotility and stricture, duodenal loop dilation, small-bowel malabsorption pattern, and large diverticula.

○ Hand X-rays show terminal phalangeal tuft resorption, subcutaneous calcification, and joint space narrowing and erosion.

○ Pulmonary function studies show decreased diffusion and vital capacity and restrictive lung disease.

○ Skin biopsy may show changes consistent with the disease's progress, such as marked thickening of the dermis and occlusive vessel changes.

○ Urinalysis shows proteinuria, microscopic hematuria, and casts (with renal involvement).

Complications

○ Arrhythmias
○ Decreased food intake and weight loss
○ Dyspnea
○ Esophageal or intestinal obstruction or perforation
○ Malignant hypertension
○ Pulmonary fibrosis
○ Raynaud's phenomenon
○ Renal failure
○ Respiratory failure
○ Slowly healing ulcerations on fingertips or toes leading to gangrene.

Treatment

○ Immunosuppressants, such as chlorambucil, are a common palliative measure.

○ Corticosteroids and colchicine seem to stabilize symptoms; D-penicillamine may be helpful.

○ Digital plaster cast may be used for chronic digital ulcerations to immobilize the area, minimize trauma, and maintain cleanliness.

○ Surgical debridement may be needed for chronic digital ulcerations.

○ Antacids, cimetidine, periodic esophageal dilation, and a soft, bland diet are recommended for esophagitis with stricture.

Scleroderma: How it happens

Scleroderma is an uncommon connective tissue disorder marked by inflammatory, degenerative, and fibrotic changes of many body organs.

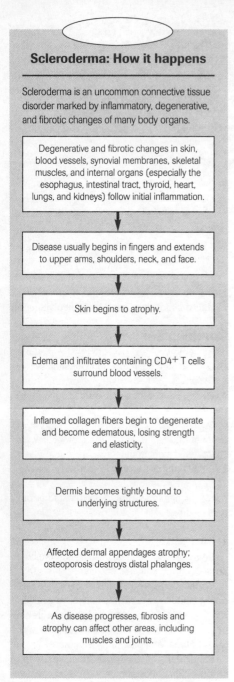

Degenerative and fibrotic changes in skin, blood vessels, synovial membranes, skeletal muscles, and internal organs (especially the esophagus, intestinal tract, thyroid, heart, lungs, and kidneys) follow initial inflammation.

↓

Disease usually begins in fingers and extends to upper arms, shoulders, neck, and face.

↓

Skin begins to atrophy.

↓

Edema and infiltrates containing CD4+ T cells surround blood vessels.

↓

Inflamed collagen fibers begin to degenerate and become edematous, losing strength and elasticity.

↓

Dermis becomes tightly bound to underlying structures.

↓

Affected dermal appendages atrophy; osteoporosis destroys distal phalanges.

↓

As disease progresses, fibrosis and atrophy can affect other areas, including muscles and joints.

○ Physical therapy maintains function and promotes muscle strength, and heat therapy relieves joint stiffness.

○ Vasodilators and antihypertensive agents (such as methyldopa or calcium channel blockers), intermittent cervical sympathetic blockade or, rarely, thoracic sympathectomy are used to treat Raynaud's phenomenon.

○ Dialysis, antihypertensives, and calcium channel blockers may be necessary to treat kidney complications (with malignant hypertension and impending renal failure).

○ Broad-spectrum antibiotics, such as erythromycin or tetracycline, counteract bacterial overgrowth in the duodenum and jejunum related to hypomotility.

 COLLABORATIVE MANAGEMENT
An interdisciplinary approach to care is needed to help the patient with scleroderma preserve normal body functions and minimize complications. The primary care provider diagnoses the disorder and devises the care plan. Referrals may be made to other specialists, such as a cardiologist, gastroenterologist, or dermatologist. The dietitian assesses the patient's nutritional status and makes dietary recommendations, such as vitamin supplements or soft foods that can be easily swallowed. The nurse educates the patient and plans interventions to reduce symptoms and minimize complications. The occupational therapist helps the patient protect fingers and hands and develop energy conservation techniques. The physical therapist teaches gentle range-of-motion exercises to maintain joint mobility and muscle tone and strength.

Special considerations

○ Assess the patient's motion restrictions, pain, vital signs, intake and output, respiratory function, and daily weight.
○ Because of compromised circulation, warn against fingerstick blood tests.
○ Remember that air conditioning may aggravate Raynaud's phenomenon.
○ Help the patient and her family adjust to the patient's new body image and to the limitations and dependence that these changes cause.
○ Encourage the patient and her family to express their feelings and help them cope with their fears and frustrations by offering informa-

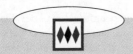

KEY TEACHING POINTS

Teaching about scleroderma

Remember these key points when teaching your patient and her family about scleroderma:

● Teach about the disease process, including its symptoms, complications, and treatments.

● Teach about prescribed medications, including their names, indications, dosages, adverse effects, and special considerations.

● Discuss warning signs of complications that require immediate medical attention, such as flexion contractures, abnormal bleeding or bruising, and any nonhealing abrasions.

● Teach the patient to avoid fatigue by pacing activities and organizing schedules to include necessary rest.

● Teach the patient to assess her skin for changes.

● Discuss the need to avoid cold weather and cigarette smoking.

● Talk about dietary changes to ease swallowing.

● Reinforce the need for follow-up care.

tion about the disease, its treatment, and relevant diagnostic tests.

○ Whenever possible, let the patient participate in treatment by measuring her own intake and output, planning her own diet, assisting in dialysis, giving herself heat therapy, and doing prescribed exercises.

○ Direct the patient to seek out support groups, which can be found in every state. Instruct the patient to call 1-800-722-HOPE or go to www.scleroderma.org (if possible) to determine the closest location.

○ Provide patient education. (See *Teaching about scleroderma*.)

Applicable patient-teaching aids

○ Coping with problems in systemic sclerosis
○ Limbering up your hands and feet
○ Living with Raynaud's syndrome
○ Performing facial exercises

Scoliosis

Scoliosis is a lateral curvature of the spine that may occur in the thoracic, lumbar, or thoracolumbar spinal segment. The curve may be convex to the right (more common in thoracic curves) or to the left (more common in lumbar curves). Rotation of the vertebral column around its axis occurs and may cause rib cage deformity. Scoliosis is commonly associated with kyphosis (roundback) and lordosis (swayback).

Causes

Scoliosis may be functional or structural. Functional (postural) scoliosis usually results from a discrepancy in leg lengths rather than from a fixed deformity of the spinal column; it corrects when the patient bends toward the convex side. Structural scoliosis results from a deformity of the vertebral bodies, and it doesn't correct when the patient bends to the side. Structural scoliosis may be:

○ *congenital:* usually related to a congenital defect, such as wedge vertebrae, fused ribs or vertebrae, or hemivertebrae; may result from trauma to zygote or embryo

○ *paralytic or musculoskeletal:* develops several months after asymmetrical paralysis of the trunk muscles due to polio, cerebral palsy, or muscular dystrophy

○ *idiopathic (the most common form):* may be transmitted as an autosomal dominant or multifactorial trait. This form appears during the growing years in a previously straight spine and is caused by equilibrium dysfunction, familial tendency, or asymmetric growth.

Idiopathic scoliosis can be classified as *infantile,* which affects mostly male infants between birth and age 3 and causes left thoracic and right lumbar curves; *juvenile,* which affects both sexes between ages 4 and 10 and causes varying types of curvature; or *adolescent,* which generally affects girls between age 10 and achievement of skeletal maturity and causes varying types of curvature.

Pathophysiology

In scoliosis, the vertebrae rotate, forming the convex part of the curve. As the spine curves

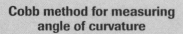

Cobb method for measuring angle of curvature

The Cobb method measures the angle of curvature in scoliosis. The top vertebra in the curve (T6 in the illustration) is the uppermost vertebra whose upper face tilts toward the curve's concave side. The bottom vertebra in the curve (T12) is the lowest vertebra whose lower face tilts toward the curve's concave side. The angle at which perpendicular lines drawn from the upper face of the top vertebra and the lower face of the bottom vertebra intersect is the angle of the curve.

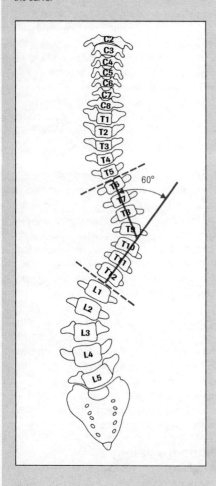

laterally, compensatory curves develop to maintain body balance and mark the deformity. The rotation causes rib prominence along the thoracic spine and waistline asymmetry in the lumbar spine. The severity of spinal deformity dictates physiological impairment. Differential stress on vertebral bone causes an imbalance of osteoblastic activity; thus the curve progresses rapidly during adolescent growth spurt. Without treatment, the imbalance continues into adulthood.

Assessment findings

The most common curve arises in the thoracic segment, with convexity to the right, and compensatory curves (S curves) in the cervical segment above and the lumbar segment below both with convexity to the left. (See *Cobb method for measuring angle of curvature.*)

Scoliosis rarely produces subjective symptoms until it's well established; when symptoms do occur, they include backache, fatigue, and dyspnea. The patient or parent may report that hemlines appear uneven, pant legs appear unequal in length, or one hip appears higher than the other. Physical examination reveals unequal shoulder heights, elbow levels, and heights of the iliac crests. Muscles on the convex side of the curve may be rounded; those on the concave side, flattened, producing asymmetry of paraspinal muscles.

Diagnosis

○ Anterior, posterior, and lateral spinal X-rays, taken with the patient standing upright and bending, confirm scoliosis and determine the degree of curvature (Cobb method) and flexibility of the spine.
○ A scoliometer can be used to measure the angle of trunk rotation.

Complications

○ Change in appearance
○ Debilitating back pain
○ Degenerative arthritis of the spine
○ Disk disease
○ Dyspnea
○ Kyphosis
○ Sciatica

Treatment

○ Spinal bracing can successfully halt progression of a curve in approximately 70% of cooperative patients. Exercises must be done daily, both in and out of the brace, to maintain muscle strength.

○ Spinal fusion and internal stabilization may be necessary for relentless curve progression (usually curves over 40°) or significant curve progression despite bracing.

○ Anterior spinal fusion corrects curvature with vertebral staples and an anterior stabilizing cable.

 COLLABORATIVE MANAGEMENT
Care of the patient with scoliosis involves several members of the health care team. The primary care provider or orthopedist refers the patient for a brace and monitors the degree of scoliosis. The surgeon is consulted if bracing doesn't halt the progression of curvature. The nurse educates and provides support to the patient and family. The physical therapist assists in assuring a proper fit for the brace and with exercise to strengthen muscles. A social worker or therapist can help the patient with body image and self-esteem issues. If the patient is being discharged with a rod and cast and must have bed rest, the visiting nurse provides home care.

Special considerations

○ Provide emotional support in addition to meticulous skin care.

If the patient needs traction or a cast before surgery:

○ Check the skin around the cast edge daily. Keep the cast clean and dry and the edges of the cast petaled.

○ Warn the patient not to insert or let anything get under the cast and to immediately report cracks in the cast, pain, burning, skin breakdown, numbness, or odor.

After corrective surgery:

○ Check sensation, movement, color, and blood supply in all extremities every 2 to 4 hours for the first 48 hours and then several times a day, for signs of neurovascular deficit, a

Cast syndrome

Cast syndrome is a serious complication that sometimes follows spinal surgery and application of a body cast. Characterized by nausea, abdominal pressure, and vague abdominal pain, cast syndrome probably results from hyperextension of the spine. This hyperextension accentuates lumbar lordosis, compressing the third portion of the duodenum between the superior mesenteric artery anteriorly and the aorta and vertebral column posteriorly. High intestinal obstruction produces nausea, vomiting, and ischemic infarction of the mesentery.

After removal of the cast, treatment includes gastric decompression and I.V. fluids, with nothing by mouth. Antiemetics should be given sparingly because they may mask symptoms of cast syndrome, which, if untreated, may be fatal.

Teach patients who are discharged in body jackets, localizer casts, or high hip spica casts how to recognize cast syndrome, which may manifest several weeks or months after application of the cast.

serious complication following spinal surgery. Logroll the patient often.

○ Measure intake, output, and urine specific gravity to monitor effects of blood loss, which is usually substantial.

○ Monitor abdominal distention and bowel sounds.

○ Encourage deep-breathing exercises to avoid pulmonary complications.

○ Medicate for pain, especially before activity.

○ Promote active range-of-motion arm exercises to help maintain muscle strength. Encourage the patient to perform quadriceps-setting, calf-pumping, and active range-of-motion exercises of the ankles and feet.

○ Watch for skin breakdown and signs of cast syndrome. (See *Cast syndrome*.)

○ Offer emotional support to help prevent depression that may result from altered body image and immobility.

○ If you work in a school, screen children routinely for scoliosis during physical examinations.

○ Provide patient teaching. (See *Teaching about scoliosis.*)

Applicable patient-teaching aids

○ Adjusting to your brace

○ Caring for your cast *

◯ Sickle cell anemia

A congenital hemolytic anemia that occurs primarily but not exclusively in blacks, sickle cell anemia results from a defective hemoglobin (Hb) molecule (HbS) that causes red blood cells (RBCs) to roughen and become sickle-shaped. Such cells impair circulation, resulting in chronic ill health (fatigue, dyspnea on exertion, swollen joints), periodic crises, long-term complications, and premature death.

Prompt antibiotic treatment can decrease morbidity and mortality from bacterial infections. Half of patients with sickle cell anemia die by their early 20s; few live to middle age.

Sickle cell anemia is most common in tropical Africans and in persons of African descent; about one in 10 American blacks carries the abnormal gene. However, sickle cell anemia also appears in other ethnic populations, including people of Mediterranean and East Indian ancestry.

Causes

Sickle cell anemia results from homozygous inheritance of the gene that produces HbS (chromosome 11). It's inherited as an autosomal recessive trait. Heterozygous inheritance of this gene results in sickle cell trait, generally an asymptomatic condition.

If two parents who are both carriers of sickle cell trait (or another hemoglobinopathy) have offspring, each child has a 25% chance of developing sickle cell anemia. (See *Inheritance patterns in sickle cell anemia.*) Overall, 1 in every 400 to 600 black children has sickle cell anemia. The defective HbS-producing gene may have persisted because, in areas where malaria is endemic, the heterozygous sickle cell trait provides resistance to malaria and is actually beneficial.

Pathophysiology

Sickle cell anemia results from substitution of the amino acid valine for glutamic acid in the HbS gene encoding the beta chain of Hb. Abnormal hemoglobin S, found in the RBCs of patients, becomes insoluble during hypoxia. As a result, these cells become rigid, rough, and elongated, forming a crescent or sickle shape. The sickling produces hemolysis. The altered cells also pile up in the capillaries and smaller blood vessels, making the blood more viscous. Normal circulation is impaired, causing pain, tissue infarctions, and swelling. Symptoms usually don't develop until after age 6 months because large amounts of fetal Hb protect infants for the first few months after birth.

Each patient with sickle cell anemia has a different hypoxic threshold and different factors that trigger a sickle cell crisis. Illness, exposure to cold, stress, acidotic states, or a pathophysiologic process that pulls water out of the sickle cells precipitates a crisis in most patients. The blockages then cause anoxic changes that lead to further sickling and obstruction. (See *Understanding sickle cell crisis,* page 300.)

Assessment findings

Characteristically, sickle cell anemia produces tachycardia, cardiomegaly, systolic and diastolic murmurs, pulmonary infarctions (which may result in cor pulmonale), chronic fatigue, unexplained dyspnea or dyspnea on exertion, hepatomegaly, jaundice, pallor, joint swelling, aching bones, chest pains, ischemic leg ulcers (especially around the ankles), and increased susceptibility to infection.

During early childhood, palpation may reveal splenomegaly, but, as the child grows older, the spleen shrinks.

Crises in a patient with sickle cell anemia may produce pale lips, tongue, palms, or nail beds; lethargy; listlessness; sleepiness with difficulty awakening; irritability; severe pain; a fever over 104° F (40° C); or a fever of 100° F (37.8° C) that persists for 2 days. (See *Managing sickle cell crisis*, page 301.)

Diagnosis

○ Positive family history and typical clinical features suggest sickle cell anemia. Hb electrophoresis showing HbS or other hemoglobinopathies can also confirm the diagnosis. Electrophoresis should be done on umbilical

Inheritance patterns in sickle cell anemia

When both parents are carriers of sickle cell trait, each child has a 25% chance of developing sickle cell anemia, a 25% chance of being a normal noncarrier, and a 50% chance of being a carrier of sickle cell trait.

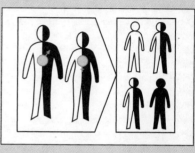

When one parent has sickle cell anemia and one is healthy, all offspring will be carriers of sickle cell trait.

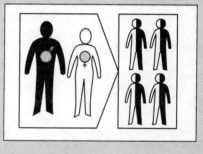

KEY
☐ Healthy, noncarrier
◧ Healthy, carrier of sickle cell trait
■ Sickle cell anemia (affected with sickle cell disease)

cord blood samples at birth to provide sickle cell disease screening for all neonates at risk.
○ Laboratory studies may show a low RBC count, elevated white blood cell and platelet counts, decreased erythrocyte sedimentation rate, increased serum iron, decreased RBC survival, reticulocytosis, and a low or normal Hb.

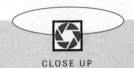

CLOSE UP

Understanding sickle cell crisis

Infection, exposure to cold, high altitudes, overexertion, or other situations that cause cellular oxygen deprivation may trigger a sickle cell crisis. The deoxygenated, sickle-shaped red blood cells (RBCs) stick to the capillary wall and each other, blocking blood flow and causing cellular hypoxia. The crisis worsens as tissue hypoxia and acidic waste products cause more sickling and cell damage. With each new crisis, organs and tissues are slowly destroyed, especially the spleen and kidneys.

A *painful crisis* (*vaso-occlusive crisis, infarctive crisis*), the most common crisis and the hallmark of the disease, usually appears periodically after age 5. It results from blood vessel obstruction by rigid, tangled sickle cells, which causes tissue anoxia and possible necrosis. This type of crisis is characterized by severe abdominal, thoracic, muscular, or bone pain and, possibly, dark urine, low-grade fever, and worsening jaundice.

Autosplenectomy, in which splenic damage and scarring is so extensive that the spleen shrinks and becomes impalpable, occurs in patients with long-term disease. This can lead to increased susceptibility to *Streptococcus pneumoniae* sepsis, which can be fatal without prompt treatment. Infection may develop after the crisis subsides (in 4 days to several weeks), so watch for lethargy, sleepiness, fever, or apathy.

An *aplastic crisis* (*megaloblastic crisis*) results from bone marrow depression and is associated with infection, usually viral. It's characterized by pallor, lethargy, sleepiness, dyspnea, possible coma, markedly decreased bone marrow activity, and RBC hemolysis.

In infants between age 8 months and 2 years, an *acute sequestration crisis* may cause sudden massive entrapment of RBCs in the spleen and liver. This rare crisis causes lethargy and pallor and, if untreated, commonly progresses to hypovolemic shock and death.

A *hemolytic crisis* is quite rare and usually occurs in patients who also have glucose-6-phosphate dehydrogenase deficiency. It probably results from complications of sickle cell anemia, such as infection, rather than from the disorder itself. Hemolytic crisis causes liver congestion and hepatomegaly as a result of degenerative changes. It worsens chronic jaundice, although increased jaundice doesn't always point to a hemolytic crisis.

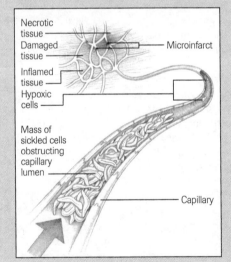

Complications
○ Chronic obstructive pulmonary disease
○ Delayed puberty and small for age
○ Heart failure
○ Infection and gangrene
○ Nephropathy
○ Retinopathy
○ Stroke

Treatment
○ Prophylactic penicillin treatment begins before age 4 months.

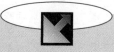

ACUTE EPISODE

Managing sickle cell crisis

If your patient experiences a sickle cell crisis, follow these guidelines:

● Administer blood components, as ordered, to correct hypovolemia and improve oxygenation.

● Provide supplemental oxygen to reduce hypoxia and sickling of red blood cells.

● Encourage oral fluid intake and administer prescribed I.V. fluids to ensure fluid balance and renal perfusion and to prevent vessel occlusion.

● Apply warm compresses to painful areas, and cover the patient with a blanket. (Never use cold compresses because they aggravate the condition.)

● Administer an analgesic, such as meperidine or morphine sulfate, if the patient is in pain.

● Maintain bed rest to reduce workload on the heart and to reduce pain.

● Give antibiotics, as ordered, to treat infection according to culture and sensitivity reports.

○ Transfusion of packed RBCs is given if the patient's Hb drops suddenly or if his condition deteriorates rapidly.

○ Folic acid supplementation is recommended to prevent megaloblastic crisis.

○ Hydroxyurea, which causes an increase in the synthesis of fetal Hb and a significant reduction in crises, is being used for some patients to reduce the frequency of painful crises and episodes of acute chest syndrome. It also decreases the need for blood transfusions.

○ Bone marrow transplantation offers the only cure for sickle cell anemia.

○ Gene therapy (replacing HbS with normal HbA) may be the ideal treatment, but it's very difficult to perform.

 COLLABORATIVE MANAGEMENT

Care of the patient with sickle cell anemia involves several members of the interdisciplinary team. A hematologist who specializes in the care of patients with

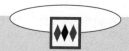

KEY TEACHING POINTS

Teaching about sickle cell anemia

Remember these key points when teaching your patient and his family about sickle cell anemia:

● Teach about the disease process, including its signs and symptoms, treatments, and patterns of inheritance.

● Explain the importance of adequate rest.

● Teach about prescribed medications, including their names, indications, dosages, adverse effects, and special considerations.

● Advise the patient to avoid tight clothing that restricts circulation.

● Warn against strenuous exercise, vasoconstricting medications, cold temperatures (including drinking large amounts of ice water and swimming), unpressurized aircraft, high altitude, and other conditions that provoke hypoxia.

● Stress the importance of normal childhood immunizations, meticulous wound care, good oral hygiene, regular dental checkups, and a balanced diet as safeguards against infection.

● Emphasize the need for prompt treatment of infection.

● Discuss the need to increase fluid intake to prevent dehydration.

● Teach about complications, including their signs and symptoms, and the need to seek prompt medical attention.

● Stress the importance of wearing medical identification and of informing all health care providers about the disorder.

● Warn women that they may have increased obstetrical risks and to seek qualified obstetric or gynecologic health care.

● To encourage normal mental and social development, warn parents against being overprotective.

● Discuss genetic counseling with the patient and his family.

sickle cell anemia typically diagnoses and treats the disorder. Because complications affect a wide range of body systems, other specialists may include a cardiologist, pulmonologist, ophthalmologist, or gastroenterologist. The nurse educates the patient and family, monitors for complications, and cares for the patient during crises. The genetic counselor educates the patient and family about the risk of transmitting the disorder to offspring and offers testing to identify carriers. The dietitian helps the patient and family prepare well-balanced meals that are high in folic acid. The social worker addresses financial and psychosocial concerns and may provide vocational counseling. The psychologist counsels parents of children with sickle cell anemia to help them cope with feelings of guilt.

Special considerations
○ Encourage the patient to talk about his fears and concerns.
○ Provide a diet with foods rich in folic acid.
○ Encourage adequate fluid intake.
○ Apply warm compresses, warmed thermal blankets, and warming pads to painful areas, unless the patient has neuropathy.
○ Administer analgesics and antipyretics, as necessary.
○ Give prescribed prophylactic antibiotics.
○ Administer oxygen and blood transfusion, as needed.
○ If the patient requires general anesthesia for surgery, make sure the surgeon and the anesthesiologist know that the patient has sickle cell anemia. Provide a preoperative transfusion of packed RBCs, as needed.
○ Provide patient education. (See *Teaching about sickle cell anemia,* page 301.)

Applicable patient-teaching aids
○ Learning about blood transfusions
○ Managing vaso-occlusive crisis *

◯ Sjögren's syndrome

The second most common autoimmune rheumatic disorder after rheumatoid arthritis

(RA), Sjögren's syndrome is characterized by diminished lacrimal and salivary gland secretion (sicca complex). Sjögren's syndrome may be a primary disorder or it may be associated with connective tissue disorders, such as RA, scleroderma, systemic lupus erythematosus, and polymyositis. In some patients, the disorder is limited to the exocrine glands (glandular Sjögren's syndrome); in others, it also involves other organs, such as the lungs and kidneys (extraglandular Sjögren's syndrome).

Sjögren's syndrome occurs mainly in females (90% of patients); the mean age of onset is between ages 40 and 50.

Causes
The cause of Sjögren's syndrome is unknown, but genetic and environmental factors probably contribute to its development. Viral or bacterial infection or perhaps exposure to pollen may trigger Sjögren's syndrome in a genetically susceptible individual.

Pathophysiology
Sjögren's syndrome is an autoimmune rheumatic disorder characterized by lymphocytic infiltration of exocrine glands, causing tissue damage resulting in xerostomia and dry eyes. Lymphocytic infiltration may be classified as benign, malignant, or pseudolymphoma (nonmalignant, but tumorlike aggregates of lymphoid cells).

Assessment findings
The patient may report rapidly progressive and severe oral and ocular dryness, in many cases accompanied by periodic parotid gland enlargement. Ocular dryness (xerophthalmia) leads to foreign body sensation (gritty, sandy eye), redness, burning, photosensitivity, eye fatigue, itching, mucoid discharge, and the sensation of a film across the field of vision. Oral dryness (xerostomia) leads to difficulty swallowing and talking; abnormal taste or smell sensation or both; thirst; ulcers of the tongue, buccal mucosa, and lips (especially at the corners of the mouth); and severe dental caries. Dryness of the respiratory tract leads to epistaxis, hoarse-

ness, chronic nonproductive cough, recurrent otitis media, and increased incidence of respiratory infections. Other effects may include dyspareunia and pruritus (associated with vaginal dryness), generalized itching, fatigue, recurrent low-grade fever, and arthralgia or myalgia.

Lymph node enlargement may be the first sign of malignant lymphoma or pseudolymphoma. Specific extraglandular findings include interstitial pneumonitis; interstitial nephritis, which results in renal tubular acidosis in 25% of patients; Raynaud's phenomenon (20%); and vasculitis, usually limited to the skin and characterized by palpable purpura on the legs (20%). About 50% of patients show evidence of hypothyroidism related to autoimmune thyroid disease. A few patients develop systemic necrotizing vasculitis.

Diagnosis

○ Detection of two of the following three conditions is diagnostic of Sjögren's syndrome: xerophthalmia, xerostomia (with salivary gland biopsy showing lymphocytic infiltration), and an associated autoimmune or lymphoproliferative disorder.
○ Tests must be performed to rule out other causes of oral and ocular dryness, including sarcoidosis, endocrine disorders, anxiety or depression, cancer, and effects of therapy such as radiation to the head and neck. Review of the patient's medical history may reveal the use of drugs that produce dry mouth as an adverse effect.
○ Laboratory test results include elevated erythrocyte sedimentation rate in most patients, mild anemia and leukopenia in 30% of patients, and hypergammaglobulinemia in 50% of patients.
○ Autoantibodies are common, including anti-Sjögren's syndrome-A (anti-Ro) and anti-Sjögren's syndrome-B (anti-La), which are antinuclear and antisalivary duct antibodies.
○ Rheumatoid factor is positive in 75% to 90% of patients; 90% of patients also test positive for antinuclear antibodies.

○ Schirmer's tearing test and slit-lamp examination with rose bengal dye measure eye involvement.
○ Salivary gland involvement is evaluated by measuring the volume of parotid saliva and by secretory sialography and salivary scintigraphy.
○ Lower-lip biopsy shows salivary gland infiltration by lymphocytes.

Complications

○ Corneal ulceration or perforation
○ Deafness
○ Epistaxis
○ Otitis media
○ Renal tubular necrosis
○ Splenomegaly

Treatment

○ Moistening the mouth using a methylcellulose swab or spray and by drinking plenty of fluids, especially at mealtime, can relieve mouth dryness.
○ Meticulous oral hygiene is essential, including regular flossing, brushing, at-home fluoride treatment, and frequent dental checkups.
○ Artificial tear instillation as often as every half hour may prevent eye damage (corneal ulcerations and corneal opacifications) from insufficient tear secretions.
○ Eye ointment administration at bedtime or twice-per-day or use of sustained-release cellulose capsules (Lacrisert) may also relieve symptoms.
○ Antibiotics are given to treat infection.
○ Local heat and analgesics treat parotid gland enlargement.
○ Corticosteroids may be administered for pulmonary and renal interstitial disease.
○ Chemotherapy, surgery, or radiation treat accompanying lymphoma.

 COLLABORATIVE MANAGEMENT Care of the patient with Sjögren's syndrome involves several members of the interdisciplinary team. The rheumatologist commonly diagnoses and manages the disorder. The dentist, dermatologist, and ophthalmologist may also consult. The nurse educates the patient about the disorder and plans

KEY TEACHING POINTS

Teaching about Sjögren's syndrome

Remember these key points when teaching your patient about Sjögren's syndrome:
- Teach about the disease process, including its signs and symptoms, complications, and treatments.
- Teach about prescribed medications, including their names, indications, dosages, adverse effects, and special considerations.
- Demonstrate how to instill eyedrops and ointments properly.
- Discuss warning signs of complications that require immediate medical attention.
- Stress the need to humidify home and work environments to help relieve respiratory dryness.
- Advise the patient to avoid drugs that decrease saliva production, such as atropine derivatives, antihistamines, anticholinergics, and antidepressants.

- If mouth lesions make eating painful, suggest high-protein, high-calorie liquid supplements to prevent malnutrition.
- Tell the patient to avoid sugar, which contributes to dental caries, as well as tobacco; alcohol; and spicy, salty, or highly acidic foods, which cause mouth irritation.
- Suggest normal saline solution drops or aerosolized spray for nasal dryness.
- Advise the patient to avoid prolonged hot showers and baths and to use moisturizing lotions to help ease dry skin.
- Suggest K-Y lubricating jelly as a vaginal lubricant.
- Recommend the use of sunglasses to protect the patient's eyes from dust, wind, and strong light; moisture chamber spectacles may also be helpful.

---

interventions to increase comfort and prevent complications. The dietitian can help with meal planning if mouth dryness and lesions make eating difficult.

Special considerations
○ Instill artificial tears as often as every 30 minutes to prevent eye damage, and instill an eye ointment at bedtime.
○ Provide plenty of fluids, especially water, for the patient to drink, as well as sugarless chewing gum or candy.
○ Refer the patient to the Sjögren's Syndrome Foundation for additional information and support.
○ Provide patient education. (See *Teaching about Sjögren's syndrome.*)

Applicable patient-teaching aids
○ Administering eyedrops
○ Examining your lymph nodes
○ Living with Raynaud's syndrome

⬭ Squamous cell carcinoma

Squamous cell cancer of the skin is an invasive tumor with metastatic potential that arises from the keratinizing epidermal cells. Any change in an existing skin lesion, such as a wart or mole, or the development of a new lesion that ulcerates and doesn't heal may indicate skin cancer. If caught and detected early, there's a high cure rate. However, if squamous cell cancer is allowed to spread, it can result in diabetes or death. (See *How squamous cell cancer develops.*)

Squamous cell cancer usually occurs in fair-skinned white males older than age 60. Outdoor employment and residence in a sunny, warm climate (southwestern United States and Australia, for example) greatly increase the risk of developing squamous cell cancer.

Causes

Predisposing factors associated with squamous cell cancer include overexposure to the sun's ultraviolet rays, the presence of premalignant lesions (such as actinic keratosis or Bowen's disease), X-ray therapy, ingestion of herbicides containing arsenic, chronic skin irritation and inflammation, exposure to local carcinogens (such as tar and oil), and hereditary diseases (such as xeroderma pigmentosum and albinism). (See *Premalignant skin lesions,* page 306.) Rarely, squamous cell cancer may develop on the site of smallpox vaccination, psoriasis, or chronic discoid lupus erythematosus.

Pathophysiology

Transformation from a premalignant lesion to squamous cell cancer may begin with induration and inflammation of a preexisting lesion. When squamous cell cancer arises from normal skin, the nodule grows slowly on a firm, indurated base. If untreated, the cancerous nodule eventually ulcerates and invades underlying tissues. Metastasis can occur to the regional lymph nodes. Lesions on sun-damaged skin tend to be less invasive and less likely to metastasize than lesions on unexposed skin. Notable exceptions to this tendency are squamous cell lesions on the lower lip and the ears. These are almost invariably markedly invasive metastatic lesions with a generally poor prognosis.

Assessment findings

Squamous cell cancer commonly develops on the skin of the face, the ears, the dorsa of the hands and forearms, and other sun-damaged areas. (See *Squamous cell cancer nodule,* page 307.) Metastasis produces characteristic systemic symptoms of pain, malaise, fatigue, weakness, and anorexia.

Diagnosis

○ Excisional biopsy provides definitive diagnosis of squamous cell cancer.
○ Other appropriate laboratory tests depend on systemic symptoms.

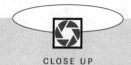

CLOSE UP

How squamous cell cancer develops

Squamous cell cancer is an invasive tumor with metastatic potential that arises from the keratinizing epidermal cells. It begins as a firm, red nodule or scaly, crusted flat lesion that may remain confined to the epidermis for a period of time. It eventually spreads to the dermis; untreated, it will spread to regional lymph nodes.

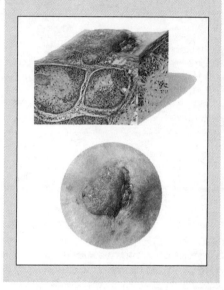

Complications

○ Lymph node involvement
○ Visceral metastasis

Treatment

○ Wide surgical excision is performed to remove the lesion.
○ Electrodesiccation and curettage offer good cosmetic results for small lesions.
○ Radiation therapy is generally recommended for older or debilitated patients.
○ Chemosurgery is reserved for resistant or recurrent lesions.

Premalignant skin lesions

Early detection and treatment of premalignant skin lesions may prevent progressive skin cancer.

Disease	Cause	Patient	Lesion	Treatment
Actinic keratosis	Solar radiation	White men with fair skin (middle-age to elderly)	Reddish brown lesions 1 mm to 1 cm in size (may enlarge if untreated) on face, ears, lower lip, bald scalp, dorsa of hands and forearms	Topical 5-fluorouracil, cryosurgery using liquid nitrogen, or curettage by electrodesiccation
Bowen's disease	Unknown	White men with fair skin (middle-age to elderly)	Brown to reddish-brown lesions, with scaly surface on exposed and unexposed areas	Surgical excision, topical 5-fluorouracil
Erythroplasia of Queyrat	Bowen's disease of the mucous membranes	Men (middle-age to elderly)	Red lesions with a glistening or granular appearance on mucous membranes, particularly the glans penis in uncircumcised males	Surgical excision
Leukoplakia	Smoking, alcohol use, chronic cheek-biting, ill-fitting dentures, misaligned teeth	Men (middle-age to elderly)	Lesions on oral, anal, and genital mucous membranes that vary in appearance from smooth and white to rough and gray	Elimination of irritating factors, surgical excision, or curettage by electrodesiccation (if lesion is still premalignant)

COLLABORATIVE MANAGEMENT Care of the patient with squamous cell cancer involves several members of the interdisciplinary team. The oncologist and dermatologist diagnose the disorder and determine the treatment plan. The surgeon excises tumors. The nurse provides education and screening and monitors for adverse effects of therapy. The dietitian ensures that the patient is receiving adequate nutrition and hydration.

Special considerations
○ Keep the wound dry and clean and change the dressings as ordered.
○ Be prepared for problems that accompany a metastatic disease (pain, fatigue, weakness, anorexia).

○ Help the patient and his family set realistic goals and expectations.
○ Encourage verbalization of feelings and provide emotional support.
○ Provide small, frequent meals and a high-protein, high-calorie diet.
○ Assess the patient for pain and administer analgesics, as indicated.
○ Provide patient education. (See *Teaching about squamous cell cancer.*)

Applicable patient-teaching aids
○ Changing a dry dressing
○ Minimizing sun exposure *

Squamous cell cancer nodule

An ulcerated nodule with an indurated base and a raised, irregular border is a typical lesion in squamous cell cancer.

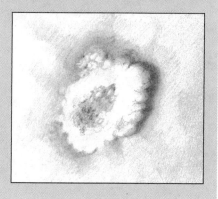

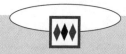

KEY TEACHING POINTS

Teaching about squamous cell cancer

Remember these key points when teaching your patient about squamous cell carcinoma:
• Teach about the disease process, including its symptoms, complications, and treatments.
• Teach about prescribed medications, including their names, indications, dosages, adverse effects, and special considerations.
• Discuss warning signs and symptoms of complications that require immediate medical attention.
• Discuss the importance of regular follow-up care for screening.
• Explain the importance of avoiding excessive sun exposure, wearing protective clothing, and using a strong sunscreen.
• Teach the patient to periodically examine the skin for precancerous lesions; have any removed promptly.

◯ Stroke

A stroke, also called *cerebrovascular accident* or *"brain attack,"* is a sudden impairment of cerebral circulation in one or more of the blood vessels supplying the brain. A stroke interrupts or diminishes oxygen supply and commonly causes serious damage or necrosis in brain tissues. The sooner circulation returns to normal after a stroke, the better chances are for complete recovery. However, about half of those who survive a stroke remain permanently disabled and experience a recurrence within weeks, months, or years. Rehabilitation can help people regain functions that were lost.

Causes

Factors that increase the risk of stroke include history of transient ischemic attacks, atherosclerosis, hypertension, kidney disease, arrhythmias (specifically atrial fibrillation), electrocardiogram changes, rheumatic heart disease, diabetes mellitus, postural hypotension, cardiac or myocardial enlargement, high serum triglyceride levels, lack of exercise, use of hormonal contraceptives, cigarette smoking, and family history of stroke. (See *Transient ischemic attack,* page 308.)

Thrombosis is the most common cause in middle-age and elderly people, who have a higher incidence of atherosclerosis, diabetes, and hypertension. The risk increases with obesity, smoking, or the use of hormonal contraceptives. Cocaine-induced ischemic stroke is now being seen in younger patients.

Embolism, the second most common cause of stroke, can occur at any age, especially among patients with a history of rheumatic heart disease, endocarditis, posttraumatic valvular disease, myocardial fibrillation and other cardiac arrhythmias, or after open-heart surgery.

Hemorrhage, the third most common cause of stroke, may, like embolism, occur suddenly, at any age, and affects more women than men.

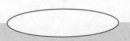

Transient ischemic attack

A transient ischemic attack (TIA) is a recurrent episode of neurologic deficit, lasting from seconds to hours, that clears within 12 to 24 hours. It's usually considered a warning sign of an impending thrombotic stroke. In fact, TIAs have been reported in 50% to 80% of patients who have had a cerebral infarction from such thrombosis. The age of onset varies. Incidence rises dramatically after age 50 and is highest among blacks and men.

most distinctive characteristics of TIAs are the transient duration of neurologic deficits and complete return of normal function. The symptoms of TIA easily correlate with the location of the affected artery. These symptoms include double vision, speech deficits (slurring or thickness), unilateral blindness, staggering or uncoordinated gait, unilateral weakness or numbness, falling because of weakness in the legs, and dizziness.

Causes

In TIA, microemboli released from a thrombus probably temporarily interrupt blood flow, especially in the small distal branches of the arterial tree in the brain. Small spasms in those arterioles may impair blood flow and also precede TIA. Predisposing factors are the same as for thrombotic strokes. The

Treatment

During an active TIA, treatment aims to prevent a completed stroke and consists of aspirin or anticoagulants to minimize the risk of thrombosis. After or between attacks, preventive treatment includes carotid endartectomy or cerebral microvascular bypass.

Hemorrhage results from chronic hypertension or aneurysms, which cause sudden rupture of a cerebral artery.

Pathophysiology

Regardless of the cause, the underlying event is deprivation of oxygen and nutrients. Normally, if the arteries become blocked, autoregulatory mechanisms help maintain cerebral circulation until collateral circulation develops to deliver blood to the affected area. If the compensatory mechanisms become overworked or cerebral blood flow remains impaired for more than a few minutes, oxygen deprivation leads to infarction of brain tissue. The brain cells cease to function because they can neither store glucose or glycogen for use nor engage in anaerobic metabolism. (See *Understanding stroke*.)

A thrombotic stroke causes ischemia in brain tissue supplied by the affected vessel as well as congestion and edema; the latter may produce more clinical effects than thrombosis itself, but these symptoms subside with the edema.

Embolic stroke is an occlusion of a blood vessel caused by a fragmented clot, a tumor, fat,

bacteria, or air. It usually develops rapidly — in 10 to 20 seconds — and without warning. When an embolus reaches the cerebral vasculature, it cuts off circulation by lodging in a narrow portion of an artery, most commonly the middle cerebral artery, causing necrosis and edema.

Both thrombotic and embolic stroke result in cerebral infarction, in which tissue injury triggers an inflammatory response that in turn increases intracranial pressure (ICP). Injury to the surrounding cells disrupts metabolism and leads to changes in ionic transport, localized acidosis, and free radical formation. Calcium, sodium, and water accumulate in the injured cells, and excitatory neurotransmitters are released. Consequent continued cellular injury and swelling set up a vicious cycle of further damage.

When hemorrhage is the cause, impaired cerebral perfusion causes infarction, and the blood itself acts as a space-occupying mass, exerting pressure on the brain tissues. The brain's regulatory mechanisms attempt to maintain equilibrium by increasing blood pressure to maintain cerebral perfusion pressure. The increased ICP forces cerebrospinal fluid

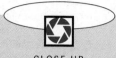

CLOSE UP

Understanding stroke

Strokes are typically classified as ischemic or hemorrhagic, depending on the underlying cause. In either type of stroke, the patient is deprived of oxygen and nutrients.

Ischemic stroke

This type of stroke results from a blockage or reduction of blood flow to an area of the brain. The blockage may result from atherosclerosis or blood clot formation.

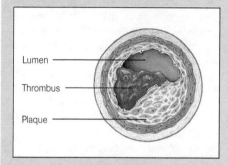

Lumen

Thrombus

Plaque

COMMON SITES OF PLAQUE FORMATION

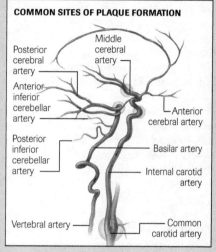

Posterior cerebral artery

Middle cerebral artery

Anterior inferior cerebellar artery

Anterior cerebral artery

Posterior inferior cerebellar artery

Basilar artery

Internal carotid artery

Vertebral artery

Common carotid artery

Hemorrhagic stroke

This type of stroke is caused by bleeding within and around the brain. Bleeding that fills the spaces between the brain and the skull (called *subarachnoid hemorrhage*) is caused by ruptured aneurysms, arteriovenous malformation, and head trauma. Bleeding within the brain tissue itself (known as *intracerebral hemorrhage*) is primarily caused by hypertension.

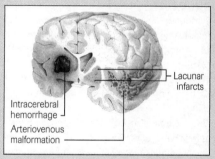

Lacunar infarcts

Intracerebral hemorrhage

Arteriovenous malformation

out, thus restoring the balance. If the bleeding is heavy, ICP increases rapidly and perfusion stops. Even if the pressure returns to normal, many brain cells die.

Initially, the ruptured cerebral blood vessels may constrict to limit the blood loss. This vasospasm further compromises blood flow, leading to more ischemia and cellular damage. If a clot forms in the vessel, decreased blood flow also promotes ischemia. If the blood enters the subarachnoid space, meningeal irritation occurs. The blood cells that pass through the vessel wall into the surrounding tissue also may break down and block the arachnoid villi, causing hydrocephalus.

Assessment findings

Disability following stroke depends on the affected cerebral artery:
○ *Middle cerebral artery:* aphasia, dysphasia, visual field cuts, and hemiparesis on affected side

(more severe in the face and arm than in the leg)

○ *Carotid artery:* weakness, paralysis, numbness, sensory changes, and visual disturbances on affected side; altered level of consciousness (LOC), bruits, headaches, aphasia, and ptosis

○ *Vertebrobasilar artery:* weakness on affected side, numbness around lips and mouth, visual field cuts, diplopia, poor coordination, dysphagia, slurred speech, dizziness, amnesia, and ataxia

○ *Anterior cerebral artery:* confusion, weakness, and numbness (especially in the leg) on affected side, incontinence, loss of coordination, impaired motor and sensory functions, and personality changes

○ *Posterior cerebral arteries:* visual field cuts, sensory impairment, dyslexia, coma, and cortical blindness; typically, paralysis is absent.

Generalized symptoms of an acute stroke include headache, unilateral limb weakness, speech difficulties, numbness on one side, vision disturbances, vomiting, mental impairment, seizures, coma, nuchal rigidity, fever, and disorientation. (See *Managing acute stroke.*)

Diagnosis

○ Computed tomography scan shows evidence of hemorrhagic stroke immediately but may not show evidence of thrombotic infarction for 48 to 72 hours.

○ Magnetic resonance imaging may help identify ischemic or infarcted areas and cerebral swelling.

○ Electrocardiogram can help diagnose underlying heart disorders.

○ Carotid duplex may detect carotid artery stenosis.

○ Angiography outlines blood vessels and pinpoints occlusion or rupture sites; it's mainly used if surgery is considered.

○ EEG helps to localize the damaged area.

Complications

○ Cognitive problems, including anosognosia, neglect, short attention span, short-term memory deficits, apraxia, and learning difficulties

○ Emotional problems, such as depression, anxiety, anger, grief, and personality changes

○ Language difficulties, such as expressive aphasia, receptive aphasia, global aphasia, amnesic aphasia

○ Motor control problems, including hemiplegia, hemiparesis, ataxia, and dysphagia

○ Sensory impairments, such as inability to feel touch, pain, temperature, or position; paresthesia; chronic pain syndromes; loss of urinary and bowel control

Treatment

○ Ticlopidine, an antiplatelet drug, may be more effective than aspirin in preventing stroke and reducing the risk of recurrent stroke.

○ Antilipemics and a diet low in saturated fats control hyperlipidemia.

○ Antihypertensives and a sodium-restricted diet control hypertension.

○ Insulin or oral hypoglycemics, dietary measures, weight loss, and exercise control blood glucose levels in the patient with diabetes.

○ Smoking cessation is essential to reduce the risk of future strokes.

○ Rehabilitation helps the patient regain his maximal level of functioning.

 COLLABORATIVE MANAGEMENT
An interdisciplinary approach involving several members of the interdisciplinary team is vital to helping the stroke survivor regain lost skills and functioning. The primary health care provider formulates the rehabilitation plan and provides care to reduce the risk of recurrent strokes and to maintain the patient's general health. The nurse coordinates the rehabilitation plan, educates the patient about regaining lost functions, and plans interventions to prevent stroke recurrence. The physical therapist helps the patient regain motor strength and function. The occupational therapist helps the patient relearn activities of daily living and to use assistive devices, if necessary. The speech therapist helps the patient with communication skills and to swallow safely. The dietitian recommends a diet to help the patient swallow safely and maintain his nutritional status. The vocational counselor helps the patient return to work or learn new skills. The social worker helps with financial concerns and in obtaining medical equipment.

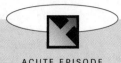

ACUTE EPISODE

Managing acute stroke

If your patient suffers an acute stroke, follow these guidelines:

● Administer tissue plasminogen activator to the patient with an ischemic stroke within 3 hours of the onset of symptoms. In other circumstances, heparin and warfarin may be used, as well as aspirin and other antiplatelet drugs.

● Begin intracranial pressure (ICP) management, induce hyperventilation (to decrease partial pressure of arterial carbon dioxide, which lowers ICP), and administer osmotic diuretics (to reduce cerebral edema) and corticosteroids (to reduce inflammation and cerebral edema).

● Give stool softeners to prevent straining, which increases ICP.

● Administer anticonvulsants, as ordered, to treat or prevent seizures.

● Prepare the patient for surgery, if indicated.

● Assess the patient's pain level, and administer analgesics to relieve the headache that typically follows hemorrhagic stroke.

● Secure and maintain the patient's airway and anticipate endotracheal intubation and mechanical ventilation.

● Monitor oxygen saturation levels via pulse oximetry and serial arterial blood gas studies; administer supplemental oxygen, as indicated.

● Turn the patient frequently using the lateral position to allow secretions to drain naturally or suction secretions, as needed.

● Assess the patient's neurologic status frequently, monitor for seizures, and observe for signs and symptoms of increasing ICP.

● If cerebral edema is suspected, maintain ICP sufficient for adequate cerebral perfusion but low enough to avoid brain herniation. Elevate the head of the bed 20 to 30 degrees; institute moderate fluid restriction; and administer osmotic diuretics, as ordered.

● Assist with insertion of a pulmonary artery catheter, if indicated, and assess hemodynamic status frequently, including central venous pressure and pulmonary artery pressure.

● Monitor vital signs frequently and report abnormal findings.

● If antihypertensive therapy is indicated, titrate the prescribed drug to maintain blood pressure within acceptable ranges without inducing hypotension.

● Begin continuous cardiac monitoring to detect arrhythmias.

● Monitor fluid intake and output and electrolyte balance; administer I.V. fluids as ordered.

● If the patient is alert and awake, check him for gag reflex before offering small oral feedings of semi-solid foods. If oral feedings aren't possible, administer enteral or parenteral nutrition, as ordered.

● Provide careful mouth care.

● Provide meticulous eye care. Instill eyedrops as ordered and patch the patient's affected eye if he can't close the lid.

● Position the patient and align his extremities correctly. Use high-topped sneakers to prevent footdrop and contracture and convoluted foam, flotation, or pulsating mattresses, or sheepskin, to prevent pressure ulcers.

● To prevent pneumonia, turn the patient at least every 2 hours.

● Establish and maintain communication with the patient.

Special considerations

○ Help the patient and family set realistic short- and long-term goals.

○ Involve the patient's family in his care when possible, and explain his deficits and strengths.

○ Encourage independence with activities of daily living and assist when needed.

○ Assess the patient's ability to swallow and provide an appropriate diet.

○ Refer the patient for physical and occupational therapy to build and maintain muscle

Teaching about stroke

Remember these key points when teaching your patient about stroke:

● Teach about the disease process, including types of strokes and their signs and symptoms and treatments.

● Teach about prescribed medications, including their names, indications, dosages, adverse effects, and special considerations.

● Discuss warning signs of complications that require immediate medical attention.

● Discuss risk factors for stroke, and help the patient identify those risk factors he can alter to reduce his risk of further stroke.

● If the patient is having surgery, explain the procedure and what he can expect in the preoperative and postoperative periods.

● Teach the importance of following a low-cholesterol, low-salt diet; achieving and maintaining an ideal weight; increasing activity; avoiding smoking and prolonged bed rest; and minimizing stress.

● Warn the patient or his family to seek prompt medical attention in an emergency department for any premonitory signs of a stroke, such as severe headache, drowsiness, confusion, and dizziness.

● Emphasize the importance of regular follow-up visits.

● Stress the importance of continuing rehabilitation to minimize deficits.

● Discuss alternate communication techniques, if indicated.

● Review dietary adjustments, such as semi-soft foods for dysphagia and the use of assistive feeding devices.

● Review the safe use of a cane or walker and home safety tips.

him to inspect that side of his body for injury and to protect it from harm.

○ Develop alternative communication techniques, if necessary.

○ Provide for the patient's safety, as indicated.

○ Assist the patient with range-of-motion exercises for both the affected and unaffected sides.

○ Provide patient education. (See *Teaching about stroke.*)

Applicable patient-teaching aids

○ Coping with depression
○ Cutting down on cholesterol *
○ Cutting down on salt *
○ Giving yourself a subcutaneous insulin injection *
○ Learning about canes *
○ Learning about daily food choices
○ Learning about walkers *
○ Learning to communicate without speech *
○ Maintaining a safe level of activity
○ Making eating easier
○ Performing active range-of-motion exercises*
○ Performing passive range-of-motion exercises
○ Preventing diabetic complications *
○ Taking anticoagulants *
○ Taking your blood pressure*
○ Testing your blood glucose level
○ Using dressing aids*
○ Walking with a cane

strength and tone and to relearn or compensate for lost skills.

○ If the patient fails to recognize that he has a paralyzed side (called *unilateral neglect*), teach

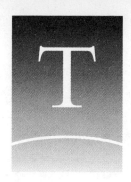

Thalassemia

Thalassemia, a hereditary group of hemolytic anemias, is characterized by defective synthesis in the polypeptide chains necessary for hemoglobin (Hb) production. Consequently, red blood cell (RBC) synthesis is also impaired.

Thalassemia is the most common form of this disorder, resulting from defective beta polypeptide chain synthesis. It occurs in three clinical forms: major, intermedia, and minor. The resulting anemia's severity depends on whether the patient is homozygous or heterozygous for the thalassemic trait. The prognosis for thalassemia varies. People with thalassemia major seldom survive to adulthood; children with thalassemia intermedia develop normally into adulthood, although puberty is usually delayed; people with thalassemia minor can expect a normal life span.

Thalassemia is most common in people of Mediterranean ancestry (especially Italian and Greek), but it also occurs in blacks and in people from southern China, southeast Asia, and India.

Causes

Thalassemia major (also known as *Cooley's anemia*, *Mediterranean disease*, and *erythroblastic anemia*) and thalassemia intermedia result from homozygous inheritance of the partially dominant autosomal gene responsible for this trait. Thalassemia minor results from heterozygous inheritance of the same gene.

Pathophysiology

Total or partial deficiency of beta polypeptide chain production impairs hemoglobin synthesis and results in continual production of fetal hemoglobin, lasting even past the neonatal period. Normally, immunoglobulin synthesis switches from gamma- to beta-polypeptides at the time of birth. This conversion doesn't happen in thalassemic infants. Their red cells are hypochromic and microcytic. (See *Understanding thalassemia,* page 314.)

Assessment findings

In thalassemia major, the neonate is well at birth but develops severe anemia, bone abnormalities, failure to thrive, and life-threatening complications. (See *Skull changes in thalassemia major,* page 315.) In many cases, the first signs are pallor and yellow skin and scleras in infants ages 3 to 6 months. Later clinical features include severe anemia; splenomegaly or hepatomegaly, with abdominal enlargement; frequent infections; bleeding tendencies (especially toward epistaxis); and anorexia.

Children with thalassemia major typically have small bodies and large heads and may also be mentally retarded. Infants may have mongoloid features because bone marrow hyperactivity has thickened the bone at the base of the nose. As these children grow older, they become susceptible to pathologic fractures as a result of expansion of the marrow cavities with thinning of the long bones. They're also subject to cardiac arrhythmias, heart failure, and other complications that result from iron deposits in

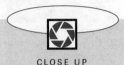

CLOSE UP

Understanding thalassemia

A hereditary group of hemolytic anemias, thalassemia is characterized by defective synthesis in the polypeptide chains of the protein component of hemoglobin. Consequently, red blood cell (RBC) synthesis is also impaired.

In thalassemia major, survival to adulthood seldom occurs. In thalassemia minor, a normal lifespan is expected. Severity depends on whether the patient is homozygous or heterozygous for the thalassemic trait.

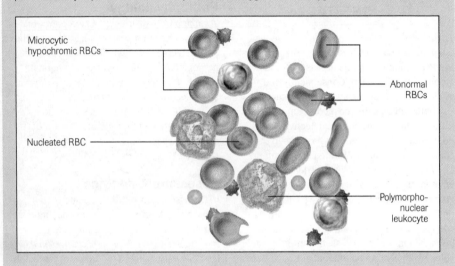

the heart and in other tissues from repeated blood transfusions.

Patients with thalassemia intermedia show some degree of anemia, jaundice, and splenomegaly and, possibly, signs of hemosiderosis due to increased intestinal absorption of iron.

Thalassemia minor may cause mild anemia, but it usually produces no symptoms and is commonly overlooked.

Diagnosis

Diagnostic testing in thalassemia major reveals the following:

○ Laboratory results show lowered RBC count and Hb level, microcytosis, and elevated reticulocyte, bilirubin, and urinary and fecal urobilinogen levels.

○ Serum folate level is reduced and indicates increased folate utilization by the hypertrophied bone marrow.

○ Peripheral blood smear reveals target cells, microcytes, pale nucleated RBCs, and marked anisocytosis.

○ X-rays of the skull and long bones show thinning and widening of the marrow space because of overactive bone marrow. The bones of the skull and vertebrae may appear granular; long bones may show areas of osteoporosis. The phalanges may also be deformed (rectangular or biconvex).

○ Quantitative Hb studies show a significant rise in HbF and a slight increase in HbA$_2$.

○ Serum iron and ferritin levels are normal or increased.

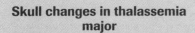

Skull changes in thalassemia major

X-rays show a characteristic skull abnormality in thalassemia major: diploetic fibers extending from the internal lamina.

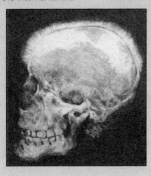

Diagnostic testing in thalassemia intermedia reveals the following:

○ Laboratory results show hypochromia and microcytic RBCs, but the anemia is less severe than that in thalassemia major.

Diagnostic testing in thalassemia minor reveals the following:

○ Laboratory results show hypochromia and microcytic RBCs.

○ Quantitative Hb studies show a significant increase in HbA_2 levels and a moderate rise in HbF levels.

Complications
○ Cardiac arrhythmias
○ Death
○ Heart failure
○ Iron overload from RBC transfusions
○ Liver failure
○ Pathologic fractures

Treatment
○ Antibiotics treat infection.
○ Folic acid supplements help maintain folic acid levels in the face of increased requirements.

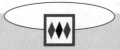

Teaching about thalassemia

Remember these key points when teaching your patient about thalassemia:

● Teach about the disease process, including its various types, mode of inheritance, signs and symptoms, and treatments.

● Teach about prescribed medications, including their names, indications, dosages, adverse effects, and special considerations.

● Discuss warning signs of complications that require immediate medical attention.

● Stress the importance of good nutrition, meticulous wound care, periodic dental checkups, and other measures to prevent infection.

● Discuss with the parents of a young patient various options for healthy physical and creative outlets. Such a child must avoid strenuous athletic activity, but he may participate in less stressful activities.

● Teach parents to watch for signs of hepatitis and iron overload, which are always possible with frequent transfusions.

● Explain the role of genetic counseling.

○ Transfusions of packed RBCs raise Hb levels but must be used judiciously to minimize iron overload.

○ Chelation therapy may be required for patients who receive significant numbers of blood transfusions to remove iron from the body.

○ Bone marrow transplantation is being investigated as a treatment, with success found mostly in children.

○ No treatment is generally needed for thalassemia intermedia and thalassemia minor.

○ Iron supplements are contraindicated in all forms of thalassemia.

 COLLABORATIVE MANAGEMENT
Care of the patient with thalassemia involves several members of the interdisciplinary team. The hematologist typically diagnoses and treats the disorder. The nurse

educates the patient and family and monitors for complications. The dietitian makes dietary recommendations and educates the patient about avoiding foods high in iron. The genetic counselor educates the patient and family about genetic transmission of the disorder. The social worker addresses financial concerns.

Special considerations

○ During and after RBC transfusions for thalassemia major, watch for adverse reactions—shaking, chills, fever, rash, itching, and hives.
○ Provide a low-iron diet and encourage oral fluid intake.
○ Provide emotional support and encourage verbalization of concerns and feelings.
○ Refer the patient and family for genetic counseling.
○ Provide patient education. (See *Teaching about thalassemia,* page 315.)

Applicable patient-teaching aids

○ Giving children medication by mouth *
○ Learning about blood transfusions

○ Trigeminal neuralgia

Trigeminal neuralgia, also called *tic douloureux,* is a painful disorder of one or more branches of the fifth cranial (trigeminal) nerve that produces paroxysmal attacks of excruciating facial pain precipitated by stimulation of a trigger zone. It can subside spontaneously, and remissions may last from several months to years.

Trigeminal neuralgia occurs mostly in people older than age 40, in women more commonly than men, and on the right side of the face more commonly than the left. Incidence is 4 to 5 cases per 100,000 people.

Causes

Although the cause remains undetermined, trigeminal neuralgia may reflect an afferent reflex in the brain stem or in the sensory root of the trigeminal nerve. Such neuralgia may also be related to compression of the nerve root by posterior fossa tumors, middle fossa tumors, or vascular lesions (subclinical aneurysm), although such lesions usually produce simultaneous loss of sensation. Occasionally, trigeminal neuralgia is a manifestation of multiple sclerosis or herpes zoster.

Pathophysiology

The trigeminal nerve has multiple branches. The pain of trigeminal neuralgia is probably produced by an interaction or short-circuiting of touch and pain fibers. Paroxysmal attacks of excruciating facial pain result. (See *Trigeminal nerve function and distribution.*)

Assessment findings

Typically, the patient reports a searing or burning pain that occurs in lightning-like jabs and lasts from 1 to 15 minutes (usually 1 to 2 minutes) in an area innervated by one of the divisions of the trigeminal nerve, primarily the superior mandibular or maxillary division. The pain rarely affects more than one division and seldom the first division (ophthalmic) or both sides of the face. It affects the second (maxillary) and third (mandibular) divisions of the trigeminal nerve equally.

These attacks characteristically follow stimulation of a trigger zone, usually by a light touch to a hypersensitive area, such as the tip of the nose, the cheeks, or the gums. Although attacks can occur at any time, they may follow a draft of air, exposure to heat or cold, eating, smiling, talking, or drinking hot or cold beverages. The frequency of attacks varies greatly, from many times a day to several times a month or year. Between attacks, most patients are free from pain, although some have a constant, dull ache.

To ward off a painful attack, the patient commonly holds his face immobile when talking. When asked where the pain occurs, he points to—but never touches—the affected area.

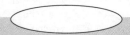

Trigeminal nerve function and distribution

Function
- Motor: chewing movements
- Sensory: sensations of face, scalp, and teeth (mouth and nasal chamber)

Distribution
I   ophthalmic
II maxillary
III mandibular

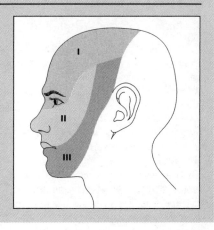

Diagnosis
○ Pain history is the basis for diagnosis because trigeminal neuralgia produces no objective clinical or pathologic changes.
○ Physical examination shows no impairment of sensory or motor function.
○ Skull X-rays, computed tomography scan, and magnetic resonance imaging rule out sinus or tooth infections and tumors; with trigeminal neuralgia, these test results are normal.

Complications
○ Depression
○ Excessive weight loss
○ Social isolation

Treatment
○ Carbamazepine or phenytoin taken orally may temporarily relieve or prevent pain.
○ Opioids may be helpful during the pain episode.
○ Percutaneous electrocoagulation of nerve rootlets under local anesthetic may be performed when medical measures fail or the attacks become increasingly frequent or severe.

○ Percutaneous radio frequency is a new treatment that causes partial root destruction and relieves pain.
○ Microsurgery may be performed for vascular decompression of the trigeminal nerve.

 COLLABORATIVE MANAGEMENT
Care of the patient with trigeminal neuralgia involves several members of the interdisciplinary team. The neurologist diagnoses and manages the disorder. The nurse educates the patient, performs pain relief measures, and provides support. The dietitian may be consulted if the patient fails to eat because he fears triggering an attack. The therapist may be helpful to help the patient cope with the condition.

Special considerations
○ Observe and record the characteristics of each attack, including the patient's protective mechanisms.
○ Provide adequate nutrition in small, frequent meals served at room temperature.
○ Avoid jarring the bed and causing increased discomfort.

Teaching about trigeminal neuralgia

Remember these key points when teaching your patient about trigeminal neuralgia:
- Teach about the disease process, including its symptoms and treatments.
- Teach about prescribed medications, including their names, indications, dosages, adverse effects, and special considerations.
- Warn the patient taking carbamazepine to immediately report fever, sore throat, mouth ulcers, easy bruising, or petechial or purpuric hemorrhage because these may signal thrombocytopenia or aplastic anemia and require discontinuation of drug therapy.
- Remind the patient taking carbamazepine that liver function and complete blood count need to be monitored periodically.
- Tell the patient receiving phenytoin to report ataxia, skin eruptions, gingival hyperplasia, and nystagmus.
- Discuss warning signs and symptoms of complications that require immediate medical attention.
- Reinforce the patient's natural avoidance of stimulation (air, heat, and cold) or trigger zones (lips, cheeks, and gums).

After resection of the first branch of the trigeminal nerve:
- Tell the patient to avoid rubbing his eyes and using aerosol spray.
- Advise him to wear glasses or goggles outdoors and to blink often.

After surgery to sever the second or third branch of the trigeminal nerve:
- Tell the patient to avoid hot foods and drinks, which could burn his mouth, and to chew carefully to avoid biting his mouth.
- Advise the patient to place food in the unaffected side of his mouth when chewing, to brush his teeth and rinse his mouth often, and to see the dentist twice a year to detect cavities because he won't experience pain from cavities in the area of the severed nerve.

○ If the patient is receiving carbamazepine, watch for cutaneous and hematologic reactions (erythematous and pruritic rashes, urticaria, photosensitivity, exfoliative dermatitis, leukopenia, agranulocytosis, eosinophilia, aplastic anemia, and thrombocytopenia) and, possibly, urine retention and transient drowsiness.
○ For the first 3 months of carbamazepine therapy, complete blood count and liver function should be monitored weekly, then monthly thereafter.
○ After surgery to sever the second or third branch, the patient may require puréed food, possibly through a straw.
○ After surgical decompression of the root or partial nerve dissection, check the patient's neurologic and vital signs often.
○ Provide emotional support, and encourage the patient to express his feelings.
○ Promote independence through self-care and maximum physical activity.
○ Provide patient education. (See *Teaching about trigeminal neuralgia*.)

Applicable patient-teaching aids
○ Coping with depression
○ Taking carbamazepine
○ Taking phenytoin

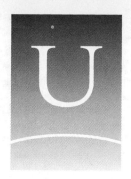

Ulcerative colitis

Ulcerative colitis is an inflammatory, usually chronic disease that affects the mucosa of the colon. It invariably begins in the rectum and sigmoid colon and commonly extends upward into the entire colon; it rarely affects the small intestine, except for the terminal ileum. Ulcerative colitis produces edema (leading to mucosal friability) and ulcerations. Severity ranges from a mild, localized disorder to a fulminant disease that may cause a perforated colon, progressing to potentially fatal peritonitis and toxemia.

Ulcerative colitis occurs primarily in young adults, especially in women. It's also more prevalent among those of Jewish ancestry, indicating a possible familial tendency. The incidence of the disease is unknown; however, some studies indicate that as many as 10 to 15 out of 100,000 persons have the disease. Onset of symptoms seems to peak between ages 15 and 30; another peak occurs between ages 50 and 70.

Causes

Although the etiology of ulcerative colitis is unknown, it's thought to be related to abnormal immune response in the GI tract, possibly associated with food or bacteria such as *Escherichia coli.* Stress was once thought to be a cause of ulcerative colitis, but studies show that although it isn't a cause, it does increase the severity of the attack.

Pathophysiology

Ulcerative colitis usually begins as inflammation in the base of the mucosal layer of the large intestine. The colon's mucosal surface becomes dark, red, and velvety. Inflammation leads to erosions that coalesce and form ulcers. The mucosa becomes diffusely ulcerated, with hemorrhage, congestion, edema, and exudative inflammation. Ulcerations are continuous. Abscesses in the mucosa drain purulent exudate, become necrotic, and ulcerate. Sloughing causes bloody, mucus-filled stools. As abscesses heal, scarring and thickening may appear in the bowel's inner muscle layer. As granulation tissue replaces the muscle layer, the colon narrows, shortens, and loses its characteristic pouches (haustral folds).

Assessment findings

The hallmark of ulcerative colitis is recurrent attacks of bloody diarrhea, in many cases containing pus and mucus, interspersed with asymptomatic remissions. The patient may have as many as 15 to 20 liquid, bloody stools daily. Other symptoms include spastic rectum and anus, abdominal pain, irritability, weight loss, weakness, anorexia, nausea, and vomiting.

Diagnosis

○ Sigmoidoscopy showing increased mucosal friability, decreased mucosal detail, and thick inflammatory exudate suggests ulcerative colitis. Biopsy, performed during colonoscopy, can confirm the diagnosis.

○ Colonoscopy may be required to determine the extent of the disease and to evaluate strictured areas and pseudopolyps.

○ Barium enema can assess the extent of the disease and detect complications, such as strictures and carcinoma.

○ A stool sample may be cultured and ana-lyzed for leukocytes, ova, and parasites.
○ Laboratory values may show decreased serum levels of potassium, magnesium, hemo-globin, and albumin as well as leukocytosis and increased prothrombin time. An elevated ery-throcyte sedimentation rate correlates with the severity of the attack.

Complications

○ Anal fissure or fistula
○ Anemia
○ Ankylosing spondylitis
○ Arthritis
○ Cancer
○ Cholangiocarcinoma
○ Cirrhosis
○ Coagulation defects
○ Erythema nodosum on the face and arms
○ Hemorrhage
○ Nutritional deficiencies
○ Perforation of the colon
○ Pericholangitis, sclerosing cholangitis
○ Perineal sepsis
○ Perirectal abscess
○ Pseudopolyps, stenosis, and perforated colon leading to peritonitis and toxemia
○ Pyoderma gangrenosum on the legs and ankles
○ Strictures
○ Toxic megacolon
○ Uveitis

Treatment

○ Supportive treatment includes bed rest, I.V. fluid replacement, and a clear-liquid diet.
○ Total parenteral nutrition (TPN) may be nec-essary to rest the intestinal tract. It decreases stool volume and restores positive nitrogen balance.
○ Blood transfusions or iron supplements may be needed to correct anemia.
○ Immunomodulators or 5-aminosalicylates may be used to decrease the frequency of at-tacks.
○ Steroids may be given to control inflamma-tion.

○ Antispasmodics and antidiarrheals are used only in patients whose ulcerative colitis is un-der control but who have frequent, loose stools.
○ Surgery, such as proctocolectomy with ileostomy, ileoanal pull-through, or pouch ileostomy (*Kock pouch* or *continent ileostomy*), is the last resort if the patient has toxic mega-colon, fails to respond to drugs and supportive measures, or finds symptoms unbearable.

 COLLABORATIVE MANAGEMENT
Care of the patient with ulcerative colitis involves several members of the interdisciplinary team to control inflamma-tion, replace nutritional losses and blood vol-ume, and prevent complications. The primary health care provider or gastroenterologist di-agnoses and manages the disorder. The sur-geon may be consulted if the patient fails to respond to drugs and supportive measures, or if she finds symptoms unbearable. The nurse educates the patient about the disorder, devel-ops a therapeutic relationship, cares for the patient during exacerbations, and performs preoperative and postoperative teaching. The enterostomal therapist teaches the patient and family about care of and adjustment to the stoma. The social worker can help with finan-cial issues and in obtaining supplies. The di-etitian can assist with nutritional issues and management of GI symptoms such as flatus.

Special considerations

○ Accurately record intake and output, particu-larly the frequency and volume of stools. Watch for signs of dehydration and electrolyte imbal-ances, especially signs and symptoms of hypo-kalemia (muscle weakness and paresthesia) and hypernatremia (tachycardia, flushed skin, fever, and dry tongue).
○ Monitor hemoglobin level and hematocrit, and give blood transfusions as ordered.
○ Provide good mouth care for the patient who's allowed nothing by mouth.
○ After each bowel movement, thoroughly clean the skin around the rectum.
○ Provide an air mattress or sheepskin to help prevent skin breakdown.
○ Administer medications, as ordered.

○ Watch for adverse effects of prolonged corticosteroid therapy (moon face, hirsutism, edema, and gastric irritation). Be aware that corticosteroid therapy may mask infection.

○ If the patient needs TPN, change dressings as ordered, assess for inflammation at the insertion site, and check capillary blood glucose levels every 4 to 6 hours.

○ Take precautionary measures if the patient is prone to bleeding.

○ Watch closely for signs of complications, such as a perforated colon and peritonitis (fever, severe abdominal pain, abdominal rigidity and tenderness, and cool, clammy skin) and toxic megacolon (abdominal distention and decreased bowel sounds).

For the patient requiring surgery:

○ Carefully prepare the patient for surgery, and inform him about ileostomy.

○ Do a bowel preparation, as ordered.

○ After surgery, provide meticulous supportive care and continue teaching correct stoma care.

○ Keep the nasogastric tube patent. After removal of the tube, provide a clear-liquid diet and gradually advance to a low-residue diet, as tolerated.

○ After a proctocolectomy and ileostomy, provide good stoma care.

○ After a pouch ileostomy, uncork the catheter every hour to allow its contents to drain. After 10 to 14 days, gradually increase the length of time the catheter is left corked until it can be opened every 3 hours. Then remove the catheter and reinsert it every 3 to 4 hours for drainage.

○ Encourage the patient to have regular physical examinations.

○ Provide patient education. (See *Teaching about ulcerative colitis*.)

Applicable patient-teaching aids

○ Applying an ostomy pouch *
○ Draining an ostomy pouch
○ Preparing for a sigmoidoscopy or colonoscopy *
○ Removing an ostomy pouch *

KEY TEACHING POINTS

Teaching about ulcerative colitis

Remember these key points when teaching your patient about ulcerative colitis:

● Teach about the disease process, including its symptoms, complications, and treatments.

● Teach about prescribed medications, including their names, indications, dosages, adverse effects, and special considerations.

● Discuss warning signs of complications that require immediate medical attention.

● Discuss the need to avoid GI stimulants, such as caffeine, alcohol, and smoking.

● If the patient is having a colostomy, teach him and his family about the procedure and proper care of a colostomy bag and the surrounding skin.

● Explain to the patient's family the importance of their positive reactions to the patient's adjustment.

● If the patient is having a pouch ileostomy, teach him to insert the catheter and care for the stoma.

● Discuss any dietary changes or restrictions.

● Tell the patient to avoid heavy lifting.

● Recommend a structured, gradually progressive exercise program to strengthen abdominal muscles.

● Reinforce the importance of yearly screening and testing to detect colorectal cancer.

● Review signs and symptoms of complications, such as intestinal obstruction and anemia.

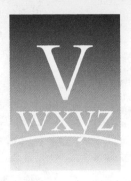

Varicose veins

Varicose veins are dilated, tortuous veins, engorged with blood and resulting from improper venous valve function. They can be primary, originating in the superficial veins, or secondary, occurring in the deep veins.

Primary varicose veins tend to be familial and to affect both legs; they are twice as common in females as in males. They account for approximately 90% of varicose veins; about 10% to 20% of Americans have primary varicose veins. Usually, secondary varicose veins occur in one leg. Both types are more common in middle adulthood.

Without treatment, varicose veins continue to enlarge. Although there's no cure, certain measures, such as walking and using compression stockings, can reduce symptoms. Surgery may remove varicose veins, but the condition can occur in other veins.

Causes

Primary varicose veins can result from congenital weakness of the valves or venous wall; conditions that produce prolonged venous stasis or increased intra-abdominal pressure, such as pregnancy, obesity, constipation, or wearing tight clothes; occupations that necessitate standing for an extended period; and a family history of varicose veins.

Secondary varicose veins can result from deep vein thrombosis, venous malformation, arteriovenous fistulas, trauma to the venous system, and occlusion.

Pathophysiology

Veins are thin-walled, distensible vessels with valves that keep blood flowing in one direction. Any condition that weakens, destroys, or distends these valves allows blood backflow to the previous valve. If a valve can't hold the pooling blood, it can become incompetent, allowing even more blood to flow backward. As the volume of venous blood builds, pressure in the vein increases and the vein becomes distended. As the veins are stretched, their walls weaken and they lose their elasticity. As the veins enlarge, they become lumpy and tortuous. As hydrostatic pressure increases, plasma is forced out of the veins and into the surrounding tissues, resulting in edema.

People who stand for prolonged periods may also develop venous pooling because there's no muscular contraction in the legs, forcing blood back up to the heart. If the valves in the veins are too weak to hold the pooling blood, they begin to leak, allowing blood to flow backward.

Assessment findings

In the patient with varicose veins, assessment reveals dilated, tortuous, purplish, ropelike veins, particularly in the calves. The patient may report edema of the calves and ankles, leg heaviness that worsens in the evening and in warm weather, and dull aching in the legs after prolonged standing or walking or during menses.

Diagnosis

◌ A manual compression test detects a palpable impulse when the vein is firmly occluded at least 8″ (20 cm) above the point of palpation, indicating incompetent valves in the vein.

○ Trendelenburg's test (*retrograde filling test*) detects incompetent deep and superficial vein valves.

○ Photoplethysmography characterizes venous blood flow by noting changes in the skin's circulation.

○ Doppler ultrasonography detects the presence or absence of venous backflow in deep or superficial veins.

○ Venous outflow and reflux plethysmography detects deep venous occlusion; this test is invasive and not routinely used.

○ Ascending and descending venography demonstrates venous occlusion and patterns of collateral flow.

Complications
○ Blood clots
○ Chronic venous insufficiency
○ Venous stasis ulcers

Treatment
○ Treat the underlying cause, such as an abdominal tumor or obesity, if possible.

○ Antiembolism stockings or elastic bandages counteract swelling by supporting the veins and improving circulation.

○ Regular exercise promotes muscular contraction to force blood through the veins and reduce venous pooling.

○ Sclerotherapy, the injection of a sclerosing agent into small to medium-sized varicosities, is an alternative to surgery.

○ Surgical stripping and ligation may be necessary for severe varicose veins.

○ Phlebectomy, removing the varicose vein through small incisions in the skin, may be performed.

 COLLABORATIVE MANAGEMENT
Care of the patient with varicose veins involves several members of the interdisciplinary team. The primary health care provider diagnoses the disorder and develops the treatment plan. The surgeon consults for cosmetic reasons or to prevent venous complications. The nurse educates the patient about proper skin care and measures to reduce venous stasis. The physical therapist helps the patient plan a regular exercise program.

Special considerations
○ After stripping and ligation or after injection of a sclerosing agent, administer analgesics, as ordered, to relieve pain.

○ Frequently check circulation in toes (color and temperature), and observe elastic bandages for bleeding. When ordered, rewrap bandages at least once per shift, wrapping from toe to thigh, with the leg elevated.

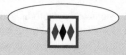
KEY TEACHING POINTS

Teaching about varicose veins

Remember these key points when teaching your patient about varicose veins:

● Teach about the disease process, including its signs and symptoms, complications, and treatments.

● Teach about prescribed medications, including their names, indications, dosages, adverse effects, and special considerations.

● Discuss warning signs of complications that require immediate medical attention.

● Tell the patient to avoid wearing constrictive clothing.

● Explain the importance of weight loss to the obese patient.

● Explain the importance of resting with the legs elevated above the heart when possible and to avoid prolonged standing or sitting.

● Demonstrate how to apply elastic, antiembolism, or compression stockings before getting out of bed in the morning.

● Discuss how to avoid injury to the lower legs, ankles, and feet. Also discuss the need to observe for altered skin integrity of those areas and to report problems.

○ Watch for signs and symptoms of complications, such as sensory loss in the leg (which could indicate saphenous nerve damage), calf pain (which could indicate thrombophlebitis), and fever (a sign of infection).
○ Provide patient education. (See *Teaching about varicose veins,* page 323.)

Applicable patient-teaching aids
○ Applying antiembolism stockings
○ Care and prevention of leg ulcers *
○ Taking steps toward healthier legs

Patient-teaching aids

Part two

◯ Adding fiber to your diet

Dear Patient:
Here are four easy ways to add fiber to your diet.

EAT WHOLE-GRAIN BREADS AND CEREALS

For the first few days, eat one serving daily of whole-grain breads (1 slice), cereal (½ cup), pasta (½ cup), or brown rice (⅓ cup). Examples of whole-grain breads are whole wheat and pumpernickel. Examples of high-fiber cereals are bran or oat flakes and shredded wheat. Gradually increase to four or more servings daily.

EAT FRESH FRUITS AND VEGETABLES

Begin by eating one serving daily of raw or cooked, unpeeled fruit (one medium-size piece; ½ cup cooked) or unpeeled vegetables (½ cup cooked; 1 cup raw). Gradually increase to four servings daily. Examples of high-fiber fruits include apples, oranges, and peaches. Some high-fiber vegetables are carrots, corn, and peas.

EAT DRIED PEAS AND BEANS

Begin by eating one serving (⅓ cup) per week. Increase to at least two to three servings per week.

EAT UNPROCESSED BRAN

Add bran to your food. Start with 1 teaspoon per day, and over a 3-week period work up to 2 to 3 tablespoons per day. Don't use more than this. Remember to drink at least six 8-ounce glasses of fluid per day.

A small amount of bran can be beneficial, but too much can irritate your digestive tract, cause gas, interfere with mineral absorption, and even lodge in your intestine.

Crisp fresh fruits and vegetables, cooked foods with husks, and nuts must be chewed thoroughly so that large particles don't pass whole into the intestine and lodge there, causing problems.

A SAMPLE MENU

Breakfast
½ grapefruit
Oatmeal with milk and raisins
Bran muffin
8 ounces of liquid

Lunch
Cabbage slaw
Tuna salad sandwich on whole wheat bread
Fresh pear with skin
8 ounces of liquid

Dinner
Vegetable soup
Broiled fish with almond topping
Baked potato with skin
Carrots and peas
Canned crushed pineapple
8 ounces of liquid

Snack
Dried fruit and nut mix
8 ounces of lquid

⊃ Adjusting to a total hip replacement

Dear Patient:
Your new artificial hip should eliminate hip pain and help you get around better. But go easy at first.

To give your hip time to heal and to avoid too much stress on it, follow these "do's and don'ts" for the next 3 months or for as long as your health care provider orders.

Do's

● Sit only in chairs with arms that can support you when you get up. When you want to stand up, first ease to the edge of your chair. Place your affected leg in front of the unaffected one, which should be well under your chair. Now, grip the chair's arms firmly, and push up with your arms — not with your legs. You should be supporting most of your weight with your arms and your unaffected leg.

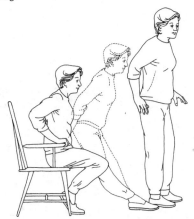

● Wear your support stockings (except when you're in bed at night).
● Keep your affected leg facing forward, whether you're sitting, lying down, or walking.
● Exercise regularly as ordered. Stop exercising immediately, however, if you feel severe hip pain.
● Lie down and elevate your feet and legs if they swell after walking.

● Obtain a raised toilet seat for use at home, and use public toilets designated for the disabled.
● Turn in bed only as directed.

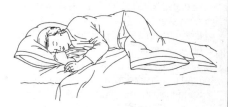

● Place a pillow between your legs when you lie on your side and when you go to bed at night. (This keeps your leg from twisting and dislodging your new hip.)
● Sit on a firm pillow when riding in a car, and keep your affected leg extended. (If your knee suddenly hits the dashboard, your hip prosthesis could be dislodged.)

DON'TS

● Don't lean far forward to stand up.
● Don't sit on low chairs or couches.
● Don't reach far when picking up objects or tying your shoes. (To pick up dropped objects, position yourself as your therapist taught you.)
● Don't cross your legs or turn your hip or knee inward or outward. This could dislodge your hip. Avoid this by placing a pillow between your knees.
● Don't scrub your hip incision.
● Don't take tub baths.
● Don't lift heavy items.

(continued)

Adjusting to a total hip replacement *(continued)*

- Don't have sexual intercourse until your health care provider says you can.
- Don't play tennis, run, jog, or do other strenuous activities.
- Don't drive a car.
- Don't reach to the end of the bed to pull the blankets up.

WHAT TO REPORT

- Redness, swelling, or warmth around your incision
- Drainage from your incision
- Fever or chills
- Severe hip pain uncontrolled by prescribed pain medicine
- Sudden sharp pain and a clicking or popping sound in your joint
- Leg shortening, with your foot turning outward
- Loss of control over leg motion or complete loss of leg motion

AN IMPORTANT PRECAUTION

You'll need to take an antibiotic just before and after tooth extractions, dental procedures other than routine fillings, any other surgery, and some diagnostic procedures.

◯ Applying an ostomy pouch

Dear Patient:
The nurse will show you how to apply the ostomy pouch. You can use this patient-teaching aid to help you remember the steps. Choose a one-piece disposable pouch, a two-piece disposable pouch, or a two-piece reusable pouch.

APPLYING A ONE-PIECE DISPOSABLE POUCH

1. Measure your stoma to determine the correct size of the pouch opening, as shown.

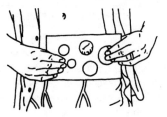

2. If the pouch opening is *precut,* remove the paper backing from the pouch, press the pouch to your abdomen, and seal well. Attach the tail closure (a small clip that secures the pouch bottom for later drainage). If you *custom-cut* your pouch, cut the opening to the correct size, remove the paper backing, and then apply as above.

APPLYING A TWO-PIECE DISPOSABLE POUCH

1. Measure your stoma to determine the correct size of your faceplate opening.
2. Cut the faceplate to the correct size, remove the paper backing, press the faceplate to your abdomen, and seal well. Secure the pouch to the faceplate and attach the tail closure.

APPLYING A TWO-PIECE REUSABLE POUCH

1. Measure your stoma to determine the size of your faceplate opening.
2. Follow the manufacturer's directions to apply new adhesive to the faceplate or to your skin with each change. First, peel off one side of the adhesive disk's paper backing. Then center the disk over the faceplate and press firmly to expel bubbles from between the faceplate and the adhesive.
3. Next, peel the remaining paper backing off the adhesive disk. Center the faceplate over your stoma. Gently press around the stoma so the adhesive sticks to your abdomen.

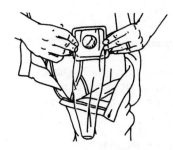

Secure the pouch to the faceplate, attach the supporting O-ring around the faceplate collar, and attach the tail closure.

◯ Avoiding asthma triggers

Dear Patient:
To make it easier for you to live with asthma, try to avoid common asthma triggers such as those listed here.

AT HOME

- Food such as nuts, chocolate, eggs, shell-fish, and peanut butter
- Beverages such as orange juice, wine, beer, and milk
- Mold spores and pollens from flowers, trees, grass, hay, and ragweed (If pollen is the offender, install a bedroom air condition-er with a filter.)
- Dander from rabbits, cats, dogs, ham-sters, gerbils, and chickens (Consider find-ing a new home for the family pet, if neces-sary.)
- Feather or hair-stuffed pillows, down comforters, wool clothing, and stuffed toys (Use smooth, not fuzzy, washable blankets on your bed.)
- Insect parts, such as those from dead cockroaches and house mites
- Medicines such as aspirin
- Vapors from cleaning solvents, paint, paint thinners, and liquid chlorine bleach
- Fluorocarbon spray products, such as fur-niture polish, starch, cleaners, and room de-odorizers
- Scents from spray deodorants, perfumes, hair sprays, talcum powder, and cosmetics
- Cloth-upholstered furniture, carpets, and draperies that collect dust (Hang light-weight, washable cotton or synthetic-fiber curtains, and use washable, cotton throw rugs on bare floors. Cover pillows and mat-tresses with impermeable covers, and wash blankets and sheets in very hot water week-ly. Use unscented laundry soap, and avoid fabric softeners.)
- Brooms and dusters that raise dust (Instead, clean your bedroom daily by damp dusting and damp mopping. Keep the door closed.)
- Dirty filters on hot-air furnaces and air conditioners that blow dust into the air
- Dust from vacuum cleaner exhaust

IN THE WORKPLACE

- Dust, vapors, or fumes from wood prod-ucts (western red cedar, some pine and birch woods, and mahogany); flour, cereals, and other grains; coffee, tea, or papain; met-als (platinum, chromium, nickel sulfate, sol-dering fumes); and cotton, flax, and hemp
- Mold from decaying hay

OUTDOORS

- Cold air, hot air, or sudden temperature changes (when you go in and out of air-conditioned stores in the summer)
- Excessive humidity or dryness
- Changes in seasons
- Smog
- Automobile exhaust
- High pollen counts

ANYPLACE

- Overexertion, which may cause wheezing
- Common cold, flu, and other viruses
- Fear, anger, frustration, laughing too hard, crying, or an emotionally upsetting situation
- Smoke from cigarettes, cigars, and pipes (Don't smoke and don't stay in a room with people who do.)
- Fumes from perfume, cologne, and after-shave

(continued)

Avoiding asthma triggers *(continued)*

PREVENTIVE MEASURES

Remember to:
- drink enough fluids — six to eight glasses daily
- take all prescribed medications exactly as directed
- tell your health care provider about all medications you take — even nonprescription ones
- schedule only as much activity as you can tolerate, taking frequent breaks on busy days
- avoid sleeping pills or sedatives to help you sleep because of a mild asthma attack. These medications may slow down your breathing and make it more difficult. Instead, try propping yourself up on extra pillows while waiting for your antiasthma medication to work.

◯ Avoiding burnout: Aid for the caregiver

Dear Caregiver:

Caring for a person who needs full-time supervision and care makes you a prime candidate for burnout. Seemingly endless responsibilities can leave you feeling emotionally and physically drained, with virtually no time for yourself. If you feel inadequate to handle an unexpected crisis, you and the patient suffer.

How can you cope? Start by learning the warning signs of burnout so you'll know if you're reaching your physical and emotional limits. Ask yourself the following questions:

- Do I have trouble getting organized?
- Do I cry for no reason?
- Am I short-tempered?
- Do I feel numb and emotionless?
- Are everyday tasks getting harder to accomplish?
- Do I feel constantly pressed for time?
- Do I feel that I just can't do anything right?
- Do I feel that I have no time for myself?

If you answered "yes" to any of these questions, you're probably suffering from burnout or heading toward it. If so, the tips below will help you meet your own needs so you can give better patient care.

GET ENOUGH REST

Exhaustion magnifies pressures and reduces your ability to cope. The first step in combating burnout is getting a good night's sleep every night, if possible. Here's how:

- First, decide how much sleep you usually need — say 7 hours — and set aside this much time. Then when you go to bed, try not to replay the day in your mind. This isn't the time to solve problems.
- To help control disturbing thoughts, practice relaxation techniques, such as deep breathing, reading, or listening to soft music. Try dimming the bathroom lights and taking a warm bath or shower to relieve muscle tension and help you wind down.

- Strenuous activity earlier in the day (not near bedtime) can promote sleep by tiring you physically. It also increases your physical stamina, improves your self-image, brightens your outlook, and gets you out of the house.
- If possible, hire a relief caretaker so you can attend aerobics classes, go for a brisk walk, or get some kind of exercise for at least 1 hour three times per week. In addition, try to schedule three or four short breaks during the day.

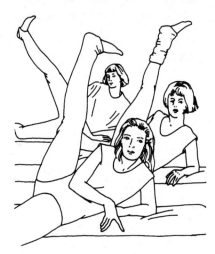

- Resting for 10 minutes with your feet up and your eyes closed can rejuvenate you and counteract the cycle of frantic activity that's probably keeping you up at night.
- Use sleeping pills or tranquilizers only as a last resort and only temporarily. These drugs have side effects that can cause more

(continued)

Avoiding burnout: Aid for the caregiver *(continued)*

problems for you in the long run. Instead, to induce drowsiness, try drinking a glass of warm milk.

EAT WELL

Eating regular, well-balanced meals helps you keep up your energy and increases your resistance to illness.

Skipping meals or eating on the run can cause vitamin and mineral deficiencies — such as anemia (a shortage of iron in the blood) — that deplete your strength and make you feel exhausted.

Choose foods from the five food groups every day, avoid empty calories and, unless you're overweight and your health care provider advises it, don't diet. You need increased calories to fuel your increased activity.

DON'T TRY TO BE SUPERHUMAN

After you've been giving home care for several weeks, reappraise your earlier plans. How much can you really do? How much time do you need for yourself?

Now delegate tasks. If possible, hire extra caretakers or someone to help with housework and shopping. Contact local support agencies for help. Send your laundry out. Remember that you don't have to do it all today, or accomplish everything on your list. Do only what's absolutely necessary, and learn to set priorities.

Remember to save some time for pleasurable activities. If you have 15 minutes of free time, listen to music or take a walk. If you want to have friends over for dinner, go ahead; just ask everyone to bring a course.

CONFIDE IN SOMEONE

A family member or close friend can help you resolve conflicts, be a sounding board for your anger and frustration, and offer emotional support. A support group can accomplish this and can offer practical hints for patient care.

SCHEDULE SOME QUALITY TIME ALONE

Free time won't happen automatically; you have to schedule it. In fact, your patient also needs time for himself. Allow yourself and your patient some personal space and private time. If you don't, you'll become too dependent on each other.

Try to keep your life as normal as possible. Continue to do things that you enjoy, either by yourself or with your friends. Remember: Meeting your own needs isn't selfish, even if the patient is homebound. If you continue to feel guilty about taking some time for yourself, go for counseling.

How much time alone is necessary? The answer depends on you. At the very least, you need to take the time to attend to your important personal needs, such as bathing, washing your hair, and dressing. You might want or need to have a part-time or full-time job. If so, arrange for a caregiver to take care of the patient while you're working away from home. Make sure that this arrangement fits your needs and your relationship with the patient.

Your goal is to provide the best quality of life for the patient without sacrificing your own. How you accomplish this is up to you. If you feel happy with the arrangement and the patient seems to be reasonably content, it's probably working.

⬭ Avoiding excessive bleeding

Dear Patient:
Because you have a tendency to bleed easily and for a longer time than normal, you may need to change your daily activities and modify your living habits. Observe these general do's and don'ts to help you function safely and avoid excessive bleeding.

DO'S	DON'TS
• Use an electric razor.	• Avoid shaving, cutting paper, or removing paint with a straight-edged razor blade.
• Wear gloves when washing dishes, raking, or gardening.	• Never go barefoot. Always protect your feet with shoes.
• Take your temperature only by mouth or ear.	• Avoid leaving knives, scissors, thumbtacks, or other sharp objects on countertops or tables where they could accidentally cut you. Store them in protective containers instead.
• Wear socks and shoes that fit properly. Footwear that's too large can cause abrasions; footwear that's too small can pinch the blood vessels in your feet.	
• Regularly check your urine, stool, and sputum for blood.	• Steer clear of contact sports and general roughhousing.
• Use a thimble while sewing on a button or stitching a hem.	• If possible, turn down intramuscular or subcutaneous injections.
• Wear a medical identification necklace or bracelet that identifies your bleeding disorder.	• Avoid plucking your eyebrows.
• Inform all health care workers of your condition before undergoing any procedure, including routine dental care.	• Reject substances that increase your risk of bleeding; for example, alcohol, nicotine, caffeine, or products containing aspirin or ibuprofen.
• Use a nasal spray containing normal saline solution or run a vaporizer to moisturize your breathing passages and prevent nosebleeds.	
• Use a soft toothbrush and floss gently unless advised otherwise.	
• Take stool softeners as needed. Eat sensibly to avoid constipation and subsequent straining and bleeding.	
• Keep your head elevated when lying down.	

⬭ Avoiding infection

Dear Patient:
If you have an increased risk of getting an infection, here are some simple steps you can take to protect yourself.

FOLLOW ALL DIRECTIONS

- Be sure to take all your medications exactly as prescribed. Don't stop taking your medication unless you're told to do so.
- Keep all medical appointments so your health care provider can monitor your progress and the drug's effects.
- If you need to go to another health care provider or to a dentist, tell them if you're receiving an immunosuppressant drug.
- Wear a medical identification tag or bracelet that says you're taking an immunosuppressant drug.

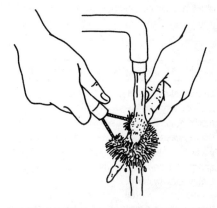

AVOID SOURCES OF INFECTION

- To minimize your exposure to infections, avoid crowds and people who have colds, the flu, chickenpox, shingles, or other contagious illnesses.
- Check with your health care provider before you get immunizations, especially livevirus vaccines. These contain weakened but living viruses that can cause illness in anyone who's taking an immunosuppressant drug. Also, avoid contact with anyone who has recently been vaccinated.
- Examine your mouth and skin daily for lesions, cuts, or rashes.
- Wash your hands thoroughly before preparing food. To avoid ingesting harmful organisms, thoroughly wash and cook all food before you eat it.

RECOGNIZE HAZARDS

- Learn to recognize and promptly report the early signs and symptoms of infection: sore throat, fever, chills, fatigue, and sluggishness. Call your health care provider immediately if you think you're coming down with an infection.
- Treat minor skin injuries with a triple antibiotic ointment such as Neosporin. If the injury is deep or becomes swollen, red, or tender, call your health care provider at once.

PERFORM ROUTINE HYGIENE

- Practice good oral and personal hygiene, especially hand washing. Report mouth sores or ulcerations.
- Don't use commercial mouthwashes if they have high alcohol and sugar content because they may irritate your mouth and promote bacterial growth.

◯ Calling for help during a myasthenic crisis

Dear Caregiver:

In a person with myasthenia gravis, the symptoms usually remain fairly well controlled. Sometimes, however, a person may require immediate medical attention if she experiences a sudden worsening of her condition. This may involve severe muscle weakness that affects her breathing. It's called a *myasthenic crisis.*

WHAT CAN TRIGGER A CRISIS?

Emotional stress, infection, surgery, or accidental injury can cause a crisis. A change in medicine or an overdose of medicine can also lead to extreme muscle weakness. Then if the weakness becomes severe enough, the person may experience a crisis that can involve many body systems.

IMPORTANT PHONE NUMBERS

Health care provider:

Hospital:

Police:

Keep these instructions in a handy place near the telephone.

WARNING SYMPTOMS

If the person in your care has *any* of the following symptoms — *especially if they occur within 1 hour after she takes her medicine* — seek immediate medical attention:

- blurred vision
- difficulty breathing
- difficulty chewing or swallowing
- difficulty speaking or pronouncing words
- inability to cough
- increased secretion of saliva
- twitching around the mouth or eyes
- nausea and vomiting
- pounding or fluttering heartbeat
- muscle spasms
- severe stomach cramps or diarrhea
- severe weakness in any muscle
- cold, moist skin and sweating
- extreme restlessness or anxiety
- confusion
- seizures
- fainting.

◯ Care and prevention of leg ulcers

Dear Patient:
You can help your leg ulcer heal and prevent new ulcers from forming by learning about your condition and its required care.

WHAT IS A LEG ULCER?

A leg ulcer is an area of dying skin. An ulcer can form wherever an artery becomes blocked or constricted. When this happens, not enough blood gets to the skin and the tissue beneath it to nourish the area. Instead, blood tends to pool in your leg veins — sometimes from a condition called *venous insufficiency.*

Pressure then builds up in these congested leg vessels, and the blood supply to the tissues decreases. As the condition worsens, the skin becomes fragile, and an infection may develop from injury, pressure, and irritation. As a result, leg ulcers may develop.

IMPROVING YOUR CIRCULATION

To improve circulation in your legs, wear elastic support stockings. Called *antiembolism stockings,* these hose will help to return blood to your heart. They'll improve circulation to your existing ulcer and may help to keep new ones from forming.

Put your feet up. Rest and elevate your legs for as long and as often as your health care provider directs. This will reduce your legs' needs for nutrients and oxygen and help to promote healing. Always raise your lower leg above heart level. Don't cross your legs.

PROMOTING HEALING

Follow these measures to help your ulcer heal:
● Keep your ulcer clean to prevent infection. Always wash your hands before and after changing your dressing or touching the wound. This keeps the area germ-free.
● Follow instructions exactly when changing your dressing and applying ointments or other medications.
● Be patient. Your ulcer may take 3 months to 1 year to heal.
● Inform your health care provider if your ulcer grows larger, feels increasingly painful, or becomes foul-smelling.

PREVENTING ULCERS

Follow these measures to prevent ulcers:
● Watch for signs and symptoms of new ulcers. These signs include leg swelling, pain, and discolored skin that looks brownish or dark blue.
● Wear support stockings to help prevent ulcers and to help heal existing ones.
● Be careful to avoid injury to your leg, which can lead to ulcer development. For example, avoid activities that involve rugged physical contact, such as roughhousing with children or dogs.
● Prevent falls by installing safety rails or a grab bar and placing a nonskid mat in your bathtub.
● Wear low, nonskid footwear whenever possible.

◯ Caring for your cast

Dear Patient:
Think of your new cast as a temporary body part — one that needs the same attentive care as the rest of you. While you wear your cast, follow these guidelines.

SPEEDING UP DRYING TIME

Your health care provider may apply a cast made of plaster, fiberglass, or a synthetic material. The wet material must dry thoroughly and evenly for the cast to support your broken bone properly. (At first, your wet cast will feel heavy and warm, but don't worry — it will get lighter as it dries.)

To speed drying, keep the cast exposed to the air. (Fiberglass and synthetic casts dry soon after application, but plaster casts don't. A plaster arm or leg cast dries in about 24 to 48 hours.)

When you raise the cast with pillows, make sure that the pillows have rubber or plastic covers under the linen case. Use a thin towel placed between the cast and the pillows to absorb moisture. Never place a wet cast directly onto plastic.

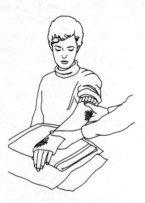

DRYING EVENLY

To make sure that the cast dries evenly, change its position on the pillows every 2 hours — using your palms, not your fingertips.

You can have someone else move the cast for you.

To avoid creating bumps inside the cast — bumps that could cause skin irritation or sores — don't poke at the cast with your fingers while it's wet. Also, be careful not to dent the cast while it's still wet.

KEEPING YOUR CAST CLEAN

After your cast dries, you can remove dirt and stains with a damp cloth and powdered kitchen cleaner. Use as little water as possible, and wipe off moisture that remains when you're done.

PROTECTING YOUR CAST

Avoid knocking your cast against a hard surface. To protect the foot of a leg cast from breakage, scrapes, and dirt, place a piece of used carpet (or a carpet square) over the bottom of the cast. Slash or cut a "V" shape at the back so the carpet fits around the heel when you bring it up toward the ankle.

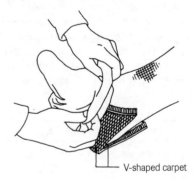

V-shaped carpet

(continued)

Caring for your cast *(continued)*

Hold the carpet in place with a large sock or slipper sock. Extending the carpet out beyond the toes a little will also help prevent bumped or stubbed toes.

PREVENTING SNAGS

To keep an arm cast from snagging clothing and furniture, make a cast cover from an old nylon stocking. Cut the stocking's toe off, and cut a hole in the heel.

Then pull the stocking over the cast to cover it.

Extend your fingers through the cut-off toe end, and poke your thumb through the hole you cut in the heel. Trim the other end of the stocking to about $1\frac{1}{2}''$ (4 cm) longer than the cast, and tuck the ends of the stocking under the cast's edges.

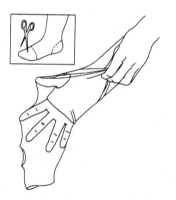

CARING FOR YOUR SKIN

Wash the skin along the cast's edges every day, using a mild soap. Before you begin, protect the cast's edges with plastic wrap. Then use a washcloth wrung out in soapy water to clean the skin at the cast's edges and as far as you can reach inside the cast. Avoid getting the cast wet. Afterward, dry the skin thoroughly with a towel. Then massage the

skin at and beneath the cast's edges with a towel or pad saturated with rubbing alcohol. This helps toughen the skin. To help prevent skin irritation, remove loose plaster particles you can reach inside the cast.

RELIEVING ITCHING

No matter how itchy the skin under your cast may feel, never try to relieve the itch by inserting a sharp or pointed object into the cast. This could damage your skin and lead to infection. Also don't put powder or lotion in your cast or stuff cotton or toilet tissue under the cast's edges. This may reduce your circulation.

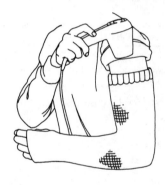

Here's a safe technique to relieve itching. Set a handheld blow-dryer on "cool," and aim it at the problem area.

STAYING DRY

If you have a plaster cast, you'll need to cover it with a plastic bag before you shower, swim, or go out in wet weather. You can use a garbage bag or a cast shower bag, which you can buy at a drugstore or medical supply store. Above all, *don't get a plaster cast wet.*

(continued)

Caring for your cast　*(continued)*

Moisture will weaken or even destroy it. If the cast gets a little wet, let it dry naturally, such as by sitting in the sun.

Don't cover the cast until it's dry. If you have a fiberglass or synthetic cast, check with your health care provider to find out if you may bathe, shower, or swim. If he does allow you to swim, he'll probably tell you to flush the cast with cool tap water after swimming in a chlorinated pool or a lake. Make sure that no foreign material remains trapped inside the cast. To dry a fiberglass or synthetic cast, first wrap the cast in a towel. Then prop it on a pad of towels to absorb remaining water. The cast will air-dry in 3 to 4 hours; to speed dry it, use a handheld blow-dryer.

SIGNING THE CAST

Family members and friends may want to sign their names or draw pictures on the cast. That's okay, but don't let them paint over large cast areas because this could make those areas nonporous and damage the skin underneath.

⌣ Caring for your hair and scalp during cancer treatment

Dear Patient:

Some hair loss is inevitable during chemotherapy or radiation therapy. But sometimes you can help minimize hair loss by keeping your hair and scalp clean and treating them gently. Just follow these suggestions.

IF YOU'RE HAVING CHEMOTHERAPY

- Shampoo regularly — every 2 to 4 days. (Shampooing every day may be too harsh.)
- Use a mild *protein-based* shampoo — for example, Appearance, an apple pectin shampoo. (Baby shampoo isn't necessarily mild.) You may want to talk with a hairdresser to determine which shampoo is best for you.

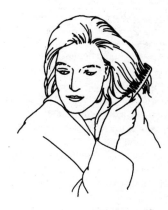

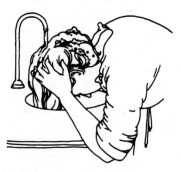

- Use a conditioner after shampooing.
- Gently pat your hair dry.
- If your scalp is very dry and flaky, try massaging it with mineral oil, castor oil, or vitamin A and D ointment after shampooing and rinsing your hair.
- Brush and comb your hair very gently, using a soft-bristled brush and a pliable, wide-toothed comb.
- Avoid harsh chemicals, permanents, and dyes. Also avoid tight curls or braids. Don't use a curling iron, hair dryer, or hot rollers. And don't sleep with curlers in your hair.

- To minimize friction on your hair, try sleeping on a satin pillowcase. And to keep your hair from shedding, try using a hair net.
- Wear a hat to protect your scalp from sunburn.

IF YOU'RE HAVING RADIATION THERAPY

- Don't use anything on your scalp except Eucerin or Aquaphor cream. You can buy these products at your local pharmacy without a prescription.
- When your hair starts to grow back, follow the hair and scalp care instructions listed above.

○ Caring for your nephrostomy tube

Dear Patient:

A nephrostomy tube allows urine to drain from your kidney into a drainage bag. This bag is attached to the tube's free end with a length of tubing. Because the nephrostomy tube goes directly into your kidney, you'll need to take proper care of the tubing and bag each day to prevent infection.

HOW TO CHANGE THE TUBING AND DRAINAGE BAG

1. Gather your equipment: a clean drainage bag, connecting tube, and alcohol swabs. Wash your hands.

Important: Always keep the drainage bag lower than the nephrostomy tube.

2. Disconnect the nephrostomy tube from the used tubing and drainage bag. Don't use your fingernails to disconnect the tubing. Clean the end of the nephrostomy tube with an alcohol swab. Also clean the end of the tubing that connects the new drainage bag to the nephrostomy tube.

3. Attach the ends of the nephrostomy tube and the connecting tube securely. Don't touch the end of either tube. Check the tubing periodically for kinks.

HOW TO CLEAN THE BAG AND TUBING

1. Wash the used bag and tubing with a weak detergent solution daily. Avoid a biodegradable or chlorine product because it may erode the bag.

2. Twice weekly, wash the bag and tubing with a weak vinegar solution (one part vinegar and three parts water) to prevent crystalline buildup. Rinse the bag and tubing with plain water and hang them on a clothes hanger to air-dry.

HOW TO CHANGE THE DRESSING

Change the dressing daily as your health care provider orders.

1. Gather the necessary equipment: absorbent powder, sterile gauze pads, and adhesive tape. Then wash your hands and remove the old dressing.

2. Gently wash around the tube with soap and water. Inspect the skin around the tube. Is redness present? If so, apply absorbent powder.

If you notice white, yellow, or green drainage, with or without odor, suspect infection, and report it to your health care provider. If you see drainage that looks or smells like urine, the tube may be displaced. Report this to your health care provider.

3. Next, fold several sterile gauze pads in half and place them around the tube's base. Cover with an unfolded gauze pad. Apply adhesive tape to secure the gauze pads to your skin. If your skin is sensitive, you can use a protective barrier wipe or a skin preparation under the tape.

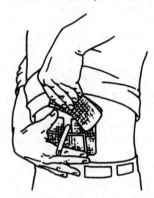

⬭ Caring for your urinary catheter

Dear Patient:
Your catheter is a tube that will continually drain urine from your bladder so you won't need to urinate. To care for your catheter, follow these guidelines.

EMPTY THE DRAINAGE BAG

How often? Usually, every 4 to 8 hours will do. First, unclamp the drainage tube and remove it from its sleeve, without touching the tip.

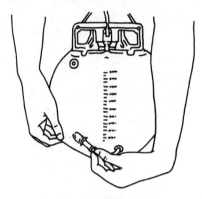

Then let the urine drain into the toilet or into a measuring container, if required. When the bag is completely empty, clean the end of the drainage tube with an alcohol swab.

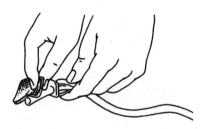

Reclamp the tube and reinsert it into the sleeve of the drainage bag.

To maintain good drainage from the catheter, frequently check the drainage tubing for kinks and loops. Never disconnect the catheter from the drainage tubing for any reason.

Also, keep the drainage bag below your bladder level, whether you're lying down, sitting, or standing.

CARE FOR YOUR SKIN

Use soap and water to wash the area around your catheter twice per day.

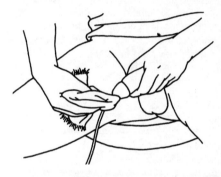

Also wash your rectal area twice per day and after each bowel movement.

Periodically check the skin around the catheter for signs of irritation, such as redness, tenderness, or swelling.

REPORT PROBLEMS EARLY

Contact your health care provider immediately if you have problems, such as urine leakage around the catheter, pain and fullness in your abdomen, scanty urine flow, or blood in your urine.

Above all, *never* pull on your catheter or try to remove it yourself.

◯ **Catheterizing yourself: For men**

Dear Patient:
Follow these instructions to perform catheterization:

1. Gather the equipment: catheter, lubricant (water-soluble), basin for collecting urine, clean washcloth, soap and water, paper towels, and plastic bag. Then wash your hands thoroughly. During the procedure, touch only the catheter equipment to avoid spreading germs.

2. Wash your penis and the surrounding area with soap and water. Be sure to pull the foreskin back while cleaning. Then pat dry.

3. Open the tube of lubricant and squeeze a generous amount onto a paper towel. Then roll the first 7″ to 10″ (18 to 25 cm) of the catheter in the lubricant.

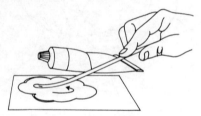

4. Put one end of the catheter in the basin or toilet. Hold your penis at a right angle to your body, grasp the catheter as you would a pencil, and slowly insert it into the urethra. If you meet resistance, breathe deeply. As you inhale, continue advancing the catheter 7″ to 10″ until urine begins to flow. Allow all urine to drain into the basin or toilet.

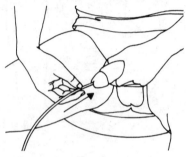

5. If the catheter isn't disposable and you plan to reuse it, boil it in water for 20 minutes and then wrap it in a clean cloth until the next use.

⬭ Catheterizing yourself: For women

Dear Patient:
Follow these instructions to perform catheterization:

1. Gather the equipment: catheter (preferably disposable), lubricant (water-soluble), basin, clean washcloth, soap and water, paper towels, and plastic bag. Then wash your hands thoroughly. During the procedure, be sure to touch only the catheter equipment to avoid spreading germs.

2. Separate the folds of your vulva with one hand and, using the washcloth, thoroughly clean the area between your legs with warm water and mild soap. Use downward strokes (front to back) to avoid contaminating the area with fecal matter. Now, pat the area dry with a towel.

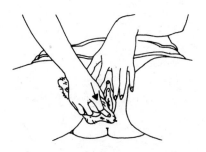

3. Open the lubricant and squeeze a generous amount onto a paper towel. Then roll the first 3" (7.6 cm) of the catheter in it.

4. Spread the lips of the vulva with one hand, and, using the other hand, insert the catheter in an upward and backward direction about 3" into the urethra (located above the vagina). You may need a mirror to help you see better. If you meet resistance, breathe deeply. As you inhale, advance the catheter, angling it upward slightly. Stop when urine begins to drain from it. Allow all urine to drain into the toilet.

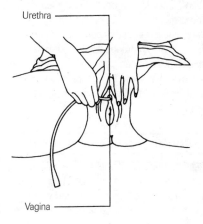

Urethra

Vagina

5. If the catheter isn't disposable and you plan to reuse it, boil it in water for 20 minutes and then wrap it in a clean cloth until the next use.

◯ Choosing iron-rich foods

Dear Patient:

Although many everyday foods contain large amounts of iron, your body typically absorbs only a small portion of it. Therefore, you'll need to choose foods that contain lots of iron. However, which ones should you choose? First, pick foods from all of the four major groups: milk and dairy, meat, bread and cereal, and fruit and vegetable. Then modify the amount from each group by considering your other dietary needs. For instance, if you need to cut back on cholesterol, don't pick liver.

SELECT WISELY

Keep in mind that the iron in grains and vegetables isn't absorbed as readily as the iron in meat, fish, and poultry. On the other hand, eating meat, fish, or poultry *along with* grains and vegetables increases iron absorption. So does eating a food that contains vitamin C — for example, an orange, tomato, or potato. In fact, eating a tomato with a hamburger quadruples iron absorption. (On the other hand, drinking tea with the same meal lowers iron absorption.)

KNOW HOW MUCH IRON YOU NEED

Recommended amounts are 15 milligrams per day for women age 50 and younger and 10 milligrams per day for men and women older than age 50. Your health care provider will tell you exactly how much iron you should consume. Consult the chart at right to find the foods highest in iron.

FOOD	QUANTITY	IRON (Mg)
Oysters	3 ounces	13.2
Beef liver	3 ounces	7.5
Prune juice	½ cup	5.2
Clams	2 ounces	4.2
Walnuts	½ cup	3.75
Ground beef	3 ounces	3
Chickpeas	½ cup	3
Bran flakes	½ cup	2.8
Pork roast	3 ounces	2.7
Cashew nuts	½ cup	2.65
Shrimp	3 ounces	2.6
Raisins	½ cup	2.55
Navy beans	½ cup	2.55
Sardines	3 ounces	2.5
Spinach	½ cup	2.4
Lima beans	½ cup	2.3
Kidney beans	½ cup	2.2
Turkey, dark meat	3 ounces	2
Prunes	½ cup	1.9
Roast beef	3 ounces	1.8
Green peas	½ cup	1.5
Peanuts	½ cup	1.5
Potato	1	1.1
Sweet potatoes	½ cup	1
Green beans	½ cup	1
Egg	1	1
Turkey, light meat	3 ounces	1

◯ Choosing the right wheelchair

Dear Patient:

To help maintain your mobility and independence, a health care professional has ordered a wheelchair for you. Depending on your condition, you may use the wheelchair for all or part of the day.

Choose your wheelchair as carefully as you would a new car. Wheelchairs come in two types — standard, which is suitable if you have some shoulder motion and upper body strength, and motorized, which is recommended if your arms and hands are weak. Both types combine many optional features to meet your special needs. Before you decide, consult your health care provider or physical therapist for suggestions and ask yourself the following questions.

IS THE CHAIR THE RIGHT SIZE?

First, check to make sure that the seat is wide and deep enough to support your thighs and allow you to sit comfortably. The seat should be low enough so that your feet touch the floor, but high enough so you can transfer easily from your bed to the chair. Next, check to see if the chair's back is tall enough to support your upper body. Consider adding an adapter to the back of the seat to support your head and neck.

WILL THE CHAIR MEET YOUR NEEDS?

You'll need a wheelchair that's easy to operate when you're weak. For instance, to compensate for upper body weakness, you may want a wheelchair with a semireclining back or a higher backrest for more support and comfort.

Think about a motorized wheelchair if you have little or no arm strength. These chairs operate in several ways — for example, by a toggle switch, a mouthpiece, or a chin control. A wheelchair with a toggle switch is hand controlled — you simply push the switch in the direction you want to move. A mouthpiece control allows you to propel the wheelchair by blowing into a tube that connects from your mouth to the motor. A chin control lets you use your chin to push a lever in the direction you want to move.

IS THE CHAIR SAFE?

All wheelchairs have safety features such as brakes that lock the wheels while you transfer to and from your bed or car. Some safety features can be modified for your special needs; for example, seatbelts can be attached at the waist, hip, or chest.

You may also want a chair with removable or swing-away footrests to help you transfer safely from the chair to your bed or car.

DOES IT SUIT YOUR LIFESTYLE?

If you spend a lot of time outdoors, you may want a wheelchair with pneumatic tires that let you maneuver more easily over soft or uneven ground. If you work at a low desk or table, consider fitting the chair with desk arms or adjustable armrests.

⬭ Controlling an asthma attack

Dear Patient:

Usually, an asthma attack is preceded by warning signs that give you time to take action. Stay alert for:

- chest tightness
- coughing
- awareness of your breathing
- wheezing.

After you've had a few asthma attacks, you'll have no trouble recognizing these early warning signs. Above all, *don't ignore them.* Instead, follow these steps:

1. Take your prescribed medicine with an oral inhaler, if directed, to prevent the attack from getting worse.

2. As your medicine starts to work, try to relax. Although you may be understandably nervous or afraid, remember that these feelings only increase your shortness of breath.

breath. Then relax these muscles and repeat this exercise with the muscles in your arms and hands, legs, and feet. Finally, let your body go limp.

3. Regain control of your breathing by doing the pursed-lip breathing exercises you've been taught. *Don't gasp for air.* Continue pursed-lip breathing until you no longer feel breathless.

4. If the attack triggers a coughing spell, you'll need to control your cough so that it effectively brings up mucus and helps clear your airways. To do so, lean forward slightly, keeping your feet on the floor. Next, breathe in deeply and hold that breath for a second or two. Cough twice, first to loosen mucus and then to bring it up. Be sure to cough into a tissue.

5. If, even after you've followed these steps, the attack gets worse, call your health care provider right away.

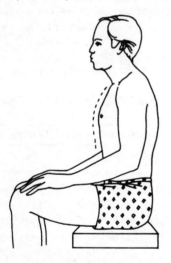

To help relax, sit upright in a chair, close your eyes, and breathe slowly and evenly. Then begin consciously tightening and relaxing the muscles in your body. First, tighten the muscles in your face and count to yourself: one-1,000; two-1,000. Be sure not to hold your

⬭ Controlling the side effects of chemotherapy

Dear Patient:
Your health care provider has ordered chemotherapy to treat your cancer. In addition to treating cancer, these therapies commonly cause unpleasant side effects. Fortunately, you can sometimes prevent or minimize them. Other times you can do things to make yourself more comfortable. Just follow the advice below.

MOUTH SORES

• Keep your mouth and teeth clean by brushing after every meal with a soft toothbrush.
• Don't use commercial mouthwashes that contain alcohol because they may irritate your mouth during chemotherapy. Instead, rinse with water or water mixed with baking soda, or use a suspension of sucralfate (Carafate), if directed. Floss daily, and apply fluoride if your dentist recommends it. If you have dentures, be sure to remove them often for cleaning.
• Until your mouth sores heal, avoid foods that are difficult to chew, such as apples, or irritating to your mouth, such as acidic citrus juices. Also avoid drinking alcohol, smoking, and eating extremely hot or spicy foods.
• Eat soft, bland foods, such as eggs and oatmeal, and soothing foods, such as popsicles. Your health care provider might also prescribe medication for mouth sores.

DRY MOUTH

• Frequently sip cool liquids and suck on ice chips or sugarless candy.
• Inquire about artificial saliva. Use water, juices, sauces, and dressings to soften your food and make it easier to swallow. Don't smoke or drink alcohol, which can further dry your mouth.

NAUSEA AND VOMITING

• Before a chemotherapy treatment, try eating a light, bland snack, such as toast or crackers. Or don't eat anything — some patients find that fasting controls nausea better.
• Keep unpleasant odors out of your dining area. Avoid strong-smelling foods. Also, brush your teeth before eating to refresh your mouth.
• Eat small, frequent meals and avoid lying down for 2 hours after you eat. Try small amounts of clear, unsweetened liquids, such as apple juice, and then progress to crackers or dry toast. Stay away from sweets and fried or other high-fat foods. It's best to eat bland foods.
• Take antiemetic drugs as prescribed. Be sure to report severe or persistent vomiting (lasting longer than 24 hours), less frequent urination, weakness, or dry mouth.

DIARRHEA

• Eat low-fiber foods, such as bananas, rice, applesauce, toast, or mashed potatoes. Avoid high-fiber foods, such as raw vegetables and fruits and whole-grain breads. Also avoid milk products and fruit juices. Cabbage, coffee, beans, and sweets can increase stomach cramps.
• Because potassium may be lost when you have diarrhea, eat high-potassium foods, such as bananas and potatoes. You may need a potassium supplement.

(continued)

Controlling the side effects
of chemotherapy *(continued)*

- After a bowel movement, clean your anal area gently and apply petroleum jelly (Vaseline) to prevent soreness.
- Inquire about antidiarrheal medications. Report persistent diarrhea, less frequent urination, dry mouth, or weakness.

CONSTIPATION

- Eat high-fiber foods unless directed otherwise. They include raw fruits and vegetables (with skins and washed well), whole-grain breads and cereals, and beans. If you aren't used to eating high-fiber foods, start gradually to let your body get accustomed to the change — or else you could develop diarrhea.
- Drink plenty of liquids unless directed not to.
- If changing your diet doesn't help, inquire about stool softeners or laxatives. Check with your health care provider before using enemas.

HEARTBURN

- Avoid spicy foods, alcohol, and smoking. Eat small, frequent meals.
- After eating, don't lie down right away. Avoid bending or stooping.
- Take oral medications with a glass of milk or a snack.
- Use antacids as your health care provider orders.

MUSCLE ACHES OR PAIN, WEAKNESS, NUMBNESS, OR TINGLING

- Take acetaminophen (Tylenol) or acetaminophen with codeine as directed.
- Apply heat where it hurts or feels numb.

- Report symptoms that don't go away and pain that focuses on one area.
- Be sure to rest. Also, avoid activities that aggravate your symptoms.

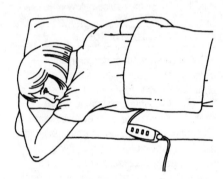

HAIR LOSS

- Wash your hair gently with a mild shampoo, and avoid frequent brushing or combing.
- Get a short haircut to make thinning hair less noticeable.
- Consider wearing a wig or toupee during therapy. Buy one before your chemotherapy

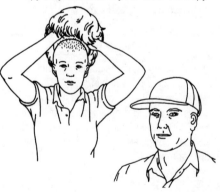

(continued)

Controlling the side effects
of chemotherapy *(continued)*

begins. You can also use a hat, scarf, or tur-
ban to cover your head during therapy.

SKIN PROBLEMS

- For sensitive or dry skin, inquire about the
most effective lotion.
- Use cornstarch to absorb moisture, and
avoid tight clothing over the treatment area.
Be sure to report blisters or cracked skin.
- Stay out of the sun during the course of
therapy. You may have to avoid the sun for
several months afterward, especially if you're
planning a vacation to a sunny area. When
you can go out in the sun, wear light clothes
over the treated area and wear a hat. Cover
all exposed skin with a strong sunblock lotion (skin protection factor 15 or above).

TIREDNESS

- Limit activities, especially sports.
- Get more sleep.
- Try to reduce your work hours until the
end of treatments. Discuss your therapy
schedule with your employer.
- If possible, schedule chemotherapy treatments at your convenience.
- Ask for help from your family and friends,
whether it's pitching in with daily chores or
driving you to the hospital. Most people are
glad to help out — they just need to be
asked.
- If you lose interest in sex during treatments, either because you're too tired or because of hormonal changes, bear in mind
that sexual desire usually returns after the
treatments end.

RISK OF INFECTION

You're more likely to get an infection during
therapy, so follow these tips:
- Avoid crowds and people with colds and
infections.
- Use a soft toothbrush. It will help you
avoid injuring your gums—a frequent site of
infection.

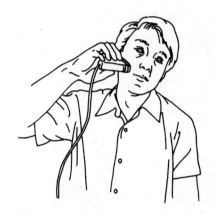

- Use an electric shaver instead of a razor.
- Report fever, chills, bruising, or unusual
bleeding.

⬭ Coping with a fall from a wheelchair

Dear Patient:
Despite all the safety features you have chosen for your wheelchair, you can still fall. As long as you have strength and movement in your arms and upper body, you probably can return to your chair without help.

SURVEY THE ROOM

Look around for a low, sturdy piece of furniture, such as a coffee table, that you can use for support.

MOVE TOWARD THE WHEELCHAIR

Place your hands, palms down, beside your hips. Push down with your hands and lift your buttocks off the floor. Inch yourself toward the chair. As you get closer to it, grasp the armrest.

POSITION YOURSELF

Position yourself at the table's opposite side with your back to the table. Now, reach back and place both hands on the table. Push down and lift your buttocks off the floor and onto the table. Then slide back on the table so your back faces the front of the wheelchair.

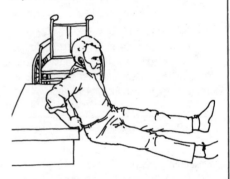

GET INTO THE WHEELCHAIR

Now, reach back and place your hands on the wheelchair's seat. Push down with both hands, and lift yourself onto the chair. Then slide back into the seat and position yourself comfortably.

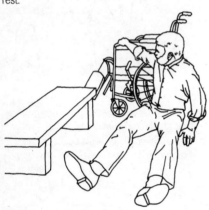

POSITION THE WHEELCHAIR

Now unlock the wheelchair's brakes, if necessary. Then inch your way over to the coffee table, pushing or pulling the wheelchair with you.

When you reach the table, move the footrests aside and position the wheelchair so the front of the seat faces the table. *Lock the wheelchair's brakes.*

⬭ Cutting down on cholesterol

Dear Patient:

By changing your diet, you can help lower your cholesterol level and ensure better health. You also need to reduce the amount of saturated fats you eat. This means cutting down drastically on eggs, dairy products, and fatty meats. Rely instead on poultry, fish, fruits, vegetables, and high-fiber breads.

Use this list as a basis for your new diet. If you do a lot of home baking, adapt your recipes by using modest amounts of unsaturated oils. Remember that one whole egg can be replaced with two egg whites.

FOOD	ELIMINATE	SUBSTITUTE
Bread and cereals	Breads with whole eggs listed as a major ingredient	Oatmeal, multigrain, and bran cereal; whole-grain breads; and rye bread
	Egg noodles	Pasta and rice
	Pies, cakes, doughnuts, biscuits, and high-fat crackers and cookies	Angel food cake, low-fat cookies, crackers, and home-baked goods
Eggs and dairy products	Whole milk, 2% milk, and imitation milk	Fat-free milk, 1% milk, buttermilk
	Cream, half-and-half, most nondairy creamers, and whipped toppings	Low-fat or nonfat whipped cream, evaporated fat-free milk, and light cream
	Whole-milk yogurt and cottage cheese	Nonfat or low-fat yogurt and cottage cheese
	Cheese, cream cheese, sour cream, light cream cheese, and light sour cream	Cholesterol-free sour cream alternative and fat-free cream cheese
	Egg yolks	Egg whites
	Ice cream	Sherbet, frozen tofu, fat-free frozen yogurt, and popsicles
Fats and oils	Coconut, palm, and palm kernel oils and oils that have been hydrogenated or partially hydrogenated	Unsaturated vegetable oils (corn, olive, canola, safflower, sesame, soybean, and sunflower)
	Butter, lard, and bacon fat	Unsaturated margarine and shortening and diet margarine
	Dressings made with egg yolks	Mayonnaise and unsaturated or low-fat salad dressings
	Chocolate	Baking cocoa
Meat, fish, and poultry	Fatty cuts of beef, lamb, or pork	Lean cuts of beef, lamb, or pork
	Organ meats, spare ribs, cold cuts, sausage, hot dogs, and bacon	Poultry
	Sardines and roe	Sole, salmon, and mackerel

◯ Cutting down on salt

Dear Patient:
Your health care provider may recommend cutting down on salt because too much salt can affect your health. Reducing your salt intake isn't hard to do. The following information and suggestions will help you get started.

FACTS ABOUT SALT

- Table salt is about 40% sodium.
- Americans consume about 20 times more salt than their bodies need.
- About three-fourths of the salt you consume is already in the foods you eat and drink.
- One teaspoon of salt contains about 2 grams of sodium.
- You can reduce your intake to one teaspoon per day simply by not salting your food during cooking or before eating.

TIPS FOR REDUCING SALT INTAKE

Reducing your salt intake to a teaspoon or less per day is easy if you:
- read labels on medications and foods.
- put away your salt shaker or, if you must use salt, use "light salt," which contains half the sodium of ordinary table salt.
- buy fresh meats, fruits, and vegetables instead of canned, processed, and convenience foods.
- substitute spices and lemon juice for salt.
- watch out for sources of hidden sodium — for example, carbonated beverages, nondairy creamers, cookies, and cakes.
- avoid salty foods, such as bacon, sausage, pretzels, potato chips, mustard, pickles, and some cheeses.

KNOW YOUR SODIUM SOURCES

Canned, prepared, and fast foods are loaded with sodium; so are condiments such as ketchup. Some foods that don't taste salty contain high amounts of sodium. Consider the values below.

FOOD	SODIUM CONTENT (IN MG)
2½ ounces dried chipped beef	3,052
1 teaspoon salt	1,955
1 cup canned spaghetti	1,236
3 ounces lean ham	1,128
1 dill pickle	928
1 can tomato soup	872
1 slice pepperoni pizza	817
1 cheeseburger	709
1 hot dog	639
1 cup corn flakes	256
1 tablespoon ketchup	156

Other high-sodium sources include baking powder, baking soda, barbecue sauce, bouillon cubes, celery salt, chili sauce, cooking wine, garlic salt, onion salt, softened water, and soy sauce.

Surprisingly, many medications and other nonfood items contain sodium, such as alkalizers for indigestion, laxatives, aspirin, cough medication, mouthwash, and toothpaste. Be sure to note which medications you're taking. If you're unsure of their sodium content, ask your pharmacist.

⬭ Dietary do's and don'ts for cirrhosis

Dear Patient:
Because you have cirrhosis, you need to pay special attention to your diet. Healthful eating habits will help damaged liver cells regenerate and prevent harm to the remaining cells. Follow this list of do's and don'ts when planning your daily meals.

Do's

- Ask your health care provider or dietitian for help in planning your diet. They can advise you about how many calories you need and how to best meet your nutritional requirements. If you're used to eating fast foods, they can help you choose the most nutritious items on a fast-food menu.
- Eat small, frequent meals. Instead of the traditional three meals, try eating five or six lighter ones. This may relieve the bloated or sick feeling that cirrhosis can cause.
- Keep a food diary. After each meal, write down the foods you ate, the time of day, and how you feel.

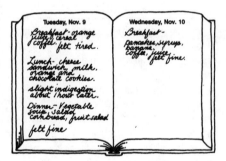

After a week, study your food diary for patterns. For example, did certain foods disagree with you? If so, avoid them. What time of day were you hungriest? Plan to eat your biggest meal then. Use the diary to make smarter choices about what and when to eat.

- Weigh yourself daily and keep a chart. If your weight goes up more than 5 lb, call your health care provider — you may be retaining fluid.
- Set an attractive table. To perk up your appetite, use nice tableware, add a colorful garnish to your plate, and set an appropriate mood with relaxing music or conversation.

Don'ts

- Avoid drinking alcoholic beverages, even occasionally. Alcohol destroys liver cells, so abstain completely.
- Stay away from coffee and tea. Avoid all caffeine-containing beverages and foods, which can cause indigestion.
- Steer clear of spicy foods, which may upset your stomach.
- Eliminate salt while cooking and don't salt your food heavily. Too much salt may make you retain fluid. Ask your health care provider if you should follow a special salt-restricted diet.
- Don't go on a quick-weight-loss diet. If you've gained weight because of fluid buildup in your body, eating less won't help you. Remember, good nutrition is essential to repair your liver.

Diet-conscious tips for dining out

Dear Patient:
When you're trying to lose weight or maintain your ideal weight, dining out may pose a dilemma. It doesn't have to. Just keep these tips in mind.

PLAN AHEAD

If you can, check the restaurant's menu a day or two before you eat there so you'll know your choices. If the menu doesn't list anything you want, choose another restaurant.

Before you leave home, eat raw vegetables or an apple to take the edge off your appetite. That way you'll be less inclined to overeat.

CHOOSE HEALTHFUL FOODS

Select an entrée of broiled, poached, or steamed (rather than sautéed or fried) chicken or fish, or choose pasta (with sauce on the side). If you want beef, order a lean cut. Because most restaurant portions are at least 6 ounces, eat only half of what you're served. Your portion should be no larger than a deck of cards. You can ask to take the other half home.

Complement the entrée with a baked or boiled potato and a salad. Choose fresh fruit, sherbet, or angel food cake for dessert. If you're very hungry, have clear soup or raw vegetables as an appetizer.

Choose a calorie-free dinner beverage, such as seltzer, water, black coffee, or tea, and limit yourself to one cocktail. Better yet, avoid alcohol entirely. Its effects may undermine your willpower.

SKIP FATTY FOODS

Trim visible fat from meats. Add little or no margarine to your baked potato. Stay away from gravies and cream sauces. Ask for salad dressing to be served on the side so you can control the amount you use, or create your own with vinegar or lemon juice and oil.

At salad bars, watch out for calorie-packed toppings, such as bacon, nuts, croutons, and cheese.

BE FIRM

Tell the waiter you're dieting. Ask him to recommend dishes that are prepared without butter, oil, or sauces. Remember, many people are health- and diet-conscious, and your waiter is probably accustomed to such requests. Don't hesitate to return food that isn't prepared the way you asked. After all, you're paying for the meal.

SPECIAL TIPS

● Think twice before you order such "diet platters" as a hamburger and a scoop of cottage cheese. These foods are loaded with fat and calories.

● If you wish to cut down on portion sizes, choose an appetizer as the main course, order a la carte, or share food with a companion.

● Don't rush through your meal. Your brain doesn't know you're full until about 20 minutes after you really are. Eating slowly allows you time to feel full without overeating.

● If you do decide to splurge, don't blame yourself. Just go back to your diet and avoid the temptation to continue overeating.

⬭ Dressing with confidence after a mastectomy

Dear Patient:

Now that your operation is over, you can begin dealing with everyday concerns. One concern may be your wardrobe. Your clothes may not fit or look the way they did before your surgery. Don't be discouraged. You can look just as fashionable after a mastectomy as before. Just summon up your creativity — everyone has some — and select a few new styles.

Maybe you'll look for comfort, maybe for flair. Whatever you look for, here are some tips to consider.

CHOOSE LOOSE, UNCONSTRICTING STYLES

- Choose soft, medium-weight fabrics that don't cling.
- Look for textured or patterned materials, which reveal less.
- Soften your line by selecting blouses and dresses with pleats, tucks, and gathers at the shoulder or neckline.
- Avoid form-fitting garments tailored with bust darts.

DIVERT THE FASHION FOCUS

- Create an optical illusion with asymmetrical, diagonal, or vertical prints to make differences less obvious.
- Look for curved lines if you want a more feminine look.
- Select a garment with sleeves that provide comfort but look decorative.
- Choose necklines that focus your attention on your face. Avoid deep "V" or scooped necklines.
- Accessorize. Add spice and color with scarves, jewelry, and belts.
- Look for swimwear that highlights the waist, hips, or the shoulder of your unaffected side. (Avoid bare shoulders.) High necklines, asymmetrical or wide shoulder straps, and blouson tops add fashion variety.

SHOP IN SPECIALTY STORES

Some women's shops carry clothing and prostheses especially for women who have had mastectomies. Or join the millions of catalog and Internet shoppers. Some clothing manufacturers make garments especially for women with mastectomies.

◯ Examining your skin

Dear Patient:

It's a good idea to examine your skin every month because persistent sun exposure or photo-sensitivity reactions can lead to skin cancer. Report suspicious-looking changes in the size, texture, or color of a mole or sore that doesn't heal to your health care provider. Detected early, most skin cancers are curable.

Check your skin right after a bath or shower. Stand before a full-length mirror in a well-lighted room. Keep a small mirror handy for seeing behind you and for examining hard-to-see spots. Note freckles, moles, blemishes, and birthmarks, remembering where they are and what they look like. Then proceed:

3. Examine your legs, checking the fronts, backs, and sides. Look between your buttocks and around the genital area.

4. Next, move close to the mirror to look carefully at your neck, face, lips, eyes, ears, nose, and scalp. Part your hair with a comb to see better.

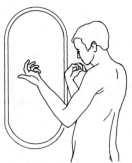

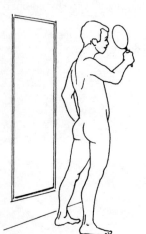

5. Now, sit down. Bend your knees to bring your feet close to you. Examine your soles, insteps, ankles, and between your toes.

1. Standing unclothed in front of the mirror, check the front of your body. Turn to each side and look over your shoulder to see behind you. Also use your hand mirror. Then lift your arms and examine the sides of your body.

2. Inspect your arms and hands. Check the backs of your hands, your palms, your fingers, and both sides of your forearms and upper arms.

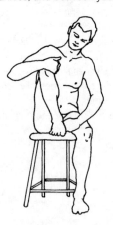

◯ **Exercising safely**

Dear Patient:
The following tips will help you to exercise safely. Remember that your goal is to pace yourself, not to overdo it. Consistency is most important, no matter which activity you enjoy.

WHAT YOU SHOULD DO

If you've been inactive for a long time, check with your health care provider before starting your exercise program, and return to exercise gradually. Take part in fitness activities, such as walking and swimming, rather than competitive sports such as tennis.

Wait 2 to 3 hours after a heavy meal before exercising. A light snack warrants a 1- to 2-hour wait. Also, avoid hot or cold showers immediately before and after exertion.

Wear comfortable, lightweight clothing and shoes with adequate support. Dress in layers and remove articles of clothing as you warm up.

Be sure to drink water before, during, and after exercising.

WHAT YOU SHOULDN'T DO

Don't exercise in extreme heat or cold, windy weather, high humidity, or heavy pollution or at high altitudes. Don't exercise if you have a fever or if you don't feel well.

WHEN TO SLOW DOWN

You may be exercising too hard if you have chest pain, muscle cramps, a side stitch, or excessive shortness of breath or fatigue. Slow down.

WHEN TO STOP EXERCISING

Stop exercising and check with your health care provider immediately if you experience chest pain, a cold sweat, dizziness, nausea or vomiting, heart palpitations or fluttering, unusual shortness of breath, or an abnormal heart rhythm.

Gaining mobility with portable oxygen equipment

Dear Patient:

Special equipment may offer you greater freedom of movement while you're breathing extra oxygen. For instance, a portable liquid oxygen unit or portable oxygen tank will let you move around freely and leave your home. A wheeled carrier or extension tubing for your regular equipment will allow for a greater range of movement inside your home. Use these guidelines, along with specific manufacturer's instructions, to operate portable oxygen equipment.

CHECKING THE OXYGEN SUPPLY

A portable liquid oxygen unit has a built-in scale that indicates the oxygen level each time you hold the unit by its carrying strap. Check the oxygen level often, and refill it when necessary. Your supplier will give you specific instructions for your model.

A portable oxygen tank has a contents gauge, a flowmeter, and a knob to turn on the oxygen. To check the tank, turn the knob until you see the needle on the flowmeter move. Then turn the knob off.

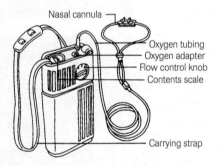

Nasal cannula

Oxygen tubing
Oxygen adapter
Flow control knob
Contents scale

Carrying strap

ATTACHING THE TUBING

Connect one end of the oxygen tubing to the nasal cannula or mask. Then connect the other end to the oxygen adapter on the liquid oxygen unit or the oxygen tank.

Make sure that the tubing connects securely and isn't kinked.

SETTING THE FLOW RATE

Now, turn the flowmeter knob to deliver oxygen at the prescribed rate. You should feel oxygen flowing from the prongs of the cannula or mask. If you don't feel oxygen flowing, briefly turn up the flow rate.

Then turn the knob back to the prescribed level. Make sure that the knob on a liquid oxygen unit clicks into position, or oxygen won't flow.

CARRYING THE PORTABLE TANK

Slip the carrying strap over your shoulder and adjust it for a comfortable fit. Try carrying the tank on each side of your body to determine which is most comfortable. Now, put on the nasal cannula or mask and begin breathing oxygen.

Giving children medication by mouth

Dear Parent or Caregiver:
Giving your child a medication doesn't have to be a problem for you or your child. With patience and care, you can make sure that your child gets medication in a calm and careful way.

TAKE A POSITIVE APPROACH

● Make sure that you're giving the right medication and dose at the right time to the right child.
● Approach your child in a matter-of-fact but friendly manner to put him at ease. Act as though you expect his cooperation, and praise him when he cooperates.
● Give an older child choices, if possible, to give him a sense of control. For example, offer him a choice of beverage to take with (or after) his medication (unless the health care provider tells you not to give the medication with certain beverages or foods).
● Taste a liquid medication (just a drop) before giving it to your child. This gives you an idea of how the medication will taste and whether you'll have to change the taste with flavoring. (Of course, don't taste a medication if you think you may be sensitive to it.)
● Explain the relation between illness and treatment to an older child. He may be more cooperative if he realizes that the medication will help him get better.
● Place a tablet or capsule near the back of your child's tongue, and give him plenty of water or flavored drink to help him swallow it. Then make sure that he swallows it.
● Encourage your child to tip his head *forward* when swallowing a tablet or capsule. Throwing his head back increases the risk of inhaling the medication and choking.
● Give medication to an infant in a manner similar to feeding. Giving medication through a bottle's nipple, for example, takes advantage of the infant's natural sucking reflex. To make sure that the infant gets the full dose, don't mix the medication with formula.

● Closely observe your child to see if the medication has the intended effect or any side effects.

BE HONEST AND CAREFUL

● Never try to trick a child into taking medication. Doing so may make him resist you the next time he has to take it and may cause him to distrust you.
● Never tell a child that medication is candy. He may try to take more than the prescribed dose. Or he may not trust you when he learns it isn't candy.
● Don't promise that the medication will taste good if you've never tasted it or if you know that it won't taste good.
● Never threaten, insult, or embarrass your child if he doesn't cooperate. These actions can lead to resistance.
● Keep medication away from a place where your child or others could accidentally take it.
● Don't force your child to swallow his medication or try to hold his nose or mouth shut to promote swallowing. Doing so may cause choking.
● *Warning:* Don't try to give medication to a crying child; he could choke on it. The medication may come in another form that your child can tolerate.

Giving yourself a subcutaneous insulin injection

Dear Patient:
To transfer insulin from the medication vial to the syringe and then give yourself an insulin injection, follow these guidelines.

GETTING READY

1. Wash your hands. Then assemble your equipment in a clean area:
• sterile syringe and needle
• sharps container
• insulin
• alcohol swabs or wipes (or rubbing alcohol and cotton balls).

2. Check the labels on the syringe and bottle of insulin to make sure that they match. (If you're using U-100 insulin, you must use a U-100 syringe.) Also check that you have the correct type of insulin, such as NPH or Lente. (If your insulin is the cloudy-looking type, roll the bottle between your hands to mix it, as shown below.)

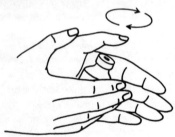

3. Mix gently to prevent large air bubbles from forming in the insulin.

4. Clean the top of the insulin bottle with an alcohol swab or wipe with a cotton ball and rubbing alcohol.

CLEANING THE SKIN AND PREPARING THE SYRINGE

1. Select an appropriate injection site.

2. Pull the skin taut. Then, using a circular motion, clean the skin with an alcohol swab or wipe with a cotton ball soaked in alcohol.

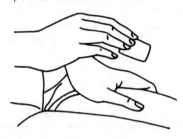

3. Remove the needle cover. To prevent possible infection, don't touch the needle; touch only the barrel and plunger of the syringe.

4. Pull back the plunger to the prescribed number of insulin units. This draws air into the syringe.

5. Insert the needle into the rubber stopper on the insulin bottle, and push in the plunger. This pushes air into the bottle and prevents a vacuum.

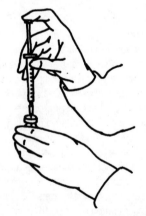

(continued)

Giving yourself a subcutaneous insulin injection *(continued)*

6. Hold the bottle and syringe together in one hand, and then turn them upside down so the bottle is on top. You can hold the bottle between your thumb and forefinger and the syringe between your ring finger and little finger, against your palm.

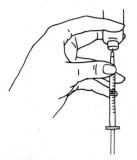

INJECTING INSULIN

1. Pull back on the plunger until the top, black portion of the barrel corresponds to the line that indicates you have withdrawn your correct insulin dose.

2. Remove the needle from the bottle. If air bubbles appear in the syringe after you fill it with insulin, tap the syringe and push lightly on the plunger to remove them.

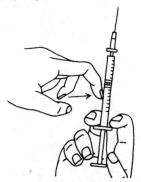

3. Draw up more insulin if necessary.

4. Using your thumb and forefinger, pinch the skin at the injection site. Then quickly

plunge the needle (up to its hub) into the subcutaneous tissue at a 90-degree angle.

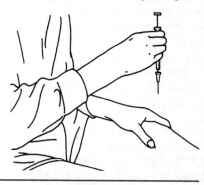

CLEANING UP

1. Place an alcohol swab or cotton ball over the injection site.

2. Press down on the swab or cotton ball lightly as you withdraw the needle. Don't rub the injection site when withdrawing the needle.

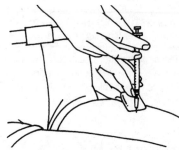

3. Dispose of the needle and syringe in a sharps container.

ADDITIONAL POINTS

● If you travel, keep a bottle of insulin and a syringe with you at all times.

● Keep insulin at room temperature. Don't refrigerate it or place it near heat (above 90° F [32.2° C]).

⬭ Helping a person into or out of a wheelchair

Transfer belt

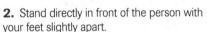

Dear Caregiver:

Before you help the person in your care transfer from his wheel-chair to his bed or into a car, you'll want to ensure his safety and yours. You may need a transfer board; you will need a transfer belt. Made of a nylon, canvas, or leather strap, this belt is about 3′ (1 m) long, with side and back handles.

The person wears the belt around his waist during transfers so that you can grip the handles to support him and prevent falls. Help him to put on the belt for either a standing or sitting transfer. Keep these safety points in mind:

- Make sure that the person can see the surface he's transferring to.
- Make sure that the person wears hard-soled shoes or slippers to prevent falls.
- Never risk injuring the person by pulling his arms or shoulders. Balance and steer him by the transfer belt's handles.
- During the transfer, remember to keep your back straight, and bend from your knees and hips.

Now you're ready to begin the transfer.

ASSISTING WITH A STANDING TRANSFER

1. Place the transfer belt around the person's waist while he sits on the edge of the bed. Place the wheelchair next to the bed and *lock its wheels.*

2. Stand directly in front of the person with your feet slightly apart.

3. Bend your hips and knees down to the person's level. Grasp his transfer belt with your hands and help him to a standing position by straightening your hips and knees. Tell him to lean forward against you for support. If his knees are weak, brace them with your own knees.

4. When the person is standing, turn him so that his back faces the wheelchair, as shown.

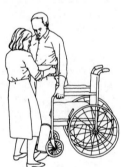

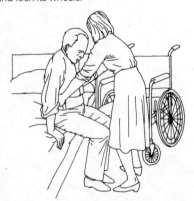

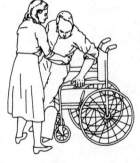

Tell him to use his arm to hold onto an armrest for support. Then, ease him into a comfortable sitting position, as shown.

(continued)

Helping a person into or out of a wheelchair *(continued)*

ASSISTING WITH A SITTING TRANSFER

1. Help the person sit on the edge of the bed, with his feet on the floor. Help him put on his transfer belt. Then position the wheelchair sideways next to the bed, and remove the armrest and footrest closest to the bed. *Lock the wheels.*

2. Grip the person's transfer belt with your hands, and angle him toward the wheelchair.

3. Slip one end of a transfer board under his buttocks, and place the other end on the wheelchair seat. To lift his buttocks, pull up on the transfer belt. Then gently slide him along on the transfer board. You may need to repeat this step several times, slowly inching him toward the chair.

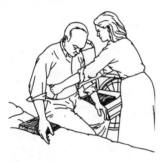

4. When he's in the chair, remove the transfer board and ease him into the proper position. Help him to lean forward, and move him into place by pushing against his knees with yours. Attach the armrest and footrest.

TRANSFERRING TO AND FROM A CAR

1. Park the car on a level surface, making sure that there's enough room for the wheelchair on the right side of the car. After you open the front passenger door as far as possible, move the person in the wheelchair over to the car. Position the left side of the wheelchair next to the car seat. Move the wheelchair's left armrest and both footrests out of the way. *Lock the chair's wheels.*

2. Position yourself facing the person. Bending your hips and knees, move down to the person's level. Grasp his transfer belt with your hands. Help him to a standing position by straightening your hips and knees. Ask him to lean forward against you for support. If his knees are weak, brace them with your own knees.

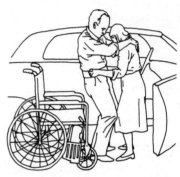

3. When he's standing, turn him so that his back faces the car seat.

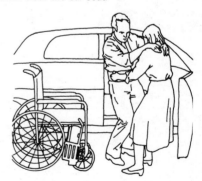

(continued)

Helping a person into or out of a wheelchair *(continued)*

4. Ease him down into a sitting position.

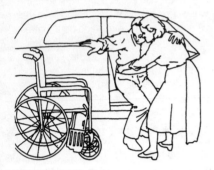

5. Place your hands under his knees and lift his legs into the car. Position him comfortably, and fasten his seat belt.

⬭ Helping a seizure victim

Dear Caregiver:
A person with a seizure disorder may have an attack at any time, in any place. During a seizure, he may lose consciousness and fall down. You can prepare yourself to help him by reading the following instructions.

DURING THE SEIZURE

1. Turn the person on his side and remove hard or sharp objects from the area. Loosen restrictive clothing, such as a collar or a belt, and place something soft and flat under the person's head.

Never force anything into the person's mouth, especially your fingers. Ask onlookers to leave the area.

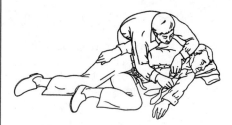

2. If you suspect the person has swallowed or inhaled his own vomit, call for medical assistance immediately.

AFTER THE SEIZURE

1. Allow the person to lie quietly. As he awakens, gently call him by name, and reorient him to his surroundings and to recent events.
2. If the person has an injury, such as a badly bleeding tongue, take him to his health care provider's office or to the hospital emergency department.
3. Write an accurate description of the seizure as soon as you can. The health care professional may request certain information, including the seizure's duration and the victim's activity immediately before, during, and after the seizure.

○ Helping your pacemaker help you

Dear Patient:
A pacemaker has been inserted in your chest to produce the electrical impulses that help your heart beat correctly. Follow these guidelines to make sure that your new pacemaker works correctly.

CHECK YOUR PACEMAKER DAILY

To check your pacemaker, count your pulse beats for 1 minute after you've been resting for at least 15 minutes — a good time to count is first thing in the morning. Ask your health care provider what your normal heart rate should be. Report if you detect an abnormal rate or if you feel faint or have chest pain, dizziness, shortness of breath, prolonged hiccups, or muscle twitching.

FOLLOW ORDERS

Take your heart medication as prescribed to ensure a regular heart rhythm. Also follow specific orders about diet and physical activity. Exercise every day, but *don't overdo it,* even if you think you have more energy than you did before getting your pacemaker. Avoid rough horseplay or lifting heavy objects. Be especially careful not to stress the muscles near the pacemaker.

Keep all follow-up appointments. Your pacemaker will need to be checked regularly at the cardiologist's office or over the telephone to make sure that it's in good working order.

Remember that pacemaker batteries have to be changed and that battery life varies, depending on usage.

TAKE PRECAUTIONS

Always carry your pacemaker emergency card. The card lists your primary health care provider, cardiologist, hospital, type of pacemaker, and date of implantation.

Don't get too close to gasoline engines or electric motors unless they are properly grounded, and don't lean over running engines or motors. Also, the strong magnet in the magnetic resonance imaging machine used by hospitals for diagnostic testing can permanently damage your pacemaker. You should also keep a safe distance from high-voltage fields created by overhead electric lines. (*Note:* Your microwave oven won't affect your pacemaker.)

If you need dental work or surgery, mention beforehand that you have a pacemaker. You may need an antibiotic to prevent infection.

If you're traveling by plane, you must pass through an airport metal detector. Before doing so, let the airport authorities know you have a pacemaker.

If you have a nuclear pacemaker and plan to travel abroad, the Nuclear Regulatory Commission requires that you tell the pacemaker manufacturer of your travel itinerary, means of travel, and the name of your health care provider.

◯ How to detect – and prevent – infection

Dear Patient:

Your condition makes you an easy target for infection. That's one reason why you need to stay alert for warning signs of infection and to take steps to prevent infection.

WARNING SIGNS

Infection can quickly grow worse. Call your health care provider at once if any of these signs develop:

- fever
- a cough that produces foul-smelling or colored (green, yellow, brown, pink, or red) sputum
- unusual fatigue or weakness
- increasing breathing difficulties
- confusion, decreased alertness, or memory loss
- cuts or scrapes that appear red or swollen, feel tender, or begin draining.

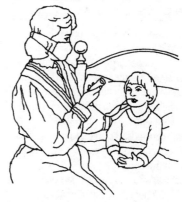

PREVENTIVE STEPS

To help prevent infection, follow these steps:

- Eat well-balanced, nutritious meals. Eat regularly. Don't skip meals or eat extra ones.
- Drink at least six 8-ounce glasses of water per day unless your health care provider directs otherwise.
- Get 7 to 8 hours of sleep at night and take frequent, brief rest breaks during the day.
- Take your medicine *exactly* as your health care provider directs.
- If possible, avoid anyone who has a cold or the flu. Stay away from crowds. If you can't avoid a sick person, wear a disposable surgical mask when you're around that person. You can usually obtain disposable masks from a local drugstore.

- Check with your health care provider about getting a flu shot (influenza vaccine).
- Avoid exposure to inhaled pollutants – for example, cigarette smoke, noxious industrial fumes, and car exhaust.
- Carefully wash your hands before meals. Also wash them after touching tissues soiled with mucus and before and after using the bathroom, handling money, or petting an animal.
- Take care to avoid cuts and other accidental injuries. If you do cut or scrape yourself, wash the area with soap and water, and cover it with a dry, sterile bandage. If healing doesn't occur within a few days, call your health care provider.

◯ How to measure fluid intake and output

Dear Patient:
Your health care provider wants you to keep a daily record of your intake and output. This record can help him judge your progress and response to treatment.

WHAT ARE INTAKE AND OUTPUT?

Intake includes everything you drink, such as water, fruit juice, and soda. It also includes foods that become liquid at room temperature, such as gelatin, custard, and ice cream. Intake even includes fluids, liquid medicines, and solutions delivered through tubing into one of your veins (I.V.) or into your stomach.

Output includes everything that leaves your body as a fluid, including urine, drainage from a wound, diarrhea, and vomit.

Because your intake should balance your output, you need to keep very accurate records. Whenever possible, *measure* fluids. Don't guess.

MEASURING INTAKE

1. Measure and record the amount of fluid you have with each meal, with medicine, and between meals. Pour liquid into a measuring cup or other graduated container before serving it in a glass or cup. Also keep in mind that labels on cans and bottles indicate exact amounts. Don't forget to subtract amounts you don't drink. The difference, of course, is your intake amount.
2. If you're receiving medicine or nutrition through an I.V. line or a stomach tube, record the amount of fluid you use.

MEASURING OUTPUT

1. Before throwing away urine from a bedpan, urinal, or portable toilet, measure and record the amount (or ask your caregiver to do this). Keep a measuring container handy for this purpose.

2. If you have a drainage bag in place, you or your caregiver should measure and record the amount of fluid in the bag before discarding it.
3. Measure and record vomit or liquid bowel movements as output.

COMMON MEASURES

Your health care provider may want you to measure your fluid intake and output metrically. To convert your household measure, use the information here:

HOUSEHOLD	METRIC
1 quart (32 oz)	1,000 ml
1 pint (16 oz)	500 ml
1 measuring cupful (8 oz)	240 ml
1 tablespoon (1 oz)	30 ml

To convert fluid ounces to the metric equivalent of milliliters, multiply by 30. To convert milliliters to ounces, divide by 30.

Keeping a food diary

Dear Patient:

Keeping a food diary can help you recognize and change poor eating habits. After keeping a diary, you may find that you eat because you associate food with certain feelings or activities. Some people, for instance, eat chocolate when they're lonely or ice cream when they watch TV.

Begin your food diary by following these steps. Remember to show this record to your health care provider.

WHAT TO INCLUDE

Record what, when, and where you eat every day for 1 week. Include how much you eat and how you feel at the moment. Rate your hunger and jot down the names of the people you're eating with, or make a note if you're eating alone.

RECOGNIZING PATTERNS

At the end of a week, review your diary. Look for patterns of overeating or other trends:
- Does the record show that you eat when you feel angry, anxious, or bored?
- Does the diary reveal that you snack during events such as talking on the phone?
- Do you tend to eat more when you're around certain people?

CHANGING PATTERNS

After you identify what prompts you to eat — even when you aren't hungry — take steps to change your responses in these situations. After you see a pattern of overeating, plan ways to modify or eliminate it.

Pace yourself for success by changing one habit at a time. Don't try to change too many bad habits at once.

Use the following sample diary page as a guide to recording your eating habits.

DAY & TIME	LOCATION	OTHER PEOPLE PRESENT	MY MOOD	FOOD EATEN (INCLUDE SNACKS)	AMOUNT	DEGREE OF HUNGER
Monday 10 a.m.	Home	Alone	Annoyed	Cookies Nuts Grapes	3 Handful Bunch	Not hungry
12:30 lunch	Janet's house	Janet and Mary	Cheerful	Club sandwich Potato chips Coke Ice cream	1 Handful Glass Bowl	Moderate

◯ Keeping a headache log

Dear Patient:
What triggers your headaches? Environmental factors? Foods? Stress? A headache log can help you identify such triggers. The log can also help you learn the most effective ways to relieve a headache when it starts.

    Record the details of each of your headaches in a diary or small notebook.

HOW TO PROCEED

Using the log below as a guide, note the date and time of the headache and any warning signs. Next, put a check mark in the appropriate box for the headache's intensity. Then do the same for the headache's duration.

    Do you have other signs or symptoms, such as nausea or vomiting or sensitivity to light? If you do, check the appropriate box.

Continue by checking the steps you took to relieve the headache (for example, medication, biofeedback, and rest) as well as the effectiveness of these measures.

    To complete the log, think carefully about the events that occurred before the headache. For instance, was your headache triggered by emotional stress, by drinking a cup of coffee, or by something else? Write down the details of such potential triggers in your log.

Dates and time headache began: _____

WARNING SIGNS	ASSOCIATED SIGNS AND SYMPTOMS
❑ Flashing lights	❑ Upset stomach
❑ Blind spots	❑ Nausea or vomiting
❑ Colors	❑ Dizziness
❑ Zigzag patterns	❑ Sensitivity to light
❑ None	❑ Sensory, motor, or speech disturbances
❑ Other	❑ Other

INTENSITY

❑ Mild   ❑ Severe
❑ Moderate   ❑ Disabling

MEASURES FOR RELIEF

❑ Medication   ❑ Biofeedback
❑ Rest   ❑ Ice pack
❑ Sleep   ❑ Relaxation exercises

DURATION

❑ 4 hours or less
❑ 4 to 8 hours
❑ 8 to 12 hours
❑ 12 to 24 hours
❑ More than 1 day
❑ More than 2 days

EXTENT OF RELIEF

❑ None
❑ Mild
❑ Moderate
❑ Marked
❑ Complete

POSSIBLE TRIGGERS:

◯ Learning about ACE inhibitors

Dear Patient:

The medication you've been prescribed is called an *angiotensin-converting enzyme (ACE) inhibitor.* This medication will help improve your heart function.

TAKING YOUR MEDICATION

- Take your medication exactly as directed. Take it at the same time each day, so you'll be less likely to forget it.
- If you miss a dose of medication, take it as soon as possible. If you're close to taking your next dose, however, don't take the skipped dose.

SOME RESTRICTIONS

- Before taking over-the-counter medications, check with your health care provider or pharmacist.
- Be sure to report if you experience light-headedness, facial swelling, difficulty breathing or sleeping at night, or signs of infection such as fever. Also report wheezing, a rash, or a very slow heart rate.

SPECIAL INSTRUCTIONS

- This medication can cause a dry, persistent, tickling cough. Be sure to report this so that the dosage may be adjusted.
- Avoid sudden position changes, which may cause temporary light-headedness.
- Tell all health care providers about the medication you're taking.
- Store this medication in a cool, dry place. Avoid storing it in direct light. Be sure to keep it out of the reach of children.
- If you become pregnant, report it at once.

Learning about an electrocardiogram

Dear Patient:
An electrocardiogram (ECG) has been ordered for you. This test tells how well your heart works.

How your heart beats

Your heart is a pump that has its own built-in pacemaker. This pacemaker is actually a group of special cells in the upper right part of the heart.

About every second, this natural pacemaker releases an electrical impulse that travels down a path of muscle fibers and spreads throughout your heart.

This impulse makes your heart contract and pump blood through its chambers and into the rest of the body through the blood vessels.

How an ECG works

An ECG records the electrical impulses that travel through your heart. The ECG machine then converts these impulses to pencil-like tracings that print on long strips of graph paper. By looking at these tracings, your health care provider can tell whether your heart is healthy or has a problem.

Before the test

You'll be asked to lie on your back, with the skin of your chest, arms, and legs exposed. Lie perfectly still and relax. (Don't even talk.) The test is painless and only takes a few minutes.

During the test

Electrodes, which resemble small stickers, will be placed on your chest, arms, and legs. Wires attached to the ECG machine will then be connected to the electrodes, and the machine will be prompted to record.

After the test

When the test is over, the electrodes will be removed. You'll be able to resume your usual activities. Your health care provider will inform you of the test results.

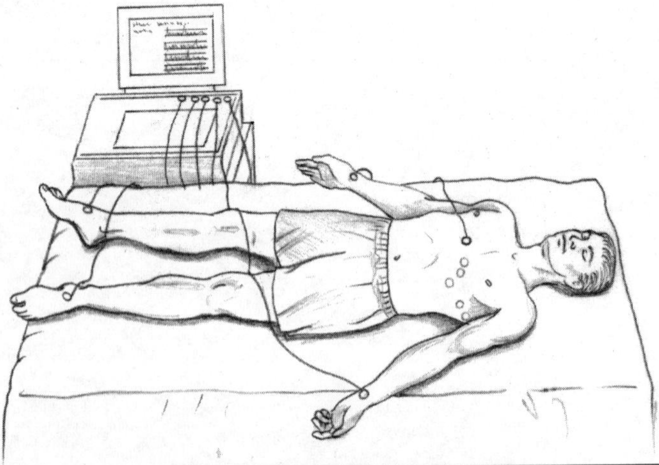

⟳ Learning about beta-adrenergic blockers

Dear Patient:
The medication you're taking is classified as a beta-adrenergic blocker. This medication has been prescribed to help improve your heart function.

TAKING YOUR MEDICATION

Take this medication exactly as the label directs. Take it at the same time each day, so you'll be less likely to forget it.

Take your pulse once per day, preferably before the first dose. If your pulse is less than 60 beats per minute, don't take the next dose. Instead, contact the prescribing health care professional as soon as possible. Don't skip more than one dose.

SOME RESTRICTIONS

Before taking over-the-counter cold medications, check with your health care provider or pharmacist.

Be sure to report if you feel depressed or dizzy or can't sleep at night. Also report if you have trouble breathing, start wheezing, develop a rash, or have a very slow heart rate.

SPECIAL INSTRUCTIONS

● To increase absorption, take the drug with meals.

● Don't stop taking this drug suddenly — doing so may distress your heart.

● To minimize dizziness, rise slowly from a sitting or lying position and avoid sudden position changes.

● Don't permit others to take your medication, and don't try theirs.

● Store your medication in a cool, dry area. Avoid keeping it in the bathroom medicine chest.

● Throw away the unused portion of your medication that's several years old.

● To prevent insomnia, take the drug no later than 2 hours before bedtime.

◯ Learning about canes

Dear Patient:
You may need a cane if you have weakness on one side of your body or if you have poor balance. A health care professional will help you select the cane that's best for you.

   Hold the cane in the hand opposite your weaker side, and flex your elbow at a 30-degree angle. If the cane is made of aluminum, you can adjust it by pushing in the metal button on the shaft and raising or lowering the shaft. If the cane is wooden, you or a helper can remove the rubber safety tip, saw off any excess wood, and replace the tip. Available in several types, canes can be standard, straight-handled, or broad-based.

STANDARD CANES

Your health care provider will recommend a standard cane if you often go up and down stairs. Made of wood or metal, a standard cane commonly comes in 34″ to 42″ (86.5- to 106.5-cm) sizes. It features a single foot and a half-circle handle. It's usually inexpensive and easy to use and hooks onto your belt or arm when you're going up or down stairs and onto the back or arm of a chair when you sit down.

   Choose a cane with a wooden or plastic handle rather than a metal one. If your hand perspires, you may lose your grip on a metal handle. A metal handle may also feel uncomfortable in hot or cold weather.

STRAIGHT-HANDLED CANES

Your health care provider will recommend a straight-handled cane if your hand is weak. Made of wood, plastic, or metal, a straight-handled cane has an easy-to-hold handgrip and a rubber safety tip. If you're selecting one, make sure that the handgrip isn't too thick or too thin for you to hold comfortably and that the cane is the proper height. Because this cane doesn't hook over railings or chair arms, you can place it near you on the floor when you sit down.

BROAD-BASED CANES

This lightweight, metal cane has three or four prongs or legs that provide a sturdy supportive base. The height can be adjusted, and extra-long handles and child sizes are also available. A broad-based cane stands upright when not in use.

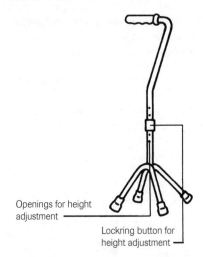

Openings for height adjustment

Lockring button for height adjustment

   Cane bases range from narrow to wide. A narrow broad-based cane fits on the standard stair step in the normal cane position, whereas a wide broad-based cane fits on the step if you turn the cane sideways. Usually, the narrower the cane's base, the less you tend to rely on it for support.

◌ Learning about cystoscopy

Dear Patient:

Your health care provider has scheduled you for cystoscopy. During this procedure, he can look inside your bladder through an instrument called a *cystoscope.* He'll insert the cystoscope through your urethra (the opening through which you urinate).

Cystoscopy allows the health care provider to diagnose and, sometimes, treat your urinary disorder. The test may be done in a hospital or in the health care provider's office. It usually takes 15 to 45 minutes.

WHAT TO EXPECT BEFORE THE TEST

You may receive a local anesthetic before the procedure. This means that the health care provider will numb the area around the urethra before inserting the cystoscope.

Alternatively, you may have general anesthesia. In this case, don't eat or drink anything after midnight on the night before the procedure. If the health care provider plans to take X-rays of your bladder during the cystoscopy, he may prescribe medication that will clean your bowels to ensure sharper, clearer images.

Just before the procedure begins, you'll have an intravenous line inserted in your arm to deliver fluids and medications if you need them. You'll also receive a sedative to help you relax.

WHAT TO EXPECT DURING THE TEST

After the anesthetic takes effect, you'll be positioned on your back. Then the health care provider will insert the cystoscope. Take deep breaths and try to relax. This will allow the test to proceed smoothly.

If you received a local anesthetic, you may feel a strong urge to urinate as the instrument is inserted and removed. If the health care provider instills an irrigant into your bladder, you may feel some pressure. Again, try to relax. If you experience pain or feel your heart beating irregularly, report it immediately.

WHAT TO EXPECT AFTER THE TEST

Your condition will be monitored until you're fully alert. If you received a local anesthetic, you'll be awake but you may feel weak, so don't chance walking by yourself. Wait for someone to assist you.

For several days after the cystoscopy, you may void blood-tinged urine. You may also have bladder spasms, a feeling that your bladder is full, or a burning sensation when you urinate. Take acetaminophen (Tylenol), drink plenty of fluids, and lie in a tub of warm water to obtain relief.

WHAT TO REPORT

Call your health care provider if you have heavy bleeding or blood clots in your urine, bladder pain or spasms that aren't relieved by medication, or burning and a frequent urge to urinate that persists for more than 24 hours. Notify your health care provider at once if you can't urinate within 8 hours after the test.

◯ Learning about digoxin

Dear Patient:

You've been prescribed digoxin (the label may also read Lanoxin or Lanoxicaps) to strengthen your heart's ability to pump blood. This drug also slows down your pulse and regulates your heart rate.

Be sure to take digoxin exactly as the label directs. Take it at the same time each day. That way, you'll be less likely to forget it. However, if you do forget a dose, you can make up for it within 12 hours of your scheduled administration time. Don't take two doses at the same time.

CHECK YOUR PULSE

Once a day, preferably in the morning *before* taking digoxin, check your pulse. If your pulse rate is less than 60 beats per minute or if your pulse rhythm isn't regular, inform your health care provider.

REPORT SIDE EFFECTS

Because digoxin is one of the oldest drugs, a lot is known about its effects. Report if you feel tired, drowsy, or dizzy or get a headache.

Also, report if you lose your appetite, vomit or feel like vomiting, or notice changes in your vision such as seeing halos.

WATCH YOUR DIET

Some food can change the way digoxin works. High-fiber foods, for instance, can reduce your body's absorption of digoxin. So, be sure to cut back on these foods. They include bran, raw and leafy vegetables, and most fruits.

ASK ABOUT OTHER DRUGS

Before you take *any other drug,* talk to your pharmacist or health care provider. Some drugs change the way digoxin works. Avoid antacids, antidiarrhea drugs (such as Kaopectate), and laxatives.

A FEW REMINDERS

- Don't take another person's digoxin tablets, and don't let anyone else take yours.
- Don't change the brand of digoxin you've been taking. Another brand may have a different effect.
- Store your digoxin in a cool, dry area. Don't keep it in your bathroom medicine cabinet. Keep it out of the reach of children.
- Throw away the digoxin that's unused or several years old.

⬭ **Learning about heparin**

Dear Patient:
The directions below will help you safely use heparin to control blood clotting. Review them at any time to refresh the instructions you were given when you learned to inject this drug.

INJECTING HEPARIN

Wash your hands and clean the injection site. Refer to the illustration below as you choose an area on your stomach between the hip bones.

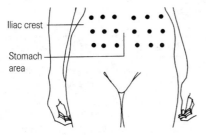

Pinch your skin gently and insert the needle deep into the underlying fat layer. Slowly inject the drug. Leave the needle in place for 10 seconds before you withdraw it. *Don't* massage or rub the area. Change your injection site each time you take this medicine.

ENSURING THE RIGHT DOSE

Inject heparin exactly as directed. If you miss a dose, take it as soon as possible. If it's almost time for your next dose, however, forget the missed dose and don't double the next one. Instead, go back to your regular schedule.

REPORTING ADVERSE EFFECTS

Report at once if you cough up blood or have bleeding gums; nosebleeds; bruises; bloody (red-tinged) urine; black, tarry stools; or bloody or coffee-ground vomitus. If you're female, also report if you bleed unusually heavily during your period.

Also report if you have pain or swelling in your joints or stomach, unusual backaches, constipation, dizziness, or a severe or persistent headache.

WATCHING YOUR DIET

Eat cheese, eggs, liver, and leafy green vegetables in moderation. These foods may reduce heparin's effectiveness. Inform your health care provider if you take vitamins C or E. In large amounts, they may interfere with your medicine.

If you drink alcohol, limit yourself to one or two drinks a day.

TAKING PRECAUTIONS WITH OTHER DRUGS

Check with your health care provider or pharmacist before taking other drugs, especially aspirin, which may cause bleeding.

PROTECTING YOURSELF FROM INJURY

- Don't engage in contact sports.
- Don't put toothpicks or sharp objects into your mouth. Don't walk barefoot. Avoid power tools and rough sports.
- Wear a medical identification tag that indicates you take an anticoagulant.
- Report a fall or another activity in which you accidentally hit your head.
- Don't cut corns and calluses yourself. Consult a podiatrist.
- Tell your other health care professionals and your dentist that you're taking heparin.

◯ Learning about laparoscopy

Dear Patient:

Your health care provider has scheduled you for a laparoscopy. This procedure lets him see your reproductive and upper abdominal organs through a slender, telescope-like instrument. Laparoscopy allows for diagnosis and, sometimes, treatment of your disorder during the same procedure.

Laparoscopy takes about 1 hour. It's performed in the operating room, and you'll probably receive a general anesthetic. Usually, you can go home the same day.

GETTING READY

Beforehand, a few routine laboratory tests will be done to assess your general health. These tests include a complete blood count, blood chemistry studies, and urinalysis.

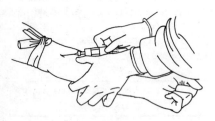

Because you'll be receiving an anesthetic, don't eat or drink anything after midnight on the night before the procedure. If you're a smoker, don't smoke for about 12 hours before surgery. Remove eye makeup and nail polish beforehand.

DURING THE PROCEDURE

When the anesthetic takes effect, the health care provider will make a small incision in the lower part of your navel. Then he'll insert a needle through the incision and inject carbon dioxide or nitrous oxide into your pelvic area. This inflates the area. It creates a viewing space by lifting the abdominal wall away from the organs below.

Next, the health care provider will insert a thin, flexible, optical instrument called a *laparoscope* through the incision. This instrument magnifies the view of your organs.

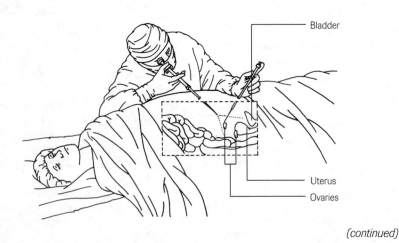

Bladder

Uterus

Ovaries

(continued)

Learning about laparoscopy *(continued)*

REMOVING IMPLANTS DURING LAPAROSCOPY

If the laparoscopic findings confirm endometriosis, the health care provider may decide to remove the implants and adhesions.

To remove them, the health care provider will make a second, smaller incision just above your pubic hairline. Then he'll insert a special instrument for moving your internal organs aside. He may also insert a blunt instrument called a *cannula* through your vagina and into your uterus to move your uterus. The implants and adhesions will be removed by inserting instruments through the laparoscope.

Next, the health care provider will release the gas through the incision and remove the laparoscope. Then he'll close the incision and apply an adhesive bandage.

AFTER THE PROCEDURE

After laparoscopy, you'll go to the postanesthesia care unit, where nurses will monitor you until you're fully alert. If necessary, you'll receive an analgesic for minor discomfort in the incisional area when the anesthetic wears off. Expect vaginal bleeding similar to a menstrual period for a few days.

TIPS FOR RECOVERY

When you get home, keep these points in mind:
- Wait until the day after surgery to remove your bandage and to bathe or shower.
- Eat lightly because some gas will remain in your abdomen; you'll probably belch or feel bloated for 1 or 2 days.
- Take acetaminophen (Tylenol) or ibuprofen to relieve shoulder pain. Called *referred pain*, this results from the remaining gas in your abdomen, which can irritate your diaphragm and cause a pain in your shoulders.
- Expect to resume your normal activities after 1 or 2 days, but avoid strenuous work or sports for about 1 week.
- Resume sexual activity when the bleeding stops or when your health care provider gives approval.

WHEN TO CALL THE HEALTH CARE PROVIDER

In rare instances, a laparoscopy may be complicated by infection, hemorrhage, or a burn or a small cut on an organ. Call the health care provider if you experience any of the following:
- a fever of 100.4° F (38° C) or higher
- persistent or excessive vaginal bleeding
- severe abdominal pain
- redness, puffiness, or drainage from your incision
- nausea, vomiting, or diarrhea.

◯ Learning about potassium-rich foods

Dear Patient:

If you're taking medication that decreases the level of potassium in your body, your health care provider may recommend adding potassium to your diet.

HOW MUCH POTASSIUM DO YOU NEED?

Health care providers recommend 300 to 400 milligrams of potassium daily. Not enough potassium can cause leg cramps, weakness, paralysis, and spasms. Too much can cause heart problems and fatigue.

The chart below lists potassium-rich foods along with their potassium content (the number of milligrams in a 3½-ounce [about 100-gram] serving). Because some of these foods are also high in calories, check with your health care provider or dietitian if you're on a weight-reduction diet.

MEATS	FISH & SEAFOOD	VEGETABLES	FRUITS	JUICES
Chicken (411)	Sardines, canned (590)	Potatoes (407)	Dates (648)	Tomato (227)
Turkey (411)	Halibut (525)	Lima beans (394)	Bananas (370)	Orange, fresh (200)
Liver (380)	Scallops (476)	Carrots (341)	Raisins (355)	Orange, reconstituted (186)
Beef (370)	Salmon (421)	Spinach (324)	Plums (299)	**OTHER FOODS**
Pork (326)	Haddock (348)	Radishes (322)	Nectarines (294)	Milk, dry (1,745)
Lamb (290)	Flounder (342)	Sweet potatoes (300)	Apricots (281)	Molasses, light (917)
Veal (50)	Tuna (301)	Brussels sprouts (295)	Prunes (262)	Peanuts (674)
	Perch (284)	Endive (294)	Peaches (202)	Peanut butter (670)
	Bass (256)	Asparagus (238)	Oranges (200)	Gingersnap cookies (462)
	Oysters (203)	Cabbage (233)	Figs (152)	Graham crackers (384)
		Peppers (213)		Oatmeal cookies with raisins (370)
				Ice milk (195)

⬭ Learning about walkers

Dear Patient:
Your health care provider has ordered a walker for you to help you get around. Depending on your needs, you may be using a stationary walker, a reciprocal walker, or a hemiwalker.

STATIONARY WALKER

Usually lightweight, inexpensive, and very stable, a stationary walker consists of an adjustable metal frame with two handgrips and four legs. Most stationary walkers have no movable parts, although some models are available with small front wheels. Some models also fold up for travel and easy storage.

RECIPROCAL WALKER

A reciprocal walker consists of a metal frame with two handgrips, four legs, and a hinge mechanism that allows one side to be advanced ahead of the other. Its height is usually adjustable from 27" to 37" inches (68.5 to 94 cm), and some models fold up for storage and travel. The reciprocal walker is flexible and "walks" with you.

Stationary walker

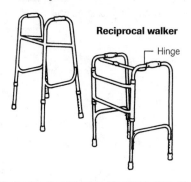

Reciprocal walker

— Hinge

HEMIWALKER

Like the walkers above, a hemiwalker also has four legs, but it has just one handgrip, not two. You'll hold the handgrip with your strong

hand as you would with a cane. To walk, move your affected leg forward first, transfer your weight to the walker and the affected leg, and then move your strong leg forward.

FEELING COMFORTABLE WITH YOUR WALKER

Put on the shoes you'll be wearing when you use the walker. Then stand up straight with your feet close together. Relax your shoulders, and put the walker in front of and partially around you. Now, grasp the sides of the walker and look at the position of your elbows — they should be nearly straight. If they aren't, adjust the walker's height by pushing in the button on each of the walker's legs and sliding the tubing up or down as appropriate. Make sure that the button locks back into place and that you have adjusted the legs to the same height.

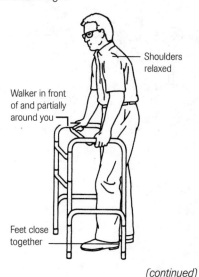

Shoulders relaxed

Walker in front of and partially around you —

Feet close together —

(continued)

Learning about walkers *(continued)*

Now, try the walker. You should be able to move it without bending over. If you still don't feel comfortable, try adjusting the height again.

COPING WITH A FALL

If you fall while using a walker, first call for help *before* you try to get up. If no help is available, use the following method to help yourself up.

1. Look around the room for a low, sturdy piece of furniture such as a coffee table. Inch backward toward the table by pushing your hands down on the floor and lifting up your buttocks. As you do this, pull the walker with one hand.

2. When you get to the table, place your walker near it. Then reach back and place both hands on the tabletop. Next, press down on the tabletop and lift your buttocks onto the table.

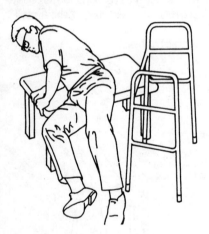

3. Place the walker in front of you, and raise yourself to a standing position by pushing your hands down on the hand grips.

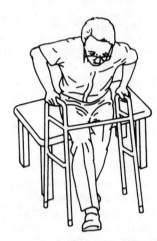

Remember: It's normal to feel a little dizzy when you first stand up. Take a moment to gain your balance before walking. If dizziness doesn't go away or seems excessive, lower yourself back onto the table and call for help. You may wish to sit for awhile before attempting to stand up.

◯ Learning to communicate without speech

Dear Caregiver:
As the person in your care weakens, his speech may become impaired. To prevent isolation, you'll need to find new ways for him to communicate, such as by lip-reading or using a communication board or a talking computer. Whichever method you choose, begin to practice it with the person before he must rely on it totally.

LIP-READING

Lip-reading is one of the most effective ways to communicate without speech; however, it will take you time and effort to learn. Here are some tips to make lip-reading easier:

● Tell the person in your care to pause after forming each word with his lips. Then repeat the word aloud to make sure that you understood him. If you can't make out the word, ask him to spell it by forming each letter with his lips.

● Ask simple questions that require a yes-or-no answer. For example, ask, "Would you like to sit outside now?" rather than, "What do you feel like doing this afternoon?"

● Try to anticipate the person's needs so you can communicate more efficiently. Pay attention to nonverbal cues. For instance, if he looks bored or depressed while watching television, suggest a game of cards or a visit with a neighbor to cheer him up.

● Don't put words in the person's mouth. Give him the opportunity to express himself in his own way, even if it takes more time.

COMMUNICATION BOARDS

With a communication board, a person can express his thoughts by pointing to words, letters, pictures, or phrases on the board. Communication boards come in various forms, including manual versions and ones that operate on a home computer.
When using a communication board:

● Make sure that the person can see it clearly.

● Decide how the person will identify the figure or character on the board. If he can't lift his arm to point, perhaps you can point for him. Alternatively, think about getting a special pointer that requires only slight hand or arm movement.

● Talk to a speech pathologist, who can help you decide which board best suits the person's needs and teach you how to use it.

TALKING COMPUTERS

If you own or wish to purchase a home computer, you may want to investigate "talking software." These programs provide a mechanical voice for the person, who controls the program through a computer keyboard. Ask your speech specialist for information.

◯ Learning to do controlled coughing exercises

Dear Patient:
Learning how to do controlled coughing exercises will help you save energy and remove mucus from your airways. Here's what to do:

1. Sit on the edge of your chair or bed. Rest your feet flat on the floor, or use a stool if your feet don't touch the floor. Lean slightly forward.

2. To help stimulate your cough reflex, slowly take a deep breath. Place your hands on your stomach. Breathe in through your nose, letting your stomach expand as far as it can.

3. Next, purse your lips and slowly breathe out through your mouth, as shown. Concentrate on pulling your stomach inward. Try to exhale twice as long as you inhaled.

4. Cough *twice* with your mouth slightly open. Once isn't enough: The first cough loosens mucus; the second cough helps remove it.

5. Pause for a moment. Then breathe in through your nose by sniffing gently. Don't breathe deeply. If you do, the mucus you brought up may slide back into your lungs.

6. Use a tissue or handkerchief to collect any mucus. Be sure to wash your hands when you're finished.

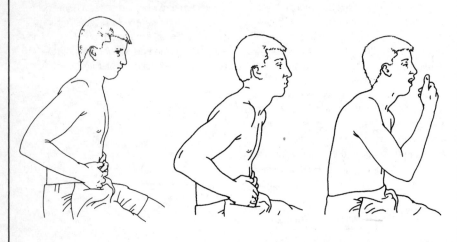

⬭ Living with heart failure

Dear Patient:

Recognizing the common early symptoms of your condition is one way for you to monitor yourself and help prevent complications. Keep your health care provider posted on the symptoms you experience. Then follow any directions you're given. Of course, continue to follow your diet, activity, and medication regimens as directed.

Common early symptoms of heart failure appear below. You'll also find tips for living with them.

BREATHING DIFFICULTIES

You may have difficulty breathing when blood and fluids don't move fast enough through your lungs. Shortness of breath may occur with exertion, such as climbing the stairs or lifting a child. If you feel short of breath, stop what you're doing and steady yourself. Then rest until you feel better.

If you feel short of breath when you're resting or lying down, try raising your head with several pillows. Or, if you're short of breath when you get up after a nap or a night's sleep, try sitting up, dangling your legs over the bedside, and wiggling your feet and ankles. You can also stand up and walk around to promote circulation.

SWELLING

You may have swelling if your body doesn't get rid of extra salt and fluid. You probably have some swelling if you press your finger to your skin and the impression remains briefly.

You may also notice puffiness in your hands, ankles, or feet. Or, you may see marks on your skin from the elastic in your socks or rings on your fingers. Try elevating your feet, ankles, or hands above the level of your heart. This may help reduce the swelling.

Be sure to weigh yourself every day at about the same time. Use the same scale and wear about the same amount of clothing. If you notice a sudden, unexplainable gain (2 lb [0.9 kg] or more in a day or 5 lb [2.3 kg] in 1 week), report it to your health care provider, who may prescribe medication or recommend other relief measures.

OTHER SYMPTOMS

Other symptoms to report include:
- a dry cough
- frequently getting up during the night to urinate
- increased weakness and fatigue
- upper abdominal pain or a bloated feeling.

WARNING

Immediately report if you can't breathe at all, if your heart is pounding, or if you cough up pink, frothy sputum.

◯ Making a medication clock

Dear Patient or Caregiver:

As a reminder of when medication is due, you can make a simple device called a *medication clock.* Using or copying the sample clocks shown below, write a.m. in the center of one clock and p.m. in the center of the other clock. Use a different-colored ink to label each clock so you can easily tell them apart.

The rest is simple: Just write the names of the medications to be taken in the appropriate hour. Then be sure to check the clock often during the day.

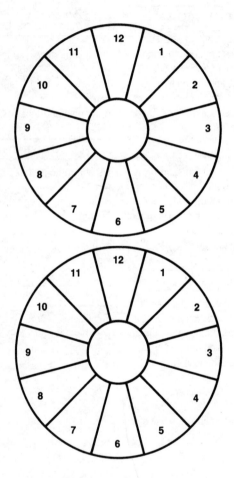

◌ Managing vaso-occlusive crisis

Dear Caregiver:

Because the person that you're caring for has sickle cell anemia, he's at risk for a serious complication called *vaso-occlusive crisis*. If this crisis occurs, the tips below can help you treat it and may prevent it from recurring.

WHAT GOES WRONG?

In sickle cell anemia, some *(not all)* red blood cells change from a normally round shape to a sickle shape. When this happens, the sickled cells clog small blood vessels and keep blood from reaching vital organs. This condition, called vaso-occlusive crisis, causes pain and, possibly, cell damage.

Some things that cause a crisis are:
- infection, such as a cold or the flu
- dehydration — from not drinking enough fluid or from sweating, vomiting, or having diarrhea
- low oxygen levels — for example, from a visit to the mountains
- temperature extremes.

RECOGNIZING A CRISIS

Suspect a crisis if the person has:
- pain, especially in the stomach area, chest, muscles, or bones
- paleness, usually around the lips, tongue, and fingernails
- unusual sleepiness or irritability
- a low-grade fever that lasts 2 days
- dark urine.

RESPONDING TO A CRISIS

First, call your health care provider and describe the person's symptoms. For a mild crisis, the health care provider may suggest home care. Here's how to help the person at home:
- Apply warm, moist compresses to painful areas. Cover the person with a blanket to prevent a chill. *Never* use ice packs or cold compresses. These could be harmful.
- Ease pain with acetaminophen, according to your health care provider's directions.
- Tell the person to stay in bed. Let him sit up if that's more comfortable.
- Make sure that the person drinks lots of fluids so he doesn't get dehydrated.
- Report persistent or worsening symptoms.

PREVENTING A CRISIS

Although these precautions aren't foolproof, they may help to prevent another crisis. Discuss these do's and don'ts with the person in your care.

DO'S

- Stay up-to-date with immunizations.
- Prevent infections: Take meticulous care of wounds, eat well-balanced meals, have regular dental checkups, and learn proper tooth and gum care.
- Seek treatment for any infection.
- Drink fluids at the first sign of a cold or other infection.

DON'TS

- Avoid tight clothing, which could block circulation.
- Never exercise strenuously or excessively. This could trigger a crisis.
- Avoid drinking lots of ice water or exposing yourself to sizzling hot or freezing cold temperatures.
- Avoid mountain climbing, unpressurized aircraft, and high altitudes.

◯ Minimizing sun exposure

Dear Patient:

The easiest way to prevent skin cancer is to reduce your exposure to the sun. Although most skin cancers appear after age 50, the sun's damaging effects begin early — in childhood.

Fortunately, it's never too late to start protecting yourself from skin cancer. Here's how.

WEAR SUNSCREEN

Protect your skin with a lotion or cream containing para-aminobenzoic acid or other sunscreen.

Sunscreens are related to strength according to sun protection factor (SPF). Choose a sunscreen with an SPF of 15 or higher — especially if you have fair skin and burn easily.

Apply sunscreen at least 15 minutes before you go outside; reapply it every 2 or 3 hours. Apply sunscreen more frequently if you perspire heavily or after you swim or exercise. Consider using a water-resistant sunscreen.

Get in the habit of applying a sunscreen routinely before you go outside because the sun's rays can damage your skin whether you're on your way to school or lounging at the pool.

Consider storing your sunscreen in a safe place near your front or back door. Keep an extra container in your car.

COVER UP

Wear protective clothing, such as a wide-brimmed hat, long sleeves, and sunglasses. Keep in mind that flimsy, lightweight clothes may not protect against sunburn because the sun's rays can penetrate them.

Don't rely on a shady tree, an umbrella, or a cloudy day to prevent sunburn. Remember that burning ultraviolet rays penetrate overcast skies and a canopy of leaves as well.

Also, keep in mind that sun reflected from water, snow, or sand can burn your skin even more intensely than direct sunlight, so carry a cover-up with you when you go out.

ADJUST YOUR SCHEDULE

Avoid outdoor activities when the sun's rays shine their strongest — between 10 a.m. and 3 p.m. (11 a.m. and 4 p.m. daylight savings time). Schedule outdoor activities at other times. For example, play tennis in the early morning or mow the lawn in the late afternoon.

ADDITIONAL POINTS

- Remember: No matter how attractive, a suntan isn't healthful.
- Don't use oils or a reflector device to promote suntan.
- Check with your health care provider or pharmacist about possible phototropic (sensitizing) effects related to prescription or over-the-counter medicines that you take.
- Avoid artificial ultraviolet light. Don't use sunlamps, and stay out of tanning parlors or booths.

⬭ Mixing insulins in a syringe

Dear Patient:

Your health care provider has prescribed regular and either intermediate or long-acting insulin to control your diabetes. To avoid giving yourself separate injections, you can mix these two types of insulin in a syringe and administer them together.

PREPARING THE INSULIN

1. Wash your hands. Then prepare the mixture in a clean area. Make sure that you have alcohol swabs for both types of insulin and the proper syringe for your prescribed insulin concentration. Then mix the contents of the intermediate or long-acting insulin by rolling it gently between your palms.

2. Using an alcohol swab, clean the rubber stopper on the vial of intermediate or long-acting insulin. Then draw air into the syringe by pulling the plunger back to the prescribed number of insulin units. Insert the needle into the top of the vial. Make sure that the point doesn't touch the insulin, as shown below left.

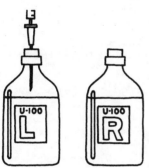

INSERTING THE NEEDLE

1. Push in the plunger, and remove the needle from the vial. Clean the rubber stopper on the regular insulin vial with an alcohol swab. Then pull back the plunger on the syringe to the prescribed number of insulin

units. Insert the needle into the top of the vial, and inject air into the vial. With the needle still in the vial, turn the vial upside down. Withdraw the prescribed dose of regular insulin.

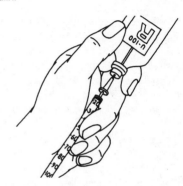

2. Clean the top of the intermediate or long-acting insulin vial. Then insert the needle into it without pushing the plunger down. Invert the vial and withdraw the prescribed number of units for the total dose. For example, if you have 10 units of regular insulin in the syringe and you need 20 units of intermediate or long-acting insulin, pull the plunger back to 30 units.

ADDITIONAL POINTS

● Never change the order in which you mix insulins.

● Always administer the insulin immediately to prevent loss of potency.

◯ Performing active range-of-motion exercises

Dear Patient:
Review these guidelines before you begin active range-of-motion exercises.

- Do your exercises daily to get the most benefit from them.
- Repeat each exercise three to five times or as often as your health care provider recommends. (As you get stronger, your activity may be increased.)
- Impose order on your routine. If you're exercising all your major joints, begin at your neck and then work toward your toes.
- Move slowly and gently so you don't injure yourself. If an exercise is painful, *stop doing it.* Then ask your health care provider if you should keep doing that particular exercise.
- Take a break and rest after an exercise that's especially tiring.
- Consider spacing your exercises over the day if you prefer not doing them in a single session.

3. After you do the recommended number of counterclockwise circles, reverse the exercise, doing an equal number of clockwise circles.

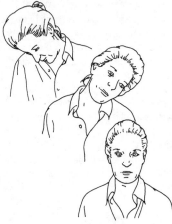

NECK EXERCISE

1. Slowly tilt your head as far back as possible. Next, move it to the right, toward your shoulder.
2. With your head still to the right, lower your chin as far as it will go toward your chest. Then move your head toward your left shoulder. Complete a full circle by moving your head back to its usual upright position.

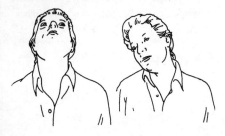

SHOULDER EXERCISE

1. Raise your shoulders as if you were going to shrug. Next, move them forward, down, then up, in a single circular motion.
2. Now move them backward, down, then up again in a single circular motion.
3. Continue to alternate forward and backward shoulder circles throughout the exercise.

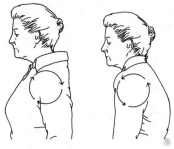

(continued)

Performing active range-of-motion
exercises *(continued)*

ELBOW EXERCISE

1. Extend your arm straight out to your side. Open your hand, palm up, as if to catch a raindrop.

2. Now, slowly reach back with your forearm so that you touch your shoulder with your fingers. Then slowly return your arm to its straight position. Now repeat with your other arm.

3. Continue to alternate arms throughout the exercise.

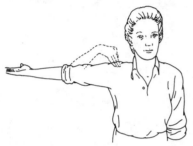

WRIST AND HAND EXERCISE

Extend your arms, palms down and fingers straight. Keeping your palms flat, slowly raise your fingers and "point" them back toward you. Then slowly lower your fingers and "point" them as far downward as you comfortably can.

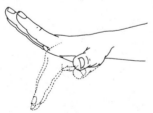

FINGER EXERCISE

Spread the fingers and thumb on each hand as wide apart as possible without causing discomfort.

Then bring the fingers back together into a fist.

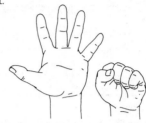

LEG AND KNEE EXERCISE

1. Lie on your bed or on the floor. Bend one leg so the knee is straight up and the foot is flat on the bed or floor.

2. Raise your foot, bend the other leg, and slowly bring your knee as far toward your chest as you can without discomfort.

3. Then straighten this leg slowly while you lower it.

4. Repeat this exercise with your other leg.

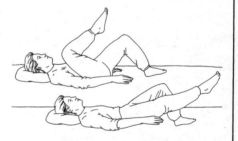

ANKLE AND FOOT EXERCISE

1. Raise one foot and point your toes away from you. Move this foot in a circular motion — first to the right, then to the left.

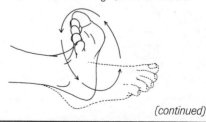

(continued)

Performing active range-of-motion
exercises *(continued)*

2. Point your toes back toward you. With your foot in this position, make a circle with it, first right, then left.

3. Now do the same exercise with your other foot.

TOE EXERCISE

---

1. Sit in a chair or lie on your bed. Stretch your legs out in front of you, with your heels resting on the floor or the bed. Slowly bend your toes down and away from you.

2. Bend your toes up and back toward you.

3. Spread out your toes so that they're totally separated. Then squeeze your toes together.

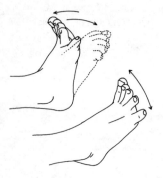

◯ Performing relaxation breathing exercises

Dear Patient:

Relaxation breathing can help you cope with stress or pain. You can use it anywhere and at any time. You can also combine it with other techniques to help control pain. Try to practice these simple breathing techniques daily. Now, get yourself comfortable and begin.

1. Close your eyes. Inhale slowly and deeply through your nose as you count silently: "In, 2, 3, 4." Notice how your stomach expands first, then your rib cage, and finally your upper chest.

Now exhale slowly through your mouth as you count silently: "Out, 2, 3, 4, 5, 6." Pretend you're breathing out through a straw to lengthen exhalation. Let your shoulders drop slightly as your upper chest, rib cage, and stomach gently deflate. Repeat this exercise four or five times.

A FEW TIPS

Use these breathing exercises for as long as you need to during painful periods. You may vary the rhythm, but always exhale for 2 to 4 seconds longer than you inhale.

If you feel light-headed or your fingers tingle, you may be breathing too deeply or too fast. Reduce the depth and speed of your breathing, or breathe into a paper bag until the feeling goes away.

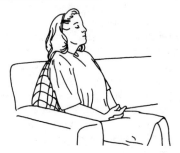

2. Inhale for 4 seconds. Hold your breath for the count of 4, but don't strain. Then exhale through your mouth for 6 to 8 seconds. Practice this exercise four or five times.

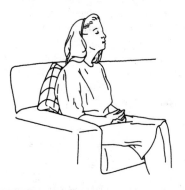

◯ Personalizing your exercise program

Dear Patient:
You can make your exercise program suit your individual needs by determining your aerobic training level, adjusting your pace accordingly, and allowing adequate time to warm up and cool down.

FINDING YOUR PACE

How do you determine the aerobic training level that's best for you? Your target heart rate provides a guideline for achieving the greatest benefits during exercising while reducing risk.

First, find your maximum heart rate. To do this, subtract your age from 220. To determine your target heart rate, calculate 75% of your maximum rate (multiply your maximum rate by 0.75). For example, if your maximum rate is 180, your target rate is 135 beats per minute.

To determine your heart rate range, calculate the range between 70% and 80% of your maximum heart rate. By monitoring your pulse and staying in this range, you'll achieve the greatest benefits from aerobic exercise. The chart below provides heart rate ranges according to age.

HEART RATE RANGE

AGE	MINIMUM	TARGET	MAXIMUM
20	140	150	160
25	137	146	156
30	133	143	152
35	130	139	148
40	126	135	144
45	123	131	140
50	119	128	136
55	116	124	132
60	112	120	128
65	109	116	124
70	105	113	120

Keep in mind, however, that these numbers provide a measure of what a healthy heart can do. Gradually slow down if you begin to experience pain. Ask your health care provider to help you determine an appropriate target heart rate. Some cardiac medications may not allow you to reach your target heart rate because of their specific action on the heart.

WARMING UP

Before starting any kind of demanding physical activity, you'll want to perform warm-up exercises to stretch muscles and loosen joints. This will lessen the risk of muscle strain or ligament damage and raise your heart rate slowly. A good warm-up offers psychological benefits as well. Use this time to focus on the activities ahead and to get rid of tension. First, take your pulse, and then do 5 to 10 minutes of stretching exercises and light calisthenics.

ADJUSTING THE PACE

Gradually work toward your optimal aerobic training level. During your exercise period, take your pulse two or three times as directed. Adjust your pace according to your pulse rate and how you feel. If you exceed your target rate or if you have chest discomfort, breathlessness, or palpitations, slow down *gradually*. Don't stop suddenly unless signs or symptoms persist or worsen.

(continued)

Personalizing your exercise program (continued)

COOLING DOWN

Never stop exercising abruptly. If you do, the amount of blood circulating back to the heart, which is still beating rapidly, won't be adequate to meet your body's needs. You need a cooldown period much as a horse needs to be walked after a race.

Gradually decrease the pace of your exercise for 5 to 10 minutes. This will lower your heart rate and blood pressure slowly. Then do 5 minutes of light calisthenics and simple stretching exercises. At this point, your pulse should be no more than 15 beats above your resting pulse. If you feel dizzy or faint after exercising, you may need a longer cooldown period.

KEEP RECORDS

Keep an exercise diary. List the date and time, the activity and its duration, your heart rate, and any symptoms you experience. Tracking your progress will help you keep your motivation, and the record will give your health care provider valuable information.

⬭ Planning a calcium-rich diet

Dear Patient:
Your body needs calcium for strong bones and teeth. Eating calcium-rich foods is one way to make sure that your body gets enough of this vital mineral. Here are some things to consider.

WHAT'S ENOUGH?

The amount of calcium you need changes throughout your lifetime. For example, teenagers need extra calcium to meet the needs of their rapidly growing bones. Women need more calcium to prevent osteoporosis after menopause, during pregnancy, and while breast-feeding.

Ask your nurse or health care provider to help you determine how much calcium you need each day.

WHERE TO GET CALCIUM

Dairy products (milk, cheese, yogurt, and ice cream) are potent calcium sources. If you're avoiding cholesterol or watching your weight, you can still have 1% or nonfat powdered milk and nonfat yogurt.

If you have trouble digesting milk, you may still be able to eat yogurt, hard cheeses, acidophilus milk, or lactose-reduced milk. (Ask your grocery store manager to order a product, such as Lactaid, if your store doesn't carry it.) Or, ask your pharmacist about adding lactobacillus acidophilus to regular milk. Also called by such trade names as *Bacid* and *Lactinex,* this substance makes milk easier to digest.

Certain green, leafy vegetables, such as collards, turnip greens, and broccoli, contain lots of calcium. Oysters, salmon, sardines, legumes, liver, nuts, and tofu are other foods with high calcium content.

OTHER TIPS

Some foods, especially very fibrous foods, can interfere with your body's uptake of calcium. To get the most calcium from the foods you eat, avoid calcium- and fiber-rich foods at the same meal.

You should also eat less red meat, chocolate, peanut butter, rhubarb, sweet potatoes, and fatty foods. Cut down on alcohol as well as caffeine-containing drinks, such as coffee, tea, and colas.

Calcium is most effective when your body has enough vitamin D. Spending just 15 minutes in the sunshine every day will fulfill your daily vitamin D requirement. Most manufacturers add vitamin D to milk and cereals. Egg yolks, saltwater fish, and liver also have this vitamin.

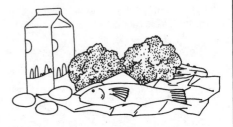

Keep in mind that too much vitamin D may do more harm than good. Avoid taking a vitamin D supplement unless your health care provider specifically tells you to do so.

⬭ Planning home care

Dear Caregiver:

Taking care of a person with Alzheimer's disease requires a great deal of patience and understanding. It also requires you to look at the person's typical daily routine and his environment with new eyes and make necessary changes to help him function at the highest possible level. The following tips can help you plan your daily care.

REDUCE STRESS

Too much stress can worsen the patient's symptoms. Try to protect him from potential sources of stress, including:

● a change in routine, caregiver, or environment; fatigue; excessive demands; overwhelming, misleading, or competing stimuli; illness and pain; and over-the-counter (nonprescription) medications.

ESTABLISH A ROUTINE

Keep the patient's daily routine stable so he can respond automatically. Adapting to change may require more thought than the patient can handle. Even eating a different food or going to a strange grocery store may overwhelm him.

Ask yourself: What are the patient's daily activities? Then make a schedule:

● List the activities necessary for his daily care and include ones that he especially enjoys such as weeding in the garden. Designate a time frame for each activity.

● Establish bedtime rituals — especially important to promote relaxation and a restful night's sleep for both of you.

● Stick to your schedule as closely as possible (for example, breakfast first, then dressing) so the patient won't be surprised or need to make decisions.

● Keep a copy of the patient's schedule to give to other caregivers. To help them give better care, include notes and suggestions about techniques that work for you; for instance, "Speak in a quiet voice" or "When helping Mitchell dress or take a bath, take things one step at a time and wait for him to respond."

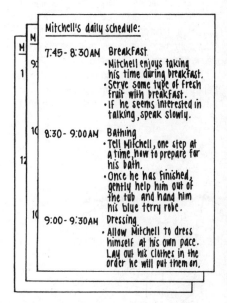

Mitchell's daily schedule:

7:45 - 8:30 AM   Breakfast
- Mitchell enjoys taking his time during breakfast.
- Serve some type of fresh fruit with breakfast.
- If he seems interested in talking, speak slowly.

8:30 - 9:00 AM   Bathing
- Tell Mitchell, one step at a time, how to prepare for his bath.
- Once he has finished, gently help him out of the tub and hand him his blue terry robe.

9:00 - 9:30 AM   Dressing
- Allow Mitchell to dress himself at his own pace. Lay out his clothes in the order he will put them on.

PRACTICE REALITY ORIENTATION

In your conversations with the patient, orient him to the day and the activity he'll perform. For instance, say "Today is Tuesday, and we're going to have breakfast now." Do this every day.

This keeps the patient aware of his immediate environment and tells him what to ex-

(continued)

Planning home care *(continued)*

pect without challenging him to remember events.

SIMPLIFY THE SURROUNDINGS

The patient will eventually lose the ability to interpret correctly what he sees and hears. Protect him by trying to decrease the noise level in his environment and by avoiding busy areas, such as shopping malls and restaurants.

Does the patient mistake pictures or images in the mirror for real people? If so, remove the photos and mirrors. Also, avoid rooms with busy patterns on wallpaper and carpets because they can overtax his senses.

To avoid confusion and encourage the patient's independence, provide cues. For example, hang a picture of a toilet on the bathroom door.

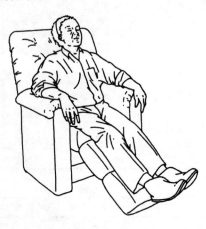

AVOID FATIGUE

The patient will tire easily, so plan important activities for the morning when he's functioning best. Save less demanding ones for later in the day. Remember to schedule breaks — one in the morning and one in the afternoon.

About 15 to 30 minutes of listening to music or just relaxing is sufficient in the early stages of Alzheimer's disease. As the disease progresses, schedule longer, more frequent breaks (perhaps 40 to 90 minutes). If the patient naps during the day, have him sleep in a reclining chair rather than in a bed to prevent him from confusing day and night.

DON'T EXPECT TOO MUCH

Accept the patient's limitations. Don't demand too much from him — this forces him to think about a task and causes frustration. Instead, offer help when needed, and distract him if he's trying too hard. You'll feel less stressed, too.

PREPARE FOR ILLNESS

If the patient becomes ill, expect his behavior to deteriorate and plan accordingly. He'll have a low tolerance for pain and discomfort.

Never rely on the patient to take his own medicine. He may forget to take it or miscount what he has taken. Always supervise him.

USE THE SENSE OF TOUCH

Because the patient's visual and auditory perceptions are distorted, he has an increased need for closeness and touching. Remember to approach the patient from the front. You don't want to frighten him or provoke him into becoming belligerent or aggressive.

Respect the patient's need for personal space. Limit physical contact to his hands and arms at first; then move to more central

(continued)

Planning home care *(continued)*

parts of his body, such as his shoulders or head.

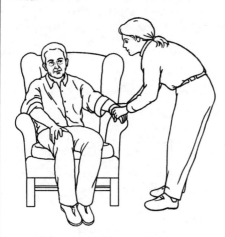

Using long or circular motions, lightly stroke the patient to help relieve muscle tension and give him a sense of his physical self. Physical contact also expresses your feelings of intimacy and caring.

Allowing the patient to touch objects in the environment can help relieve stress by providing information. Let him handle or shake objects — for example, a handbag, a brush, or a comb. Make sure that they're unbreakable and can't harm him.

HANDLE PROBLEM BEHAVIOR

If the patient becomes restless or agitated, divert his attention with an appropriate activity. Good choices include walking, rocking in a rocking chair, sanding wood, folding laundry, or hoeing the garden.

These repetitive activities don't require any particular sequence or planning. A warm bath, a drink of warm milk, or a back massage can also be calming.

Although problem behavior can be taxing for you, try to remember that the patient can't help himself. Your understanding and compassion can increase his sense of security.

⬭ Preparing for a CT scan

Dear Patient:
Your health care provider has scheduled you for a computed tomography (CT) scan. This test uses X-rays and a computer to create detailed images of the body part being scanned. It involves the use of a large machine called a *CT scanner.* The test is painless and takes between 30 and 60 minutes.

BEFORE THE TEST

You may receive an injection of a contrast dye in your arm. This substance highlights certain areas of your body. If the test requires this dye, don't eat or drink anything for 4 hours before the test.

Tell your health care provider if you have ever had an allergic reaction to X-ray contrast material or if you're allergic or sensitive to shellfish or iodine-containing solutions. Also, report other allergies.

Remove all metal objects and jewelry, such as a watch, hairpins, and earrings. Also remember to remove objects that might obstruct the X-ray beam, such as glasses, dentures, and a hearing aid. Wear loose, comfortable clothing or a hospital gown. You may be given a mild sedative to help you relax.

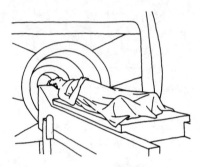

If you received contrast material, you may develop a headache, have a salty taste in your mouth, or feel warm or flushed and nauseous. These reactions usually subside rapidly, but be sure to mention them to the technician.

AFTER THE TEST

You may resume your usual activities and diet. If you received a contrast dye, drink plenty of fluids for the rest of the day to help flush it from your system. Report nausea or vomiting; also report if you have a headache after the test.

Within 1 to 2 days, your health care provider will review the scan and discuss the results with you.

DURING THE TEST

A technician will position you on an X-ray table. Then the table will slide into the tubelike scanner, which looks like a giant thermos bottle lying on its side. Every few seconds, the table will move a small distance and an X-ray image will be taken. You'll hear clicking or buzzing noises from the scanner as it revolves, obtaining images from many angles.

Remember to lie still. To prevent blurring of the X-ray images, your body will be steadied with straps or a support. You'll be alone in the scanner room during the test, but you can talk to the technician through a two-way intercom.

◯ Preparing for a sigmoidoscopy or a colonoscopy

Dear Patient:

Your health care provider wants you to undergo a flexible sigmoidoscopy. (Continue reading if you're scheduled for a colonoscopy because the two tests are similar. The differences are listed at the end of this patient-teaching aid.)

A sigmoidoscopy allows the health care provider to see inside the *lower* part of the large bowel, which includes the sigmoid colon, rectum, and anus. To do this, the health care provider will gently insert a flexible fiber-optic tube called an *endoscope* into the rectum.

WHY IS THIS TEST NECESSARY?

Sigmoidoscopy allows for careful examination of the lower bowel and rectum for disease. (These areas are difficult to visualize in X-rays.) If needed, this test will also enable the health care provider to take a biopsy specimen for further testing or to remove polyps.

WILL I NEED TO PREPARE FOR THE TEST?

Yes. Be sure to follow your health care provider's directions for diet and bowel preparation. Stay on a liquid diet for 48 hours beforehand. You may drink clear juices without pulp, broth, tea, gelatin, and water, and you may continue to take prescription medicine.

Take a laxative the evening before the test and give yourself an enema (for example, a Fleet enema) the morning of the test or as directed by your healthcare provider. If the test is scheduled for early morning, don't consume anything past midnight.

Just before the test, you'll take off your clothes and put on a hospital gown. Leave your socks on for warmth. Also, empty your bladder.

WHAT CAN I EXPECT DURING THE TEST?

The test is done by the health care provider and an assistant in an office or a special procedures room. It will last about 15 to 30 minutes. Before the test begins, the assistant will

POSITIONING FOR SIGMOIDOSCOPY OR COLONSCOPY

BOWEL SEGMENTS

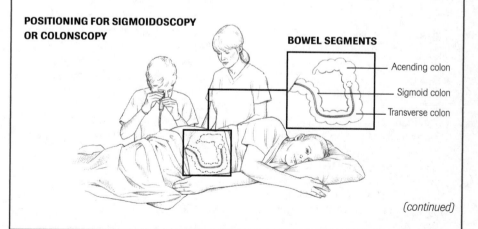

- Acending colon
- Sigmoid colon
- Transverse colon

(continued)

Preparing for a sigmoidoscopy or a colonoscopy *(continued)*

help you lie on your left side with your knees flexed and drape you with a sheet.

When you're in position, the health care provider will gently insert a well-lubricated, gloved finger into the anus to examine the area and dilate the rectal sphincter.

Next, the health care provider will gently insert the endoscope through the anus into the rectum. As it passes through the rectal sphincter, you may feel some lower abdominal discomfort and the urge to move your bowels. Bear down gently when the endoscope is first inserted. Also, breathe slowly and deeply through your mouth to help you relax. This will help ease the passage of the endoscope through the sphincter. The health care provider will gradually advance the endoscope through the rectum into the lower bowel.

Sometimes air is blown through the endoscope into the bowel to distend it and permit better viewing. If you feel the urge to expel some air, try not to control it and don't be embarrassed. The passing of air is expected and necessary. You may hear and feel a suction machine removing liquid that obscures the health care provider's view during the test. This machine is noisy but painless.

The health care provider will advance the endoscope slowly about 24 inches into the lower bowel. Continue to breathe slowly and deeply through your mouth to help the test go smoothly.

The health care provider may remove biopsy specimens or polyps from the lining of the bowel at any time during the test. These procedures are also painless because the bowel lining doesn't sense pain.

Toward the end of the test, the health care provider may insert a rigid anoscope into the lower rectum. This instrument will provide a clearer view of the anal wall, revealing any abnormalities that the flexible endoscope might miss.

WHAT CAN I EXPECT AFTERWARD?

The assistant will monitor your vital signs for about an hour afterward. Because air was introduced into your bowel, you'll begin to pass large amounts of gas. In addition, you may have slight rectal bleeding if the health care provider removed tissue specimens. Notify the health care provider or assistant immediately if you experience heavy, bright red bleeding; fever; abdominal swelling; or tenderness after the test.

HOW DOES A COLONOSCOPY DIFFER FROM A SIGMOIDOSCOPY?

The two tests are similar except a colonoscopy allows the health care provider to visualize *all* of your large bowel.

To prepare for a colonoscopy, follow the health care provider's directions for a clear liquid diet and bowel preparation. The bowel preparation is one of two kinds: You may be instructed to drink a large amount of an electrolyte solution (GoLYTELY or Co-Lyte). This solution will clear your bowel in about 4 hours, so plan to stay at home after drinking it. Alternatively, you may be asked to take a laxative for 2 nights before the test and give yourself enemas the morning of the test.

Just before a colonoscopy, you'll receive a sedative to help you relax and ease any discomfort you may experience as the health care provider advances the endoscope past the curves of the bowel.

⬭ Preparing for bone marrow aspiration and biopsy

Dear Patient:

Your health care provider has ordered a bone marrow aspiration and biopsy. This test will evaluate your bone marrow, which is the soft tissue inside your bone.

An *aspiration biopsy* involves withdrawing a fluid sample containing bone marrow particles from the marrow. A *needle biopsy* involves removing a core of solid cells from the marrow. Either test will take about 10 to 20 minutes.

The bone marrow sample will be examined under a microscope to determine whether the marrow produces enough normal blood cells and how mature they are. You'll usually know the results in 1 or 2 days.

BEFORE THE TEST

● You may continue your usual diet and fluid intake. However, you may wish to eat lightly before the test.
● Expect to have a blood sample taken.
● You may be given a mild sedative an hour before the test to help you relax.

DURING THE TEST

The most common biopsy site is the back of the hip (called the *posterior superior iliac crest*). Other sites include the spine, a leg bone (epiphysis), or the breastbone.

A marrow sample will be taken from the back of the hip while you lie on your stomach as still as you can. The skin around the site will be draped and the skin cleaned with an antiseptic solution. A local anesthetic will then be injected, which may cause brief discomfort before the area becomes numb.

For *aspiration biopsy:* An aspiration needle will be inserted through the skin, the tissue below, and the cortex of the bone in a twisting motion until it reaches the bone marrow. Then the metal core from the needle will be removed and a bone marrow sample will be drawn into the syringe.

For *needle biopsy:* A biopsy needle will be inserted through the skin and underlying tissue and into the bone. Next, the core of the needle will be removed. The needle will then be advanced and rotated in both directions, forcing a tiny core of bone into the needle.

As the bone marrow sample is collected, you'll feel a pulling or grinding sensation or a brief, sharp pain. After the needle is withdrawn, pressure will be applied to the biopsy site for several minutes to stop bleeding. Finally, a bandage will be applied to the wound.

AFTER THE TEST

● Rest for several hours.
● Report bleeding that completely soaks the dressing or continues for more than 24 hours.
● Reinforce the dressing if needed, but don't remove it for at least 24 hours.
● If you have discomfort, take medication as directed.

◯ Preparing for bronchoscopy

Dear Patient:

Here are some facts you'll want to know about the bronchoscopy your health care provider has scheduled for you.

This test permits your health care provider to examine your airway (windpipe and lungs) with a thin, flexible instrument called a *bronchoscope.*

By looking through the instrument's eyepiece, your health care provider can see abnormalities and obstructions. With another part of the instrument, your health care provider can obtain tiny tissue samples to help diagnose your illness or remove foreign bodies or excess mucus.

BEFORE THE TEST

Don't eat for 8 hours before the test, and don't drink alcoholic beverages for 24 hours beforehand. Food and alcohol can cause test complications and create problems with any sedatives you're given.

Continue to take prescribed drugs unless you're told not to.

Just before the test, you'll receive a local anesthetic to numb the back of your throat and to stop you from gagging. This helps the bronchoscope slide easily inside your trachea. You'll receive a sedative to help you relax.

DURING THE TEST

The test takes 30 to 60 minutes. You'll lie on your back or sit upright. After the anesthetic takes effect, the end of the bronchoscope will be inserted through your nose or mouth.

As the instrument is advanced, small amounts of liquid anesthetic will be flushed through it to decrease any coughing and wheezing you might have. The instrument will slide through your major airways. You may experience some discomfort with breathing. Remember to stay calm. If necessary, you'll be given extra oxygen.

When the examination is over, your health care provider will remove the bronchoscope.

AFTER THE TEST

You'll lie comfortably with your head raised and will be monitored closely for 1 to 2 hours. Until the anesthetic wears off and your gag reflex returns, you won't be allowed to eat, drink, or take oral medications. You may be hoarse and may have a sore throat, but this is only temporary. When your gag reflex returns, you'll be able to gargle or suck on throat lozenges.

Soon after the test, you'll have a chest X-ray to make sure that you're doing well.

Your sedative may not have worn off by the time you're ready to go home, so arrange for someone to take you home from the hospital or clinic.

Immediately report bloody mucus, difficulty breathing, wheezing, or chest pain.

⬭ Preparing for cardiac catheterization

Dear Patient:

You've been scheduled for cardiac catheterization, a procedure that looks at the inside of your heart. First, a small incision is made in a blood vessel near your elbow or groin, and then a long, thin, flexible tube called a *catheter* is inserted into the vessel.

The catheter is then slowly threaded through your bloodstream into your heart. When the catheter is in place, certain tests may be performed that require the injection of a special dye. The test results will guide further treatment designed to improve the function of your heart.

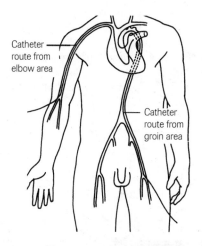

Catheter route from elbow area

Catheter route from groin area

Cardiac catheterization usually takes 1 to 2 hours. You'll be awake throughout the procedure, although you may receive medication to help you relax. Some patients even doze off. You may feel pain in your chest, flushing, or nausea during catheterization, but these sensations should pass quickly.

DURING THE PROCEDURE

First, a local anesthetic will be injected at the catheter insertion site to numb the area before the catheter is inserted. When the catheter is going in, you may feel a little pressure but no pain. You may receive nitroglycerin during the test to enlarge your heart's blood vessels and help provide a better view of your heart.

If the catheter's passage is blocked — for example, because of a narrowed blood vessel — the catheter will be removed, and a different insertion site will be used.

When the catheter enters your heart, you may feel a fluttering sensation. Report this sensation, but don't worry — this is a normal reaction. You'll probably also feel a warm sensation, some nausea, or the urge to urinate if dye is injected, but these feelings will quickly pass. Throughout the catheterization, remember to let someone know if you have chest pain.

BEFORE THE PROCEDURE

If your catheterization is scheduled for early morning, you probably won't be allowed to eat or drink anything after midnight the day before the test.

The area where the incision will be made may be shaved. Before you go to the catheterization laboratory, you'll be asked to urinate and then to put on a hospital gown. You may also have an I.V. line started in your arm.

When you reach the catheterization laboratory, you'll be placed on a padded table and probably be strapped to it. During the test, the table may be tilted to permit viewing of your heart from different angles. The straps will keep you from slipping out of position. Special foam pads, called *electrodes,* may be put on your chest to monitor your heartbeat.

(continued)

Preparing for cardiac catheterization *(continued)*

During the test, you may be given oxygen and asked to cough or to breathe deeply.

When the test is finished, the catheter will be removed, and a special bandage will be placed on your arm or groin. You may need a few stitches at the insertion site. Because the anesthetic will still be working, you shouldn't feel anything.

AFTER THE PROCEDURE

You'll be taken to a recovery area, where you'll be monitored for a short time. You'll be placed on a cardiac monitor to check your heart rhythm, and an electrocardiogram may be done. Your vital signs will be taken frequently during this time, and your bandage site will be checked for bleeding.

Your bandaged arm or leg must stay completely still for up to 8 hours. To help keep you from moving, your arm may be splinted or your leg may be weighed down with a sandbag. The site will be checked frequently for swelling and inadequate blood flow. You'll be asked to wiggle your toes or fingers once per hour or more.

As your anesthetic wears off, you'll probably feel some pain at the insertion site. Pain medication may be ordered.

As soon as the test results are available, you and your family will be informed of them. Don't hesitate to ask any questions that you may have.

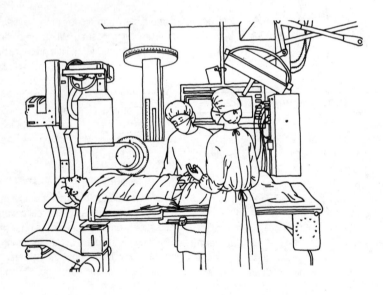

⬭ Preparing for ERCP

Dear Patient:

You're about to undergo endoscopic retrograde cholangiopancreatography — called *ERCP* for short. This procedure uses a dyelike substance, a flexible tube called an *endoscope,* and X-rays to outline your gallbladder and pancreatic structures.

ERCP is performed in the radiology department and may take up to 1 hour to complete. Read the information below to help you prepare.

BEFORE THE TEST

The day before ERCP, you can eat and drink as usual. After midnight before the procedure, don't eat or drink anything unless your health care provider directs otherwise. He may tell you to continue taking certain medications. Before you enter the test room, be sure to urinate because an ERCP can cause you to retain urine.

DURING THE TEST

You'll lie on an X-ray table for this test. The nurse will take your temperature, blood pressure, and pulse rate. An I.V. line will be inserted into your hand or arm to administer medication. You'll receive a sedative to relax you and to ease the discomfort of the procedure.

The health care provider will spray your throat with a bitter-tasting anesthetic, which will make your mouth and throat feel swollen and numb. Because you'll have difficulty swallowing, you may be given a device to suction your saliva.

Next, a mouthguard will be placed in your mouth to keep your mouth open and to protect your teeth during the ERCP. You'll be unable to talk but won't have trouble breathing. When the health care provider passes the endoscope down your throat, you may gag a little, but this reflex is normal.

As the tube reaches the duodenum (small intestine), the health care provider may inject air through the tube. You'll also receive medication through your I.V. line to relax the duo-denum. Next, the health care provider will thread a thinner tube through the endoscope to the biliary structures and the duodenum.

When the second tube is in place, dye will be injected and X-ray images will be taken quickly from several angles. After the images are viewed and a tissue sample obtained, the endoscope, tube, and mouthguard will be gently removed.

AFTER THE TEST

The nurse will check your blood pressure, pulse rate, and temperature frequently for several hours.

When you regain feeling in your throat and your gag reflex returns, you'll be allowed to have a light meal and liquids. You can resume your regular diet the next day.

Expect to have a sore throat for a few days. Call the health care provider if you can't urinate or if you experience chills, abdominal pain, nausea, or vomiting.

⊙ Preparing for needle aspiration of the breast

Dear Patient:
Your health care provider wants to perform needle aspiration on your breast lump or cyst. This procedure involves inserting a needle into the lump to remove fluid that may be present.

Needle aspiration may sound scary, but it's actually quick, safe, and almost always painless.

HOW SHOULD I PREPARE FOR NEEDLE ASPIRATION?

Before the procedure, you'll need a mammography or ultrasonography. These tests help pinpoint the lump's location and characteristics.

You'll be asked to remove your clothing from the waist up, and you'll be given a hospital gown to wear.

WHAT HAPPENS DURING THE PROCEDURE?

Usually, the health care provider can do the procedure in his office. It takes 5 to 10 minutes. You'll be asked to lie on an examination table.

The health care provider will clean the skin on your breast with an antiseptic solution. You may receive a local anesthetic to numb the area. Except for a brief sting when the anesthetic is injected, you should feel little or no discomfort during the procedure.

The health care provider will use one hand to steady the lump between his fingers. With his other hand, he'll quickly insert a small, hollow needle into the lump, as shown in the illustration.

If it's a cyst, he'll remove the fluid. The amount will be anywhere from a few drops to several ounces. After the cyst is aspirated, it usually disappears. Your health care provider should send a sample of the fluid to the laboratory for analysis.

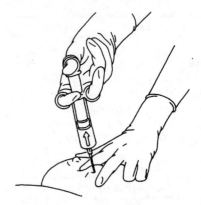

WHAT CAN I EXPECT AFTERWARD?

The health care provider will withdraw the needle and apply a bandage.

Be sure to keep all appointments for follow-up visits. Typically, your health care provider will want to examine your breasts again 1 month and 6 months after the aspiration. Sometimes, a cyst recurs or a new one forms. If this happens, you may need to undergo another aspiration.

If the health care provider was unable to remove fluid during the aspiration, he may order more tests to evaluate the lump.

○ Preparing for pulmonary function tests

Dear Patient:
Pulmonary (or lung) function tests have been ordered for you. These tests measure how well your lungs work. Here's what to expect.

HOW THE TESTS WORK

You'll be asked to breathe as deeply as possible into a mouthpiece that's connected to a machine called a *spirometer.* This measures and records the rate and amount of air inhaled and exhaled.

You may also sit in a small, telephone booth–like enclosure for a test called *body plethysmography.* Again, you'll be asked to breathe in and out, and the measurements will be recorded.

BEFORE THE TESTS

Avoid smoking for at least 4 hours before the tests. Eat lightly, and don't drink a lot of fluid. Wear loose, comfortable clothing. Remember to use the bathroom.

To make the tests go quickly, give your full cooperation. Tell the technician if you don't understand the instructions. If you wear dentures, keep them in — they'll help you keep a tight seal around the spirometer's mouthpiece.

DURING THE TESTS

During spirometry, you'll sit upright, and you'll wear a noseclip to make sure you breathe only through your mouth. During body plethysmography, you won't need a noseclip.

If you feel too confined in the small chamber, keep in mind that you can't suffocate. You can talk to the nurse or technician through a window.

The tests have several parts. For each test, you'll be asked to breathe a certain way — for example, to inhale deeply and exhale completely or to inhale quickly. You may need to repeat some tests after inhaling a bronchodilator to expand the airways in your lungs. A blood sample may be obtained from an artery in your arm. This sample will be used to measure how well your body uses the air you breathe.

HOW WILL YOU FEEL?

During the tests, you may feel tired or short of breath. However, you'll be able to take rest breaks between measurements.

Tell the technician right away if you feel dizzy, begin wheezing, or have chest pain, a racing or pounding heart, an upset stomach, or severe shortness of breath. Also tell him if your arm swells or if you're bleeding from the spot where a blood sample was taken or experience weakness or pain in that arm.

AFTER THE TESTS

When the tests are over, rest if you feel like it. Resume your usual activities when you regain your energy.

⬭ Preparing for the patient's homecoming

Dear Caregiver:

Most people don't realize how dangerous or inconvenient their homes can be — especially for someone recovering from an illness. Use this list to pinpoint household areas that you need to adapt to the patient's needs.

BATHROOM

- Install grab bars in the shower and tub.
- Obtain a tub seat if the tub is hard to enter and exit.
- Buy a shower chair for sitting instead of standing to bathe.
- Install a raised toilet seat.
- Put nonskid strips or a tub mat in the bathtub to prevent falls.
- Attach a handheld shower head for easy rinsing.
- Install easy-to-turn faucet handles.
- Hang mirrors, shelves, and racks at wheelchair level.
- Set the water heater temperature no higher than 120° F (48.9° C) to prevent burns.

BEDROOM

- Keep a commode chair, urinal, or bedpan close to the bed.
- Provide a hospital-type bed (with side rails and attached trapeze).
- Install a bedside telephone.
- Provide a night-light or a bedside flashlight.
- Install a fire escape or portable ladder.

KITCHEN

- Provide a working fire extinguisher.
- Reorganize storage areas.
- Install easy-to-reach stove controls.

LIVING ROOM

- Provide cushions to raise the seating level if the person has trouble rising from a low chair or sofa.
- Arrange furniture to permit free access.
- Remove electrical cords and wires from walkways.
- Provide a conveniently located telephone (either stationary or portable) with a secured long cord (perhaps on a desk or table).

ALL AREAS

- Install smoke or heat detectors.
- Cover exposed heating pipes and radiators to prevent burns.
- Keep the indoor temperature no higher than 80° F (26.7° C) for maximum comfort.
- Provide good lighting.
- Install handrails along walls for support while walking.
- Provide low-pile carpeting for easy movement.
- Remove area and throw rugs, and keep floors clutter-free.
- Tape down loose carpet edges to prevent accidental trips and falls.
- Repair holes and rough floor areas.
- Install ramps over raised doorsills.
- Secure stair banisters and railings.
- Brightly tape step edges.
- Widen door frames to at least 27" (68.6 centimeters) to accommodate a wheelchair.
- Provide a ramp leading into the house, and repair uneven spots on the steps and sidewalk.

◯ Preventing adrenal crisis

Dear Patient:

Even though you follow your treatment plan carefully, unexpected situations can create stress and worsen your condition. Because your adrenal glands can't respond to increased demands, you'll need to prepare for stressful situations and know what to do to prevent adrenal crisis.

TAKE PRECAUTIONS

- Always wear or carry medical identification with your name, the name of your disorder, and the phone numbers of your health care provider and a responsible person.
- Always carry a clearly labeled emergency kit, especially when you travel. Double-check to make sure that the kit contains a syringe and needle, 100 milligrams of hydrocortisone, and instructions for use.

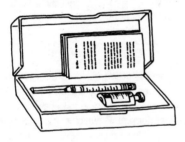

- Avoid strenuous physical activity in hot, humid weather. If you begin to perspire heavily, drink more fluids and add salt to your food.
- Follow your health care provider's directions for increasing your daily doses of prescribed steroids during stressful times — emotional crisis, overexertion, infection, illness, or injury.

WATCH YOUR DIET AND GET ADEQUATE REST

- Eat regularly. Don't skip meals or go for a long time without food.

- Be sure to follow a high-carbohydrate, high-protein diet with up to 8 grams of salt (sodium) daily — more if you perspire a lot.
- Balance active periods with rest.

RECOGNIZE WARNING SIGNS

Notify your health care provider immediately (or go directly to the nearest hospital emergency department) if you have any of these warning signs of adrenal crisis:

- apathy or restlessness, apprehensiveness, confusion, dizziness, headache
- pallor or cool, clammy skin
- fever
- increased breathing and pulse rates
- unusual fatigue or weakness
- loss of appetite, stomach cramps, diarrhea, nausea, and vomiting
- dehydration or reduced urine output.

If you can't reach your health care provider or get to a hospital at once, give yourself a subcutaneous injection of 100 milligrams of hydrocortisone. Then seek medical help.

PLAN AHEAD

Instruct a family member or a friend to give you a subcutaneous injection of 100 milligrams of hydrocortisone if he finds you unconscious or physically unable to take your medicine by mouth. He should then seek medical help immediately.

◯ Preventing diabetic complications

Dear Patient:
There's no way around it. Controlling your diabetes means checking your blood glucose level daily and making the following good health habits a way of life.

CARE FOR YOUR HEART

Because diabetes raises your risk of heart disease, follow these American Heart Association guidelines:
- Maintain your normal weight.
- Exercise regularly, following your health care provider's recommendations.
- Help control your blood pressure and cholesterol levels by eating a low-fat, high-fiber diet.

CARE FOR YOUR EYES

Have your eyes examined by an ophthalmologist at least once per year. He may detect damage, which could cause blindness, before symptoms appear. Early treatment may prevent further damage.

CARE FOR YOUR TEETH

Schedule regular dental checkups and follow good home care to minimize dental problems, such as gum disease and abscesses, which may occur with diabetes. Report bleeding, pain, or soreness in your gums or teeth to the dentist immediately. Brush your teeth after every meal and floss daily. If you wear dentures, clean them thoroughly every day and make sure that they fit properly.

CARE FOR YOUR SKIN

Breaks in your skin can increase the risk of infection, so check your skin daily for cuts and irritated areas. See your health care provider if necessary. Bathe daily with warm water and a mild soap, and apply a lanolin-based lotion afterward to prevent dryness. Pat your skin dry thoroughly, taking extra care between your toes and in other areas where skin surfaces touch. Always wear cotton underwear to allow moisture to evaporate and help prevent skin breakdown.

CARE FOR YOUR FEET

Diabetes can reduce blood flow to your feet and dull their ability to feel heat, cold, or pain. Follow your health care provider's instructions on daily foot care and necessary precautions to prevent foot problems.

CHECK YOUR URINE

Because symptoms of kidney disease usually don't appear until the problem is advanced, your health care provider will check your urine routinely for protein, which can signal kidney disease. Don't delay telling your health care provider if you have symptoms of a urinary tract infection (burning, painful, or difficult urination or blood or pus in the urine).

HAVE REGULAR CHECKUPS

Regular checkups help ensure the early detection and prompt treatment of complications.

Preventing infection – and recognizing its symptoms

Dear Patient:

Because acquired immunodeficiency syndrome damages your immune system and impairs your body's ability to fight infections, preventing infections is extremely important.

However, if you do come down with an infection, remember that early recognition and treatment are equally important.

Appropriate and timely treatment may prevent your condition from getting worse.

PREVENTING INFECTION

To help prevent infection, review these guidelines and follow them whenever possible:

- Avoid crowds and people with known infections, such as herpes, influenza, mononucleosis, and cytomegalovirus. You should also stay away from people who have minor colds.
- Get adequate sleep at night, and rest often during the day.
- Eat small, frequent meals, even if you have lost your appetite and have to force yourself to eat.
- Practice good hygiene, especially good oral hygiene. Don't use commercial mouthwashes because their high alcohol and sugar content may irritate your mouth and provide a medium for bacterial growth.
- Don't use unprescribed intravenous drugs, and don't share needles with anyone.
- Avoid traveling to foreign countries. If you must travel, however, consider drinking only bottled or boiled water and avoiding raw vegetables and fruits to prevent a possible intestinal infection.
- Wear a mask and gloves to clean bird cages, fish tanks, or cat litter boxes.
- Keep rooms clean and well ventilated, and keep air conditioners and humidifiers cleaned and repaired so they don't harbor infectious organisms.

RECOGNIZING SIGNS AND SYMPTOMS OF INFECTION

Immediately report any of these signs and symptoms:

- persistent fever or nighttime sweating not related to a cold or the flu
- swollen lymph nodes in your neck, armpits, or groin that last more than 2 months and aren't related to other illness
- profound, persistent fatigue unrelieved by rest and not related to increased physical activity, longer work schedules, drug use, or a psychological disorder
- loss of appetite and weight loss
- open sores
- a dry, persistent, unproductive cough
- persistent, unexplained diarrhea
- a white coating or spots on your tongue or throat, possibly accompanied by soreness, burning, or difficulty swallowing
- blurred vision or persistent, severe headaches
- confusion, depression, uncontrolled excitement, or inappropriate speech
- a persistent or spreading rash or skin discoloration
- unexplained bleeding or bruising.

◯ Preventing infection with antibiotics

Dear Patient:
If you're recovering from infective endocarditis or rheumatic fever, you need to avoid getting another infection, which could harm your heart valves. By taking an antibiotic drug, you can protect yourself from infection.

WHEN TO TAKE AN ANTIBIOTIC

Take your antibiotic drug exactly as directed. This lets the drug do its job of fighting infection. If you've been exposed to an infection, an antibiotic helps your body defend itself by killing bacteria before they multiply and make you sick.

You may also be told that you need to take antibiotics before you have dental work or any kind of surgery. Dental work, for instance, may allow germs to enter your bloodstream through your gums. Let your dentist or other health care provider know you have a heart valve disorder *before* treatment.

IF YOU FORGET YOUR ANTIBIOTIC

If you forget to finish or renew your prescription, tell your health care provider right away. You'll be told whether you need to continue your medicine.

WHAT TO REPORT

Report a break in your skin or if you feel sick because a cut, a puncture, a rash, or an abscess can introduce germs. A sore throat, fever, cold, or flu means that germs are already at work.

Stay alert for signs and symptoms that your heart valves may be infected again. These include:
- shortness of breath
- fever
- fatigue
- weakness
- swollen ankles
- sudden weight gain, such as 2 lb (0.9 kg) in 1 day or 5 lb (2.3 kg) in 1 week.

Report these signs or symptoms to your health care provider right away or go to the nearest emergency department.

AN IMPORTANT REMINDER

Get a card from your local American Heart Association that tells dentists (and other health care providers) which antibiotics you need to prevent heart valve infection. Always carry the card with you. Each year, have the card checked to make sure that you're carrying accurate information.

◯ Preventing infection with proper hand washing

Dear Patient:

Everyday activities, such as petting your dog and sorting money, leave unwanted germs on your hands. These germs may enter your body and cause an infection. To prevent this, wash your hands several times daily and always before meals. Here's how.

HOW TO WASH

1. Wet your hands under lots of running water. This carries away contaminants.

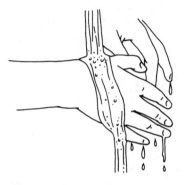

2. Lather your hands and wrists with an antibacterial soap. Rub your hands together, paying particular attention to the areas between your fingers and under your nails.

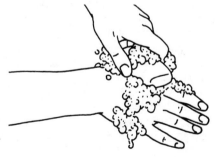

3. Thoroughly rinse your hands in running water. Make sure that your fingers point downward so that water flows away from your fingers.

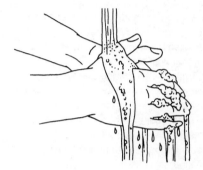

4. If you're at home, dry your hands with a clean cloth or paper towel. Don't dry off with a used towel, which may put germs right back on your hands. If you're in a public place, a hot-air hand dryer is best, but clean paper towels will do.

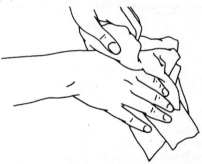

SKIN CARE

● If your hands become dry or itchy from frequent hand washing, soothe them with hand lotion.

● Don't use strong soaps. (They aren't needed for good hand hygiene, and they may cause drying and even allergic reactions.)

◯ Preventing peritonitis

Dear Patient:

Because you'll be using peritoneal dialysis at home, you must guard against peritonitis — an infection that occurs when harmful bacteria enter the dialysis system. Follow these tips to help prevent peritonitis.

AVOID CONTAMINATION

● Wash your hands with soap and water before opening the dialysis system, handling the dialysis solution, or changing the dressing over your catheter.

● Change the dressing over your catheter every day and whenever it becomes wet or soiled.

● Cover your mouth or nose with a surgical mask whenever you open the dialysis system — for example, to perform a solution exchange.

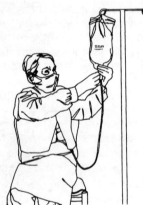

● Perform solution exchanges in a clean, dry room with the doors and windows closed. Don't do them in the bathroom.

● Check dialysate drainage for cloudiness or particles — possible signs of infection.

● Always make sure that you have the equipment you'll need to do the exchange before you get started.

● Ask your family to handle phone calls and other interruptions while you're doing your exchange. Otherwise, ignore distractions until you're done.

● Don't use fresh dialysate solution that has excessive moisture on the outside of the bag. This could indicate a leak in the bag and possible contamination.

● Take showers instead of tub baths to prevent bacteria from entering the dialysis system. Tape a plastic cover over the insertion site to prevent contamination of the connections.

● Follow other instructions or restrictions recommended by your nurses and health care providers.

WHEN TO SEEK HELP

● Call your continuous ambulatory peritoneal dialysis (CAPD) unit or health care provider if the skin around the peritoneal catheter becomes red, warm, or painful or if you note drainage. Also report leakage around the catheter insertion site.

● Follow the instructions you were given for care of the dialysate tubing spike should it become contaminated by contact with your hand or some other surface. This will necessitate a tubing change, which is usually done in the CAPD unit.

● Notify your CAPD unit or health care provider if you detect signs of peritonitis, such as abdominal distention or pain, cloudy dialysate, fever, chills, nausea, vomiting, or diarrhea.

◯ Promoting patient safety

Dear Caregiver:

A person with Alzheimer's disease requires intensive physical care and almost constant supervision to keep him from hurting himself. This means removing potential safety hazards from his environment and installing assistive devices where needed.

You can purchase many of these devices from large pharmacies or medical supply stores. You can also use childproofing devices, such as safety caps for electrical outlets, soft plastic corners for furniture, and doorknob covers. They're available from catalogs and where baby products are sold.

Use these guidelines to help you provide a safe environment for the person in your care.

REMOVE POTENTIAL SAFETY HAZARDS

● Move knives, forks, scissors, and other sharp objects beyond the patient's reach.
● Taste the patient's food before serving it so he won't burn his mouth or skin if he spills it.
● Serve the patient's food on unbreakable dishes.
● Remove the knobs from the stove and other potentially hazardous kitchen appliances. Put dangerous small appliances, such as food processors and irons, out of reach.
● Adjust your water heater to a lower temperature (no higher than 120° F [48.9° C]) to prevent accidental burns.
● Cover unused electrical outlets, especially those above waist level, with safety caps.
● Remove mirrors or install ones with safety glass in rooms the patient uses.
● Remove throw rugs and cover slippery floors with large area rugs. Place pads under the rugs, and secure them so they don't slide.
● Keep floors and stairways clear of toys and other objects that can trip the patient.
● Lock doors or camouflage them with murals or posters so they don't look like exits. Install a lock at the base of the door as an extra security measure, or install a childproofing device over the knob.
● Barricade stairways with high gates.

● Remove breakable wall hangings and pictures, and attach curtains to the wall with Velcro.
● Keep traffic patterns open by moving unsafe furniture to the walls.
● Store all medications out of the patient's reach, preferably in a locked container.

INSTALL ASSISTIVE DEVICES

● Pad sharp furniture corners with masking tape or plastic corners.
● Provide a low bed for the patient.
● Keep the house well illuminated during waking hours. Keep a night-light in the bathroom.
● If the patient uses the stairs, mark the edges with strips of yellow or orange tape to compensate for poor depth perception.
● Encourage the patient to use the bathroom by making a "path" of colored tape leading in that direction.
● Attach safety rails in the bathtub, near the toilet, and on stairways.
● Glue nonskid strips in the bathtub and by the toilet.
● Provide an identification bracelet for the patient, listing his name, address, phone number, and medical problems.
● Give the local police a photograph and description of the patient, in case he's found wandering in the streets.

Protecting your joints

Dear Patient:
You can help protect your joints from injury by following these guidelines.

USING YOUR STRENGTHS

Use your largest and strongest joints. When stirring a pot, for example, use your elbow and whole arm instead of just relying on your wrist and hand to do the work. Support weak or painful joints as much as possible.

When using stairs, lead with your stronger leg going up and your weaker leg going down.

If you carry a purse, place its strap over your shoulder rather than grasping it in your hand. This will help protect a painful elbow or wrist or painful fingers.

SITTING AND STANDING

Sit in a straight-backed chair that's high enough for your feet to remain flat on the floor. This will help relieve joint stress. Consider buying a raised seat for your toilet so you can get up more easily.

Avoid bending, stooping, or holding the same position for a long time. When you have to stand for longer than a few minutes, put one foot on a stool or step, switching legs periodically.

PUSHING

Push open a heavy door with the side of your arm, not with your hand and outstretched arm.

GRASPING AND LIFTING

When grasping an object, put your hands near the center of your body. This will let you draw strength from your whole body, not just from your hands and arms.

When lifting an object that's low or on the ground, bend your knees and lift with your back straight. This spreads the weight of the object over many joints, instead of just relying on your hands, wrists, and elbows. Whenever possible, slide objects instead of lifting them.

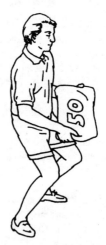

Carry heavy loads in your arms instead of gripping them with your fingers or hands. Use both palms to lift and hold cups, plates, pots, and pans, rather than gripping them with your fingers or only one hand.

STRAIGHTENING

Keep your fingers stretched out, instead of bent in, as much as possible. This will help prevent exaggerating deformities. Bend your knuckles as briefly as possible to hold objects.

Spread your hand flat over a sponge or rag instead of squeezing it with your fingers.

⬯ Protecting your skin

Dear Patient:

Exposure to the sun, or even to fluorescent lights, may make your condition worse. Excessive exposure, in fact, may cause rashes, fever, arthritis, and even damage to the organs inside your body.

However, you don't need to spend your waking hours in the dark to be safe. Just follow the precautions below.

PREPARE FOR GOING OUTDOORS

Wear a wide-brimmed hat or visor to shield yourself from the sun's rays. Protect your eyes by wearing sunglasses. Put on a long-sleeved shirt and trousers to filter out harmful rays. In hot weather, choose clothing made of light-weight, loosely woven fabrics such as cotton.

Buy a sunscreen containing PABA (para-aminobenzoic acid) with a skin protection factor of 30 to 45. If you're allergic to PABA, choose a PABA-free product offering equivalent sun protection.

Before you go outside, rub the sunscreen onto unprotected parts of your body, such as your face and hands. Read the label to determine how often to reapply it. Usually, you'll use more after swimming or perspiring.

AVOID STRONG SUNLIGHT

Try to stay indoors during the most intense hours of sunlight, from 10 a.m. to 3 p.m. The ideal time to garden, take a walk, play golf, or do other outdoor activity is just after sunrise or just before sunset.

REMOVE FLUORESCENT LIGHT

At home, replace fluorescent fixtures or bulbs with incandescent ones. At work, however, avoiding fluorescent light may be difficult. Consider asking your supervisor about moving to a work area closer to a window, so you can use natural light. If you have a fluorescent light above your desk, turn it off and request a lamp that uses incandescent bulbs.

BE CAREFUL WITH SOAPS AND DRUGS

Certain toiletries, including deodorant soaps, may increase your skin's sensitivity to light, so try switching to nondeodorant or hypoaller-genic soaps. Certain drugs, including tetracy-clines and phenothiazines, also make you more sensitive to light.

Always check with your health care provider or pharmacist before taking a new medication.

RECOGNIZE AND REPORT RASHES

Stay alert for the key sign of a photosensitivity reaction: a red rash on your face or other exposed area. Report suspicious rashes or other reactions to light. Remember that prompt treatment can prevent damage to the tissues beneath your skin.

◯ Recognizing warning signs of ulcer complications

Dear Patient:
You shouldn't have serious complications from your ulcer if you follow your treatment plan, but just in case, get to know the warning signs of complications. Make sure that you get prompt medical attention if any of these signs occur.

SIGNS OF BLEEDING

If you've ever bumped a scab off a cut finger, you know it can bleed. At times, an ulcer can affect the blood vessels in your stomach lining in much the same way. Contact your health care provider or go to the hospital if you have:
- bloody or black, tarry stools
- vomit that looks like coffee grounds
- chills, sweating, or both
- dizziness
- paleness
- restlessness and anxiety
- breathing problems.

SIGNS OF PERFORATION

If you've ever stepped on a nail or a pin, you know it hurts and leaves a little hole in your skin. An ulcer can leave a hole and hurt, too. What's more, the hole lets what's in your stomach leak out to cause infection and other problems. Contact your health care provider or go to the hospital if you have:
- severe pain in your stomach or shoulder (or both) that's relieved if you bend at your waist or pull your knees up to your chest
- a rigid, boardlike stomach
- a flushed, sweaty sensation
- fever and dizziness
- breathing problems.

SIGNS OF OBSTRUCTION

If you've ever had a plumbing problem — perhaps your sink has backed up or your washing machine overflowed — you know that an obstruction must be fixed to allow normal function again. Likewise, an obstruction that results from an ulcer needs attention. Contact your health care provider or go to the hospital if you have:
- a swollen stomach or an extremely full feeling that gets worse after meals or at night
- wavelike stomach tremors that you can see
- constipation
- a foul taste in your mouth and on your tongue
- loss of appetite, nausea, or foul-smelling vomit
- unusual thirst
- weight loss.

◯ Relieving reflux and heartburn with diet

Dear Patient:

A change in the timing, size, and content of your meals can help relieve the reflux and heartburn symptoms of a hiatal hernia.

Keeping your weight within normal range can help, too. Being overweight not only contributes to the development of a hiatal hernia, but also aggravates the condition. That's because extra body fat means more weight to push upward when you're sitting, lying down, or bending.

Follow the guidelines below to prevent reflux and heartburn or to help make them less severe.

EAT SMALL, FREQUENT MEALS

This means four to six small meals daily. Eating *frequently* prevents the stomach from becoming totally empty, thereby decreasing the acid it secretes during digestion. Eating *small meals* reduces stomach bulk, which also helps relieve your symptoms.

PREVENT REFLUX

Eat slowly to reduce stomach secretions, and sit up while you're eating. Keep in mind that while you're sitting up, gravity helps drain acid back into the stomach if it refluxes. Gravity can't help if you're lying down.

To decrease nighttime distress, eat your evening meal (a small one) at least 3 hours before bedtime. Also drink water after eating to clean the esophagus.

AVOID CERTAIN FOODS

Don't drink beverages that may intensify your symptoms — acidic juice (for example, orange juice), caffeinated coffee or tea, alcohol, and carbonated beverages.

Eliminate raw fruits and highly seasoned foods (chili) from your diet. Also avoid foods high in fat (fatty meats, eggs, potato chips) or carbohydrates (beans).

Instead, consume easily digested foods, such as skim milk rather than whole milk or broiled chicken with the skin removed instead of fried chicken.

Stay away from extremely hot or cold foods and fluids because they can cause gas.

Keep track of what you eat. Avoid foods that seem to cause discomfort.

LOSE WEIGHT (IF YOU NEED TO)

If you're overweight, ask your health care provider about an appropriate weight-loss program. If you've gone on a diet before, think about what strategies worked best for you. Also ask yourself what strategies and diets didn't work.

Losing weight will help you feel better — and look better too.

Relieving symptoms of carpal tunnel syndrome

Dear Patient:

If you're having symptoms of carpal tunnel syndrome, you know how disabling they can be. You know, too, that strain on your wrist nerve triggers your discomfort. To get relief and prevent permanent damage, you need to *stop* or *cut back* on the activity producing the strain.

Of course, that's easier said than done. If the activities that produce strain are related to your job or hobbies, stopping or decreasing them takes careful planning. Use the following suggestions to help.

MAKE CHANGES AT WORK

Modify your work habits and work area. If you work on an assembly line, do piece work, or have a repetitive job, ask your supervisor to help you change or eliminate activities that strain your wrist. For example:

● Make sure that the tools you use fit your hand correctly so you don't need to twist your wrist too much when turning, gripping, or squeezing objects.

● If you must lift and move objects, use both hands rather than the hand with carpal tunnel syndrome.

● Install a padded armrest at your workstation to relieve stress on your hands, wrists, and shoulders.

● Arrange to rotate your duties, or find a different technique for doing your job that puts less stress on your wrist.

● If you work at a typewriter, computer, or another type of terminal, try lowering the height of your work table to decrease the angle of wrist flexion.

● Raise your chair or sit on a pillow if you can't adjust your work table. Just be sure to support your feet to promote good posture and good circulation in your lower legs.

WEAR A RESTRAINING DEVICE

Wear a splint or a specially designed glove when you perform repetitive activities — or all the time, if your health care provider advises.

These devices are available by prescription from medical supply stores.

SLOW DOWN

Slow down when performing repetitive activities with your hands. For example, if knitting causes symptoms, you can knit at a slower pace. But, if you do piece work or if you work on an assembly line and a machine paces your work, discuss the problem with your supervisor or union representative.

DO HAND EXERCISES

Your health care provider will teach you special exercises to strengthen all your hand and wrist muscles. If all your muscles are strong, you'll put less strain on one particular muscle or group of muscles.

REDUCE SWELLING

If fluid retention aggravates your symptoms, ask your health care provider about taking diuretics to relieve some of the swelling in the carpal tunnel. Or drink plenty of fluids. Coffee and tea are natural diuretics. Elevating your hand may also help relieve swelling temporarily.

⬭ **Removing an ostomy pouch**

Dear Patient:
Be sure to change your pouch on a regular schedule. This will help prevent skin irritation and leakage.

HOW OFTEN SHOULD YOU CHANGE THE POUCH?

This depends on your type of ostomy, your activities, and the type of pouch you wear. Keep in mind that you may need to change the pouch more often in hot, humid weather. Avoid changing it daily because this can cause skin stripping and irritation. If you think the pouch may need changing daily, contact the enterostomal therapy nurse or your health care provider for guidelines.

REMOVING THE POUCH

1. Gather a washcloth, a towel or paper towels, adhesive solvent and an eyedropper (if needed to apply the solvent), karaya powder or Stomahesive Protective Powder, protective-film wipes, and karaya or pectin-based skin barriers.

2. Remove your old pouch by gently pulling up on the adhesive with one hand while carefully pushing down on the skin with the other. Most disposable pouches will come off easily without a solvent. If the pouch you're using requires a solvent, follow the product directions. Make sure that the solvent is completely removed from your skin before applying the new pouch. If you're using a reusable pouch, set it aside to clean after you apply your new pouch.

3. Wash your skin well with warm water and pat dry. Soap is usually not needed, but if you choose to use it, *rinse your skin thoroughly.* Soap residue will interfere with pouch adhesion and may irritate your skin.

4. Check your skin for redness or irritation. The most common causes of irritation are stool leakage under the seal or an overly large pouch opening, which allows stool to come in contact with the skin and cause irritation. Measure the stoma routinely to ensure that the stomal opening on your pouch is correct.

If your skin is red but intact, use a protective-film wipe to provide a clear, thin film between the adhesive and your skin.

If your skin is weeping, dust the affected area lightly with karaya powder or Stomahesive powder. Wipe off excess powder and cover the skin with a protective skin barrier. This may be either a karaya wafer or pectin-based wafer cut to fit the stoma. Apply your pouch over this wafer. Many disposable pouches have a protective wafer as part of the system itself.

Skin irritation will usually clear in a few days. If it doesn't, notify your enterostomal therapist or health care provider.

◯ Removing and applying an eye shield

Dear Patient:
Your health care provider wants you to remove the eye shield (and the patch) that he placed on your eye after surgery. For the next 4 to 6 weeks, he wants you to protect your eye with the eye shield at night. This will prevent rubbing or bumping your eye during sleep.

REMOVING THE SHIELD AND PATCH	APPLYING THE SHIELD

1. Wash your hands thoroughly with soap and water.

1. Before using the eye shield at bedtime, wash your hands.

2. Use a downward motion to peel the tape off your forehead. Gently remove the shield and patch from your eye and continue to peel the tape downward to your cheek. Now, remove the tape from the shield and discard the patch.

2. Place the shield over the affected eye. Then secure it with two parallel strips of hypoallergenic tape, taping from the middle of your forehead to your cheekbone. Make sure that you leave a space between the strips of tape so that you can see through the shield.

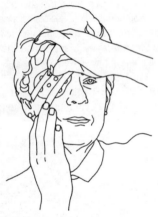

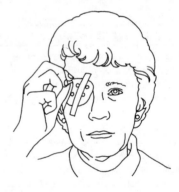

3. If your health care provider has ordered eyedrops, insert them now.

3. When you get up in the morning, carefully remove the shield. Keep it in a convenient place ready to apply again the next night or anytime you lie down.

◯ Restoring strength and relieving pain in arthritis

Dear Patient:

Don't underestimate the benefits of exercise. Done regularly, it can help you to overcome the pain and stiffness of rheumatoid arthritis, restore and maintain strength, and limber up your joints. It can also improve your circulation.

Develop a routine. Perform 5 to 10 repetitions of selected exercises once or twice each day. Move in a slow, steady manner. Don't bounce. If a joint is inflamed, gently move it as much as you comfortably can. Have someone help you, if necessary.

Don't hold your breath while exercising. Instead, slowly breathe in and out. You may count out loud.

SHOULDER EXERCISES

Try these two exercises for your shoulders.
1. Lie on your back. Raise one arm over your head, keeping your elbow straight and your arm close to your ear. Then return your arm slowly to your side. Repeat with your other arm.

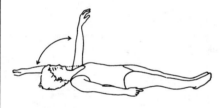

2. While standing, place your hands behind your head. Move your elbows back as far as you can. As you move your elbows back, tilt your head back (as shown). Return to the starting position and repeat.

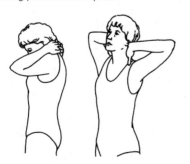

KNEE AND HIP EXERCISES

Try these five exercises for your knees and hips.
1. Lie on your back with one knee bent. Keep the other leg as straight as possible. Now bend the knee of the straight leg and bring it toward your chest. Push the leg into the air and then lower it to the floor. Repeat, using the other leg.

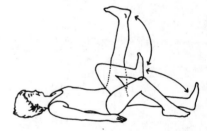

2. Lie on your back with your legs as straight as possible, about 6″ (15 cm) apart. Keep your toes pointed up. Roll one hip and knee from side to side, keeping your knees straight. Repeat with your other hip and knee.
3. To strengthen your knees even more, try this. While lying on your back with both legs out straight, try to push the back of your knee against the floor. Then tighten the muscle on the front of your thigh. Hold it tight and slowly count to 5. Relax. Repeat with the other knee.

(continued)

Restoring strength and relieving pain in arthritis *(continued)*

4. Lie on your back with your legs straight and about 6″ (15 cm) apart. Point your toes up. Slide one leg out to the side and return. Try to keep your toes pointing up. Repeat with your other leg.

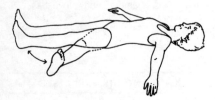

5. Sit in a chair that's high enough for you to swing your leg. Keep your thigh on the chair and straighten your knee. Hold a few seconds. Then bend your knee back as far as possible. Repeat with the other knee.

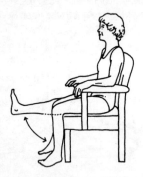

ANKLE EXERCISE

While sitting, keep your heels on the floor and lift your toes as high as possible. Then lower your toes to the floor and lift your heels as high as possible. Lower your heels and repeat.

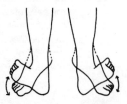

THUMB EXERCISE

Open your hand and straighten your fingers. Reach your thumb across your palm until it touches the base of your little finger. Stretch your thumb out and repeat. Repeat with the other thumb.

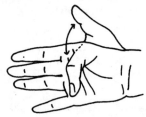

FINGER EXERCISE

Open your hand, with fingers straight. Bending all the finger joints except the knuckles, touch the top of your palm with your fingertips. Open your hand and repeat.

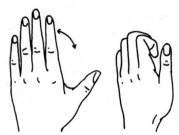

Speeding your recovery after prostate surgery

Dear Patient:

Here's what you can expect after prostate surgery, along with directions for caring for yourself.

EXPECT TROUBLE URINATING

At first, you may have a feeling of heaviness in the pelvic area, burning during urination, a frequent need to urinate, and loss of some control over urination. Don't worry, these symptoms will disappear with time.

If you notice blood in your urine during the first 2 weeks after surgery, drink fluids and lie down to rest. The next time you urinate, the bleeding should decrease.

Let your health care provider know right away if you continue to see blood in your urine or if you can't urinate at all.

Also let your health care provider know immediately if you develop a fever.

PREVENT CONSTIPATION

Eat a well-balanced diet and drink 12 eight-ounce glasses of fluid daily, unless your health care provider directs otherwise. Don't strain to have a bowel movement. If you become constipated, take a mild laxative.

Don't use an enema or place anything, such as a suppository, into your rectum for at least 4 weeks after surgery.

CUT BACK ON ACTIVITIES

Take only short walks and avoid climbing stairs as much as possible. Don't lift heavy objects. Also, don't drive for at least 2 weeks, and don't exercise strenuously for at least 3 weeks.

STRENGTHEN YOUR PERINEAL MUSCLES

Perform this exercise to strengthen your perineal muscles after surgery: Press your buttocks together, hold this position for a few seconds, and then relax. Repeat this 10 times.

Perform this exercise as many times daily as your health care provider orders.

WAIT TO HAVE SEX

Don't have sex for at least 4 weeks after surgery because sexual activity can cause bleeding.

When you have sex, most of the semen (the fluid that contains sperm) will pass into your bladder rather than out through your urethra. This won't affect your ability to have an erection or an orgasm. However, it will decrease your fertility.

Don't be alarmed if the semen in your bladder causes cloudy urine the first time you urinate after intercourse.

ASK ABOUT WORK

During your next appointment with your health care provider, ask when you can return to work. The timing will vary depending on the type of surgery you had, the kind of work you do, and your general health.

SCHEDULE AN ANNUAL CHECKUP

Continue to have an annual examination so your health care provider can check the prostate area that wasn't removed during surgery.

◯ Taking another person's blood pressure

Dear Caregiver:
You can use a standard blood pressure cuff and stethoscope to take the blood pressure of the person in your care. Just follow these steps:

1. Ask the person to sit comfortably and to relax for about 2 minutes. Tell him to rest his arm on a table so it's level with his heart. (Use the same arm in the same position each time you take his blood pressure.) While the person relaxes, hang the stethoscope around your neck.

2. Push up the person's sleeve, and wrap the cuff around his upper arm (just above the elbow) so you can slide only two fingers between the cuff and his arm.

3. Using your middle and index fingers, feel carefully for a pulse in the wrist near the person's thumb. When you find this pulse, turn the bulb's screw counterclockwise to close the screw; then squeeze the bulb rapidly to inflate the cuff. Note the reading on the gauge when you can no longer feel his pulse. (This reading, which is called *the palpatory pressure,* is your guideline for inflating the cuff.) Now you can deflate the cuff by turning the screw clockwise.

4. Place the stethoscope's ear pieces in your ears. Then place the stethoscope's diaphragm (the disc portion) over the pulse in the crook of the person's arm (this is called the *brachial pulse*).

5. Inflate the cuff 30 points higher than the palpatory pressure (the reading you obtained in step 3). Then loosen the bulb's screw to allow air to escape from the cuff. Listen for the first beating sound. When you hear it, note the number shown on the gauge; this is the *systolic* pressure (the top number of a blood pressure reading).

6. Slowly continue to deflate the cuff. When you hear the beating stop, note and record the number indicated on the gauge; this is the *diastolic* pressure (the bottom number of a blood pressure reading). Now deflate and remove the cuff. Record the blood pressure reading, date, and time. Report extreme changes in blood pressure to the health care provider.

    Remember: If you're using an aneroid model blood pressure cuff, you may need to have it calibrated every 6 months.

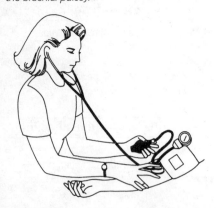

Taking anticoagulants

Dear Patient:

Your health care provider has prescribed an anticoagulant (also known as a *blood thinner*) because you have a blood clot, once had one, or are at risk for developing one. This medication will decrease the clotting ability of your blood, helping to prevent clots.

HOW TO TAKE ANTICOAGULANTS

Anticoagulants are available as tablets or injections. Read the drug label carefully, and take the drug exactly as directed. You'll need periodic blood tests to monitor the drug's effects.

WHAT TO DO IF YOU MISS A DOSE

If you miss a dose, take it as soon as possible, and then return to your normal schedule. If you don't realize that you've missed a dose until the next day, skip the missed dose. Don't take a double dose — it can increase your risk of bleeding. Keep a record of each dose you take, and report any missed doses.

WHAT TO DO ABOUT ADVERSE EFFECTS

Report immediately if you have nosebleeds; excessive bleeding from your gums or from cuts; easy bruising; blood in your urine; black, tarry stools; or coffee-ground vomitus.

Also report if your toes hurt and become blue or purple, if your urine becomes dark or cloudy, if you have trouble urinating, or if you're unusually tired. Some patients also temporarily lose their hair.

WHAT YOU MUST KNOW ABOUT ALCOHOL AND OTHER DRUGS

Don't take other prescription or over-the-counter medications while taking an anticoagulant unless approved by your health care provider. Many drugs interact with anticoagulants, including aspirin.

Limit your use of alcohol to no more than one or two drinks at a time because alcohol may affect how the anticoagulant works.

SPECIAL DIRECTIONS

- Tell all health care professionals that you're taking an anticoagulant, especially before you have a test, surgery, or dental work.
- It's important that the effects of this drug on your body be monitored. Routine blood tests will be scheduled for you. Be sure to adhere to this schedule.
- Carry identification stating that you're on an anticoagulant.
- Avoid contact sports.
- Report any falls or cuts.
- Use caution when shaving and brushing your teeth. Use an electric shaver and a soft toothbrush to decrease the risk of bleeding.
- Eat a normal, balanced diet while on this medication because changes in diet may affect the way the anticoagulant works.
- Avoid overeating green, leafy vegetables because the vitamin K in your diet interacts with oral anticoagulant medication. Be consistent in your diet so that the amount of vitamin K in your diet remains constant.

KEEP IN MIND

- Tell your health care provider if you're breast-feeding before taking this medication.
- Don't take this medication if you're pregnant, and don't become pregnant while taking it.
- Tell the prescribing health care provider if you've recently had surgery, a medical procedure, or a trauma such as falling.

◯ Taking care of your feet in diabetes

Dear Patient:

Because you have diabetes, your feet require meticulous daily care. Why? Diabetes can reduce blood supply to your feet, so normally minor injuries, such as an ingrown toenail or a blister, can lead to a dangerous infection. Because diabetes also reduces sensation in your feet, you can burn or chill them without feeling it. To prevent foot problems, follow these instructions.

ROUTINE CARE

- Wash your feet in warm, soapy water every day. To prevent burns, use a thermometer to check the water temperature before immersing your feet.
- Dry your feet thoroughly by blotting them with a towel. Be sure to dry between the toes.
- Apply oil or lotion to your feet immediately after drying to prevent evaporating water from drying your skin. Lotion will keep your skin soft. Don't put lotion between your toes.
- If your feet perspire heavily, use a mild foot powder. Sprinkle lightly between your toes and in your socks and shoes.
- File your nails even with the end of your toes. Don't cut them. Don't file the corners of your nails at a sharp angle or file them shorter than the ends of your toes. If your nails are too thick, tough, or misshapen to file, consult a podiatrist. Don't dig under toenails or around cuticles.
- Exercise your feet daily to improve circulation. Sitting on the edge of the bed, point your toes upward and then downward 10 times. Then make a circle with each foot 10 times.

SPECIAL PRECAUTIONS

- Make sure that your shoes fit properly. Buy only leather shoes (because *only* leather allows air in and out), and break in new shoes gradually, increasing wearing time by half an hour each day. Check worn shoes frequently for rough spots in the lining.

- Wear clean cotton socks each day. Don't wear socks with holes or darns that have rough, irritating seams.
- Consult a podiatrist to treat corns and calluses. Self-treatment or application of caustic agents may be harmful.
- If your feet are cold, wear warm socks or slippers and use extra blankets in bed. Avoid using heating pads and hot water bottles. These devices may cause burns.
- Check the skin of your feet daily for cuts, cracks, blisters, or red, swollen areas.
- If you cut your foot, no matter how slightly, contact the health care provider. Wash the cut thoroughly and apply a mild antiseptic. Avoid harsh antiseptics, such as iodine, which can cause tissue damage.
- Don't wear tight-fitting garments or engage in activities that can decrease circulation. Especially avoid wearing elastic garters, sitting with your knees crossed, picking at sores or rough spots on your feet, walking barefoot, or applying adhesive tape or bandages to your feet.

◯ Taking naproxen

Dear Patient:
Naproxen is usually prescribed to reduce joint pain, swelling, and stiffness caused by arthritis. The label may read Naprosyn.

HOW TO TAKE NAPROXEN

Naproxen comes in regular and extended-release tablets and an oral suspension. Check the label. Take only as prescribed.

Take each dose with a full glass (8 ounces [237 ml]) of water. Stay upright for about 30 minutes afterward.

Be sure to swallow the *extended-release tablets* whole. Don't crush or break them.

Take *regular tablets* with food or an antacid if naproxen causes heartburn. However, check with your health care provider first.

Shake the *oral suspension* well before measuring a dose; don't mix it with an antacid.

WHAT TO DO IF YOU MISS A DOSE

Take the dose as soon as you remember. However, if it's almost time for the next dose, skip the missed dose and resume your regular schedule. Don't take a double dose.

WHAT TO DO ABOUT SIDE EFFECTS

Immediately report blood in your urine or less frequent urination. Also report diarrhea, black stools, a sore throat, wheezing, dizziness, drowsiness, light-headedness, ringing in your ears, vision changes, swollen ankles, or a rash.

Headache, heartburn, indigestion, nausea, vomiting, or stomach or abdominal cramps or pain may occur. Call your health care provider if these side effects persist or become bothersome.

WHAT YOU MUST KNOW ABOUT ALCOHOL AND OTHER DRUGS

Avoid alcohol while taking this medication. The combination may make you drowsy.

Check with your health care provider before taking other medications. Many medications increase the chance for serious side effects when taken with naproxen. Avoid aspirin and steroids because these medications increase the risk of stomach or gastrointestinal (GI) side effects.

SPECIAL DIRECTIONS

Warning: Don't take this medication if you're allergic to it or to aspirin.
● Tell your health care provider your medical history, especially if you have had stomach or intestinal disease, ulcers, kidney disease, or heart or blood vessel disease.
● Avoid hazardous activities, such as driving a car, until you know how to react to naproxen because it may make you drowsy.
● Take all doses at the prescribed times.
● Keep taking naproxen even if your symptoms don't get better right away. Naproxen may take 1 month to achieve its desired effect.
● If you'll be taking this medication for a long time, your health care provider will evaluate your progress regularly.

KEEP IN MIND

● If you're pregnant, check with your health care provider before taking this medication.
● If you're an older adult, you may be more likely to have GI side effects.

◯ Taking nitroglycerin

Dear Patient:

Nitroglycerin has been prescribed to control your angina. By temporarily widening your veins and arteries, nitroglycerin brings more blood and oxygen to your heart when it needs it most. This drug is available in ointment, disk, tablet, and spray forms. To ensure its effectiveness, follow these directions for the form of medication you're taking.

OINTMENT

1. Measure the prescribed amount of nitroglycerin ointment onto the special paper.

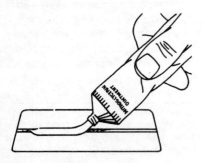

2. Spread it lightly over the area specified in the instructions — usually the upper arm or chest. Don't rub it into your skin. For best results, spread the ointment to cover an area about the size of the application paper (roughly 3½" by 2¼" [9 by 6 cm]).

3. Cover the ointment with paper and tape it in place. You may want to cover the paper (including the side edges) with plastic wrap to protect your clothes from stains. If you get a persistent headache or feel dizzy while using the ointment, call your health care provider.

DISK

1. Apply the disk to any convenient skin area — preferably on the upper arm or chest, but never below the elbow — touching only the back of the disk. If necessary, shave the site first.

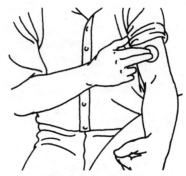

Avoid applying the disk to skin folds, scars, calluses, and damaged or irritated skin. Use a different site every day.

2. After application, wash your hands. Avoid wetting the disk. If the disk should leak or fall off, throw it away and apply a new disk at a different site.

To ensure 24-hour coverage, set a routine for applying a new disk each day. Also, apply the new disk 30 minutes before removing the old one. If you get a persistent headache or feel dizzy while using the disk, tell your health care provider.

(continued)

Taking nitroglycerin *(continued)*

SUBLINGUAL TABLETS	**SPRAY**

SUBLINGUAL TABLETS

1. Check to make sure that the medication hasn't expired. Then take a sip of water.
2. Place one tablet under your tongue, as shown, and let it dissolve. Avoid swallowing while the tablet is dissolving.

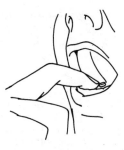

3. If your angina lasts longer than 5 minutes after taking the first tablet, take another tablet. Then take a third one after 5 more minutes, if necessary.
4. If three tablets don't provide relief, call your health care provider and have someone take you to the nearest hospital. *Never* take more than three tablets.

Get new tablets after 3 months, even if you have some left in the container.

SPRAY

1. Hold the spray canister upright as close as possible to your open mouth.

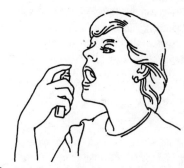

2. Press the button on the canister's top to release the spray onto or under your tongue.

Release the button and close your mouth. Avoid spraying into your eyes. Don't swallow immediately after spraying.
3. If your angina lasts longer than 5 minutes, spray again. Then spray a third time after 5 more minutes, if necessary.

Don't take more than three sprays within any 15-minute period. If your angina continues, call your health care provider and have someone take you to the nearest hospital.

◯ Taking your blood pressure

Dear Patient:
To take your own blood pressure, you can use a digital blood pressure monitor. You can also use a standard blood pressure cuff and stethoscope, but you'll probably need help from someone else to do so.

Before you begin, review the instruction booklet that comes with the blood pressure monitor. Operating steps vary with different monitors, so be sure to follow the directions carefully. They're usually also written in Spanish.

Start by taking your blood pressure in both arms. (It's common for blood pressure readings to differ by as much as 10 points from arm to arm.) If the readings stay consistently similar, your health care provider will probably suggest that you use the arm with the higher reading. Here are some guidelines:

1. Sit in a comfortable position and relax for about 2 minutes. Rest your arm on a table so it's level with your heart. Use the same arm in the same position each time you take your blood pressure.

2. Wrap the cuff securely around your upper arm, just above the elbow. (Make sure that you can slide only two fingers between the cuff and your arm.) Next, turn on the monitor.

3. Inflate the cuff, as the instruction booklet directs. When the digital scale reads 160, stop inflating. The numbers on the scale will start changing rapidly. When they stop changing, your blood pressure reading will appear on the scale.

4. Record this blood pressure reading, with the date and time. Then deflate and remove the cuff, and turn off the machine.

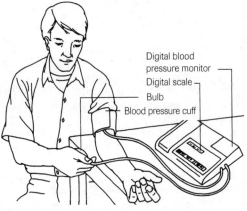

Digital blood pressure monitor —
Digital scale ⌐
Bulb
Blood pressure cuff

⬭ Taking your pulse

Dear Patient:
Your health care provider wants you to take your pulse (the number of times your heart beats per minute). Take your pulse at rest and during exercise. By comparing these two pulse rates, your health care provider can evaluate how well your heart is pumping.

TAKING YOUR PULSE AT REST

1. Don't check your resting pulse right after exercising or eating a big meal. When you're ready to take your resting pulse rate, make sure that you have a watch or a clock with a second hand.
2. Sit quietly and relax for 2 minutes.
3. Then place your index and middle fingers on your wrist, as shown here.

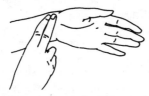

4. Count the pulse beats for 30 seconds and multiply by 2, or count for 60 seconds but don't multiply if your health care provider has so instructed because of your irregular heart rhythm.
5. Record this number and the date.

TAKING YOUR PULSE DURING EXERCISE

1. As soon as you stop exercising, find your neck (carotid) pulse. To do this, place two or three fingers on your windpipe and move them 2″ to 3″ (5 to 8 cm) to the left or right, as shown here.

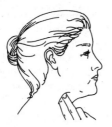

2. Feel for the pulse point low on your neck, and don't press too hard. (Pressing too hard can interrupt blood supply to the brain by applying pressure too high on the carotid artery. It may also cause an irregular heartbeat.)
3. Count the beats for 6 seconds, and then add a zero to that figure. This gives you a reliable estimate of your working heart rate for 1 minute. (Don't count your pulse for a whole minute because your heart rate slows dramatically when you rest.)
4. Record this number and the date.

ADDITIONAL POINTS

● If your heart rate during exercise is 10 or more beats above your target rate, don't exercise so hard the next time.
● If your working heart rate is lower than your target rate, exercise a little harder the next time.

⬭ Treating and preventing urinary tract infections

Dear Patient:
Here's some advice to help you treat your urinary tract infection (UTI) and prevent it from occurring again.

TREATMENT GUIDELINES

• Take your prescribed medicine exactly as your health care provider directs. *Don't* stop taking your medicine just because you feel better. Finish the prescription to kill all the infection-causing bacteria. Otherwise, you run the risk of the infection coming back.
• Lay a warm heating pad on your abdomen and sides to soothe pain and burning sensations you may have. Ask your health care provider to prescribe a pain reliever.

DIET TIPS

• Drink 10 to 14 eight-ounce glasses of fluid daily to increase urine flow and flush out bacteria.
• Eat foods and drink fluids with a high acid content. This will acidify your urine. Acidic urine inhibits urinary tract bacteria. High-acid foods include meats, nuts, plums, prunes, and whole-grain breads and cereals. High-acid drinks include cranberry and other fruit juices.
   A note of caution: If you're taking a sulfonamide drug (such as Gantrisin or Gantanol) to treat your infection, *avoid* cranberry juice because its high acid content can interfere with the action of the drug.
• Limit your intake of milk and other products with a high calcium content.
• Avoid caffeine, carbonated beverages, and alcohol because these substances irritate the bladder.

PREVENTION TIPS

• Practice sensible hygiene. For example, wipe from front to back each time you go to the bathroom. This reduces the chance that bacteria from stools will enter your urinary tract.
• Change your underpants daily.
• Wear cotton undergarments because cotton "breathes." This enhances ventilation, which deters bacteria growth.
• Avoid wearing tight slacks that prevent air circulation. Inadequate ventilation encourages bacteria to multiply and grow.
• Take showers instead of baths because bacteria in the bathwater can enter your urinary tract.
• Avoid bubble baths, bath oils, perfumed vaginal sprays, and strong bleaches and detergents in the laundry. These products can irritate your perineal area, which may trigger bacteria growth and infection.
• Urinate frequently (every 3 hours) to completely empty your bladder.
• Use the bathroom as soon as you sense the need to.
• Urinate after sexual relations. This will help rid your urinary tract of bacteria.

WHEN TO CALL YOUR HEALTH CARE PROVIDER

• Call your health care provider right away if you suspect you have a new or repeated UTI.
• Call your health care provider if you notice such symptoms as an increased urge to urinate, increased urination (especially at night), pain when you urinate, or bloody or cloudy urine.

◯ Understanding seizures and your child

Dear Parent:
You probably have many questions about seizures and how to help your child lead a normal life. Here are some answers.

WHAT CAUSES SEIZURES?

Seizures may follow a birth injury, a head injury, a high fever, or a disease that affects your child's nervous system, such as meningitis and encephalitis. However, the cause of many seizures is never known. Rest assured, however, that seizures aren't contagious. No one gave them to your child, and no one can catch them from him, either.

TAKING MEDICATION

Follow directions *exactly* for the dose of medication to give your child and when to give it. Taking medication exactly as prescribed will help control your child's seizures. *Remember:* Missing doses of medication could lead to a seizure.

When your child begins taking medication for seizures, he may seem less alert or his behavior may change. Report these side effects if they interfere with his activities and schoolwork. Your health care provider may adjust the dose or change the medication.

RESTRICTING ACTIVITIES

Has your health care provider placed restrictions on your child's activities? If so, follow all instructions. If not, take the same precautions as you would with another child. For example, caution him to wear a helmet when he's skateboarding or bicycling, and don't let him swim alone.

PROVIDING SUPPORT

Help your child deal with people who have misguided ideas about seizures. If you have other children, help them understand their brother's or sister's condition. Explain what they should do if their brother or sister has a seizure.

TELLING OTHERS

Enlist the support of your child's teacher. Tell her about your child's seizures, and explain what to do if he has one in school. She can help your child's classmates accept him as being just like them — except that he has seizures. She can also help his classmates deal emotionally with a seizure if he has one in school.

Ask the school nurse to help if your child must take medication during school hours. Also, inform camp counselors, baby-sitters, and other people who care for your child about his seizures and how to handle them.

GETTING MORE INFORMATION

Contact the Epilepsy Foundation for free information for you, your child, the rest of your family, and your child's friends. You can also call your health care provider if you have questions.

◯ Understanding the menstrual cycle

Dear Patient:
Your menstrual cycle has three distinct phases: menstrual, proliferative, and secretory.

MENSTRUAL PHASE

Starting on the first day of menstruation, your body's levels of the hormones estrogen and progesterone fall if an ovum (egg) hasn't been fertilized and implanted in the lining (endometrium) of your uterus. As a result, the tissues of the endometrium's superficial layer break down and flow through the vaginal opening and out of the body. This outflow, called the *menses* or *menstrual period,* consists of blood, mucus, and unneeded tissue.

PROLIFERATIVE PHASE

During this phase, estrogen levels rise, causing the endometrium to thicken. At the same time, follicles (containing eggs) in your ovary are maturing in preparation for possible pregnancy.

SECRETORY PHASE

During this phase, the endometrium continues to thicken by the following process: At ovulation, around day 14, one of the developing follicles ruptures, releasing an egg from the ovary. The ruptured follicle cells develop into the corpus luteum, which starts secreting progesterone as well as estrogen. These hormones prepare the endometrium for implantation and nourishment of the embryo should fertilization occur. Without fertilization, the top layer of the endometrium breaks down, and the cycle begins again.

The menstrual cycle repeats itself about every 28 days.

How your endometrium changes during your menstrual cycle

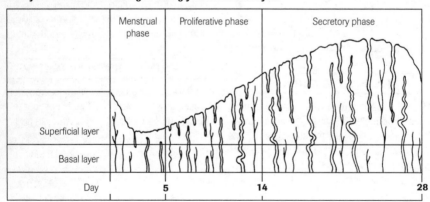

Understanding your home oxygen equipment

Dear Patient:
To relieve your shortness of breath, oxygen therapy has been ordered for you to use at home. Your first job is to become familiar with your oxygen delivery equipment.

OXYGEN OPTIONS

You'll be using a liquid oxygen container, an oxygen tank, or an oxygen concentrator.

Liquid oxygen is stored at very cold temperatures in thermoslike containers. When released, it's warmed up to breathe as oxygen gas.

Usually, a stationary liquid oxygen unit has a contents indicator that shows the amount of oxygen in the unit, a flow selector that controls the oxygen flow rate, a humidifier bottle that connects to a humidifier adapter, and a filling connector that attaches to a matching connector on the portable unit.

Oxygen tank

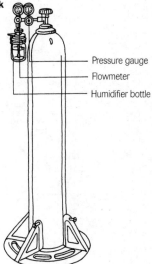

Pressure gauge
Flowmeter
Humidifier bottle

Stationary liquid oxygen unit

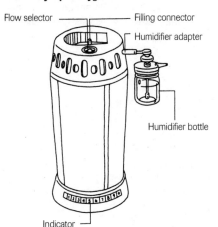

Flow selector — Filling connector
Humidifier adapter
Humidifier bottle
Indicator

An oxygen tank stores oxygen gas under pressure. It contains a pressure gauge that tells you how much oxygen is left, a flowmeter that tells you the flow rate, and a humidifier bottle.

The oxygen concentrator removes nitrogen and other components of room air, then concentrates the remaining oxygen and stores it.

Oxygen concentrators come in different models and sizes, but most have the following operating parts: a power switch and light, a flow selector that regulates the oxygen flow rate, an alarm buzzer that warns of power interruptions, and a humidifier bottle that attaches to a threaded outlet.

When using an oxygen concentrator, you must check the air inlet filter before operat-

(continued)

Understanding your home oxygen
equipment *(continued)*

ing the unit. If the filter is dirty, wash it with soap and water, rinse, and pat it dry before replacing it. Also, push the power switch once to check the alarm buzzer. If the buzzer doesn't sound, use a different oxygen source, and contact your supplier. If it does sound, push the power switch again to turn it off.

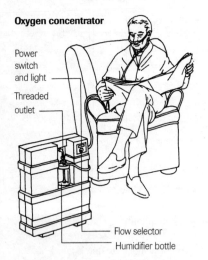

Oxygen concentrator

Power switch and light

Threaded outlet

Flow selector
Humidifier bottle

STEP-BY-STEP GUIDELINES

When using an oxygen tank, an oxygen concentrator, or liquid oxygen, be sure to follow these important guidelines:

1. Check the level of water in the humidifier bottle. If it's below the correct level, refill the bottle with sterile or distilled water or replace it with a new, prefilled bottle.

2. Attach one end of the oxygen tubing to your breathing device. Attach the other end to the humidifier nipple.

3. Set the flow rate using the appropriate method for your device. You may use one of the following methods to set the flow rate:
- Turn the dial to the correct number.
- Turn the dial until the metal ball rises to the correct level on the scale.
- Wait for the gauge needle to reach the correct level.

If you're using the liquid oxygen system, set the flow rate to turn on the oxygen. If you're using an oxygen tank, before setting the flow rate, open the tank by turning the valve counterclockwise at the top, until the needle on the pressure gauge moves. If you're using a concentrator, plug the power cord into a grounded electrical outlet and push the power switch before setting the flow rate.

Never increase the flow rate on your equipment without your health care provider's permission.

4. Put on your breathing device and breathe the oxygen for as long as your health care provider orders.

◯ Using an oral inhaler

Dear Patient:
Inhaling your medication through this metered-dose nebulizer will help you breathe more easily. Use it exactly as directed.

PREPARING THE INHALER

1. Shake the inhaler well immediately before each use.
2. Remove the cap from the mouthpiece, as shown. The strap on the cap will stay attached to the actuator. If the strap is lost, the inhaler's mouthpiece should be inspected for foreign objects.

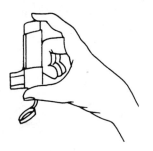

TAKING A BREATH

1. Make sure that the canister is fully and firmly inserted into the actuator.
2. Exhale fully through pursed lips. Then, holding the nebulizer upright, as shown, close your lips around the mouthpiece.

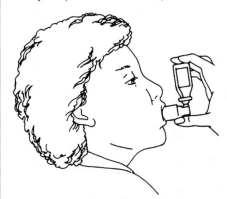

3. Tilt your head back slightly and take a slow, deep breath. As you do, slowly depress the top of the canister with your index finger.
4. Continue inhaling until your lungs feel full.

HOLDING YOUR BREATH

1. Take the mouthpiece away from your mouth, and hold your breath for several seconds. Then purse your lips and exhale slowly.
2. If your health care provider wants you to take more than one dose, wait a few minutes and then repeat.
3. When done, rinse your mouth, gargle, and drink a few sips of fluid.

CLEANING UP

1. Remember to clean the inhaler once per day by removing the canister and rinsing the plastic case and cap under warm running water for 1 minute (or immerse in alcohol). Shake off the excess fluid and allow the parts to dry. (This prevents clogging and also sanitizes the plastic case and cap.)
2. Then gently replace the canister with a twisting motion and put the cap back over the mouthpiece.

ADDITIONAL POINTS

● ***Important:*** Never overuse your oral inhaler.
● Discard the canister after you have used the labeled number of inhalations.

⬭ Using dressing aids

Dear Patient:

Does dressing yourself seem to take a long time? If so, here are some tips to make dressing faster and easier.

First, place your clothes close by, in the order in which you'll put them on. To pull your pants on or off, lie down, sit on a bed or a chair, or lean against a sturdy piece of furniture.

Also consider using the dressing aids described below.

DRESSING STICKS

A dressing stick helps you pull garments over your shoulders. Pad one end of the stick, or tip it with a rubber thimble so that your clothes will cling to the stick. Screw a small cup hook into the other end to help you manage zippers.

To help you pull garments over your feet and up, attach cup hooks (lightly taped to protect your skin) to two dowel sticks. Slip the hooks into tape loops, which you can sew inside a garment's waistband.

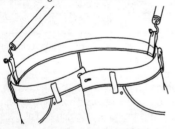

BUTTONHOOK

If you struggle with buttons, consider getting a buttonhook. Slip this aid through the buttonhole and over the button. Then pull the button back through the hole.

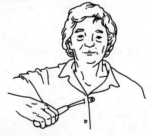

STOCKING AID

With a stocking aid, you can put on stockings without bending over. If you're using an aid like the one shown, first slide the stockings over the form. Secure the stockings, and then pull the form up your leg — along with the stocking.

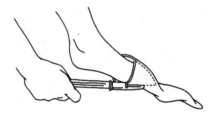

ZIPPER PULL

A large zipper pull will make opening and closing zippers easier, or attach an object, such as a key ring or a large paper clip, to a small zipper pull.

⬭ Using oxygen safely and effectively

Dear Patient or Caregiver:
Oxygen has been ordered for home administration. An oxygen concentrator, a liquid oxygen unit, or an oxygen tank will be delivered. The prescribed oxygen flow rate is _____ liters per minute for _____ hours per day.

OBTAINING EQUIPMENT

The medical equipment supplier will deliver the equipment, teach you how to set it up, check for problems, and clean it. The system will include a humidifier to warm and add moisture to the prescribed oxygen and a nasal cannula or a face mask through which to breathe the oxygen. Keep the supplier's phone number handy in case of problems. Also, get a backup system suitable to use in an emergency.

GENERAL GUIDELINES

When using an oxygen tank, an oxygen concentrator, or liquid oxygen, be sure to follow these important guidelines:
● Check the water level in the humidifier bottle often. If it's near or below the refill line, pour out any remaining water and refill it with sterile or distilled water.
● If your nose dries up, use a water-soluble lubricant such as K-Y Jelly.
● If you'll need a new supply of oxygen, order it 2 or 3 days in advance or when the register reads one-quarter full.
● Maintain the oxygen flow at the prescribed rate. If you aren't sure whether oxygen is flowing, check the tubing for kinks, blockages, or disconnection. Then make sure that the system is on. If you're still unsure, invert the nasal cannula in a glass of water. If bubbles appear, oxygen is flowing through the system. Shake off extra water before reinserting the cannula.

SAFETY TIPS

● Oxygen is highly combustible. Alert your local fire department that oxygen is in the house, and keep an all-purpose fire extinguisher on hand.
● If a fire does occur, turn off the oxygen immediately and leave the house.
● Don't smoke – and don't allow others to smoke – near the oxygen system. Keep the system away from heat and open flames such as a gas stove.
● Don't run oxygen tubing under clothing, bed covers, furniture, or carpets.
● Keep the oxygen system upright.
● Make sure that the oxygen is turned off when it isn't in use.

WHAT TO REPORT

Immediately report signs or symptoms of insufficient oxygen (difficult, irregular breathing; restlessness; anxiety; tiredness or drowsiness; blue fingernail beds or lips; confusion; or distractibility) or of excessive oxygen (headaches, slurred speech, sleepiness or difficulty waking up, or slow, shallow breathing). Above all, *never change the oxygen flow rate* unless instructed to do so.

⬭ Walking with a wide-based gait

Dear Patient:
Walking with a wide-based gait and swinging your arms will help you to maintain balance and keep moving forward. Use the following step-by-step guidelines to practice this technique. Remember to look ahead when walking and not at your feet.

1. Start by positioning your feet 8″ to 10″ (20 to 25 cm) apart. Stand as straight as you can.

2. Now lift your foot high with your toes up, taking as large a step as possible.

4. Swing your right arm forward when moving your left leg. Swing your left arm forward when moving your right leg.

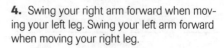

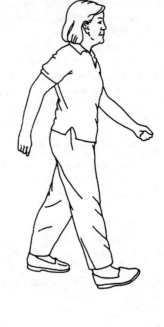

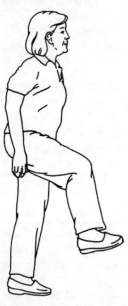

3. As you bring your foot down, place your heel on the ground first and roll onto the ball of your foot and then your toes. Perform the same steps with the other foot. Repeat these movements.

◯ Warming up before exercise

Dear Patient:

Exercising every day can help you stay healthy and feel younger. But don't just plunge into exercise. Spend 5 or 10 minutes doing the warm-up exercises below before starting a demanding physical activity. That way, you'll be more relaxed and less likely to injure yourself.

   While you're warming up, breathe normally and don't overdo it. Stretch only to the point that you feel mild tension and then relax. Repeat the exercises to cool down after your workout.

OVERHEAD STRETCH

Stand straight, extending both arms over your head. Clasp your hands and hold for 10 to 30 seconds; next, keeping your lower body straight, bend left and hold for 10 to 30 seconds. Straighten up for 10 to 30 seconds and then bend right and hold for 10 to 30 seconds. Straighten again for 10 to 30 seconds. Repeat five times.

Overhead stretch

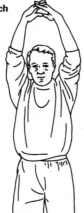

SHOULDER AND ARM STRETCH

Stand straight. Place your right elbow behind your head, touching your left shoulder with your right hand. Place your left hand on your right elbow.

   Hold for 10 to 30 seconds and then repeat the exercise with your left arm. Do this exercise five times for each arm.

Shoulder and arm stretch

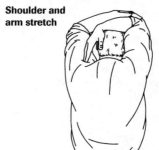

KNEE BENDS

Stand with both feet flat and about 6″ (15 cm) apart on a firm surface. Bend both knees forward slightly and hold for 10 to 30 seconds. Repeat five times.

Knee bends

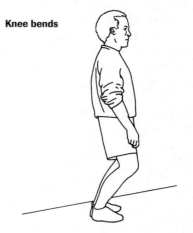

(continued)

Warming up before exercise *(continued)*

CALF STRETCH

Stand 2' or 3' (0.6 to 0.9 m) away from a wall. Place your right foot at the base of the wall, keeping your right knee flexed. Lean your head and forearms against the wall to stretch your left leg. Hold for 10 to 30 seconds, and then change feet to stretch your right leg. Do this exercise five times for each leg.

Calf stretch

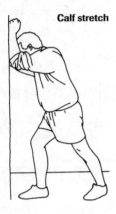

BACK STRETCH

Keeping your knees flexed, bend over slowly, and place your hands on a small footstool, box, or the bottom stair. Hold for 10 to 30 seconds and then slowly straighten up. Repeat five times.

Back stretch

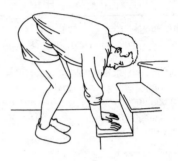

HIP FLEX

Place both hands, palms down, on a table. With your right foot 2' or 3' in front of your left, flex both knees and hold for 10 to 30 seconds. Now switch legs and repeat the exercise. Do this exercise five times for each leg.

Hip flex

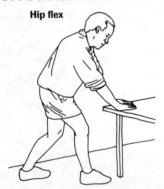

Internet resources for chronic disorders
Selected references
Index

⬭ Internet resources for chronic disorders

Administration on Aging
www.aoa.gov

Agency for Healthcare Research and Policy
www.ahcpr.gov

Al-Anon (for friends and family members of alcoholics)
www.al-anon.org

Alcoholics Anonymous
www.alcoholics-anonymous.org

Alzheimer's Association
www.alz.org

American Academy of Allergy, Asthma and Immunology
www.aaaai.org

American Academy of Ophthalmology
www.aao.org

American Association of Retired Persons
www.aarp.org

American Cancer Society
www.cancer.org

American Chronic Pain Association
www.theacpa.org

American Diabetes Association
www.diabetes.org

American Foundation for AIDS Research
www.amfar.org

American Foundation for Urologic Disease
www.afud.org

American Heart Association
www.americanheart.org

American Kidney Fund
www.akfinc.org

American Liver Foundation
www.liverfoundation.org

American Lung Association
www.lungusa.org

American Pain Society
www.ampainsoc.org

American Parkinson Disease Association
www.apdaparkinson.com

American Social Health Association
www.ashastd.org

Amyotrophic Lateral Sclerosis Association
www.alsa.org

Arthritis Foundation
www.arthritis.org

Arthritis National Research Foundation
www.curearthritis.org

Asthma and Allergy Foundation of America
www.aafa.org

Carpal Tunnel Syndrome Home Page
www.ctsplace.com

Centers for Disease Control and Prevention
www.cdc.gov

Crohn's and Colitis Foundation of America
www.ccfa.org

Cystic Fibrosis Foundation
www.cff.org

Epilepsy Foundation
www.efa.org

Food and Drug Administration
www.fda.gov

Glaucoma Research Foundation
www.glaucoma.org

Heart Life
www.heartlife.com

Leukemia & Lymphoma Society
www.leukemia.org

Lupus Foundation of America
www.lupus.org

Muscular Dystrophy Association
www.mdausa.org

Myasthenia Gravis Foundation of America
www.myasthenia.org

National Association for Home Care & Hospice
www.nahc.org

National Cancer Institute
www.cancer.gov

National Coalition for Cancer Survivorship
www.canceradvocacy.org

National Council on Alcoholism and Drug
Dependence
www.ncadd.org

National Headache Foundation
www.headaches.org

National Hemophilia Foundation
www.infonhf.org

National Hospice and Palliative Care
Organization
www.nhpco.org

National Institute of Neurological Disorders
and Stroke
www.ninds.nih.gov

National Institute on Aging
www.nih.gov/nia

National Kidney Foundation
www.kidney.org

National Marrow Donor Program
www.marrow.org

National Multiple Sclerosis Society
www.nmss.org

National Osteoporosis Foundation
www.nof.org

National Parkinson Foundation
www.parkinson.org

National Psoriasis Foundation
www.psoriasis.org

National Stroke Association
www.stroke.org

Scleroderma Foundation
www.scleroderma.org

Scoliosis Association
www.scoliosis-assoc.org

Skin Cancer Foundation
www.skincancer.org

United Ostomy Association
www.uoa.org

Selected references

Abela, G.S. *Peripheral Vascular Disease Basic Diagnostic and Therapeutic Approaches.* Philadelphia: Lippincott Williams & Wilkins, 2004.

American Diabetes Association. "Diagnosis and Classification of Diabetes Mellitus," *Diabetes Care* 28(Suppl. 1):S37-S42, January 2005.

American Psychiatric Association. *Diagnostic and Statistical Manual of Mental Disorders,* Fourth edition, Text Revision. Washington, D.C. American Psychiatric Association, 2000.

Bell, D. "Heart Failure: A Serious and Common Comorbidity of Diabetes," *Clinical Diabetes* 22(2):61-65, April 2004.

Bickley, L.S., and Szilagyi, P.G. *Bates' Guide to Physical Examination and History Taking,* 8th ed. Philadelphia: Lippincott Williams & Wilkins, 2003.

Cush, J.J., et al. *Rheumatology: Diagnosis and Therapeutics,* 2nd ed. Philadelphia: Lippincott Williams & Wilkins, 2005.

ECG Interpretation Made Incredibly Easy, 3rd ed. Philadelphia: Lippincott Williams & Wilkins, 2005.

Fischbach, F.T. *A Manual of Laboratory and Diagnostic Tests,* 7th ed. Philadelphia: Lippincott Williams & Wilkins, 2004.

Guido, M., and Rugge, M. "Liver Biopsy Sampling in Chronic Viral Hepatitis," *Seminars in Liver Disease* 24(1):89-97, February 2004.

Hickey, J. *The Clinical Practice of Neurological and Neurosurgical Nursing,* 5th ed. Philadelphia: Lippincott Williams & Wilkins, 2003.

Huether, S.E., and McCance, K.L. *Understanding Pathophysiology,* 3rd ed. St. Louis: Mosby–Year Book, Inc., 2004.

Hughes, B.W., et al. "Pathophysiology of Myasthenia Gravis," *Seminars in Neurology* 24(1):21-30, March 2004.

Kasper, D.L., et al., eds. *Harrison's Principles of Internal Medicine,* 16th ed. New York: McGraw-Hill Book Co., 2005.

Koennecke, H.C. "Secondary Prevention of Stroke: A Practical Guide to Drug Treatment," *CNS Drugs* 18(4):221-41, March 2004.

Neal, L.J., and Guillett, S.E. *Care of the Adult with a Chronic Illness or Disability: A Team Approach.* St. Louis: Mosby–Year Book, Inc., 2004.

Nursing2005 Drug Handbook, 25th ed. Philadelphia: Lippincott Williams & Wilkins, 2005.

Paul, W.E. *Fundamental Immunology,* 5th ed. Philadelphia: Lippincott Williams & Wilkins, 2003.

Porth, C.M. *Pathophysiology: Concepts of Altered Health States,* 7th ed. Philadelphia: Lippincott Williams & Wilkins, 2005.

Rakel, R.E., and Bope, E.T. *Conn's Current Therapy.* Philadelphia: W.B. Saunders Co., 2004.

Rubin, E., et al. *Rubin's Pathophysiology: Clinico-pathologic Foundations of Medicine,* 4th ed. Philadelphia: Lippincott Williams & Wilkins, 2005.

Sadock, B.J., and Sadock, V.A., eds. *Kaplan & Sadock's Comprehensive Textbook of Psychiatry,* 8th ed. Philadelphia: Lippincott Williams & Wilkins, 2004.

Smith, G.D., and Watson, R. *Gastrointestinal Nursing.* Malden, Mass.: Blackwell Scientific Pubs., 2005.

Tierney, L., et al. *Current Medical Diagnosis and Treatment,* 43rd ed. New York: McGraw-Hill Book Co., 2004.

Woods, S.L., et al. *Cardiac Nursing,* 5th ed. Philadelphia: Lippincott Williams & Wilkins, 2005.

Yamada, T., et al., eds. *Textbook of Gastroenterology,* 4th ed. Philadelphia: Lippincott Williams & Wilkins, 2003.

Zychowicz, M.E. *Orthopedic Nursing Secrets.* Philadelphia: Hanley & Belfus, 2003.

Index

A

Acetylcholine receptor antibody titer in myasthenia gravis, 229

Acid perfusion test in gastroesophageal reflux disease, 151

Acid phosphatase levels in prostate cancer, 265

Acquired immunodeficiency syndrome. *See also* Human immunodeficiency virus infection.
CD4+ T-cell count in, 176
common infections and neoplasms in, 176

Acral lentiginous melanoma, 215. *See also* Malignant melanoma.

Actinic keratosis, 306t

Acute angle-closure glaucoma, 153, 154
treatment guidelines for, 153

Acute intoxication, 8

Acute myocardial infarction, treatment guidelines for, 109

Acute respiratory failure in chronic bronchitis, 61

Acute sequestration crisis, 300

Adalimumab for rheumatoid arthritis, 282t

Addisonian crisis. *See* Adrenal crisis.

Addison's anemia. *See* Pernicious anemia.

Addison's disease. *See* Adrenal hypofunction.

Adrenal crisis, 2, 4
preventing, 413

Adrenal hypofunction, 2-6
pathophysiology of, 2-4, 3i
primary, 2-4
secondary, 2, 4
teaching points for, 5

Adrenal insufficiency. *See* Adrenal hypofunction.

Adult chorea, 180-181

Agoraphobia, panic disorder and, 253, 255

AIDS. *See* Acquired immunodeficiency syndrome.

Alanine aminotransferase levels
in anorexia nervosa, 19
in cirrhosis, 99

Albumin levels
in anorexia nervosa, 19
in celiac disease, 85
in cirrhosis, 99

Albumin levels *(continued)*
in hepatitis, 172
in ulcerative colitis, 320

Alcohol addiction, 6-10
acute episode of, 8
teaching points for, 10

Alcoholic cirrhosis, 97

Alcohol use, complications of, 9

Alcohol withdrawal, signs and symptoms of, 7t

Alkaline phosphatase levels
in ankylosing spondylitis, 16
in breast cancer, 57
in celiac disease, 85
in chronic cholelithiasis, 93
in cirrhosis, 99
in hypothyroidism, 191
in Paget's disease, 250
in prostate cancer, 265

Alzheimer's disease, 10-13
abnormal cellular structures in, 11i
teaching points for, 12

Aminotransferase levels in hepatitis, 172

Ammonia levels
in alcohol addiction, 8
in cirrhosis, 99
in hepatitis, 172

Amylase levels
in alcohol addiction, 8
in anorexia nervosa, 19
in chronic cholelithiasis, 93
in chronic pancreatitis, 252

Amyloid plaques in Alzheimer's disease, 11i

Amyotrophic lateral sclerosis, 13-16
progression of, 14i
teaching points for, 15

Androstenedione levels in polycystic ovarian syndrome, 262

Angina, types of, 108

Angiography. *See also specific type.*
in Cushing's syndrome, 116
in stroke, 310

---

i refers to an illustration; t refers to a table.

i refers to an illustration; t refers to a table.

i refers to an illustration; t refers to a table.

i refers to an illustration; t refers to a table.

i refers to an illustration; t refers to a table.

i refers to an illustration; t refers to a table.

---

i refers to an illustration; t refers to a table.

i refers to an illustration; t refers to a table.

i refers to an illustration; t refers to a table.

i refers to an illustration; t refers to a table.

i refers to an illustration; t refers to a table.

i refers to an illustration; t refers to a table.

i refers to an illustration; t refers to a table.

i refers to an illustration; t refers to a table.

---

i refers to an illustration; t refers to a table.

i refers to an illustration; t refers to a table.

PATIENT-TEACHING AIDS on CD-ROM

The CD-ROM on the inside back cover provides more than 350 patient-teaching aids in a program that allows users to identify and print the patient-teaching aids they need quickly and easily. Nurses can scroll through an alphabetical list; browse by topic, disorder, or test or treatment; or perform a search to identify a particular patient-teaching aid. Each entry provides complete instructions for the patient or caregiver, including the equipment needed and preparation guidelines.

To operate the CD-ROM, we recommend that you have the following computer equipment, at a minimum:

- IBM-compatible personal computer
- Windows®95
- Pentium® 133 MHz or higher (166 MHz recommended) processor
- 32 MB of RAM
- 40 MB of free hard-disk space
- SVGA monitor with high color (16-bit) — display area must be set to 800 × 600 and the display font size must be set to "Small Fonts"
- CD-ROM drive
- Mouse.

Installation

Before performing the installation, make sure that your monitor is set up to display high color (16-bit) or greater, your display area is set to 800 × 600, and your display font size is set to "Small Fonts." If it isn't, consult your monitor's user's manual for instructions about changing the display settings (typically found in *Start/ Settings/Control Panel/Display/Settings*). Set the color palette equal to high color (16-bit) or true color (24-bit), the display area to 800 × 600, and the font size to "Small Fonts."

To install this program onto the hard drive of your computer, follow these steps:
1. Start Windows®.
2. Place the CD in your CD-ROM drive and close the tray. After a few moments, the installation process will begin automatically.
3. Follow the on-screen instructions.
Note: If the install program doesn't automatically begin, click the "Start" menu and select "Run." Type *d:\setup.exe* (where *d:* is the letter of your CD-ROM drive) and click OK.